The Sense of Suffering

Intersections

Yearbook for Early Modern Studies

VOLUME 12 – 2008

The Sense of Suffering

Constructions of Physical Pain in Early Modern Culture

Edited by

Jan Frans van Dijkhuizen
Karl A.E. Enenkel

BRILL

LEIDEN • BOSTON
2009

Illustration on the cover: The Petrarch Master, Woodcut illustration to Petrarch's *Von der Artzney baider Glueck* [...] (Augsburg: 1532), book II, chapter 29, fol. XXXVIIIr.

This book is printed on acid-free paper.

Library of Congress Cataloging-in-Publication Data

The sense of suffering : constructions of physical pain in early modern culture / edited by Jan Frans van Dijkhuizen, Karl A.E. Enenkel.
p. ; cm. — (Intersections, ISSN 1568-1181 ; v. 12)
Includes bibliographical references and index.
ISBN 978-90-04-17247-0 (hardback : alk. paper) 1. Pain—Europe—History. 2. Pain—Religious aspects—Christianity. I. Dijkhuizen, Jan Frans van, 1970– II. Enenkel, K. A. E. III. Title. IV. Series: Intersections (Boston, Mass.) ; v. 12 . [DNLM: 1. Pain—history—Europe. 2. Christianity—history—Europe. 3. Culture—Europe. 4. History, 17th Century—Europe. 5. History, Early Modern 1451–1600—Europe. 6. Literature—history—Europe. WL 11 GA1 S478 2009]

RB127.S398 2009
306.4'61—dc22

2008042099

ISSN 1568-1181
ISBN 978 90 04 17247 0

PRINTED IN THE NETHERLANDS

CONTENTS

Acknowledgements ix
Notes on the Editors xi
List of Contributors xiii
List of Illustrations xvii

Introduction: Constructions of Physical Pain in Early Modern Culture 1
JAN FRANS VAN DIJKHUIZEN AND KARL ENENKEL

Aesthetics and Anesthetics: The Art of Pain Management in Early Modern England 19
MICHAEL SCHOENFELDT

Whipping Boys: Erasmus' Rhetoric of Corporeal Punishment and its Discontents 39
ANITA TRANINGER

Articulating Pain: Martyrology, Torture and Execution in the Works of Antonio Gallonio (1556–1605) 59
JETZE TOUBER

Pain as Persuasion: The Petrarch Master Interpreting Petrarch's *De remediis* 91
KARL A.E. ENENKEL

Green Wounds: Pain, Anger and Revenge in Early Modern Culture 165
KRISTINE STEENBERGH

Partakers of Pain: Religious Meanings of Pain in Early Modern England 189
JAN FRANS VAN DIJKHUIZEN

Colour Plates I–XVI

Passio und *Compassio*: Geisselungsrituale italienischer Bussbruderschaften im späten Mittelalter 221
Andreas Dehmer

Self-Flagellation in the Early Modern Era 253
Patrick Vandermeersch

'Esta pena tan sabrosa': Teresa of Avila and the Figurative Arts in Early Modern Europe 267
Maria Berbara

Godly Beds of Pain: Pain in English Protestant Manuals (*ca.* 1550–1650) 299
Jenny Mayhew

Experiencing Pain in John Donne's *Devotions upon Emergent Occasions* (1624) 323
Mary Ann Lund

Reading Bleeding Trees: The Poetics of other People's Pain in "The Legend of Holiness" 347
Joseph Campana

Bodies in Pain and the Transcendental Organization of History in Joost van den Vondel 377
Frans Willem Korsten

Schmerz hat nichts Gutes: Spinozas Begriff von *Tristitia* und *Dolor* 403
Anne Tilkorn

Imagining Physical Pain in a Sixteenth-Century Hungarian Poisoning Trial 423
Emese Bálint

Severing what was Joined Together: Debates about Pain in the Seventeenth-Century Dutch Republic 443
Lia van Gemert

Seeing, Feeling, Judging: Pain in the Early Modern Imagination 469
STEPHEN PENDER

Index nominum 497

ACKNOWLEDGEMENTS

The essays in this volume originated as papers for the conference "Perceptions of Pain in Early Modern Culture", organized at the University of Leiden in October 2007. This conference could not have taken place without the generous financial support of Leids Universiteits Fonds (LUF) and Pallas, Institute for Art Historical and Literary Studies.

NOTES ON THE EDITORS

Jan Frans van Dijkhuizen is lecturer in English literature and research fellow at the University of Leiden. He is the author of *Devil Theatre: Demonic Possession and Exorcism in English Renaissance Drama, 1558–1642* (Cambridge: 2007). His current project, funded by the Netherlands Organization for Academic Research (NWO), investigates perceptions of physical pain in early modern England. He is editor of the series *Proteus. Studies in Early Modern Identity Formation.*

Karl A.E. Enenkel is Professor of Neo-Latin Literature at Leiden University, director of the research project *The New Management of Knowledge in the Early Modern Period: The Transmission of Classical Latin Literature via Neo-Latin Commentaries*, funded by the Netherlands Organization for Academic Research (NWO), and director of the international research group *Discourses of Self-Reflection and Meditation in Literature and the Arts, 1300–1600* of the Netherlands Institute for Advanced Studies (NIAS). His research focuses on international Humanism, the reception of Classical Antiquity, the history of ideas, literary genres and emblem studies. He is a member of the *Royal Netherlands Academy of Arts and Sciences* and of the *Conseil international pour l'edition des oeuvres complètes d'Erasme*. He is the author of *Francesco Petrarca: De vita solitaria, Buch 1. Kritische Textausgabe und ideengeschichtlicher Kommentar* (1991), of *Kulturoptimismus und Kulturpessimismus in der Renaissance* (1995) and of a monography on Neo-Latin autobiography (*Die Erfindung des Menschen. Die Autobiographik des frühneuzeitlichen Humanismus von Petrarca bis Lipsius*, 2008). He has (co)edited and co-authored among others *Lipsius in Leiden* (1997), *Modelling the Individual. Biography and Portrait in the Renaissance* (1998), *Mundus Emblematicus. Studies in Neo-Latin Emblem Books* (2003) and *The Manipulative Mode. Political Propaganda in Antiquity* (2005), as well as a number of volumes in the *Intersections* series. He is series editor of *Proteus. Studies in Early Modern Identity Formation* and the general editor of *Intersections.*

LIST OF CONTRIBUTORS

Emese Bálint took her PhD in History at the Central European University of Budapest and in Linguistics at the Babes-Bolyai University of Cluj. Her research focuses on social and cultural history of early modern towns and on Anabaptist groups in Central and Eastern Europe.

Maria Berbara is professor of Art History at the State University of Rio de Janeiro (Brazil). She has specialized in Italian and Iberian art of the Early-Modern period. Her recent publications include an annotated translation of Michelangelo's letters in Portuguese as well as articles on Francisco de Hollanda and the artistic exchanges between Italy and Portugal in the Renaissance.

Joseph Campana teaches Renaissance literature and creative writing at Rice University. He is the author of a collection of poems, *The Book of Faces* (2005) and received a Creative Writing Fellowship from the National Endowment for the Arts. His current research focuses on *Suffering Romance: Edmund Spenser and the Pain of Reformation* and *The Child's Two Bodies*, a study of sovereignty and sexuality in the children of the Shakespearean stage and page.

Andreas Dehmer is curator at the Staatliche Kunstsammlungen of Dresden. He has studied art history, Italian literature and philosophy at the universities of Regensburg, Perugia and Hamburg and is the author of *Italienische Bruderschaftsbanner des Mittelalters und der Renaissance* (2004). He has worked at the Zentralinstitut für Kunstgeschichte in München on the project *Formen und Funktionen öffentlicher Bildwerbung zwischen Mittelalter und Früher Neuzeit*. His main research interests include Italian Painting 1200–1800, the art of religious confraternities and Renaissance papal iconography.

Lia van Gemert is professor of Historical Dutch literature at the University of Amsterdam. Her research focuses on the dynamic relations between literature and society. She has published on topics relating to genre, gender and transfer of scientific discourse. At present her research focuses on problems of identity and translation in early modern novels.

FRANS WILLEM KORSTEN is a lecturer in Literary Studies at the University of Leiden. Since May 2007 he holds the endowed chair in Literature and Society at the the Erasmus University in Rotterdam. His publications include *The Wisdom Brokers: Narrative's Interaction with Arguments in Cultural Critical Texts* (1998), *Lessen in Literatuur* (2002), and *Vondel belicht: voorstellingen van soevereiniteit* (2006).

MARY ANN LUND is Junior Research Fellow in the Humanities at Mansfield College, Oxford, and works on seventeenth-century English prose writing. Her current projects are a book on Robert Burton's *The Anatomy of Melancholy* and an edition of some of the sermons preached by John Donne at St Paul's Cathedral, to be published as one volume of *The Complete Sermons of John Donne* (Oxford U.P.).

JENNY MAYHEW studied English literature at the Oxford University and wrote her PhD thesis on *English Godly Art of Dying Manuals, c. 1590–1625.* She is currently a tutor in English at Bristol University and in Creative Writing at Oxford University's Department for Continuing Education. She is also a creative writer; her work includes the script for the film *To Kill a King.*

STEPHEN PENDER is associate professor of English and director of the Humanities Research Group at the University of Windsor (Canada). He is currently at work on the relationship between rhetoric, medicine, and emotion in early modern England, on medical thought in contemporary historiography, the history of the imagination, and laughter. He is currently finishing a monograph on *Essaying the Body: Rhetoric, Medicine, and Emotion in Early Modern England.*

MICHAEL SCHOENFELDT is Professor of English at the University of Michigan. He is the author of *Bodies and Selves in Early Modern England: Physiology and Inwardness in Spenser, Shakespeare, Herbert, and Milton* (Cambridge: 1999), the editor of *A Blackwell Companion to Shakespeare's Sonnets* (Oxford: 2006), and the co-editor of *Divisions on a Ground: Essays in Honor of Donald Friedman* (George Herbert Journal: 2008).

KRISTINE STEENBERGH is lecturer in English literature at the Vrije Universiteit Amsterdam. She specializes in early modern culture, theatre, gender and the history of the emotions. Her PhD thesis *Wild Justice* (University of Utrecht: 2007) examined the dynamics of gender and revenge in early modern English drama. In her current research, she explores early modern thinking on the transmission of affect.

ANNE TILKORN has studied philosophy and art history at the Maximilians-Universität in Munich and written her dissertation on Kant's notion of "Zufall" (*Zufallswelten. Kants Begriff modaler, teleologischer und ästhetischer Zufälligkeit*, Wilhelms Universität Münster: 2005). Currently, she works at the Herzog August Bibliothek in Wolfenbüttel. Her recent research focuses on the theory of emotions, especially in Kant's and Spinoza's works.

JETZE TOUBER studied History at the University of Groningen. He is currently completing his PhD thesis on the hagiographical writings of Antonio Gallonio at the University of Groningen. He is also a member of the editorial board of *Incontri*, journal for Italian Studies.

ANITA TRANINGER is Assistant Professor at the Department of Romance Languages and Literatures at the Freie Universität Berlin. She studied German and Japanese Literature at the Universität Wien, where she received her doctorate in 1998 for a study on the debate about universal methods of gaining and feigning knowledge (1500–1720). She is currently working on a book-length study of academic and literary cultures of conflict between scholasticism and humanism. Her research interests include the history of rhetoric, literature and knowledge, cultures of violence, and the fact/fiction divide.

PATRICK VANDERMEERSCH is Professor of Psychology of Religion at the University of Groningen. He started his academic career with research on the ethics of psychiatry and psychotherapy, before moving on to the psychology of religion. His publications include *Unresolved Questions in the Freud/Jung Debate. On Psychosis, Sexual Identity and Religion* (1991), *La chair de la Passion. Une histoire de foi: la flagellation* (2004) and *Godsdienstpsychologie in cultuurhistorisch perspectief* (with Herman Westerink, 2007).

LIST OF ILLUSTRATIONS

Colour plates I–XVI can be found following page 220.

Figure 1 (belonging to the introduction by Jan Frans van Dijkhuizen and Karl Enenkel):

Fig. 1. Gerard van Gutschoven, The perception of pain according to Descartes. From René Descartes, *Traité de l'homme* (Paris, Claude Clerselier: 1664) 27 2

Figures 1–3 (belonging to the article by Anita Traninger):

Fig. 1. Quentell workshop, *Teacher on the cathedra with pupils*, woodcut, Cologne, 1495. From Reicke E., *Der Gelehrte in der deutschen Vergangenheit* (Leipzig: 1900) 36 43

Fig. 2. Quentell workshop, *Albertus Magnus as teacher*, woodcut, Cologne, ca. 1480. From Reicke E., *Lehrer und Unterrichtswesen in der deutschen Vergangenheit* (Leipzig: 1901) 36 44

Fig. 3. [Col. pl. I] Ambrosius Holbein, *Signboard of a schoolmaster*, 1516 (Inv. Nr. 311). Spruce wood, 55.5 × 65.5 cm, Kunstmuseum Basel (Photo: Kunstmuseum Basel, Martin Bühler) 54

Figures 1–4 (belonging to the article by Jetze Touber):

Fig. 1. An inventory of ways of crucifying. From Antonio Gallonio, *Trattato de gli instrumenti di martirio, e delle varie maniere di martoriare usate da'gentili contro christiani* (Rome, Ascanio and Girolamo Donangeli: 1591) 10–11, copper engraving. Biblioteca Vallicelliana 64

Fig. 2. The bronze bull, among a number of torture methods that involve fire. From Antonio Gallonio, *Trattato de gli instrumenti di martirio, e delle varie maniere di martoriare usate da'gentili contro christiani* (Rome, Ascanio and Girolamo Donangeli: 1591) 90–91, copper engraving. Biblioteca Vallicelliana 71

Fig. 3. A martyr's entrails are cut out. Detail of an engraving depicting various forms of torture. From Antonio Gallonio, *De sanctorum martyrum cruciatibus liber quo potissimum instrumenta et modi, quibus iidem Christi martyres olim torquebantur, accuratissime tabellis expressa describuntur* (Rome, Typographia Congregationis Oratorii: 1594) 253, woodcut. Biblioteca Vallicelliana 82

Fig. 4. Gérard's heart and entrails are taken out. Detail of an engraving depicting the execution of Balthasar Gérard. From Frans Hogenberg, *Kroniek van de opstand in de Lage Landen, 1555–1609: actuele oorlogsverslaggeving uit de zestiende eeuw met 228 gravures van Frans Hogenberg*, ed. K. Kinds (Wenum – Wiesel: 1999), vol. II, 57 83

Figures 1–38 (belonging to the article by Karl Enenkel):

Fig. 1. The Petrarch Master, Woodcut illustration to Petrarch's *Von der Artzney baider Glueck* [...] (Augsburg: 1532), book II, chapter 94, fol. CXIXv 97

Fig. 2. [Col. pl. II] Gerard van Honthorst, *The Tooth-puller* (1628). Oil on canvas, 137 × 200 cm. Paris, Musée du Louvre 99

Fig. 3. [Col. pl. III] Jan Victors, *The Tooth-puller* (1654). Oil on canvas, 76 × 94.5 cm. Amsterdam, Rijksmuseum 100

Fig. 4. [Col. pl. IV] Jan Steen, *The Tooth-puller* (1651). Oil on canvas, 32.5 × 26.7 cm. The Hague, Mauritshuis 101

Fig. 5. Andries Pauli, etching after Theodoor Rombouts, *The Tooth-Puller*, 29.6 × 38.2 cm 102

Fig. 6. [Col. pl. V] "Augsburger Monatsbild", "Winter", detail with tooth-puller. Oil on canvas. Augsburg, Städtische Kunstsammlungen, Maximiliansmuseum 104

Fig. 7. Albrecht Dürer, woodcut illustration to Sebastian Brant, *Narrenschiff*, chapter 35 106
Fig. 8. The Petrarch Master, Woodcut illustration to Petrarch's *Von der Artzney baider Glueck* [...] (Augsburg: 1532), book II, chapter 107 (erroneously 112), fol. CXXXIIIIv 107
Fig. 9. Lucas van Leyden, *The Tooth-puller*. Engraving (1523), 11.6 × 7.5 cm 108
Fig. 10. The Petrarch Master, Woodcut illustration to Petrarch's *Von der Artzney baider Glueck* [...] (Augsburg: 1532), book II, chapter 94, fol. CXIXv. Detail 111
Fig. 11. Lambert Doomer, *The Tooth-puller*. Drawing, 28.7 × 40.2. Oxford, Ashmolean Museum 112
Fig. 12. Jan Steen, *The Tooth-puller* (1651). Oil on canvas, 32.5 × 26.7 cm. The Hague, Mauritshuis. Detail 113
Fig. 13. Jost Amman, The "Zanbrecher". From Hans Sachs' *Eygentliche Beschreibung Aller Staende auff Erden* [...] (Frankfurt a. M.: 1568), no. 52 114
Fig. 14. German Painter, Portrait of the Emperor Maximilian I, after Albrecht Dürer. Oil on wooden panel, 40 × 31 cm. Vienna, Kunsthistorisches Museum 116
Fig. 15. The Petrarch Master, Woodcut illustration to Petrarch's *Von der Artzney baider Glueck* [...] (Augsburg: 1532), book II, chapter 96, fol. CXXIv 122
Fig. 16. The Petrarch Master, Woodcut illustration to Petrarch's *Von der Artzney baider Glueck* [...] (Augsburg: 1532), book II, chapter 120, fol. CLVIIIr 126
Fig. 17. Dido committing suicide. Woodcut illustration in Sebastian Brant's edition of Virgil (Strasbourg: 1502), at the end of book IV 127
Fig. 18. The Petrarch Master, Woodcut illustration to Petrarch's *Von der Artzney baider Glueck* [...] (Augsburg: 1532), book II, chapter 96, fol. CXXIv. Detail 128
Fig. 19. The Petrarch Master, Woodcut illustration to Petrarch's *Von der Artzney baider Glueck* [...] (Augsburg: 1532), book II, chapter 65, fol. LXXVIv 130
Fig. 20. The Petrarch Master, Woodcut illustration to Petrarch's *Von der Artzney baider Glueck* [...] (Augsburg: 1532), book II, chapter 7, fol. VIIIv. Detail, left part of the image 132

Fig. 21. The Petrarch Master, Woodcut illustration to Petrarch's *Von der Artzney baider Glueck* [...] (Augsburg: 1532), book II, chapter 29, fol. XXXVIIIr. Detail, left part of the image 133
Fig. 22. The Petrarch Master, Woodcut illustration to Petrarch's *Von der Artzney baider Glueck* [...] (Augsburg: 1532), book II, chapter 67, fol. LXXIXr. Detail, left part of the image 134
Fig. 23. The Petrarch Master, Woodcut illustration to Petrarch's *Von der Artzney baider Glueck* [...] (Augsburg: 1532), book II, chapter 46, fol. LVv. Detail, left part of the image 135
Fig. 24. The Petrarch Master, Woodcut illustration to Petrarch's *Von der Artzney baider Glueck* [...] (Augsburg: 1532), book II, chapter 122, fol. CLXIIr 136
Fig. 25. The Petrarch Master, Woodcut illustration to Petrarch's *Von der Artzney baider Glueck* [...] (Augsburg: 1532), book II, chapter 103, fol. CXXXr. Detail, right part of the image 137
Fig. 26. The Petrarch Master, Woodcut illustration to Petrarch's *Von der Artzney baider Glueck* [...] (Augsburg: 1532), book II, chapter 60, fol. LXXIIr. Detail, left part of the image 138
Fig. 27. Fig. 20. The Petrarch Master, Woodcut illustration to Petrarch's *Von der Artzney baider Glueck* [...] (Augsburg: 1532), book II, chapter 7, fol. VIIIv. Detail, left part of the image 140
Fig. 28. [Col. pl. VI] Duccio, "Flagellation of Christ", part of his *Maestà* painted for the cathedral of Siena (1308–1311). Tempera on wood, 99.6 × 53.2 cm. Siena, Museo dell' Opera di Duomo 141
Fig. 29. [Col. pl. VII] Master of the Osservanza, "Flagellation of Christ" (ca. 1425–1450). Tempera and gold on wood, 36.5 × 45.7 cm. Vatican, Musei Vaticani 142
Fig. 30. The Petrarch Master, Woodcut illustration to Petrarch's *Von der Artzney baider Glueck* [...] (Augsburg: 1532), book II, chapter 29, fol. XXXVIIIr 145

Fig. 31. The Petrarch Master, Woodcut illustration to Petrarch's *Von der Artzney baider Glueck* [...] (Augsburg: 1532), book II, chapter 97, fol. CXXIIIIr 149
Fig. 32. "Übers Ohr hauen". Illustration from Röhrich, *Lexikon der sprichwörtlichen Redensarten*, 1113 151
Fig. 33. [Col. pl. VIII] Ascribed to Jan Joest of Kalkar, "Arrest of Christ" (ca. 1500). Altar table, 173 × 111 cm. Wittenberg, Schloßkirche 153
Fig. 34. [Col. pl. IX] Duccio, "Imprisonment of Christ", part of his *Maestà* painted for the cathedral of Siena (1308–1311). Tempera on wood, 102 × 76 cm. Siena, Museo dell' Opera di Duomo. Detail, left part of the painting 155
Fig. 35. [Col. pl. X] Anonymous, Altar of monastery Tempzin (Mecklenburg, 1411). Tempera on wood, 180 × 204 cm. Schwerin, Staatliches Museum. Detail 156
Fig. 36. Dürer, "Arrest of Christ", from the *Large Passion.* Woodcut, 39.1 × 27.7 cm 157
Fig. 37. Dürer, "Arrest of Christ", from the *Large Passion.* Woodcut, 39.1 × 27.7 cm. Detail 158
Fig. 38. The Petrarch Master, Woodcut illustration to Petrarch's *Von der Artzney baider Glueck* [...] (Augsburg: 1532), book II, chapter 97, fol. CXXIIIIr. Detail, central part of the image 159

Figure 1 (belonging to the article by Kristine Steenbergh):

Fig. 1. Henry Peacham, "Cholera". From idem, *Minerva Britanna* (London, Walter Dight: 1612) 128. Copy of Leiden University Library 182

Figures 1–3 (belonging to the article by Andreas Dehmer):

Abb. 1. [Col. pl. XI] Modenesisch, *Geißelungsritual.* Miniatur (letztes Viertel des 14. Jahrhunderts). Modena, Biblioteca Estense (Congregazione della Carità, Ms. 2) (A. Dehmer, mit freundlicher Genehmigung der Biblioteca Estense) 234

Abb. 2. [Col. pl. XII] Norditalienisch, *Thronende Madonna und Kind, Fra Raniero Fasani und Bruderschaftsrepräsentanten*. Aquarell (um 1567). Verona, Archivio di Stato (Ospedale di S. Bovo 1) 236
Abb. 3. Norditalienisch, *Imago Pietatis*. Fresko, 140 × 85 cm (Ende des 14./Anfang des 15. Jahrhunderts). Bergamo, S. Maria Maddalena (Archiv des Autors) 246

Figures 1–12 (belonging to the article by Maria Berbara):

Fig. 1. Anton Wierix, *Mystic Transverberation of St Teresa* (ca. 1622–1624). Engraving, New York, The Metropolitan Museum of Art, The Elisha Whittelsey Collection, The Elisha Whittelsey Fund, 1951 (51.501.6213). Image © The Metropolitan Museum of Art 277
Fig. 2. [Col. pl. XIII] Lorenzo Bernini, *Transverberation of St Teresa*. 1647–1652. Sculpture from marble. Rome, Santa Maria della Vittoria, Cornaro Chapel 279
Fig. 3. Lorenzo Bernini, *Transverberation of St Teresa*. Detail 280
Fig. 4. Palma il Giovane, *Transverberation of St Teresa*, 1615. Oil on canvas. Rome, Basilica di San Pancrazio 282
Fig. 5. Anton Wierix, *Transverberation of St Teresa* (ca. 1614–1622). Engraving, New York, The Metropolitan Museum of Art, Harris Brisbane Dick Fund, 1953 [53.601.19(143)]. Image © The Metropolitan Museum of Art 283
Fig. 6. [Col. pl. XIV] Gregorio de Ferrari, *Transverberation with St Francis and St Francis Xavier*, ca. 1680–90. Oil on canvas. Genoa, Church of Maria Santissima della Misericordia e di Santa Fede 284
Fig. 7. [Col. pl. XV] Peter Paul Rubens, *Vision of the Dove* (ca. 1614). Oil on canvas. Rotterdam, Museum Boijmans van Beuningen 286
Fig. 8. Juan de la Miseria, *Portrait of St Teresa*. 1576. Seville, Convent of the Discalced Carmelites. Detail ... 287
Fig. 9. Adrien Collaert and Corneille Galle, engraving, from *Vita B. Virginis Teresiae a Iesu* (Antwerp: 1613), fig. 23 289

Fig. 10. Titlepage of *Vita della M. Teresa di Giesù*, translated by Francesco Bordini (Rome, Guglielmo Facciotto: 1599) 290
Fig. 11. Page from the front matter of *Vida, virtudes y milagros de la B.V. Teresa de Jesús* (Zaragoza, Diego de Yepes: 1606) 291
Fig. 12. [Col. pl. XVI] Valdes Leal, *Maria Maddalena Pazzi.* Oil on canvas. Cordoba, Carmelite Church. Detail 296

Figures 1–5 (belonging to the article by Lia van Gemert):

Fig. 1. Johan van Beverwijck discusses his books on health with Apollo. Title page of Johan van Beverwijck, *Wercken der genees-konste, bestaende in den Schat der gesontheyt, Schat der ongesontheyt, Heel-konste* (Amsterdam, Jan Jacobsz. Schipper: 1664). Private copy 444
Fig. 2. First page of the book on wounds in *Heel-konste.* In: Johan van Beverwijck, *Wercken der genees-konste bestaende in den Schat der gesontheyt, Schat der ongesontheyt, Heel-konste* (Amsterdam, Jan Jacobsz. Schipper: 1664) 127. Private copy 449
Fig. 3. Jan Luyken, "De docter". From Jan Luyken, *Spiegel van het menselyk bedryf* (Amsterdam, Johannes en Caspaares Luiken: 1694), pages not numbered. Private copy 452
Fig. 4. Arnold Nicolai (?), Prisoner on the rack. From Joos de Damhouder, *Practycke ende handbouck in criminele zaeken* (Leuven, Wouters – Bathen: 1555) 56. Copy of Amsterdam University Library 456
Fig. 5. Gerard van Gutschoven, The perception of pain according to Descartes. From René Descartes, *Traité de l'homme* (Paris, Claude Clerselier: 1664) 27. Copy of Amsterdam University Library 464

INTRODUCTION: CONSTRUCTIONS OF PHYSICAL PAIN IN EARLY MODERN CULTURE

Jan Frans van Dijkhuizen and Karl Enenkel

What is physical pain? If this seems an obvious question to pose in the introduction to a volume of essays on pain in early modern European culture, it is worth reminding ourselves that medical views of the last four decades have increasingly come to doubt whether it can be adequately answered. 'Pure' pain does not seem to exist, both in the sense that what we think of as the singular sensation of pain is in fact a complex of physiological events, and in the sense that the experience of pain is inextricably bound up with our mental response to it. Pain, therefore, confronts us with basic questions about the relation between body and mind, and challenges common-sense dualist assumptions about the nature of physical and mental experience. This also becomes clear from the definition drawn up by the International Association for the Study of Pain (IASP), which describes pain as both a 'sensory and emotional experience'.[1]

It is therefore extremely difficult to offer any meaningful definition of physical pain as an exclusively bodily event. In his 1999 study *Pain: The Science of Suffering* Patrick Wall, best known for his contribution to the influential 'Gate Control' theory of pain, writes that 'all pain includes an affective quality that depends on the circumstances of the injury and on the character of the victim' and that 'pain is always accompanied by emotion and meaning'.[2] Recent discussions on pain have also increasingly come to emphasize that pain is a deeply *cultural* phenomenon;[3] the experience of pain is powerfully mediated by cultural and historical context. Studying pain, therefore, is a way of studying the intersections between the physical human body – the product of

[1] "Pain", "IASP Pain Terminology", <www.iasp-pain.org>, accessed 10 January 2008.

[2] Wall P., *Pain: The Science of Suffering* (London: 1999) 21; 38.

[3] See for example Melzack R., *The Puzzle of Pain* (Harmondsworth: 1973) and Porter R., "Western Medicine and Pain: Historical Perspectives", in Hinnells J.R. – Porter R. (eds.), *Religion, Health and Suffering* (London – New York: 1999) 364–381.

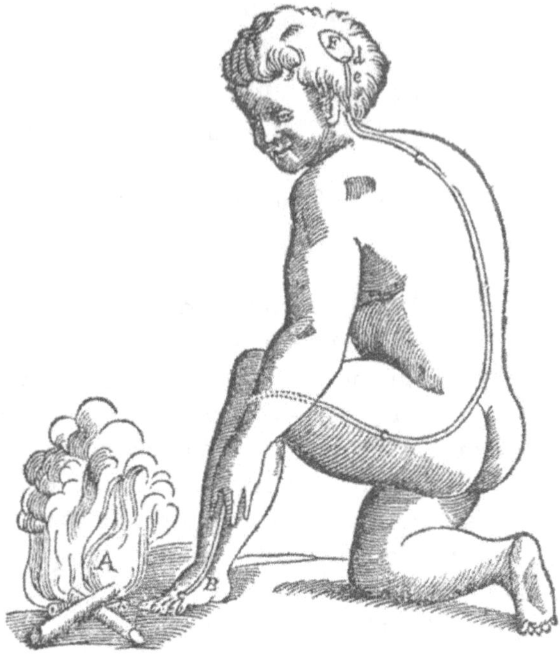

Fig. 1. Gerard van Gutschoven, The perception of pain according to Descartes. From René Descartes, *Traité de l'homme* (Paris, Claude Clerselier: 1664) 27.

evolutionary processes – and the cultural body, the human body as it is experienced and perceived by people in specific cultural and historical circumstances.

In proposing these new models of pain, contemporary pain medicine has frequently attacked what it sees as the misguided, modern dualist view of pain as divided into distinctly physical and mental categories. Moreover, it has often traced the origins of this view to the philosophy of René Descartes (1596–1650), whose obervations on pain have been an important point of reference in recent medical writings on the subject.[4] Descartes' reputation for inaugurating a dualist conception of pain seems to rest especially on the famous drawing of the kneeling boy by the fire [Fig. 1] in the *Traité de l'homme* (1664) – first published in

[4] For a useful discussion of Descartes' role as scapegoat in modern medical pain discourse, see Duncan G., "Mind-Body Dualism and the Biopsychosocial Model of Pain: What Did Descartes Really Say?", *Journal of Medicine and Philosophy* 25,4 (2000) 485–513.

1662, twelve years after Descartes' death, in a Latin translation by the Dutch physician and philosopher Florentius Schuyl (1619–1669). The drawing has been invoked, for example by Patrick Wall in *Pain*, as an illustration of Descartes' reductive view of pain as a purely mechanical bodily event.[5]

It would be inaccurate, however, to see the drawing in the *Traité* as representative of Descartes' understanding of pain.[6] His more detailed remarks about pain in the *Meditations on First Philosophy* (1641) suggest a more complex and unresolved attitude. Pain, he notes in the Sixth Meditation, confronts us with the fact that we do not just *have* bodies, but that we *are* our bodies:

> [T]here is nothing which this nature teaches me more expressly (nor more sensibily) than that I have a body which is adversely affected when I feel pain [...]. Nature also teaches me by these sensations of pain, hunger, thirst, etc., that I am not only lodged in my body as a pilot in a vessel, but that I am very closely united to it, and so to speak so intermingled with it that I seem to compose with it one whole. For if that were not the case, when my body is hurt, I, who am merely a thinking thing, should not feel pain, for I should perceive this wound by the understanding only, just as the sailor perceives by sight when something is damaged in his vessel.[7]

Pain is not seen from a distance – the metaphor of the pilot on his ship suggests that sight is characterised by its lack of direct physical contact with the world – but is felt and experienced from within.

For Descartes, then, the epistemological problem of pain lies partly in the way in which it straddles the mind-body divide. Pain also intensifies the doubts about sense perception that Descartes investigates in the *Meditations*. If vision and touch can convey inaccurate information about the *external* world, pain, for all its physical immediacy and intensity,

---

[5] Wall, *Pain* 60. Wall notes that the illustration is highly similar to the diagram in '[j]ust about every high-school biology text [...] where a finger touches a saucepan and is rapidly withdrawn'. He adds that he 'would estimate that we spend a few seconds in an entire lifetime successfully withdrawing from a threatening stimulus' (60–61). For a similar view on Descartes, see Wall P. – Melzack R., "Pain Mechanisms: A New Theory", *Science* 150 (1965) 971.

[6] See also Morris D.B., "The Challenges of Pain and Suffering", in Jensen T.S. – Wilson P.R. (eds.), *Clinical Pain Management: Chronic Pain* (London: 2003) 3–15. Morris notes that 'as the best-known proponent of mind-body dualism, Descartes has erroneously been identified as the precursor or progenitor of any theory that separates body from mind' (4).

[7] René Descartes, "Meditations on First Philosophy", in Haldane E.S. – Ross G.R.T. (trls. & eds.), *Descartes: Key Philosophical Writings* (Hertfordshire: 1997) 183.

can mislead the mind about what goes on *inside* the body, as becomes clear, Descartes argues, from the phenomenon of phantom pain. Pain therefore leads him to question the mind's ability to separate itself from the unreliable physical senses. He attempts to solve this problem in part by positing a form of divine epistemological benevolence: physical objects must exist (if not perhaps in the exact same form in which they present themselves to our perception), since God would be a deceiver if he misled us into believing that sense perceptions have their origin in physical objects, without also giving us the ability to correct these false conclusions. This is also why pain does provide information about the external world; the pain we feel when we approach a fire too closely signals 'that there is something in it, whatever it may be, which excites in me these sensations of heat or of pain' (185). The source of nociception does exist, even if our pain perception does not represent the essence of that source accurately, and pain therefore functions adequately as a warning system. On a more general level, Descartes concludes that sense perceptions are reliable enough for day-to-day living, but that they do not provide any genuinely intellectual understanding of the world around us in its cognitive essence.

That pain should play such a central role in one of the key early modern reflections on the mind-body question, and that Descartes has so often been referred to, and frequently misread, in recent medical reflections on pain, suggests that it is worth investigating early modern attitudes towards physical pain more thoroughly, and in a wider range of historical sources. If modern medical theories hold that the experience of pain is mediated by psychology and by cultural belief systems, and that there is therefore also a *history of pain*,[8] this volume aims to show that the early modern period is a particularly relevant and fascinating chapter in this history, as well as to investigate how the early modern era can serve as a kind of testing ground for modern anti-dualist views of pain.

We have seen that it is the sheer physicality of pain that troubles Descartes, and it is partly in this respect that the *Meditations* can serve as a useful entry point into early modern perceptions of pain. If pain

[8] For an example of such a history, see Roseline Rey's *The History of Pain*, trl. L.E. Wallace (Cambridge MA: 1995). Rey's chapters on the medieval and early modern periods are brief and tentative.

is partly cultural, the cultural meanings of pain in early modernity revolved to a significant extent around the *physicality* of pain. Early modern perceptions of pain are often characterized precisely by a lack of interest in what we would now see as the psychological aspects of pain, and by an attempt to locate the meaning of pain first and foremost in its overwhelmingly bodily nature. This is also the reason why the essays in this volume take physical pain as their starting point, rather than what we might now classify as mental or emotional pain: it is part of the argument of this volume that early modern discourses of pain centred around its somatic dimensions. Even evocations of physical pain that we would now tend to see as metaphorical, for example in descriptions of emotional pain, would have struck many early moderns as literal. For example, as Michael Schoenfeldt notes in the opening essay, early modern physiology sees grief as having a 'palpable, material presence in the body'. 'Flesh', he writes, 'is not a realm completely separate from the soul, but is a name for the thickening and coagulation of emotion around the intense sensations of pain and grief'. Early modern culture construes intense emotions as inherently physical; their physicality even serves as an index of their intensity. Paradoxically, then, it is precisely through the importance of the body in early modern notions of pain that the cultural dimensions of pain become clear.

In this respect, early modern conceptualizations of pain at once confirm and question modern anti-dualist views. On the one hand, they show that bodily experiences cry out for meaning: far from representing some form of mute, pre-linguistic meaninglessness (as dualist understandings of pain imply), the physicality of pain can in fact encourage the production of meaning. On the other hand, modern reconceptualizations of pain seem to show a degree of distrust of the physicality of pain, as if acknowledging the broader psychological and cultural resonance of pain somehow requires a downplaying of its somatic aspects. On the closing pages of his seminal study *The Culture of Pain*, for example, David Morris writes that 'we must begin to proliferate the meanings of pain in order that we do not reduce human suffering to the dimensions of a *mere physical problem* for which, if we could only find the right pill, there is always a medical solution'.[9] In a similar vein, Lucy Bending opens her study of pain in nineteenth-century English

[9] Morris D.B., *The Culture of Pain*, (Berkeley – Los Angeles: 1991) 289–290, italics added.

culture by observing that 'pain is not a brute given with a single, universally accepted meaning. Instead, those who suffer refer their physical discomfort to external systems of value'. She adds that her book 'is concerned not with the idea of pain as an ultimate sensation, but with arguments over the meaning and interpretation of pain'.[10] Both scholars seem to imply that investigating the meaning of pain implies a moving away from pain as sensation, that the meaning of pain is effectively located *outside* sensation; the adjective 'physical' is preceded by 'merely'. There seems to be, therefore, a subtle residual dualism at work in their analysis. Early modern perceptions of pain frequently work in precisely the opposite direction: they invoke the physicality of pain to invest other, non-bodily categories of experience with the authority and palpable reality of bodily sensation. The phrase 'constructions of physical pain' in the title of this volume, therefore, refers both to early modern interpretations of the *experience* of pain – as it presented itself for instance during illness – and to the ways in which early moderns employed the idea of physical suffering as a *rhetorical tool* in debates over other issues, for example the nature of religious experience.

The idea that the physicality of pain endowed it with a unique reality, and with a kind of rhetorical power that could be transferred to other areas of experience is effectively illustrated in Anita Traninger's essay on the role of pain in early modern education, especially in the teaching of Latin. Pain was seen by early modern educators as a helpmeet in learning and memorizing since it linked the 'weak stimulus' of the matter to be memorized to 'the intensity of physical experience'. Moreover, the beatings that were habitual in early modern education constituted a sustained *rite de passage*, an initiation into adult manhood. Drawing on Judith Butler's notions of gender and performativity, Traninger argues that in early modern education, daily beatings were an instrument in 'the fabrication of male identity'; pain served to root the elusive and contingent concept of masculinity in the concrete reality of bodily pain.

In spite of our emphasis on the physical, early modern medical culture plays a relatively modest role of in the various essays in this volume. If early moderns were preoccupied by the physicality of pain, it is striking that early modern medicine had a limited conceptual interest

---

[10] Bending L., *The Representation of Bodily Pain in Late Nineteenth-Century English Culture* (Oxford: 2000) 1.

in pain – a point also made in this volume by Michael Schoenfeldt and Mary Ann Lund. Galenic theory, certainly in its medieval and early modern incarnations, understood pain mainly as a symptom of humoral imbalance, like all bodily ailments.[11] Unlike modern medicine, with its detailed models of nociception, Galenism did not see pain as a distinct medical phenomenon with its own specific mechanisms and logic. A characteristic example is Gualterus Bruele's *Praxis medicinae* (1632), a medical manual that contains chapters on headaches, pain in the eyes, and gout. Bruele puts these pains under the larger rubric of "inward Diseases from the Head to the Foote", and he invariably locates their causes in humoral imbalance, to be redressed by an expulsion of excess matter, for example. He defines headache as

> a painefull griefe of the head, by reason of some dangerous and sad change thereof. This name is given to it, eyther in regard of the effect it worketh, as also in regard of the part affected. And it so happens, that the head is more tormented with paine then any other parte of the body: which is partly caused by the location of the head; for sharpe va[pou]rs, and swelling humours ascending from the lower Parts, doe assault the head, partly because the braine is of a cold and moyst temperature, superfluity of excrements are therein generated, which if they increase and be not avoyded by the expulsive faculty in their due season, are wont to disturbe the head with aches.[12]

The pains of gout, Bruele writes, are similarly caused by a humoral 'flux, which winds it selfe betweene the ligaments, filmes and tendones of the joynts' (380), while the 'loading [i.e. oppressive] paine' (127) that accompanies an 'Inflammation of the Eyes' (126) has its roots in a 'fulness & great store of bloud, wherewith the membrane growing close unto the eye, is filled and stretched' (127).

In addition to explaining pain in terms common to all diseases, such descriptions enhanced what might be termed the mysteriousness of pain, the sense that pain is an invisible process that goes on in the inner recesses of the body. While Galenic medicine did maintain that the accumulation of humours in particular body parts could cause pain

---

[11] In this respect, early modern medical notions of pain form an apt illustration of Mary Lindemann's remark that '*specific diseases* or *disease* entities as we normally speak of them (e.g., influenza, plague, AIDS) did not exist' (Lindemann M., *Medicine and Society in Early Modern Europe* [Cambridge: 1999] 9–10).

[12] Gualterus Bruele, *Praxis medicinae, or, the physicians practice vvherein are contained inward diseases from the head to the foote: explayning the nature of each disease, with the part affected* (London, John Norton: 1632) 1–2.

(and Bruele's *Praxis medicinae* is an example), it had no detailed model of humoral flow, or of the process of humoral corruption often evoked in early modern medical textbooks. Rather, it pictured the humours as coursing through the body in a disorganized, unpredictable manner, sometimes through locatable channels such as veins, arteries and nerves, sometimes in an unspecified process of diffusion. As Andrew Wear notes, 'although the humours could be seen (with the possible exception of black bile), what happened to them in the body was a matter of inference'.[13] In Bruele's account of headache, humours 'ascend' from the bowels to the brain in the form of 'sharpe vapours'; the clergyman Ralph Josselin wrote in his diary, in 1648, that his body, in its entirety, was 'full of cold waterish humours'.[14]

If humoral theory thought of the interior of the body as a mass of interconnected, permeable cavities and vessels, it likewise saw pain as a nameless, free-floating force inside the body. It is revealing that Andrew Wear's extensive *Knowledge and Practice in English Medicine, 1550–1680* devotes only a few pages to pain, mostly in connection to surgery rather than learned medicine, and it is worth noting that learned physicians often saw surgery as separate from, and indeed inferior to, their own profession. Inflicting pain was, of course, an unavoidable part of surgery, and as a result pain was, according to Wear, 'deeply integrated into the thinking and practice of surgeons'.[15] Surgery manuals emphasized the need of minimizing pain through proper surgical skill and by post-operation treatment, for example certain methods of bandaging and stitching. Yet, like theoretical medicine, surgery offered little in the way of an analytical perspective on pain beyond the immediate practicalities of pain management. We might add that early modern medicine also had a limited ability to mitigate pain (although some of the pain-killers it prescribed are likely to have had at least some effect), while in its emphasis on the importance of regimen, it focused as much on prevention of illness as on treatment.[16]

---

[13] Wear A., *Knowledge and Practice in English Medicine, 1550–1680* (Cambridge: 2000) 135.

[14] Bruele, *Praxis medicinae* 34. See also Wear, *Knowledge and Practice* 135, n. 66. Ralph Josslin, *The Diary of Ralph Josselin 1616–1683*, ed. Macfarlane A. (Oxford: 1976) 149, quoted in Wear, *Knowledge and Practice* 136.

[15] Wear, *Knowledge and Practice* 248.

[16] See also Lindemann M., *Medicine and Society in Early Modern Europe* 10.

It seems, then, that in early modern society, the cultural work of interpreting pain was done to a large extent *outside* the realm of medicine. In this respect, early modernity offers an enactment of modern theories of pain. Early moderns would hardly have had to be reminded that, as David Morris notes, '[m]edicine alone cannot possibly resolve all the questions raised by pain', or to be encouraged to interpret pain from non-medical perspectives. In this sense, moreover, early modernity can be seen as diametrically opposed to modern western societies in its dealings with pain.

A specific conceptual medical interest in pain began to emerge only in the second half of the seventeenth century, and in the closing essay of this volume Stephen Pender analyzes one particularly intriguing manifestation of this change, Everard Maynwaring's *Pains Afflicting Humane Bodies* (1682), which puts forward a highly specific theory of pain as an assault on the so-called *archeus*, or 'life principle'.[17] Indeed, as Pender shows, pain is central to Maynwaring's critique of Galenic theory and practice (although he is also clearly indebted to Galenism), and he sees pain as a crucial starting point for medical diagnosis.

Pender also explores what we have referred to as the invisibility of pain in early modern thought: early modern physicians, he writes, 'do not have a "*speculum matricis*" that would allow them to peer into the viscera. Pain must be judged by sensation: it can only be felt'. Diagnosis therefore depends on imagination, on 'description and redescription of something available only to feeling', and Pender investigates the implications of this idea in writings on pain by Maynwaring, Michel de Montaigne and René Descartes. Descartes' reflections on pain are also analysed by Lia van Gemert, in her overview of different understandings of pain in the seventeenth-century Dutch Republic, and by Anne Tilkorn, who traces the concept of pain in Spinoza's response to Descartes in the *Ethics*. Like Pender, Emese Balint pursues the question of how pain, as an invisible sensation inside the body, can be described. She analyses a 1572 poisoning trial in Klausenburg, and shows how the deponents described the pains of the poisoning victim in exclusively physical terms, drawing on a culturally shared set of images that revolved around bodily sensation.

---

[17] Maynwaring also published a treatise on pain in 1679, entitled *The frequent, but unsuspected progress of pains, inflammations, tumors, apostems, ulcers, cancers, gangrenes, and mortifications internal therein shewing the secret causes and course of many lingering and acute mortal diseases, rarely discerned: with a tract of fontanels or issues and setons* (London, J.M.).

Religious discourse provided one of the most important tools for interpreting pain. Indeed, it seems that in its preoccupation with the pains of Christ, late medieval and early modern religious culture was especially well suited to this task. In Catholicism, the human identification with Christ's Passion not only formed a central locus of officially sanctioned religious experience, but also served to legitimate various forms of lay spirituality. The era between 1300 and 1700 witnessed something like a *theological pain contest*. The Protestant Reformation denied the soteriological efficacy of pain, and attacked the idea that sinful humans can take part in the sufferings of the divine Christ, in this way attempting to rob the Catholic Church of one of its most potent means of propaganda. The Counter Reformation, by contrast, intensified the cultivation of physical suffering that had also characterized late medieval Catholicism, for example in a range of Jesuit writings and in the visual arts. The theological meaning of pain thus formed an important battlefield in the struggle for religious authority, and early modern debates about pain were therefore also intimately bound up with questions of power.

It is for this reason that a considerable number of contributions to this volume focus on the religious dimension of pain. Andreas Dehmer and Patrick Vandermeersch address one particularly important theme within the polico-religious controversy over pain, that of self-inflicted suffering. Dehmer shows how late medieval Italian lay confraternities developed a piety that centred around self-inflicted suffering as a way of identifying extremely closely with the suffering Christ. In this way, they sought to wrest religious experience from the control of religious authorities, and to organize their own lay spirituality around ritual experience rather than dogma or theological propositions. Patrick Vandermeersch analyses the practice of religious self-flagellation from a psychoanalytical point of view, arguing that during the sixteenth century, it came to be carried out in private, often darkened spaces, rather than in public. If in this way, self-flagellation served to create a new, private sense of self, rather than as a means of forging a public spiritual community around the suffering of Christ, pain once again served as a vital tool in the development of a religious sensibility that eludes institutional control.

Physical suffering occupies a similarly central position in the works of Teresa of Avila (1515–1582), undoubtedly one of the most famous religious writers on pain of the period. Maria Berbara shows how Teresa appropriated Catholic theologies of suffering for a highly individual understanding of mystical experience, in which intensely physical pain was both a source of spiritual pleasure and a distinctly personal privilege. Berbara also investigates the various ways in which Teresa was depicted in the visual arts of the early modern period. Although Catholic authorities downplayed Teresa's emphasis on mystical delight in their attempt to incorporate Teresa into official Catholicism (for example in the canonization bull), contemporary artists seized precisely on this aspect of her spirituality. Teresa's iconography – unlike that of sixteenth-century Carmelites such as Maddalena Pazzi or medieval mystics such as Catherine of Siena – does not stress mortification or the imitation of Christ, but rather a personal love experience symbolized by her main attribute, the arrow that pierces her heart in one of her most famous mystical experiences, captured in Bernini's celebrated sculpture.

The Protestant attempt to downplay the importance of Christ's physical suffering may have been an effective means of chipping away at a central pillar of early modern Catholicism, yet it also created a problem. The identification with the Passion had been a way of enlisting the body as a spiritual tool – of attaching meaning to bodily sensation and integrating it into an overarching theology. In disparaging this, reformers ran the risk of robbing the faithful of a crucial aspect of religious experience. As Jan Frans van Dijkhuizen shows, this tension may be observed in an intensified form in early modern England. Van Dijkhuizen investigates how early modern England dealt with the legacy of what Esther Cohen has called the 'philopassianism' of late medieval religious culture. Analysing early modern English translations of Calvin's *Institutes*, and of works by Teresa of Avila, Louis of Granada and Thomas of Villacastin S.J., he argues that in spite of its official Calvinism, early modern English religious culture was deeply hybrid in its understanding of pain. If Calvin's *Institutes* downplayed the significance of Christ's physical suffering, and emphasized his mental anguish, the emotional and bodily identification with the suffering Christ continued to have a powerful appeal. Indeed, the religious preoccupation with Christ's Passion seems to have caterered to a persistent need for both ritual and bodily religious experience, and Calvin's demotion of Christ's physical pain created a kind of cultural vacancy filled in part by Counter Reformation writers such as Louis of Granada.

If the lay confraternities of late medieval Italy cultivated a compassionate response to the divine suffering of Christ, Jenny Mayhew traces a specifically Protestant tradition of managing the human pains of illness. Mayhew maps a range of 'strategies of pain management' in a number of English Protestant godly manuals of the late sixteenth and early seventeenth centuries. She shows that the godly were encouraged to think of their symptoms in moral terms, as a sign of the 'need for the individual to mend the rift with his or her divine Maker'. Godly understandings of pain also shed light on a basic tension built into Calvinist understandings of suffering. Calvinism continued to stress the importance of suffering in the making of a true Christian, but had to reconcile this with its distrust of human free will. If Counter Reformation meditation manuals place the initiative squarely with the Christians who seek to identify with Christ's suffering, in godly manuals they can only accept the suffering that God has ordained for them: 'because the faithful have been chosen to suffer, they willingly choose to suffer'. In this sense, Mayhew also maps a Calvinist strategy for reclaiming a role for physical experience while avoiding any theological pitfalls: humans cannot *actively* choose to suffer with Christ, since this would amount to an arrogation of Christ's divinity, yet they can willingly embrace suffering when it presents itself.

Mayhew's emphasis is in part on the literary strategies – the rhetorical figures, imagery and narrative structures – employed in godly manuals. She also explores the idea that these strategies can affect the actual experience of pain; the authors she discusses certainly seem to have thought so. Mary Ann Lund similarly analyses the language of pain in John Donne's *Devotions upon Emergent Occasions, and Severall Steps in my Sicknes*, written in 1623 during a period of serious illness, and argues that the literary structuring of the experience of illness and pain, primarily through a pattern of arresting images, is central to the *Devotions*. Donne makes highly individual use of imagery drawn, for example, from the Scriptures and from Galenic and Paracelsian medicine.

As a devotional work with a deliberate literary design, the *Devotions* may be said to occupy a space between religion and literature. A number of the contributions to this volume focus on the representation of pain in texts more conventionally classified as 'literary', and investigate what specific role the literary representation of pain could take on in the interpretation of pain. Michael Schoenfeldt locates this role in the act of aesthetic representation itself. He proposes that a world with very few effective means of alleviating pain – as well as a lack of medical interest in the topic – would have have been especially 'alert to the possible anesthetic effects of literary and artistic representation'. He examines how a number of plays and poems by William Shakespeare explore the idea that the literary representation of pain, the 'aesthetic encounter with suffering', can somehow help to diminish it.

In Joseph Campana's essay on Edmund Spenser's *Faerie Queene*, the literary imagination takes on a mediating role within the changes in early modern religious attitudes towards pain discussed earlier in this introduction. Campana reads the persistent concern with physical suffering in Book I, "The Legend of Holiness", in the context of the English Reformation, investigating how Spenser employs the literary imagination to compensate for the loss of Catholic forms of affective piety, specifically the centrality of the suffering Christ. In placing pain at the centre of his conception of Holiness, Campana argues, Spenser drew on pre-Reformation religious sensibilities, re-imagining the meaning of suffering for a newly Protestant England that had pushed the bodily pain of Christ to the margins of its religious culture.

Frans Willem Korsten, by contrast, reads three plays by the seventeenth-century Dutch playwright Joost van den Vondel – *Gysbreght van Aemstel*, *Leeuwendalers* and *Noah* – as a critique of the Christian understandings of pain we have outlined. Korsten focuses on the Christian notion that both the suffering and the infliction of bodily pain are necessary for what Korsten terms 'the just organisation of history': the end of history, in both senses of that phrase, can only be realized through pain. He examines how Van den Vondel not only critically engages with this idea, but also imagines a radical alternative: a world without an ultimate end in history that, in Korsten's formulation, 'exists in time, and does not move through time', and is therefore not dependent on pain.

We noted earlier that the meaning of pain was bound up with issues of power and authority. This has also become clear in the large body of scholarship on the judicial infliction of pain in early modernity. Indeed, partly in the continuing wake of Michel Foucault's *Discipline and Punish*, torture has been a dominant topic in research on pain in the early modern period, especially the later sixteenth and seventeenth centuries.[18] As Jetze Touber shows in his contribution to this volume, the literature on this subject centres around two areas: early modern torture as punishment and as truth-finding. In punitive pain, the humiliation of the criminal, and the disintegration of his or her body (often continuing after death) served both as a public manifestation of the

[18] Jetze Touber's contribution to this volume contains a useful bibliography of the large and still expanding body of literature on this topic.

power of the state and, in Touber's words, 'as a collective vindication of the restored integrity of the social body'.

Inquisitive torture, carried out not in public but in a secluded space, operated on the assumption that only the body speaks the truth; pain is a way of bypassing the suspect's corrupt, sinful will. As Touber notes, 'the body, with its involuntary reactions, was deemed a more reliable witness than the devious mind'. In his analysis of a late sixteenth-century martyrology by the priest Antonio Gallonio, Touber argues that these two forms of torture could also be part of a single process, and that the idea of the body as a bearer of truth had a powerful ideological resonance. For Gallonio, a martyr's tortured body bore witness to the truth of the Catholic faith partly because it invested that faith with the reality and absoluteness of the body in pain. In this way, the destruction of the body and the production of (theological) truth blend into each other.

If for Gallonio the physicality of pain formed a source of rhetorical power, a kind of ultimate *enargeia*, it could also be employed to *discredit* a given ideological position, as becomes clear in Kristine Steenbergh's essay on notions of pain, anger and revenge in early modern England. She shows how the idea of pain as a bodily sensation was employed politically in early modern English controversies over the validity of anger. Seeking to denounce an aristocratic cult of righteous masculine anger, representatives of the newly centralized Elizabethan legal system defined anger as a form of self-inflicted bodily pain in which mental self-control is lost. Anger, precisely because of its physicality, 'serves no purpose but painful, uncontrollable self-destruction'. Aristocrats, by contrast, claimed that anger is an effective antidote to pain: it can 'make a valiant fighter forget his pain during combat' and therefore fosters masculine behaviour. In spite of their differences, it might be argued that both positions associate physical pain with weakness and with an undermining of masculinity.

The relation between pain and power comes to the fore in a different form in the discourse of early modern Neo-Stoicism, especially in the distinction it posits between bodily and mental pain. Neo-Stoicism locates ultimate authority in the individual – the Neo-Stoic sage who, through an extreme form of self-control, enables reason to triumph over affect. Pain management is a crucial element within this process: Neo-Stoicism construes physical pain as one of the external forces that can cause people to be overwhelmed by emotions. The Neo-Stoic sage seeks to manage pain, and to combat the power of affect, by maintaining that bodily pain is no true evil, and ultimately meaningless. Pain of the soul, by contrast, is a genuine evil, since it incapacitates reason, and makes it impossible to exercise virtue as the only true good. Reason has the fundamental ability to refuse to 'consent' to pain, in this way preventing it from penetrating into the soul. In order to keep physical pain from becoming real, mental pain, the sage must continuously repeat these principles to himself. The belittling of bodily pain requires a constant process of cultivation, daily exercise and meditation.

The Stoic individual, then, constitutes himself in part through pain; pain offers an opportunity to exercise true self-control. That the "Stoic path" played an important part in intellectual life from the mid-fourteenth until the late sixteenth century is shown by the enormous success of Petrarch's meditation manual *De remediis utriusque fortune* (first published in 1366), which forms the focus of Karl Enenkel's essay. Enenkel shows that Neo-Stoic attitudes towards pain were part of an elite humanist discourse, and had an implicit political dimension. In his illustrations to a popular early sixteenth-century German edition of *De remediis*, the so-called Petrarch Master reinterpreted Neo-Stoic discourse from a vernacular, Lutheran perspective, attaching a radically different meaning to pain. Physical pain plays a central and frequently spectacular role in these illustrations, and the Petrarch Master employs pain to propagate a range of religious and political views linked to the nascent Lutheran Reformation and at odds with Petrarch's Neo-Stoicism. This results in a striking discrepancy between word and image: while Petrarch's elite discourse revolves around a denial of the relevance of bodily pain, the Petrarch Master 'makes the viewer feel the violation, and indeed the humiliation' of the human body in pain. Pain is inflicted, moreover, on the powerless by those in power, and the Petrarch Master enlists pain in a critique of existing social hierarchies.

In early modernity, the cultural work of interpreting pain was carried out in a variety of areas. The meanings of pain were forged in religious, philosophical, judicial and political discourse, as well as in literary texts and the visual arts. Moreover, if early moderns turned, for example, to religion to make sense of pain, pain, as a powerful bodily sensation, in turn provided a tool for discussing a range of other issues, such as the nature of ritual, definitions of religious experience, notions of masculinity, selfhood and community, and the nature of political power. In order to do justice to this diversity, and to the interactions between the various ways of making sense of pain, an analysis of early modern perceptions of pain requires an interdisciplinary approach. The present volume aims to offer a first step towards such an approach, by studying the role of pain in a range of historical materials (including philosophical and medical treatises, poems, plays, paintings, engravings, martyrologies, educational manuals, ego documents, theological and mystical works, religious manuals, and trial reports), by mapping a number of the issues that were central in early modern understandings of pain, and by investigating how these issues interact.

Selective Bibliography

Bending L., *The Representation of Bodily Pain in Late Nineteenth-Century English Culture* (Oxford: 2000).

Cohen E., "Towards a History of European Physical Sensibility: Pain in the Later Middle Ages", *Science in Context* 8,1 (1995) 47–74.

Del Vecchio Good M.J. *et al.* (eds.), *Pain as Human Experience: An Anthropological Perspective* (Berkeley etc.: 1992).

Duncan G., "Mind-Body Dualism and the Biopsychosocial Model of Pain: What Did Descartes Really Say?", *Journal of Medicine and Philosophy* 25,4 (2000) 485–513.

Egmond F., "Execution, dissection, pain and infamy – a morphological investigation", in Egmond F. – Zwijnenberg F. (eds.), *Bodily Extremities: Preoccupations with the Human Body in Early Modern European Culture* (Aldershot – Burlington: 2003) 92–128.

Glucklich A., *Sacred Pain: Hurting the Body for the Sake of the Soul* (New York: 2001).

Hinnells J.R. – Porter R. (eds.), *Religion, Health and Suffering* (London – New York: 1999).

Lindemann M., *Medicine and Society in Early Modern Europe* (Cambridge: 1999).

Merback M.B., *The Thief, the Cross and the Wheel. Pain and the Spectacle of Punishment in Medieval and Renaissance Europe* (London: 1999).

Morris D.B., *The Culture of Pain* (Berkeley – Los Angeles: 1991).

Perkins J., *The Suffering Self: Pain and Narrative Representation in the Early Christian Era* (London: 1995).

Rey R., *The History of Pain*, trl. L.E. Wallace (Cambridge MA: 1995).

Scarry E., *The Body in Pain: The Making and Unmaking of the World* (Oxford: 1985).

Silverman L., *Tortured Subjects: Pain, Truth, and the Body in Early Modern France* (Chicago: 2001).

Wall P., *Pain: The Science of Suffering* (London: 1999).

Wear A., *Knowledge and Practice in English Medicine, 1550–1660* (Cambridge: 2000).

AESTHETICS AND ANESTHETICS: THE ART OF PAIN MANAGEMENT IN EARLY MODERN ENGLAND

Michael Schoenfeldt

'Pain don't hurt'
– Sparky Anderson

'Fuck Pain'
– Ishmael Reed[1]

If there is anything that unites us with early modern individuals, it is the inexorable experience of pain. Yet if there is anything that divides us, it is the available attitudes to pain, and the number of effectual measures for alleviating it. It is hard for us to think through a world which lacks ether, chloroform, and aspirin, much less the elaborate pharmacopoeia we now possess for treating pain. This was a world in which pain could be intense, unrelenting, and intractable; it is a world we have happily lost. Indeed, whereas we spend enormous amounts of money trying to relieve pain, the early modern period was more likely to expend effort to impose and enhance pain. Their extensive lexicon of implements of torture attests to this effort. People showed up in droves to watch the pain of others in public executions, and the represented pain of others in Renaissance tragedy. The predominant mode of poetry in the period – the Petrarchan sonnet sequence – was dedicated to the lyric exhibition of the prolonged agonies of unsatisfied desire (what Shakespeare in Sonnet 140 aptly characterizes as 'The manner of my pity-wanting pain'[2] and Donne, in 'The Triple Fool', irreverently terms 'whining poetry').[3]

The significant cultural productions of early modern Europe, then, were deeply invested in the cultivation and articulation of pain. Indeed,

[1] Both quotations are from Morris D., *The Culture of Pain* (Berkeley: 1993) 194 and 285, a wide-ranging exploration of the meanings of pain over time and culture.
[2] Quoted from Greenblatt S. (ed.), *The Norton Shakespeare* (New York: 1997). All subsequent citations of Shakespeare are from this edition.
[3] Quoted from Smith A.J. (ed.), *John Donne: The Complete English Poems* (London: 1971).

most evidence indicates that the culture would have distrusted and shunned the use of anesthetics had they been available. Gen. 3.16–17 suggests that suffering is God's punishment for the Fall; God tells Eve – 'I will greatly multiply thy sorowe and thy conception. In sorrow thou shalt bring forth children' – and he tells Adam: 'cursed is the ground for thy sake: in sorrow shalt thou eate of it all the dayes of thy life' [KJV]. Most commentators used this passage to suggest that pain is the compulsory condition of postlapsarian humanity; to attempt to mitigate it was seen as an abrogation of divine will (indeed, even in the nineteenth century, when ether and chloroform first became available, doctors and moralists worried about using any anesthetic, particularly around childbirth).[4] The etymology of the word *pain* from 'poenas', penalty or punishment, betrays much of the culture's attitude to pain. Embedded in the word is the notion that a person's suffering is due to some wrong for which one is being deservedly punished (this sense lingers in the legal phrase 'on pain of death'). Women are to have pain in childbirth, and all humans are to experience suffering, as a result of the Original Sin of Adam and Eve. In this theological framework, to alleviate pain is to repudiate God's will.

Pain, moreover, is the primary medium for divine-human communication in Judeo-Christian thought. Whereas the book of Job and the Davidic Psalms are extensive, lyrical meditations on divinely inspired pain, Christianity raises the level of pain several notches, suggesting that suffering is not just incidental to divine-human relations but rather is integral to salvation. Indeed, Christianity is the only religion I know in which an instrument of torture and death (the crucifix) serves as its central symbol. The image of Hell most frequently put forward by Christianity is that of a vast torture chamber. Since apostolic times, moreover, one's spiritual authenticity was continually attested by one's capacity to endure pain. In fact, what has been called the 'analgesic state' of Christian martyrs – in which they seem not to feel the horrible pains to which they are subjected – becomes the highest testament to their spiritual purity.[5]

---

[4] On the pains of childbirth, see Howard S., "Imagining the Pain and Peril of Seventeenth-Century Childbirth: Travail and Deliverance in the Making of an Early Modern World", *Social History of Medicine* 16,3 (2003) 367–382.

[5] On the analgesic state of martyrs, see Knott J.R., "John Foxe and the Joy of Suffering", *Sixteenth Century Journal* 27, 3 (Autumn, 1996) 721–734.

Very little attention, though, was paid to actual analgesics. Even medicine, a practice designed to heal, has in the early modern period few strategies of intervention that do not, inadvertently or directly, increase the pain of the patient. Most casebooks of the period simply address pain as a symptom of the body's humoral imbalance, and try to cure it by restoring that balance, usually through the imposition of uncomfortable or even painful therapeutic procedures. The typical response to pain is either bleeding the patient, or giving the patient medicines to induce vomiting or defecation, all in the effort to purge the humoral excess that in theory caused the pain. It is perhaps for this reason that Moliere was led to observe in the seventeenth century: 'Most people die of the cure, not the disease'.[6]

In the medical casebooks of John Hall, a physician in Stratford, England, who also happens to be Shakespeare's son-in-law, we are allowed to glimpse the quotidian registers of pain and its treatment in the period. Hall does record the pain of his patients; indeed, the biggest entry in the 'Alphabetical Table of Diseases and Medicines' that prefaces his casebook published under the wonderful title, *Select Observations on English Bodies* is 'Pain'. Under 'Pain' are listed: 'Of the Head, Of the teeth, Of the Shoulder, Of the Neck, Of the Breast, Of the Side, Of the Loins, Of the Back, Of the Stomach, Of the Belly'.[7] As the catalog makes clear, pain is promiscuous, located potentially in any part of the body where there are nerve endings. This entry is in fact followed by a whole range of maladies classed under 'Pain after Meat', and including 'With Indigestion, By Wind in the Stomach, With Pain and Hardness, Of the Heart, Of the Arms, Of the Thighs, of the Joynts, After delivered, Of various Parts, Of the Hemorrhoids, Of the Feet'. The observation of pain in all its myriad forms and locations, moreover, is scattered throughout the book.

A typical record of symptoms and treatment is that of John Nason, a 40-year-old Stratford barber. Nason, we are told, 'always after Meat suffered most bitter Pain of the Stomach, as also cruel Misery in the Loins, so that he had seldom any Sleep at nights'. Hall first prescribes an 'Emetick Infusion' which 'gave six Vomits and four Stools'. Such dramatic results were often imagined as proof of the efficacy of the

[6] Molière. *The Miser and Other Plays*, trans. J. Wood and J. Coward (New York: 2000) 276.

[7] John Hall, *Select Observations on English Bodies of Eminent Persons in desperate Diseases* (London, HH: 1683).

medicine! Hall then prescribes a mixture which includes hore-hound, rhubarb, aloe, and 'the Juyce of Goose dung' and concludes: 'And thus in few days he was cured'.[8] This, by the way, is Hall's concluding summary of every case, even those in which the patient was dead within the month. It is typical of the Galenic tradition to have medicines composed of numerous complex ingredients, each designed to do something that would restore the patient's humoral balance. Reading these casebooks in the context of modern medical treatment, one is struck by just how little attention is given to alleviating the pain of the patient, and how much attention is bestowed on addressing the imagined cause – some humoral imbalance – through the imposition of painful therapies.

The story is not much different for the period's surgeons. Indeed, in one of the most popular manuals of surgery in early modern England, William Clowes's *A Prooued practice for all young Chirurgians, concerning burnings with Gunpowder, and woundes made with Gunshot, Sword, Halbard, Pyke, Launce, or such other* (1588) [Verwijder London], the most unnerving thing is how incidental the attention to the pain of the surgical patient is. He writes, for example, of one patient who needs to have a limb amputated (probably the most common surgical intervention because of the widespread danger of infection in a world without penicillin):

> you shall haue a great regard to the state of his body, for evacuation and dieting. And after that his body is well prepared and purged, then the same morning that you attempt to cut off the member, be it leg or arm, let him haue some two hours before some good comfortable caudel or other broths, according vnto the direction of the Physician or Surgeon, only to corroborate and strengthen his stomach, and in any wise omit not but that he or she have ministered unto them some good exhortation by the minister or preacher.[9]

The patient is given only warm broth and moral exhortation as a preparation for the physiological torments that await. Now a caudel is in fact a warm drink consisting of thin gruel, sometimes mixed with wine or ale, sweetened and spiced, so the caudel might have had a little alcohol in it, although the analgesic effects of alcohol are not its primary goal.[10] It is unsettling that humoral preparation and moral exhortation

---

[8] Hall, *Select Observations* 62–63.

[9] William Clowes, *Selected Writing 1544–1604*, ed. F. Poynter (London: 1948) 84–85.

[10] See John Woodall, *The surgeons mate* (London, John Legate: 1655): 'a comfortable caudle made with some Wine, Spices, Sugar, and the yolk of an egge' (164).

about patience in adversity are imagined to be the only direct efforts to address the horrific pain the patient is about to feel.

In fact, the pain to be caused by the procedure is subsequently acknowledged, but only indirectly, through anxious attention to the details of preparation:

> you shall have in readiness a good, strong and steady form, and set the patient at the very end of it. Then there shall bestride the form behind him a man that is able to hold him or her fast by both arms. This done, if the leg must be taken off beneath the knee, let there be also appointed another strong man to bestride the leg that is to be cut off, and he must hold the member very fast about the place where the incision is to be made, and very steadily, without shaking; and he that doth so hold should have a large strong hand and a good fast grip, whereby he may the better stay the bleeding in the place or stead of a straight band or ligature, which band indeed is also very necessary, for, by reason of the hard and close binding, it so benumbs the part that the pain of the binding doth greatly obscure the sense and feeling of the incision.[11]

In this final detail, we get finally at some attention to the patient's excruciating pain beyond the need for strong men with steady hands to hold the patient down. The numbing effect of being bound tightly is valued, both for its minor analgesic effect, and for its ability to create a pain that distracts from the pain of the incision.

The medical practitioner here confronts something of a paradox – in order to minimize the patient's pain, the surgeon must find some way to ignore the ghastly agony he is about to cause. He must, in every sense of the phrase, be cruel to be kind:

> In like manner, there must be chosen another skilful man that has good experience in holding the leg below, for the member must not be held too high for fear of staying or choking of the saw, neither must he bear down his hand too low, for fear of fracturing the bones in the time it is a-sawing or cutting off. And he that is the Master or Surgeon who cuts off the member must be sure to have a sharp saw; also a very good catlin [a double-edged, sharp-pointed knife] and an incision knife. Then boldly, with a steady and quick hand cut the flesh round about to the bones without staying [...]. All this being orderly performed, then set your saw as near the sound flesh as well as you may, and so cut asunder the bones.[12]

---

[11] Clowes, *Selected Writings* 85–86.
[12] Clowes, *Selected Writings* 86.

Clowes also shows that he is on the cutting edge of surgical practice by advertising his knowledge of the techniques of Ambroise Pare, the innovative French surgeon: 'This done, Ambrose Pare, a man of great knowledge and experience in surgery, willeth, [...] that you then draw the sides of the wound together with four stitches that are deep in the flesh and made crosswise over the member'. Before Pare, the standard procedure for stopping the bleeding was to cauterize the wound with hot oil. Clowes, though, does not use Pare's technique himself: 'I must confess that I have cured many and yet never so stitched them'.[13] Nor does he endorse cauterization; instead, he emphasizes the use of a powder 'of my invention' which 'never causes pain, but often brings with it a perfect white digestive matter'. He mentions a time 'when there was taken off in one morning seven legs and arms, where, by the assistance and help of Almighty God, we stayed all their fluxes of blood, without any pain unto them, but only in the compression and close rolling, and tenderness of the wound excepted'.[14] This unknown powder functions as a kind of early topical analgesic.

Some effort, then, did go into the development of analgesics in the early modern period, but this work was diffuse, not sustained, and frequently under threat by the medical and religious establishment. In the sixteenth century, Paracelsus, the leading expounder of chemical medicine, experimented with the medical value of opium. One story suggests that he decided that its curative powers were of such magnitude that he called it Laudanum, from the Latin *laudare*, to praise.[15] It is hard to know exactly how widely laudanum was used, particularly in early modern England (although its addictive capacity would make it the bane of many Romantic writers). In John Manningham's *Diary* at the beginning of the seventeenth century, we learn that 'There is a certaine kinde of compound called Laudanum [...] the virtue of it is verry soveraigne to mitigate anie paine'.[16] In the later seventeenth century, the English physician Thomas Sydenham (1624–89) developed his own form of Laudanum. He recommended its use to relieve pain, to induce sleep, and to treat diarrhea and bowel obstruction. Sydenham

[13] Clowes, *Selected Writings* 86–87.

[14] Clowes, *Selected Writings* 88–89.

[15] Less colorfully, according to the *OED*, the name may come from or from *labdanum*, the term for a plant extract.

[16] Manningham J., *The Diary of John Manningham of the Middle Temple 1602–3* (Hanover, New Hampshire: 1976), 82.

praises opium fulsomely and unreservedly as the gift of a merciful deity to his suffering creatures:

> And here I cannot but break out in praise of the great God, the giver of all good things who hath granted to the human race, as a comfort in their afflications, no medicine of the value of opium; either in regard to the number of diseases that it can control, or its efficiency in extirpating them.[17]

Unlike so many in his generation and later, Sydenham imagined a deity invested in diminishing the suffering of humanity. In the *Advancement of Learning* (1605), Francis Bacon does not invoke the will of such a deity, but he does argue similarly that the goal of the healer should be the unconditional alleviation of suffering:

> I esteem it [...] to be clearly the office of a physician, not only to restore health, but also to mitigate the pains and torments of diseases; and not only when such mitigation of pain, as of a dangerous symptom, helps and conduces to recovery; but also when, all hope of recovery being gone, it serves only to make a fair and easy passage from life.[18]

Bacon is careful to distinguish between the incidental alleviation of pain in the effort to extend life, which most would support, and the intentional mitigation of pain when there is no help of recovery, which many would question. Bacon, with characteristic boldness, endorses the latter.

Such sporadic emphasis on the deliberate amelioration of suffering is so important because the experience of pain can consume one's entire being. If it is intense and unrelenting, pain inexorably invades all aspects of existence. 'Pain', writes Aristotle, one of its first theorists, 'upsets and destroys the nature of the person who feels it'.[19] It is a bodily phenomenon that affects and alters the behavior and psychological essence of those subject to it. In attempting to excuse the inexplicably rude behavior of Cornwall, King Lear invokes this principle, remarking that 'We are not ourselves / When nature, being oppressed, commands the mind / To suffer with the body' (2.2.272–4). The full and terrible truth of the transformative power of agony is unveiled over the oppressive

---

[17] Sydenham T., *Works* (London, 1848) I, 173.

[18] Francis Bacon, "Of the Dignity and Advancement of Learning", in Spedding J. – Ellis R.L. – Heath D.D. (eds.), *The works of Francis Bacon*, 14 vols. (London: 1861–1879), vol. IV, 387.

[19] Aristotle, *The Nicomachean Ethics*, transl. D. Ross (Oxford: 1980) 1119a.

course of that grueling play. The subject in intense pain can know nothing but that pain, and would instinctively do anything to end it; that is why it is so politically useful for repressive regimes to impose pain on others, as we have learned from Elaine Scarry and others.[20]

Yet Aristotle also linked the experience of pain to the exhibition of the virtue of courage, since 'courage involves pain, and is justly praised; for it is harder to face what is painful than to abstain from what is pleasant'.[21] Pain, moreover, has its salutary and even profitable aspects. Frequently a symptom of some deeper disorder, pain can be an urgent if enigmatic message delivered by illness or injury that must be read carefully. It is the body's insistent way of getting our attention when it is under duress. Without it, we would not remove our hand from a hot burner, or even notice a cut that requires bandaging and cleaning. The body that felt no pain would be a dangerous one to inhabit, as diabetic neuropathy has unfortunately taught us.

Pain, furthermore, can be considered philosophically useful in that its agonies can make visible the intrinsically invisible pleasures of health. As Michel de Montaigne, who suffered horribly from kidney stones, remarks:

> But is there anything so sweet as that sudden change, when from an extreme pain, by the voiding of my stone, I come to recover as if by lightning the beautiful light of health, so free and so full, as happens in our sudden and sharpest attacks of colic? Is there anything in this pain we suffer that can be said to counterbalance to the pleasure of such sudden improvement? How much more beautiful health seems to me after the illness, when they are so near and so contiguous.[22]

For Montaigne, the uses of corporeal adversity are truly sweet; Montaigne in fact finds an exhilarating pleasure in the health incumbent on the cessation of excruciating pain.

Montaigne, moreover, famously describes in exquisite detail his extensive ordeal with kidney stones, even as he struggles to welcome it as the occasion for the virtuous and praiseworthy exhibition of stoic forbearance:

---

[20] See Scarry E., *The Body in Pain: The Making and Unmaking of the World* (New York: 1985). 'Intense pain', asserts Scarry, 'is world-destroying' (29).

[21] Aristotle, *Nicomachean Ethics* 1117a.

[22] Michel de Montaigne, *The Complete Works*, transl. D.M. Frame (New York: 2003) 1021.

> There is pleasure in hearing people say about you: There indeed is strength, there indeed is fortitude! They see you sweat in agony, turn pale, turn red, tremble, vomit your very blood, suffer strange contractions and convulsions, sometimes shed great tears from your eyes, discharge thick, black, and frightful urine, or have it stopped up by some sharp rough stone that cruelly pricks and flays the neck of your penis; meanwhile keeping up conversation with your company with a normal countenance; jesting in the intervals with your servants, holding up your end in a sustained discussion, making excuses for your pain and mimizing your suffering. Do you remember those men of past times who sought out troubles with such great hunger, to keep their virtue in breath and in practice?[23]

Montaigne continually invokes stoic principles of forebearance in the effort to make his affliction morally useful as well as socially and ethically meaningful. Much of the immense attraction of Stoicism in the period derived from the fact that it offered a philosophical strategy for dealing with the inevitable onslaught of physical and emotional suffering. Stoicism is philosophy as anesthesia, a form of pain management. For the Stoic, pain is morally useful because it weans us from the flesh, preparing us for our ultimate separation from the flesh in death. Montaigne tries, and almost succeeds, in wringing meaning from the mundane details of his agonizing disease, taking heart, for example, in the idea that kidney stones only afflict the elderly, who have less to do with that region of the body anyway.

Caused by some disruption to the body but experienced as an assault on the soul, pain provides various early modern writers with an opportunity for exploring the philosophical conundrum of body-soul relations. Andrew Marvell's "A Dialogue between the soul and body" is a playful meditation on just this issue.[24] The poem is part of a long convention of such poems, but it is fascinating how completely Marvell imagines that the primary forms of communication between the body and soul entail the sensation of pain and the experience of coercion. The existence of the poem nevertheless attests to the necessary if agonized interdependence of the soul and the body. The soul calls the body a dungeon, and describes itself as 'inslaved' by 'bolts of bones', 'that fettered stands / In feet', and 'manacled in hands' (2–4). Etymology and assonance betray the bitter bondage of the body. Contemporaneous anatomical explorations and forms of political duress merge in the

---

[23] Montaigne, *Complete Works* 1019–20.

[24] Quoted in Smith N. (ed.), *The Poems of Andrew Marvell* (London: 2003). All subsequent citations of Marvell are from this edition.

description of the soul 'hung up, as 'twere, in chains / Of nerves, and arteries, and veins. / Tortured' (7–8). The body in turn attacks 'this tyrannic soul', complaining that it impales the body with its insistently upright posture. The body also declares that even the soul's purported gift of warmth and movement is no more than a fever could do (12). The soul responds by describing the complex processes by which pain is an experience of the body that scourges the soul: 'I feel, that cannot feel, the pain' (24). With a glance at the suffering caused by contemporary medicine, the soul complains that it is 'Constrained not only to endure / Diseases, but, what's worse, the cure' (27–28). The body in turn blames the soul for its experience of spiritual agonies, which it claims are even worse than corporal ones: 'the cramp of Hope', 'the palsy shakes of Fear', 'The pestilence of Love', 'Hatred's hidden ulcer', 'Joy's cheerful madness', and 'Sorrow's other madness' (33–38). Emotions, then, are imagined to be maladies that the Soul inflicts on the body. Marvell here plays on the deep connections among pathos, passion, and pathology intrinsic to the Stoic definition of apathy as the ideal state. The poem is a devastatingly witty account of the respective claims and complaints of body and soul. Whereas Montaigne imagines that the afflictions of the body provide a welcome opportunity for the soul to exercise virtue, Marvell wittily depicts a body and soul involved in the effort to impose mutual blame for the unquestioned fact of suffering. He shows how easily psychological and physiological agony become metaphors for each other.

Even as philosophy attempts to render suffering explicable and so bearable, there is a pronounced sense in early modern literature of the ideals of philosophy foundering before the hard facts of the body. The effort to treat pain with philosophy was one that Shakespeare and others viewed with much skepticism. In *Much Ado About Nothing*, Shakespeare betrays his fascination with the way that pained flesh defies the tenets of philosophy. Leonato protests to those who would offer him philosophical comfort: 'I will be flesh and blood, / For there was never yet philosopher / That could endure the toothache patiently, / However they have writ the style of gods, / And made a pish at chance and sufferance' (5.1. 34–8). In *King Lear*, Shakespeare famously uses the full gamut of human physical and psychological suffering to reveal the hollowness of the platitudes by which characters repeatedly attempt to comprehend and explain, if not ease, their pain. Edgar's moralization of Gloucester's blindness sounds horribly false against the myriad senseless horrors that the audience has been made to witness:

> The gods are just, and of our pleasant vices
> Make instruments to plague us.
> The dark and vicious place where thee he got
> Cost him his eyes (*King Lear* 5.3.160–3).

Edgar's words bespeak an understandable longing for some symmetry between crime and punishment. The extreme and agonizing details of the play's relentless suffering, though, belie any fiction of apparent justice.

Similarly, John Milton's *Samson Agonistes*, a closet drama, is also concerned with the ways that horrible suffering challenges any assertion of terrestrial justice or divine goodness. The chorus demonstrates a deep skepticism about the capacity of philosophical platitudes to ease suffering:

> Many are the sayings of the wise
> In ancient and in modern books enrolled;
> Extolling patience as the truest fortitude;
> And to the bearing well of all calamities,
> All chances incident to man's frail life
> Consolatories writ
> With studied argument, and much persuasion sought
> Lenient of grief and anxious thought,
> But with the afflicted in his pangs their sound
> Little prevails, or rather seems a tune,
> Harsh, and of dissonant mood from his complaint.[25]

In both *Lear* and *Samson*, the fact of unrelenting agony challenges the rationalizations that characters keep generating in a vain effort to comfort themselves and others.

The pain experienced by Montaigne and Gloucester is inexorably physical while Leonato's is primarily emotional, but this is a period that did not make a hard and fast distinction between physical and emotional pain. Indeed, the vocabularies of suffering continue to migrate between these two realms that for us designate quite separate phenomena. The word 'grief', for example, is used extensively in the period to describe both physical and emotional suffering. Derived from the Old French word, *grever*, 'to harm', grief means 'hardship, suffering, injury, both physical and social; physical as well as mental pain', as if the distinction were not worth making in the face of the agony involved. The common

[25] Quoted in Carey J. (ed.), *Milton: The Complete Shorter Poems* (London: 2007) 652–662. All subsequent citations of Milton are from this edition.

phrase 'grievous wounds' attests to the capacity of the word to bridge physical and emotional suffering. Indeed, in *The Use of Passions*, J.F. Senault explores the effects of grief on both body and soul:

> Grief is a Reall evill, which sets upon the soul, and body both at once, and makes two wounds at one blow. I know, there are some sorrows that wound only the minde, and exercise all their might upon the Noblest part of man; but if they be Violent, they work upon the body; and by a secret contagion: the pains of the Mistress, become the disease of the Slave.[26]

In the early modern physiological regime, grief is continually imagined to have a palpable, material presence in the body. Before her apparently fatal attack of grief, Shakespeare's Hermione declares to Leontes: 'But I have / That honourable grief lodged here which burns / Worse than tears drown' (*The Winter's Tale* 2.1.112–14). Discussing the death of his spouse, the moral philosopher and medical inquirer Sir Kenelm Digby eloquently portrays his internal agony as a 'corrosive masse of sorrow lying att my hart wch will not be worne away vntill it haue worne me out'.[27] Flesh is not a realm completely separate from the soul, but is a name for the thickening and coagulation of emotion around the intense sensations of pain and grief. Even our word 'disease', we should remember, derives from the idea of the intense discomfort intrinsic to illness. Hall and other physicians repeatedly treat patients for the ostensibly spiritual state of 'melancholy' with aggressive purges of their material humors.

Milton's *Samson Agonistes* is among many things an extended study in the excruciating concurrence of physical and spiritual torment. Samson complains bitterly about the way his suffering occurs in body and soul at once:

> O that torment should not be confined
> To the body's wounds and sores
> With maladies innumerable
> In heart, head, breast, and reins;
> But must secret passage find

---

[26] Senault J.F., *The Use of Passions*, trans. Henry, earl of Monmouth. (London: 1649) 477.

[27] Quoted in Evans R.C., "Lyric Grief in Donne and Jonson", in Swiss M. – Kent D.A. (eds.), *Speaking Grief in English Literary Culture: Shakespeare to Milton* (Pittsburgh: 2002) 56. The series of letters that Digby writes to his brother describing in excruciating detail his grief can be read in Gabrielli V., *Sir Kenelm Digby: Un Inglese Italianato nell'età della Controriforma* (Rome: 1957) 237–283.

To the inmost mind,
There exercise all his fierce accidents,
And on her purest spirits prey,
As on entrails, joints, and limbs,
With answerable pains, but more intense,
Though void of corporal sense.
My griefs not only pain me
As a lingering disease,
But finding no redress, ferment and rage,
Nor less than wounds immedicable
Rankle, and fester, and gangrene,
To black mortification.
Thoughts my tormenters armed with deadly stings
Mangle my apprehensive tenderest parts,
Exasperate, exulcerate, and raise
Dire inflammation which no cooling herb
Or med'cinal liquor can assuage,
Nor breath of vernal air from snowy alp.
Sleep hath forsook and given me o'er
To death's benumbing opium as my only cure (606–630).

For Samson, the 'torture of the mind' (to borrow a phrase from *Macbeth* [3.2.23]) is even crueler than the physical tortures to which it is compared because there are no available therapies of tangible relief. Indeed, the only opiate that Samson can imagine capable of relieving his fierce agony is death.

Samson finds himself experiencing the deleterious effects of physical and spiritual pain cumulatively. Others, though, imagined that one kind of pain might distract from another. Lear on the heath – another searing image of the body and soul at once in pain – finds physical suffering strangely soothing, because it distracts him from his profound mental anguish: 'where the greater malady is fixed, / The lesser is scarce felt' (*King Lear* 3.4.8–9). Lear here invokes an ancient principle of pain management – the idea that one pain distracts from another. In the *Hippocratic Writings*, we read the parallel recommendations 'Match like with like, for example pain calms pain' and 'From two pains occurring simultaneously but not in the same place, the strongest obscures the other'.[28] The idea that pain is not necessarily cumulative, but can be used as a distraction from another pain, fascinated many early modern

[28] *Epidemics V and Aphorismes II*, 46 in Littré E., *Oeuvres complètes* (Paris: 1839–1861). Cited in Rey R., *The History of Pain*, transl. L.E. Wallace, J.A. and S.W. Cadden (Cambridge: 1995) 22.

writers. Shakespeare in particular makes frequent use of the idea. In *Romeo and Juliet*, Benvolio tells Romeo: 'one fire burns out another's burning, / One pain is lessened by another's anguish [...] One desperate grief cures with another's languish. / Take thou some new infection to thy eye, / And the rank poison of the old will die' (1.2.43–8). Suffering and disease here function as a kind of homeopathic cure for suffering and disease. In *King Lear*, Edgar remarks on the sobering comfort he achieves by confronting a monarch whose even greater afflictions have brought him to the point of madness:

> When we our betters see bearing our woes,
> We scarcely think our miseries our foes.
> Who alone suffers suffers most i' the mind,
> Leaving free things and happy shows behind:
> But then the mind much sufferance doth o'erskip,
> When grief hath mates, and bearing fellowship.
> How light and portable my pain seems now,
> When that which makes me bend makes the king bow,
> He childed as I fathered! (3.6.95–103).

Edgar discovers a kind of topical relief from his own severe pain in the presence of the profound suffering of his monarch. In *Cymbeline*, a play engaged with a wide range of suffering, Belarius remarks: 'Great griefs, I see, medicine the less' (4.2.244). Like the benumbing effect of close binding identified by Clowes, discomfort can elicit the analgesic of distraction. Indeed, if the various violent purges recommended by Galenic medicine had any positive effects at all, it may have been in the production of a kind of distress that distracted one from the primary pain.

A world that had few genuine analgesics at its disposal would be more likely to cherish this minor blessing. It would also have been more alert to the possible anesthetic effects of literary and artistic representation. The paradoxically consoling effects of pain, I would argue, can occur not only in the tangible worlds of the individual body and its socio-political relations, but also in the more ethereal realm of aesthetics. In *The Rape of Lucrece*, Shakespeare's early narrative exploring the immense personal suffering caused by the personal and political violence of rape, Shakespeare explores the possibility that the aesthetic encounter with suffering can produce a kind of anesthetic effect. When the despairing Lucrece looks at a painting of the sack of Troy, she looks for a face 'where all distress is stelled' (1444), and finds it in the figure of 'despairing Hecuba':

> In her the painter had anatomized
> Time's ruin, beauty's wreck, and grim care's reign;
> Her cheeks with chaps and wrinkles were disguised;
> Of what she was no semblance did remain.
> Her blue blood changed to black in every vein,
> Wanting the spring that those shrunk pipes had fed,
> Showed life imprisoned in a body dead (1450–1456).

Hecuba of course is a figure to whom Shakespeare would return in *Hamlet*. The prince famously asks of an actor who has been brought to actual tears in playing the role: 'What's Hecuba to him or he to Hecuba?' (2.2.536). Whereas in *Hamlet*, Shakespeare is fascinated by the way that dramatic reenactment elicits an outpouring of extreme emotion that Hamlet envies, in *Lucrece* Shakespeare is preoccupied by the painter's capacity to find physical correlatives for the devastations of immense internal suffering. In both cases, he explores the potentially salutary effects of another's agony.

Lucrece, we learn, finds a particular model of emotional self-fashioning in Hecuba's extravagant grief:

> On this sad shadow Lucrece spends her eyes,
> And shapes her sorrow to the beldame's woes,
> Who nothing wants to answer her but cries
> And bitter words to ban her cruel foes.
> The painter was no god to lend her those,
> And therefore Lucrece swears he did her wrong,
> To give her so much grief and not a tongue (1457–1463).

As 'feelingly she weeps Troy's painted woes' (1492), Lucrece completely loses track of the time, or of her own tragic situation. In the words of Marvell's Soul, she finds a way 'Within another's grief to pine' (22). Shakespeare here is interested in the idea that aesthetic absorption can have anesthetic effects. Sympathetic identification with other's suffering, he suggests, offers some temporary relief from our pain.

Lucrece in fact is briefly transported from her own tragic situation by her commiserative encounter with the painting:

> Which all this time hath overslipped her thought
> That she with painted images hath spent,
> Being from the feeling of her own grief brought
> By deep surmise of others' detriment,
> Losing her woes in shows of discontent.
> It easeth some, though none it ever cured,
> To think their dolour others have endured (1576–1582).

Shakespeare here rejects any possibility of art's curative powers, but he does suggest that there is a significant, if temporary, analgesic effect achieved in compassionately viewing the suffering of others in art. Remarkably, Lucrece temporarily forgets her actual woes in her gripping encounter with the painted woes of Hecuba. She is transported beyond her own suffering through her thorough identification with another's suffering.

Lucrece, though, feels that the painter has wronged Hecuba 'To give her so much grief and not a tongue', because speaking is another way of assuaging suffering (1463). The relief involved in viewing the suffering of others is matched by the possible cathartic relief involved in the verbal articulation of one's pain. Pain and suffering, first of all, induce a series of physical manifestations which are in fact physiologically efficacious. Sighing, groaning, and weeping, for example, were for the most part encouraged in the medical literature, because they were thought to have a deeply therapeutic function. As Senault argues in *The Use of Passions*, 'a man that weeps, easeth himself, and comforts himself whilest he complains; he finds somewhat of Delight in his lamentations; [...] As Choler dischargeth it self by Railing, Sorrow being more innocent, drops away by Tears, and abandons the Heart, when it gets up into the Face'.[29] Senault here connects emotional catharsis to the Galenic purgation of excess humors.

Characters in Shakespeare's plays continually voice the need to express their inner suffering. Ross in *Richard II* complains about the weight of a heart surcharged with emotion, having no safe outlet: 'My heart is great, but it must break with silence / Ere'it be disburdened with a liberal tongue' (2.1.229–30). In *All's Well that Ends Well*, the Countess connects crying to speaking as parallel forms of catharsis: 'My heart is heavy and mine age is weak; / Grief would have tears, and sorrow bids me speak' (3.4.41–2). In *Macbeth*, Malcolm urges the distraught and stunned Macduff to utter rather than to suppress his extreme grief over the slaughter of his family: 'Give sorrow words. The grief that does not speak, / Whispers the o'er-fraught heart, and bids it break' (4.3.210–11).[30] In *The Arte of English Poesie*, George Puttenham explores the complex relief that is involved in the verbal release of intense woe:

---

[29] Senault, *Use of Passions* 485.

[30] See my essay, "'Give Sorrow Words': Emotional Loss and the Articulation of Temperament in Early Modern England", in Dufallo B. – McCracken P. (eds.), *Dead Lovers: Erotic Bonds and the Study of Premodern Europe* (Ann Arbor: 2007) 149.

'Lamenting is altogether contrary to rejoicing: every man saith so, and yet it is a piece of joy to be able to lament with ease and freely to pour forth a man's inward sorrows and the griefs wherewith his mind is surcharged'.[31] The Galenic idea of purging humoral excess provides a model for the apt expression of emotion as a way of alleviating the devastations of grief. Like art, expressive language provides a kind of topical, temporary anesthetic for suffering.

Nietzsche claimed that we engage with tragedy in order to come to terms with the truth about unredeemable suffering.[32] It is also possible that we engage with tragedy because we find in it a precious if temporary anesthesia from our own suffering. Perhaps the analgesic effect of viewing another's suffering is an early modern version of Aristotelean catharsis. In the Preface to *Samson Agonistes*, Milton gives his own particularly materialist reading of Aristotle's definition of tragedy, arguing that the genre is designed

> to be of power by raising pity and fear, or terror, to purge the mind of those and such-like passions, that is to temper and reduce them to just measure with a kind of delight, stirred up by reading or seeing those passions well imitated (3–6).

Tellingly, Milton suggests that tragedy functions therapeutically. He compares the action of tragedy to the principles of homeopathic medical therapy: 'for so in physic things of melancholic hue and quality are used against melancholy, sour against sour, salt to remove salt humours' (7–9). One reads a narrative of horrible suffering such as *Samson* in order to achieve a kind of temporary reprieve from one's own inevitable suffering.

Auden famously declared that 'about suffering they were never wrong, the old masters'. I would like to disagree. It may indeed be true that we are always necessarily oblivious to the full toll of the agony around us, that, as Auden says, suffering 'takes place / While someone else is eating or opening a window or just walking dully along'.[33] But the tendency of certain old masters to gratify and sanctify suffering is an area in which I would like to posit that they were misguided. Suffering,

---

[31] Puttenham G., *The Art of English Poesy*, ed. Whigham F. and Rebhorn W. (Ithaca: 2007) 135.

[32] Friedrich Nietzsche, *The Birth of Tragedy* (Harmondsworth: 1994).

[33] Auden W.H., "Musee des Beaux-Arts" 1, 3–4. Cited in Mendelson E. (ed.), *W.H. Auden: Collected Poems* (New York: 1991) 179.

I want to argue, is no necessary mark of virtue or sanctification. It is just pain, something to be avoided or diminished whenever possible, knowing that it is always around the corner, and always will win in the end. Indeed, the myth, inherited from the Romantics, that great art is forged in the crucible of suffering, is simply a secularization of the religious valorization of pain as necessary to salvation. The distribution of pain is so random, so widespread, and so irrational that like Edgar in *King Lear*, we are drawn out of desperation to explain it by recourse to the divine. Much of the religious and literary history of the west can be explained by the ubiquitous if understandable need for a narrative that could successfully rationalize the phenomenon of indiscriminate and purposeless suffering.

If, as Frederick Jameson asserts in *The Political Unconscious*, 'History is what hurts', then most literary and artistic production can be seen as the effort to deal with the pain of history. The end of history, moreover, would be the end of pain.[34] Here the Marxist literary critic Jameson, surprisingly, agrees completely with John of Patmos (perhaps revealing an unexpected connection between Marxist apocalypticism and Christian soteriology). In the Revelation of St. John, the end of time is imagined as the end of the sorrow and woe inaugurated by the Fall: 'God shall wipe away all tears from their eyes; and there shall be no more death, neither sorrow, nor crying, neither shall there be any more pain' (Rev. 21.4; KJV). If God is imagined to be the source of all our pain and woe in the Judeo-Christian dispensation, he will also be the agent of its amelioration at the end of time. The end of time is the end of pain, and until then, pain will not end. Until then, we need to work on developing a history, and a history of pain, that is neither a celebration of pain nor deaf to the sufferings of others. I have tried in this essay to use the sporadic early modern engagements with pain management to try to think about pain untainted by the meretricious and distorting discourses of sadism, masochism, and sanctification. 'The only end of writing' argues Dr. Samuel Johnson, a century after the writers we have been considering, 'is to enable readers better to enjoy life or better to endure it'.[35] I find some real comfort in the idea

---

[34] Jameson F., *The Political Unconscious: Narrative as Socially Symbolic Act* (Ithaca: 1981) 102.

[35] Johnson Samuel, "Review of a Free Inquiry into the Nature and Origin of Evil", in Brack O.M. Jr (ed.), *The Yale Edition of the Works of Samuel Johnson*, vol. XVII (New Haven: 2004) 421.

that literature at its best is designed to add to our small modicum of pleasure, or to help us deal with the inevitable, myriad, assaults of pain. Perhaps even with our contemporary plethora of powerful painkilling drugs, there is still a need for the subtle anesthetic effects of aesthetic phenomena.

Selective Bibliography

Aristotle, *The Nicomachean Ethics*, transl. D. Ross (Oxford: 1980).

Bacon Francis, *Of the Dignity and Advancement of Learning*, in Sedding J. – Ellis R.L. – Heath D.D. (eds.), *The works of Francis Bacon*, 14 vols. (London: 1861–1879).

Carey J. (ed.), *Milton: The Complete Shorter Poems* (London: 2007).

Clowes William, *Selected Writing 1544–1604*, ed. F. Poynter (London: 1948).

Evans R.C., "Lyric Grief in Donne and Jonson", in Swiss M. – Kent D.A. (eds.), *Speaking Grief in English Literary Culture: Shakespeare to Milton* (Pittsburgh: 2002) 42–68.

Greenblatt S. (ed.), *The Norton Shakespeare* (New York: 1997).

Hall John, *Select Observations on English Bodies of Eminent Persons in desperate Diseases* (London, HH: 1683).

Howard S., "Imagining the Pain and Peril of Seventeenth-Century Childbirth: Travail and Deliverance in the Making of an Early Modern World", *Social History of Medicine* 16,3 (2003) 367–382.

Jameson F., *The Political Unconscious: Narrative as Socially Symbolic Act* (Ithaca: 1981).

Johnson Samuel, "Review of a Free Inquiry into the Nature and Origin of Evil", in Brack O.M. Jr (ed.), *The Yale Edition of the Works of Samuel Johnson*, vol. XVII (New Haven: 2004) 421.

Knott J.R., "John Foxe and the Joy of Suffering", *Sixteenth Century Journal* 27,3 (1996) 721–734.

Manningham John, *The Diary of John Manningham of the Middle Temple 1602–3* (Hanover, New Hampshire: 1976).

Mendelson E. (ed.), *W.H. Auden: Collected Poems* (New York: 1991).

Molière, *The Miser and Other Plays*, transl. Wood J. and Coward J. (New York: 2000).

Montaigne Michel de, *The Complete Works*, transl. Frame D.M. (New York: 2003).

Morris D., *The Culture of Pain* (Berkeley: 1991).

Nietzsche Friedrich, *The Birth of Tragedy* (Harmondsworth: 1994).

Puttenham G., *The Art of English Poesy*, ed. F. Whigham and W. Rebhorn (Ithaca: 2007).

Rey R., *The History of Pain*, transl. L.E. Wallace, J.A. and S.W. Cadden (Cambridge: 1995).

Scarry E., *The Body in Pain: The Making and Unmaking of the World* (New York: 1985).

Schoenfeldt M., "'Give Sorrow Words': Emotional Loss and the Articulation of Temperament in Early Modern England", in Dufallo B. – McCracken P. (eds.), *Dead Lovers: Erotic Bonds and the Study of Premodern Europe* (Ann Arbor: 2007) 143–164.

Senault J.F., *The Use of Passions*, trans. Henry, Earl of Monmouth (London: 1649).

Smith A.J. (ed.), *John Donne: The Complete English Poems* (London: 1971).

Smith N. (ed.), *The Poems of Andrew Marvell* (London: 2003).

Sydenham T., *Works*, tr. Greenhill, 2 vols. (London: 1848, 1850).

Woodall John, *The surgeons mate* (London, John Legate: 1655).

WHIPPING BOYS: ERASMUS' RHETORIC OF CORPOREAL PUNISHMENT AND ITS DISCONTENTS

Anita Traninger

It *is* possible to teach Latin without beating the student at the same time. That, in any event, was Roger Ascham's claim in his work *Schoolmaster Or plain and perfect way of teaching children to understand, write, and speak the Latin tongue.* At the time it was written, however, this was still a minority opinion, and Ascham's claim would have seemed outlandish to most educators of the day.[1]

It is quite telling that Ascham should have plugged his method of conveying 'a sufficient ability to understand, write, and speak Latin' with the promise to succeed 'in short time, and with small pains'. For as Juan Luis Vives suggests in the *Exercitatio linguae latinae* (1538), a series of didactic dialogues meant to facilitate the learning of Latin, pain-related terminology such as *vapulare* ('being beaten') and *ferula* ('the rod') belong to the basic vocabulary related to schools and schooling. In the dialogue *Euntes ad ludum literarium* Vives lets us listen in on a conversation between Cirratus and Praetextatus, who are on their way to school, and the gallivanting Titivillitius:

Cirratus:	But why art thou then not remaining at home?
Titivillitius:	I shall return immediately, only I will now play dice a little with the son of this cobbler. Will you also come with us?
Cirratus:	We will go, please.
Praetextatus:	Certainly I shall not do so.
Cirratus:	Why not?
Praetextatus:	We don't want to get a thrashing.
Cirratus:	Ah! I had not thought of that.
Titivillitius:	You won't get thrashed.
Cirratus:	How do you know that?
Titivillitius:	Because your master lost his rod to-day.
Cirratus:	Eh! by what means did you get to know that?

[1] Ascham R., *The Schoolmaster* (1570), ed. L.V. Ryan (Ithaca, NY: 1967) 1.

Titivillitius: To-day we heard him from our house shouting out – and it was for his rod he was seeking.[2]

A dialogue about being whipped by the schoolmaster was seen as a matter of course in the sixteenth century. And more than this: in the genre of student dialogues in the late medieval and early modern period, the theme was widespread, indeed one of the most popular of all.[3] Against this backdrop, it is quite surprising that in modern handbooks of pedagogy and histories of education the historical practices are not analysed in depth. Hardly an effort is made to come to terms with the prevailing method of teaching; instead the writings of its opponents are quoted at length. That there *was* a pervasive and habitualized practice that corresponded to the thematic ubiquity of pain seems a reasonable conclusion to draw. And yet there is remarkably little reflection on the function of beatings, canings, and general maltreatment in the classroom in the early modern period. When one turns to the standard reference works, often multi-volume surveys of considerable breadth, the theme is addressed primarily at the level of theory and pedagogical writings,[4] and quite often, it has to be said, the discussion is biased

---

[2] *Tudor School-Boy Life. The Dialogues of Juan Luis Vives*, transl. F. Watson (London: 1908; reprint London: 1970) 13: 'CIR.: Quin tu igitur manes domi? TIT.: Continuo reuertar, nunc prodeo lusum talis com filio huius cerdonis. Vultis et uos uenire? CIR.: Eamus sodes. PRAET.: Minime uero id quidem. CIR.: Quid ni? PRAET. Ne uapulemus. CIR.: Vah, non memineram. TIT.: Non uapulabitis. CIR.: Qui scis? TIT.: Quia magister uester perdidit heri ferulam. CIR.: Hem quomodo nosti? TIT.: Hodie de domo nostra audiebamus eius uociferationem quaerentis ferulam'; Juan Luis Vives, *Los diálogos (Lingvae Latinae Exercitatio)*, ed. M.a Pilar García Ruiz (Pamplona: 2005) 132–134.

[3] *A Fifteenth Century School Book. From a Manuscript in the British Museum (Ms. Arundel 249)*, ed. W. Nelson (Oxford: 1956) xiii: 'All the vulgaria have much to say about beating – it seems to have been one of the major topics of conversation among Tudor schoolboys'. See the documentation in Bömer A., *Die lateinischen Schülergespräche der Humanisten* (Berlin: 1897/1899; reprint Amsterdam: 1966), as well as Bömer, "Lernen und Leben auf den Humanistenschulen im Spiegel der lateinischen Schülerdialoge", in the same volume, 1–29 (separate pagination), here 10.

[4] To name just a few works, flogging as a pedagogical practice is not acknowledged in Garin E., *L'educazione in Europa 1400/1600. Problemi e programmi* (Rome: 1976); Musolff H.-U., *Erziehung und Bildung in der Renaissance. Von Vergerio bis Montaigne* (Cologne – Weimar – Vienna: 1997); there are no pertinent entries in Benner D. – Oelkers J. (eds.), *Historisches Wörterbuch der Pädagogik* (Weinheim – Basel: 2004). Good overviews of historical practices, on the other hand, are to be found in Grendler P.F., *Schooling in Renaissance Italy. Literacy and Learning, 1300–1600* (Baltimore – London: 1989); Strauss G., *Luther's House of Learning: Indoctrination of the Young in the German Reformation* (Baltimore – London: 1978); Bowen J., *A History of Western Education. Volume Two. Civilization of Europe, Sixth to Sixteenth Century* (London: 1975). Yet even these works do not examine this theme in detail.

against corporeal punishment,[5] however understandable this may be from a modern point of view.

As a general rule, the early modern period is usually discussed by way of the reflections of prominent men such Erasmus, Vives, Montaigne, and Comenius, all of whom were well-known for their more or less rigorous denunciations of the use of physical punishment as an educational method. It is thus the ideological writings of a few which are taken to be representative, but which actually obfuscate the historical meaning of a pedagogy characterized by a violent involvement of the student's body almost unimaginable today. Yet it is true that it was precisely the daily and habitual beatings in the schools themselves that left few discursive traces behind. There is hardly a tract available to the modern scholar that interprets beatings from the perspective of its intentions or that provides it with a methodological foundation. That it was ubiquitous, however, is not least evidenced by the polemics and invectives written against it. An irrelevant phenomenon hardly would have been attacked so fervently.[6]

Flogging, of course, goes back a long way.[7] Although in Roman antiquity the beating of freemen was actually viewed as somewhat precarious in contrast to the beating of slaves, the use of violence in the classroom was a habitual practice. In the classical age, the various methods of beating were subject to a finely differentiated code of practice that not only placed significant distinctions between the situations, the participants, and the instruments in their appropriate combinations, but invested the practice with meaning as well. Freemen were punished with rods or switches (*virgae*), those in the military with clubs (*fustes*). The whip (*flagrum*, but more frequently *flagellum*), the most humiliating and least honourable of all, was reserved for the beating of slaves.[8] In the schools, finally, and in the realm of the pedagogic in general, the cane

[5] Cf. the evocative title of the German translation of de Mause's *History of Childhood* (New York: 1974), *Hört Ihr die Kinder weinen* (Frankfurt a.M.: 1980).

[6] Cunningham H., *Children and Childhood in Western Society since 1500* (London – New York: 1998) 43: 'Historians are rightly wary of assuming that advice was put into practice; we might do better to assume that the advice was necessary only because practice was to the contrary'.

[7] Cf. Marrou H.-I., *Histoire de l'éducation dans l'antiquité* (Paris: ³1955) 220–222.

[8] Saller R.P., *Patriarchy, Property and Death in the Roman Family* (Cambridge: 1996) 133–153; for the peculiarities of the beating of children within the household cf. de Bruyn T.S., "Flogging a Son: The Emergence of the *pater flagellans* in Latin Christian Discourse", *Journal of Early Christian Studies* 7,2 (1999) 249–290.

(*ferula*) was the preferred tool.[9] For the beating of children outside of the home there was a clear tendency to grant general licence: it was numbered among the typical duties of the *magistri* or the schoolmaster. On account of its pedagogical purpose, a beating by a teacher was not viewed as *iniuria*. The use of violence in the school was the expression of *potestas*, which had been invested in the schoolmaster, and not the application of illegitimate *violentia*. And thus, with no legal impediments, the cane held sway in both the elementary and the grammar schools; only very few educators appear to have completely done away with the physical disciplining of students.[10] As a consequence, both the *ferula* and the *virga* became the stock items of any European classroom. They became the insignia, the iconographical attributes of the pedagogue as well as the emblems of scholastic discipline [Fig. 1 and 2].

Hence we are dealing with a well established code of practice when, in 1529, Erasmus of Rotterdam published *De pueris statim ac liberaliter instituendis* (*A Declamation on the Subject of Early Liberal Education for Children*).[11] Although scholars do not count it among his more re-nowned or popular works, it nevertheless proved to be widely influential both during its age and beyond. The intention of the text was no less than to level the charge of scandal against the praxis of school beatings, a gesture that has since earned the humanist a place in educational research that associates him with a type of pacific humanism considered years ahead of its time.[12] Erasmus is seen as not only the greatest pedagogue of the sixteenth century (despite the fierce competition of figures such as Vives, Melanchthon, and Sturm, to name just a few), but even as a proto-feminist and an early advocate for the education of

---

[9] Fuhrmann M., "verbera", in *Paulys Realencyclopädie der Classischen Altertumswissenschaft. Supplementband IX* (Stuttgart: 1962) 1589–1597, here 1590. Cf. Garnsey P., *Social Status and Legal Privilege in the Roman Empire* (Oxford: 1970) 137.

[10] Fuhrmann, "verbera" 1596–1597, quoting Quintilian, *Institutio oratoria* I 3,14–17 and Plutarchus, *Liber educationis*, 9 A. Cf. also Ferrari L.C., "The Boyhood Beatings of Augustine", *Augustinian Studies* 5 (1974) 1–14.

[11] I will refer to the following editions: Desiderius Erasmus of Rotterdam, *Declamatio de pueris statim ac liberaliter instituendis*, ed. J.-C. Margolin (Geneva: 1966); idem, "A Declamation on the Subject of Early Liberal Education for Children. De pueris statim ac liberaliter instituendis declamatio, transl. and annotated by Beert C. Verstraete", in idem, *Literary and educational writings 4. De pueris instituendis; De recta pronuntiatione*, ed. J.K. Sowards, *Collected Works of Erasmus* 26 (Toronto – Buffalo – London: 1985) 291–346.

[12] For a sketch of the pedagogical programme see Margolin J.-C., "Pédagogie et philosophie dans le 'De pueris instituendis' d'Erasme", *Paedagogica Historica* 4,2 (1964) 370–391.

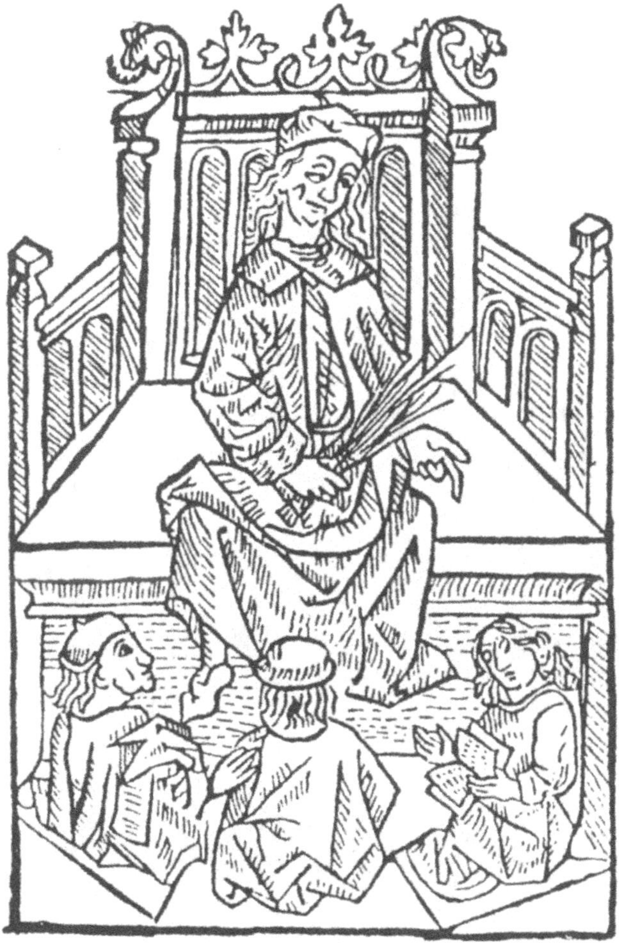

Fig. 1. Quentell workshop, *Teacher on the cathedra with pupils*, woodcut, Cologne, 1495. From Reicke E., *Der Gelehrte in der deutschen Vergangenheit* (Leipzig: 1900) 36.

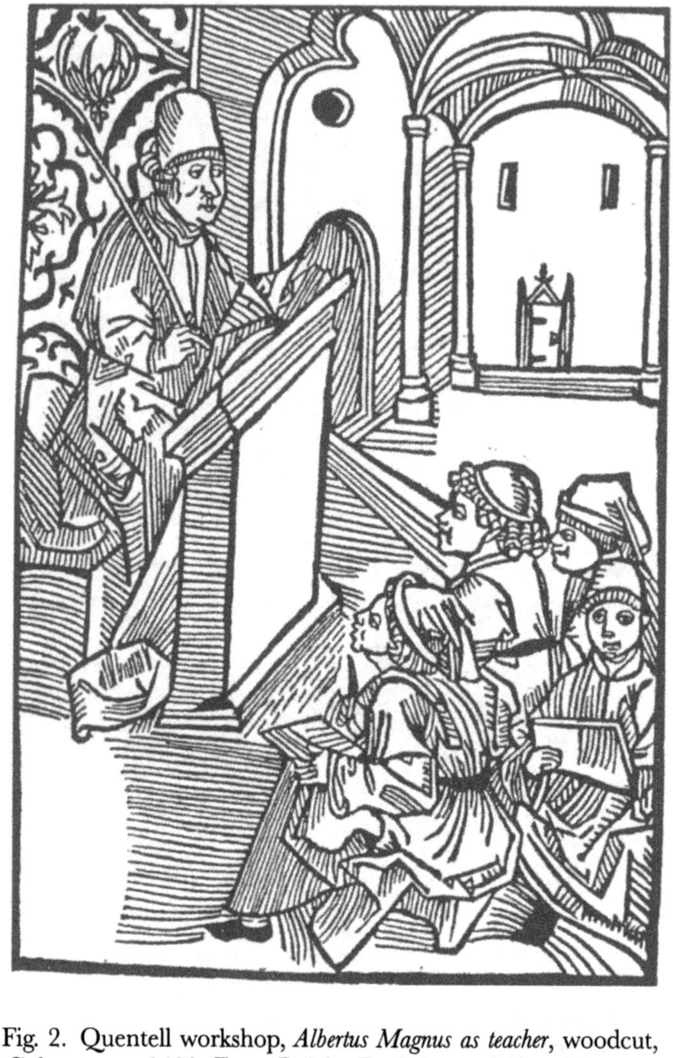

Fig. 2. Quentell workshop, *Albertus Magnus as teacher*, woodcut, Cologne, ca. 1480. From Reicke E., *Lehrer und Unterrichtswesen in der deutschen Vergangenheit* (Leipzig: 1901) 36.

women.[13] But in fact all of his important pedagogical works were written with a view to the education of boys or addressed to their teachers. The education of women was a theme in only two of his tracts, the *Christiani matrimonii institutio* of 1526 and in an open letter to Guillaume Budé. His scattered observations on erudite women, who, for Erasmus, demonstrated a learning 'beyond their sex' (the prime example being Margaret Roper, the daughter of Thomas More), should be understood, I would suggest, in the same terms as the amazement induced by a prodigy or other wonder of learning. What Erasmus' texts emphatically do not provide is an interpretation or argument in support of the education of women on the basis of equivalent intellectual talents. In sum, although *pueri* could denote either gender, the declamation is also clearly focussed on the early education of boys.

Fundamental to Erasmus' comments is an anthropology that privileged what Niklas Luhmann has termed the 'genesis of personality',[14] not only confirming the general malleability of the child, but also insisting that true humanity intrinsically depends on law and discipline:

> Trees perhaps come into existence as trees once and for all, even if they turn out wild and barren; and horses are born as horses, even if they prove to be useless. But man certainly is not born, but made man. Primitive man, living in a lawless, unschooled, promiscuous life in the woods, was not human, but rather a wild animal. It is reason which defines our humanity; and where everything is done at the whim of physical desire, reason does not hold its rightful place.[15]

What is translated here as 'unschooled' refers to the multifaceted term *disciplina*, which had always denoted both schooling and punishment. The severity of early juvenile education is necessitated by the precarious frontier between man and animal. And the precondition for the discussion is an anthropology that sees the child as a formless mass (to use the expression of Erasmus). Neglect or disregard will allow the child

[13] Sowards J.K., "Erasmus and the Education of Women", *Sixteenth Century Journal* 13,4 (1982) 77–89.

[14] Luhmann N., *Das Erziehungssystem der Gesellschaft*, ed. D. Lenzen (Frankfurt a.M.: 2002) 38.

[15] Erasmus, *De pueris*, ed. Sowards, 304. Cf. Desiderius Erasmus, *De pueris*, ed. Margolin, 389 [493b]: 'Arbores fortasse nascuntur, licet aut steriles aut agresti foetu; equi nascuntur, licet inutiles; at homines, mihi crede, non nascuntur, sed finguntur. Prisci mortales qui nullis legibus, nullis disciplinis, vago concubitu vitam agebant in nemoribus, ferae verius erant quam homines. Ratio facit hominem, ea locum non habet ubi affectuum arbitrio geruntur omnia'.

to regress to the status of a brute beast; with the proper education, however, the child's nature can become quasi-divine.

Erasmus implied what other texts of the day openly professed: that children did not have yet proper understanding or a controlling faculty of reason; rather, they were entirely subject to their emotions.[16] The passions, which had to be kept in check, presented the educator with a problem: in so far as they were the opposite of reason, children could hardly be reached by way of reason. This could lead to the conclusion, as it did in Vives' *De tradendis disciplinis* (1531), that the use of physical discipline was the only solution. According to Vives, every act that was driven by emotion and not first subject to proper reflection must be reprimanded and punished – first through words and, when necessary, through beatings as well. As with animals, so too with children: those without the power of reason must be put in their proper place through the infliction of pain.[17] It is thus indeed in-humanity that is at the root of the beating of young children, though not in the metaphorical sense of inhuman comportment of abusive adults, but rather in concrete terms with reference to the child. For this reason, in extreme cases, and just like an animal, a child can be tamed through a good thrashing.

Erasmus, in contrast, formulated his position by drawing on Plutarch and the analogous arguments of Quintilian,[18] claiming that the only proper instruments for the education of young boys were words in the form of praise and reproach – and the same, he asserts quite surprisingly, holds true for animals. As with children, so too with elephants or lions; there is a sense of optimism underwriting Erasmus' text that suggests the possibility of taming conduct through the proper encouragement. Let us remind ourselves that the underlying maxim against

---

[16] Motley M., *Becoming a French Aristocrat. The Education of the Court Nobility 1580–1715*, (Princeton, NJ: 1990) 43. Cf. also my "Im Namen des Vaters. Politik der Verheißung und Performanz der Drohung als interdependente Phänomene in der Erziehung Louis' XIII.", in Heisler E. – Koch E. – Scheffer T. (eds.), *Drohung und Verheißung. Mikroprozesse in Verhältnissen von Macht und Subjekt* (Freiburg i.Br.: 2007) 29–53.

[17] Juan Luis Vives, "De tradendis disciplinis", in: idem, *Opera omnia*, ed. G. Mayans y Síscar, 8 vols. (Valencia: 1782–90) VI, 317: 'At vero quoniam hominis ingenium ab incitatis animi morbis ad pejora deprimitur, coercendus est inconsultus ille motus, et compescendus reprehendendo, castigando verbis, et quum opus est, verberibus, ut belluarum more revocet eum dolor, cui ratio non est satis, tametsi liberalem hanc castigationem, quantum fieri possit, esse malim, non asperam, aut servilem, nisi ejusmodi sit ingenium, ut officii sui plagis sit tamquam mancipium admonendum'. English translation: Juan Luis Vives, *On Education*, transl. and ed. F. Watson (Cambridge: 1913) book III, ch. IV, 119–120.

[18] See note 10.

which Erasmus actually inveighs here is just as contrarian as it was authoritative, as simple as it was generally accepted at the time: 'Qui parcit virgae suae odit filium suum' ('He who spares the rod hates his son', *Prov.* 13:24).[19]

What Erasmus expected of the intended reader of the declamation (the fictive addressee being a young father) was not only the ability to school his child without the use of force or violence, but a degree of personal engagement in the early upbringing of the child and a measure of edification in place of the usual juvenile games. This call for the father to take part in or even to oversee the early education of his son has further implications with regard to gender relations. What the humanist is demanding here is the usurpation of the early education by the father. Up to the age of seven the raising of the young was generally left to women. Nurseries were coeducational spaces where both boys and girls could mix freely. Not even their clothing set them apart. Erasmus, however, argues not only in favour of a gentle discipline by the word, not by the rod, but his advocation of an early involvement of men in the education of boys at the same time hastens the separation of girls and boys and stresses the asymmetry of the gender dichotomy.

In his subsequent train of argumentation, Erasmus switches over to the contemporary practice of schooling, which was of course a predominantly male province. In describing school discipline, the language he uses is deliberately hyperbolic as he compares the school to a torture chamber ('non esse scholam, sed carnificinam'), where 'you hear nothing but the thudding of the stick, the swishing of the rod, howling and moaning, and shouts of brutal abuse'.[20] He thus not simply presupposes the general practice of school beatings as the precondition for an alternative method, but he stages educational techniques as excessively cruel. Employing the rhetorical device of *enargeia*, Erasmus presents the schoolroom as a space reverberating with the traces of suffering and pain. Beyond this, he says, there is nothing to hear, which is also to say,

[19] Erasmus himself quotes this verse as being a 'Hebraeorum oraculum' but attenuates his rant against a Bible verse by claiming that the passage had to be read allegorically with the rod being a metaphor for reproach. See Erasmus, *De pueris*, ed. Sowards, 332; ed. Margolin, 437–439 [507f–508a].

[20] Erasmus, *De pueris*, ed. Sowards, 325. Cf. Erasmus, *De pueris*, ed. Margolin, 427 [504b–c]: 'Dicas non esse scholam, sed carnificinam, praeter crepitum ferularum, praeter virgarum strepitum, praeter ejulatus ac singultus, praeter atroces minas nihil auditur. Quid aliud hinc discant pueri, quam odisse literas? Hoc odium ubi semel insedit teneris animis, etiam grandes facti abhorrent a studiis'.

there is nothing to learn: for without words there is no knowledge.[21] The school has evolved, he suggests, into something contrary to its original intentions; or to put it another way, it has become a *mundus inversus*, where students only learn what it means to hate to learn. All of this corresponds to the characterization of teachers as brutal, choleric, sadistic, syphilitic drunkards, or even worse, boozed-up women. Schoolmasters are portrayed as being enslaved by emotion, and thus precisely the opposite of the type of people suited to the raising of the young. In this view, the authority that had traditionally been invested in the praeceptor actually meant the transgression, the right to discipline nothing less than unrightful *violentia*.

Erasmus takes his denunciation of physical discipline one step further. While the need to form the unshapely body and mind of the young child is explained with a view to animality, the schoolchild is likened to a slave. Even though there is no space to delve into this theme, which is intricately woven into Erasmus' declamation, a few aspects should be highlighted. Already the image of the school as a torture chamber (*carnificina*), which I have mentioned before, implies slavery via its historical semantics: it evokes the *carnifex*, the Roman public slave who had to impose those punishments reserved for foreigners and other slaves. But the theme of slavery is also brought up explicitly by the *figura etymologica* drawing on *liberi* (children) and *liber* (free):

> If someone reforms his ways only out of fear of evil consequences, he has a slavish disposition. In the common usage of our language, however, we call our sons *liberi*, realizing that they should have a liberal education, which bears no resemblance to anything servile. In fact, wise masters treat their slaves kindly and with consideration so that they may lose the stigma of slavery; these masters remember that their slaves are human beings and not animals.[22]

---

[21] For Erasmus' rhetorical strategies see Rummel E., "Structure and Argumentation in Erasmus' *De pueris instituendis*", *Renaissance and Reformation* ns. 5 (1981) 127–140, here 129. The passage is echoed in Montaigne's *essai* "De l'institution des enfans" (I, 26): '[...] vous n'oyez que cris et d'enfans suppliciez, et de maistres enyvrez en leur cholere. Quelle maniere pour esveiller l'appetit envers leur leçon, à ces tendres ames et craintives, de les y guider d'une troigne effroyable, les mains armées de fouets?'; Michel de Montaigne, *Œuvres completes*, ed. A. Thibaudet – M. Rat (Paris: 1962) 144–177, here 165.

[22] Erasmus, *De pueris*, ed. Sowards, 327. Cf. Erasmus, *De pueris*, ed. Margolin, 429–431 [505d]: 'Servile est metu mali castigari, atqui publica consuetudo filios appellat liberos, quod hos deceat liberalis educatio, servili multum dissimilis: tametsi qui sapiunt hoc agunt potius, ut servi lenitate ac beneficiis exuant mancipii capillum, memores et illos esse homines, non belluas'.

In order to fashion something divine out of mortal man – and this is in essence the pedagogical goal of the Erasmian programme – it is necessary to differentiate him from animals *and* slaves by removing all traces of savagery and servitude. As a consequence, the parameters of proper education become fairly narrow. The child must not be left hostage to his emotion and take on the status of quasi-animality due to a lack of guidance or control; and yet at the same time, at no stage should he be subject to methods of discipline similar to slavery or be associated in any way with the characteristics of a slave. Instead of sharpening these distinctions, however, Erasmus blurs the lines: in stressing that even animals could be domesticated with the use of words, he undermines the traditional border between man and brute. At the same time, in likening the contemporary schooling system to the slave trade, he deliberately mingles two realms usually kept scrupulously distinct (and throws in, for good measure, a demand for more humane treatment of slaves while lamenting the fact that the practice still exists in Christian cultures). Taken together, these views of Erasmus represent an appeal to non-violent disciplinary and pedagogical techniques that went well beyond contemporary theories and stood in direct opposition to the practices of the day.[23]

Despite his radical formulation of the problem, later in the text Erasmus retreats to the more commonly acceptable position that physical discipline is a question of degree. Hitting a child too much and too often can be harmful.[24] But this of course implies the reverse, that beatings are acceptable if done in moderation. Apparently that was one of the reasons why Erasmus drew on the discourse of slavery, as it provided a referencing system for the permissible grades of discipline.

It has to be stressed that what seems intuitively reasonable to us, that children should be treated and educated humanely, required some persuasion in the early sixteenth century. Erasmus' argument is highly dependent on the imagery he himself had put before the eyes of his reader. The aim of his argument, the rejection of beating as an educational tool, could gain in plausibility only because he managed to paint schooling as a practice that included unreserved inflictment of pain. It is a rhetoric of corporeal punishment that Erasmus develops here, while

---

[23] On slavery in the Middle Ages and the early modern period cf. Davis D.B., *The Problem of Slavery in Western Culture* (Harmondsworth: 1970) 109–141.

[24] Erasmus, *De pueris*, ed. Sowards, 331–332; ed. Margolin, 437 [507e–f].

its opponents, who were the hundreds and thousands of schoolmasters in Europe, took the liberty to disagree – in practice, of course.

Given the historical perseverance of the practice, and assuming that it cannot only have fed on individual cruelty and serial transgression, I would now like to map out possible productive functions of pain inflicted by magisterial beatings in early modern schools.

Although primarily concerned with the raising of young children, Erasmus grants a surprising amount of space to the discussion of violence in student initiation rites. The *beanum exuere*, that is, the hazing of the academic freshmen or *beani*, is characterized by Erasmus as 'a barbaric custom with a barbaric name'.[25] In his view, what links this excursus to the actual theme of the declamation are instances of the excessive use of force, even though the examples he brings forward – the ordeals with faeces, salt, and vinegar and the use of a student's body as a battering ram – did not actually have a place in the daily rounds of school life.

The comments appear to lead us away from the actual theme. While the deposition was a ritual bound to a particular time and place, its beginning and end clearly circumscribed and its duration strictly regulated to last no more than a few days, the beating was, as it were, the staple of the educational system. It was an everyday act, and even when less than a daily occurrence, it was an ever-present threat. Nevertheless, Walter Ong has argued (and here, without necessarily intending it, Erasmus has left us some interesting clues) that the daily schoolroom beatings were the reverberations of a *rite de passage*.[26] Closely analogous to the rites of passage in many societies, they are to be seen as the enactment of gender segregation: in the medieval and early modern period, grammar schools and universities were exclusively male institutions. The deposition may thus be seen as a ritual that marks the exclusion of the feminine.[27] And indeed, even though the different

[25] See now Füssel M., "Riten der Gewalt. Zur Geschichte der akademischen Deposition und des Pennalismus in der frühen Neuzeit", *Zeitschrift für historische Forschung* 32,4 (2005) 605–648.

[26] Ong W.J., "Latin Language Study as a Renaissance Puberty Rite", *Studies in Philology* 56 (1959) 103–123.

[27] Karras R.M., *From Boys to Men: Formations of Masculinity in Late Medieval Europe* (Philadelphia: 2003), esp. ch. 3. In the same vein, Pierre Bourdieu stresses 'the essential effects of rites, namely that of separating those who have undergone it, not from those who have not yet undergone it, but from those who will not undergo it in any sense, and thereby instituting a lasting difference between those to whom the rite pertains and those to whom it does not pertain'. See Bourdieu P., "Rites of Institution", in idem,

procedural details make it difficult to speak in general terms, there were functionally analogous practices in the schools that signified the final leave-taking of the young boy from the guardianship of women.

The habitual beating of children in the schools begs the question of why it had been legitimated for so long specifically in this place. One aspect is certainly the transfer of authority from the absent parents to the teacher. Another is the fact that the school is a place outside of the family, where a sense of belonging bound up in blood relations no longer applies. Instead, belonging has to be continually confirmed and reproduced through specific practices. One of the central media for this type of reproduction was the Latin language. By the early modern period, Latin had died out as a native language and had assumed its role as a code of knowledge and erudition. But more important in the context of this discussion, along with the application of violence, it was one of the twin tools for the creation of scholarly identity. If we are to judge by the comments of some contemporaries, the teaching of Latin was intimately bound up with the use of violence in the classroom.[28] Witness the comments of John Locke in his *Thoughts Concerning Education*:

> Why [...] does the Learning of Latin and Greek need the Rod, when French and Italian needs it not? Children learn to Dance and Fence without Whipping; nay, Arithmetick, Drawing, & c. they apply themselves well enough to without beating [...].[29]

Or as Stephen Greenblatt put it in *Will in the World*: 'Everyone understood that Latin learning was inseparable from whipping. One educational theorist of the time speculated that the buttocks were created in order to facilitate the learning of Latin'.[30]

Serving as an exclusive code of learning meant taking on the traits of an arcane communication system, which, according to Walter Ong,

---

Language and Symbolic Power, ed. J.B. Thompson, trans. G. Raymond – M. Adamson (Cambridge, MA: 1991) 117–126, here 116.

[28] Bömer, "Lernen und Leben auf den Humanistenschulen" 10. Bömer points out that beatings were of course not confined to grammar lessons, but those were 'particularly calamitous' ('verhängnisvoll'). Significantly, disciplining beatings were administered if boys failed to speak Latin outside the classroom, e.g. during breaks and at games.

[29] John Locke, "Some Thoughts Concerning Education", in idem, *The Educational Writings of John Locke*, ed. James L. Axtell (Cambridge: 1968) 114–325, here 185, § 86.

[30] Greenblatt S., *Will in the World: How Shakespeare became Shakespeare* (London: 2004) 26.

is also one of the characteristics of a *rite de passage*.[31] Similarly, the inflicting of pain and suffering on the body is built into the initiation rituals of all societies. Pierre Bourdieu has stressed that a variety of psychological experiments have demonstrated that 'people's adherence to an institution is directly proportional to the severity and painfulness of the rites of initiation'.[32] These observations open up a perspective on the long-term function of such rituals, in both an individual and a collective sense; they also throw light on the deeper, pre-discursive foundation behind the school beatings, which were able to persist despite the steady stream of learned protest. Such practices unite those who have undergone the process of initiation with the institution and its laws and thus function as a type of socio-cultural glue, both synchronically and diachronically. Even Erasmus' own history lends itself to this reading. For as he reveals in an autobiographical anecdote in his *declamatio*, he too had been excessively caned by his teacher, to the point where his love for study had been beaten out of him.[33] Even though he would maintain more or less strained relations with universities, Erasmus' assertion is undermined by the fact that he did not lose his love for letters but came to be the most famous scholar of his age.

Since beatings in combination with the teaching of Latin are only inflicted on boys, we may also speak of a practice that aims at the performative enactment of masculinity. This refers to a notion of performativity that does not build on Austin, who conceived some speech acts – such as promising, baptizing, opening a meeting – as actual deeds. Rather, this is an observation indebted to Judith Butler's concept of a performative notion of gender that does not refer to formalized

[31] Ong, "Latin Language Study" 107.

[32] Bourdieu, "Rites of Institution" 123.

[33] Erasmus, *De pueris*, ed. Sowards, 326; ed. Margolin, 427 [504f]. Interestingly, the programme of corporeal punishment Erasmus later underwent at Montaigu College at the University of Paris, which is often quoted as the cause for his aversion towards scholasticism and the university, had only just been introduced by his very own teacher Jean Standonck whom he also mentions as an exemplar of cruelty in the *declamatio*. See Rashdall H., *The Universities of Europe in the Middle Ages*, ed. Powicke F.M. – Emden A.B., 3 vols. (Oxford: 1936) vol. III, 369. Physical discipline had been notably absent from the universities in the Middle Ages, and it would be an issue for more in-depth research why this innovation was brought about by the self-declared civilised humanists. See for a brief account Durkheim E., *L'évolution pédagogique en France* (Paris: ²1969) 182–185.

linguistic acts, but to the serialization and daily repetition of particular practices that result in the fabrication of gender identity.[34]

To achieve this, the body is treated like a kind of memory,[35] which raises another, almost technical aspect that may have contributed to the longevity of beating as a practice. Erasmus' *De pueris*, with its scenes of extreme physical discipline, all characterized by the humanist as senseless and cruel, almost forces us to overlook the practical aspirations behind the beatings. From antiquity to the early modern period, the methodical infliction of pain was conceived as a helpmeet to learning and memorising.[36] The blow rendered at the moment of taking in new subject matter is meant to couple the weak stimulus of the abstract matter – letters on paper, the teacher's words – with the intensity of physical experience and thus to emboss it on the memory. It is this idea that is behind images such as the advertisement for a Basel schoolmaster painted by Hans Holbein's brother Ambrosius [Fig. 3] which shows a boy reading Greek (which was taught much more infrequently but can in general be ascribed the same functions as Latin) and being nonchalantly brushed by his teacher.

Above all, the pedagogy of the cane, as Jörg Jochen Berns has termed it, was necessary in relation to the main method of knowledge acquisition in the early modern period: memorization or rote learning. And the basic subject of this exercise was of course Latin – the grammar, vocabulary, declensions and conjugations. It is not by accident that the iconographical symbol of grammar (which exclusively denoted Latin grammar) was the cane. Latin formed the conjunction between the perpetualized ritual of initiation and a general mnemotechnics of pain. Friedrich Nietzsche's reflections on the process of memory building, although written centuries after the period we are considering here, nonetheless get to the heart of the concept:

---

[34] Austin J.L., *How to Do Things With Words* (Cambridge, MA: ²1975); Butler J., *Bodies that Matter: On the Discursive Limits of 'Sex'* (New York – London: 1993) 230–234. For a useful discussion of the changing notions of the performative see Culler J., "Philosophy and Literature: The Fortunes of the Performative", *Poetics Today* 21,3 (2000) 48–67.

[35] Bourdieu, "Rites of Institution" 123.

[36] Berns J.J., "Liebe & Hiebe. Unvorgreifliche Gedanken zur mnemonischen Kraft christlicher Schmerzikonographie", in Hüttel B. – Hüttel R. – Kohl J. (eds.), *Re-Visionen. Zur Aktualität von Kunstgeschichte* (Berlin: 2002) 247–262, here 250.

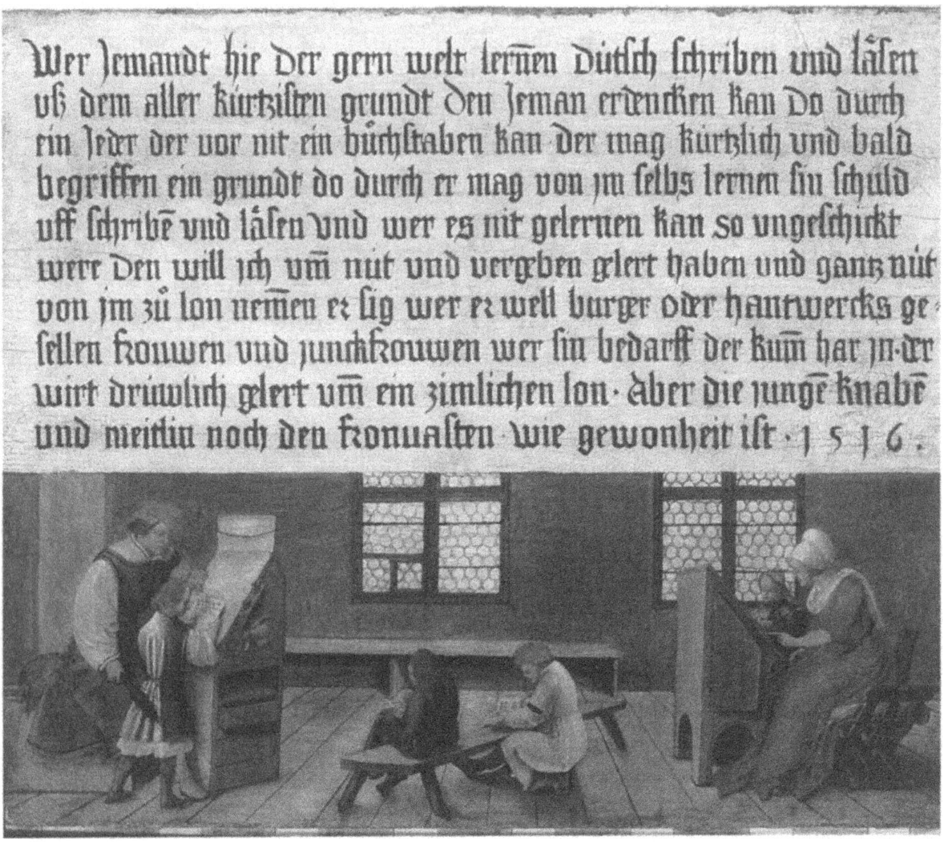

Fig. 3 [Col. pl. I]. Ambrosius Holbein, *Signboard of a schoolmaster*, 1516 (Inv. Nr. 311). Spruce wood, 55.5 × 65.5 cm, Kunstmuseum Basel (Photo: Kunstmuseum Basel, Martin Bühler).

How does one give the man-animal a memory? How does one impress something on this partly insensate, partly idiotic ephemeral understanding, this incarnated forgetfulness, so that it remains present to mind?' As we might imagine, the means employed to find a solution or answer to this ancient problem have been far from tender; there is, perhaps, nothing more frightening and more sinister in the whole prehistory of man than his *technique for remembering things*. 'Something is branded in, so that it stays in the memory: only that which hurts incessantly is remembered' – this is a central proposition of the oldest (and unfortunately also the most enduring) psychology on earth.[37]

There is ample testimony to the phenomenon of memorization through the inflicting of pain. In his 1920 compilation *Rechtsbrauch und Kinderspiel*, Eberhard von Künssberg brought together a wide range of examples. In seventeenth-century France, for instance, parents took their children along to public executions and hit them with canes while the death sentence was carried out; in the German province of Brandenburg, beatings on the borders of parishes and similar frontiers were known as 'gesetzliche Grenzstreiche' (border strokes); and in schools, it was not unusual to accompany the caning of young students with communal hymnody, keeping the rhythm of the beating in step with the rhythm of the song.[38] Thus there was a mnemotechnical impetus behind the use of force, one which the art of memory in antiquity tried to replicate by drawing on the agitating *imagines agentes.* The *art* of memory thus becomes, to quote Jörg Jochen Berns, 'the art of carefully calculated self-harm'.[39] What is imprinted at school is thus both: matter and masculinity, content and identity.

This combination was so powerful that the humanists' counter-arguments remained purely discursive and generally were not translated into practice. It is therefore a rather elegant paradox that the authoritative educational style behind the habitual beatings reveals itself as a subversive praxis that undermines and even simply ignores basic precepts

---

[37] Friedrich Nietzsche, *On the Genealogy of Morals*, trans. D. Smith (Oxford – New York: 1998) 42. Cf. also Borgards R., "Schmerz/Erinnerung. Andeutung eines Forschungsfeldes", in idem (ed.), *Schmerz und Erinnerung* (Paderborn: 2005) 9–24.

[38] Künßberg E. von, *Rechtsbrauch und Kinderspiel. Untersuchungen zur deutschen Rechtsgeschichte und Volkskunde*, Sitzungsberichte der Heidelberger Akademie der Wissenschaften, philosophisch-historische Klasse 1920, 7 (Heidelberg: 1920) 21–22.

[39] Berns J.J., "Schmerzende Bilder. Zu Machart und mnemonischer Qualität monströser Konstrukte", in Borgards R. (ed.), *Schmerz und Erinnerung* (Paderborn: 2005) 25–55, here 54. Cf. also Braungart G., "Schmerzgedächtnis – Körperschrift", in Kurz G. (ed.), *Meditation und Erinnerung in der Frühen Neuzeit* (Göttingen: 2000) 357–367.

of humanist pedagogy. And it is constant in its resistance, despite the fact that there is a relatively homogenous sequence of criticism and contrary advice reaching from Plutarch to Emile Durkheim who in his first course on pedagogy given at the Sorbonne in 1902/03 still had to contend that discipline must not be administered by physical 'torment'.[40] But in contrast to the invective, the advocacy of such beatings has not been articulated in theory but primarily through praxis – that is, through the basic use of force.

To conclude, and to return to the claim introduced at the beginning, is it even possible to learn Latin without being flogged from time to time? What proofs are there for the type of approach to teaching publicised by Roger Ascham? The one example he provides is that of a young girl, the young Lady Jane Grey, whom the English humanist encountered one day as she sat alone deeply engrossed in a Latin translation of Plato's *Phaidon* while the rest of the court was off on the hunt. According to Lady Jane, it was the kindness and the mildness of her teacher that had inspired her to seek study in solitude.[41] Thus the answer to the question is yes, it is possible to learn Latin without the accompaniment of beatings – but not for someone aspiring to be a man.

---

[40] Durkheim E., *L'éducation morale* (Paris: 1963) 12e leçon, 146–159, here 147.

[41] Ascham, *Schoolmaster* 35–36. The anecdote is discussed in Ong, "Latin Language Study" 120–121.

Selective Bibliography

ROGER ASCHAM, *The Schoolmaster (1570)*, ed. L.V. Ryan (Ithaca, NY: 1967).

BERNS J.J., "Liebe & Hiebe. Unvorgreifliche Gedanken zur mnemonischen Kraft christlicher Schmerzikonographie", in Hüttel B. – Hüttel R. – Kohl J. (eds.), *Re-Visionen. Zur Aktualität von Kunstgeschichte* (Berlin: 2002) 247–262.

BÖMER A., *Die lateinischen Schülergespräche der Humanisten* (Berlin: 1897/1899; reprint Amsterdam: 1966).

BOURDIEU P., *Language and Symbolic Power*, ed. J.B. Thompson, transl. G. Raymond – M. Adamson (Cambridge, MA: 1991).

BOWEN J., *A History of Western Education*, vol. II. *Civilization of Europe, Sixth to Sixteenth Century* (London: 1975).

BUSHNELL R.W., *A Culture of Teaching. Early Modern Humanism in Theory and Practice* (Ithaca, NY – London: 1996).

BUTLER J., *Bodies that Matter: On the Discursive Limits of 'Sex'* (New York – London: 1993).

CUNNINGHAM H., *Children and Childhood in Western Society since 1500* (London – New York: 1995).

DURKHEIM E., *L'éducation morale* (Paris: 1963).

ERASMUS DESIDERIUS, *Declamatio de pueris statim ac liberaliter instituendis*, ed. J.-C. Margolin (Geneva: 1966).

FUHRMANN M., "verbera", in *Paulys Realencyclopädie der Classischen Altertumswissenschaft*, Supplementband IX (Stuttgart: 1962) 1589–1597.

GRENDLER P.F., *Schooling in Renaissance Italy. Literacy and Learning, 1300–1600* (Baltimore – London: 1989).

KARRAS R.M., *From Boys to Men: Formations of Masculinity in Late Medieval Europe* (Philadelphia: 2003).

MARGOLIN J.-C., "Pédagogie et philosophie dans le 'De pueris instituendis' d'Erasme", *Paedagogica Historica* 4,2 (1964) 370–391.

MARROU H.-I., *Histoire de l'éducation dans l'antiquité* (Paris: [3]1955).

NIETZSCHE FRIEDRICH, *On the Genealogy of Morals*, transl. D. Smith (Oxford – New York: 1998).

ONG W.J., "Latin Language Study as a Renaissance Puberty Rite", *Studies in Philology* 56 (1959) 103–123.

RUMMEL E., "Structure and Argumentation in Erasmus' *De pueris instituendis*", *Renaissance and Reformation* ns. 5 (1981) 127–140.

STRAUSS G., *Luther's House of Learning: Indoctrination of the Young in the German Reformation* (Baltimore – London: 1978).

VIVES JUAN LUIS, *Los diálogos (Linguae Latinae Exercitatio)*, ed. M.a Pilar García Ruiz (Pamplona: 2005).

——, "De tradendis disciplinis", in: idem, *Opera omnia*, ed. G. Mayans y Síscar, 8 vols. (Valencia: 1782–1790), vol. VI, 243–437.

ARTICULATING PAIN: MARTYROLOGY, TORTURE AND EXECUTION IN THE WORKS OF ANTONIO GALLONIO (1556–1605)

Jetze Touber

Introduction

Catholic ecclesiastical scholars of the early modern period wrote extensively about early Christian martyrs.[1] In the aftermath of the Council of Trent, which confirmed the validity of the cult of the saints, relics of early Christian martyrs were regularly paraded in extensive translation ceremonies. Accompanying texts were written that reconstructed in detail the historical events that had led to the martyrs' veneration.[2] Such writings on the torments, deaths and subsequent cults of martyrs were a mixture of devotional exaltation and academic discussion, and were firmly grounded in ancient traditions of martyrological writing. In the course of the sixteenth century, the Catholic Church revised liturgical manuals, such as the *Martyrologium Romanum*, and purged them of what were seen as historically dubious elements or medieval corruptions. Clerical writings on individual martyrs had to accord with

[1] I would like to thank Catrien Santing, Albrecht Diem and Arnold Otto, as well as the editors of this volume, for their helpful comments on earlier versions of this paper. It was first presented in 'Something for the pain', a session of the International Medieval Congress 2006 of the University of Leeds, organized by Arnold Otto with support of the Oswald von Wolkenstein Gesellschaft, Frankfurt/Main, Germany. All translations are mine and are intended as 'working translations'. I am certain they can be improved upon and all mistakes in them are entirely my responsibility.

[2] Schraven M., *Festive Funerals: Funeral Apparati in Early Modern Italy, Particularly in Rome* (Groningen: 2006) 127–141; Ditchfield S., "Il mondo della Riforma e della Controriforma", in Benvenuti A. *et al.* (eds.), *Storia della santità nel cristianesimo occidentale* (Rome: 2005) 261–329; MacCulloch D., *Reformation: Europe's House Divided 1490–1700* (London: 2003) 401–404; Ghilardi M., *Subterranea civitas: quattro studi sulle catacombe romane dal medioevo all'età moderna* (Rome: 2003) 7–9; 43–75; Gregory B., *Salvation at Stake: Christian Martyrdom in Early Modern Europe* (Cambridge, MA: 1999) 250–254; 272–283; Hecht C., *Katholische Bildertheologie im Zeitalter von Gegenreformation und Barock: Studien zu Traktaten von Johannes Molanus, Gabriele Paleotti und anderen Autoren* (Berlin: 1997) 257–258; Gamrath H., *Roma sancta renovata: studi sull'urbanistica di Roma nella seconda metà del sec. XVI con particolare riferimento al pontificato di Sisto V (1585–1590)*, Analecta Romana Instituti Danici. Supplementum XIII (Rome: 1987) 115–121.

these new reference works, and *passiones* and *vitae* were thus increasingly standardized.[3] This article focuses on one of these texts: a treatise on martyrdom by the priest Antonio Gallonio, published in Rome in Italian in 1591, and in Latin in 1594.[4] The treatise discusses the torments which the early Christian martyrs underwent at the hands of their persecutors.

It does not speak for itself that the strongly conventional martyrological writings show an interest in the concrete human experience of pain. If the essence of martyrdom was a metaphorical relationship between physical disintegration and spiritual fulfilment, scholarly writings on martyrs were nevertheless also informed by perceptions of violence, both ancient and recent, that revolved around bodily destruction and pain.[5] Ecclesiastical scholars drew on classical idioms, as well as on contemporary notions of interrogation and punishment. For them, studying the philology as well as the mechanics of torture was a means of reaching an empathic understanding of martyrdom.

In what follows, I will first give a general overview of Antonio Gallonio's treatise on martyrdom. I will then address the issues of trial and punishment, martyrdom and civil authority, and the practical application of antiquarian reconstructions. Martyrdom was represented as a theatrical execution of the martyr, but it also involved elements of secluded torture. Martyrological literature was strongly conditioned by ready-made metaphors, but could nevertheless function as a way of publicising real, recent experiences. Antiquarian erudition provided the tools to convey these experiences and to articulate the ostentatious destruction of the martyrs' bodies, as well as their pain. Corporeal disintegration served to profess publicly the truth of the Catholic creed; theological truth was validated by pain.

[3] Ditchfield S., *Liturgy, Sanctity and History in Tridentine Italy: Pietro Maria Campi and the Preservation of the Particular* (Cambridge: 1995) 17–67. On the project of the revised *Martyrologium Romanum* and its successive editions: Guazzelli G.A., "Cesare Baronio e il *Martyrologium Romanum*: problemi interpretativi e linee evolutive di un rapporto diacronico", in Firpo M. (ed.), *Nunc alia tempora, alii mores. Storici e storia in età postridentina. Atti del Convegno internazionale Torino, 24–27 settembre 2003* (Florence: 2005) 47–89.

[4] Antonio Gallonio, *Trattato de gli instrumenti di martirio, e delle varie maniere di martoriare usate da'gentili contro christiani* (Rome, Ascanio and Girolamo Donangeli: 1591); Antonio Gallonio, *De sanctorum martyrum cruciatibus liber quo potissimum instrumenta et modi, quibus iidem Christi martyres olim torquebantur, accuratissime tabellis expressa describuntur* (Rome, Typographia Congregationis Oratorii: 1594).

[5] Cf. Bynum C.W., *The Resurrection of the Body in Western Christianity, 200–1336* (New York: 1995) 1–13; 43–51.

The Treatise on Martyrdom

Antonio Gallonio was a member of the Roman Oratory. This newly founded religious organisation exerted a strong influence on the culture and politics of late sixteenth-century Rome, alongside the Society of Jesus.[6] Many members of the Roman Oratory wrote works of ecclesiastical scholarship,[7] and the most famous of them was Cesare Baronio, responsible for a heavily documented history of the Latin Church, the *Annales ecclesiastici*.[8] Baronio also had a major part in the revision of the *Martyrologium Romanum*, the liturgical manual that lists all martyrs and confessors universally venerated in the Catholic Church.[9]

The treatise on martyrdom by Gallonio was in a sense an elaboration of the subject matter of the *Martyrologium Romanum*.[10] He published the Italian edition together with a series of short *vitae* of Roman virgin saints, mainly martyrs: the *Historia delle sante vergini romane*.[11] The *Martyrologium Romanum* was a major reference point for both the *Trattato de gli instrumenti del martirio* and the *Historia delle sante vergini*. Gallonio cited the *Martyrologium* but also commented on it. The treatise on martyrdom describes the various categories of torments suffered by Christian

---

[6] Gotor M., *I beati del papa. Santità, Inquisizione e obbedienza in età moderna* (Florence: 2002) 1–41; Simoncini S., "Tendenze e figure della cultura", in Pinelli A. (ed.), *Storia di Roma dall'antichità a oggi. Roma del Rinascimento* (Rome: 2001) 199–266.

[7] Bonadonna Russo M.T., "La cultura storica nella Congregazione dell'Oratorio", in Bonadonna Russo M.T. – Del Re N. (eds.), *San Filippo Neri nella realtà romana del XVI secolo* (Rome: 2000) 69–88; Zuccari A., "Politica culturale dell'Oratorio romano nella seconda metà del Cinquecento", *Storia dell'Arte* 41 (1981) 77–112.

[8] The bibliography on Cesare Baronio and the *Annales Ecclesiastici* is quite extensive; important works are: Zen S., *Baronio storico: Controriforma e crisi del metodo umanistico* (Naples: 1994); De Maio R. *et al.* (eds.), *Baronio storico e la Controriforma: atti del convegno internazionale di studi, Sora 6–10 ottobre 1979* (Sora: 1982); Jedin H., *Kardinal Caesar Baronius. Der Anfang der katholischen Geschichtsschreibung im 16. Jahrhundert* (Münster: 1978); Pullapilly C.K., *Caesar Baronius: Counter-Reformation historian* (Notre Dame – London: 1975); Calenzio G., *La vita e gli scritti del cardinale Cesare Baronio* (Rome: 1907).

[9] Guazzelli, "Cesare Baronio e il *Martyrologium Romanum*" *passim*; Ditchfield, *Liturgy, Sanctity and History* 44–54.

[10] As suggested by Baronio himself in a letter to Antonio Talpa, fellow oratorian in Naples, in 1592: 'il detto p. ms. Antonio scrive un libro delli instrumenti dei martyrii, oltra quelli che sono nell'Annotatione del Martyrologio Romano, darne altri loci reconditi' ('the aforementioned father mr. Antonio is writing a book about the instuments of martyrdom, going beyond those which are in the Annotation of the *Martyrologium Romanum*, citing other little-known sources'), cited in Zen, *Baronio storico* 119 n. 8. The 'p. ms. Antonio' is Antonio Gallonio.

[11] Antonio Gallonio, *Historia delle sante vergini romane con varie annotationi e con alcune vite breui de' santi parenti loro, e de' gloriosi martiri Papia e Mauro soldati romani* (Rome, Ascanio and Girolamo Donangeli: 1591).

martyrs: installations from which they were hung, racks on which they were stretched, instruments with which they were beaten, scorched and burnt. The chapters correspond approximately to mechanical categories: 'Of crosses and poles and ways of suspending', 'Of wheels, pulleys and the press', 'Of the wooden horse and various kinds of bonds', 'Of instruments of flogging' etcetera.[12]

Gallonio starts his treatise with a chapter on ways of suspending martyrs, since this was the category that the cross belonged to, and it was on the cross that Jesus Christ had died.[13] In this first chapter, Gallonio identified several forms of crucifying and hanging in the acts of martyrs – martyrs crucified upside down; martyrs suspended from gallows by their arms or by their hair; martyrs suspended from gallows with various kinds of weights attached to their bodies. In the next chapter, on wheels, pulleys and the press, Gallonio makes a careful distinction between large wheels on which martyrs were hoisted and their limbs subsequently broken, and small wheels that served as pulleys in contrap-

---

[12] Gallonio, *Trattato* 1 "Della Croce, e Pali, e modi di sospendere. Cap. 1."; 20 "Delle Rote, Troclee, e Torchio, instrumenti di martorio. Cap. 2."; 34 "Dell'equuleo, instrumento di martirio. Cap. 3."; 4 "De gli instrumenti, co i quali erano i Martiri flagellati. Cap. 4." etc.; *De sanctorum* 1 "De Cruce, stipitibus et modis, quibus Christiani in Christi confessione perseverantes appendebantur. Cap. primum"; 33 "De Rotis, Trochleis et Torculari, instrumentis torquendi. Cap. secundum."; 47 "De Equuleo martyrii instrumento, atque de quamplurimis vinculorum generibus. Cap. tertium."; 97 "De instrumentis, quibus martyres caedebantur", etc.

[13] Gallonio, *Trattato* 1: 'Havendo conseguito i gloriosi combattenti di Christo (le honorate imprese de'quali ho pensato in questo trattato abozzare) mercè della santissima croce, virtù di poter resistere à contrarii grandi, e di superare le forze invincibili del demonio, e de gli Imperatori Gentili, e de i Re della terra, lor ministri; per questo mi sono resoluto dalla croce principiarlo' ('Since the glorious warriors (whose honoured insignia I have wanted to sketch in this treatise) have acquired the strength to face great adversities and the invincible powers of the devil, of the pagan emperors and of the worldly kings, their servants, on account of the most holy cross; because of that I have decided to commence with the cross').

Gallonio, *De sanctorum* 1: 'Tractaturi hoc libello cum de martyrii instrumentis, tum etiam de innumerabilibus pene modis, quibus gloriosissimi atque invicti Domini nostri Iesu Christi milites pro eius honore mortem forti animo subiere; a sacrosancta cruce operis initium merito facere decrevimus: Haec enim illa fuit, in qua Salvator Orbis, aeterni Patris Filius, mortis vincula rumpens, callidum aspidem superavit et suis fortitudinem promeruit, ut maxima cum cordis laetitia essent parati ad omnia omnino ardua ac dificillima, etiam, si sic res postulaverit, usque ad sanguinis effusionem et membrorum omnium crudelissimam obtruncationem' ('In the prospect of treating in this little book the instruments of martyrdom, as well as the almost innumerable ways in which the very glorious and unbeatable soldiers of our Lord Jesus Christ met their deaths in his honour, in high spirits, we have deemed it right to commence the work with the sacrosanct cross: as it is the cross, on which the Saviour of the Earth, the Son of the eternal Father, breaking the bonds of death, defeated the crafty serpent').

tions that were used as racks. It was logical to have a next chapter on the *equuleus*, or wooden horse, one of the most common instruments of torture in classical texts, which contained just this sort of pulleys.[14] The treatise continues in the same vein, until a final chapter lists all torments that do not fit in the other categories: piercing martyrs with arrows or spears, decapitating them with swords or axes, dissecting martyrs and cooking their entrails, throwing martyrs off cliffs or drowning them in seas, lakes or rivers, banishing them or condemning them to forced labour in mines or construction works.[15]

At the end of each chapter, Gallonio added detailed illustrations, in order to clarify his reconstructions, such as his inventory of ways of crucifying [Fig. 1].[16] The martyrs in these engravings are represented with stern or even content faces. As was customary in hagiography, they are depicted as undisturbed by the cruel treatment they are undergoing, and pain hardly seems relevant to them.[17] Gallonio's treatise on martyrdom has usually been interpreted as a work of erudition in the same humanistic vein that inspired Baronio's *Annales Ecclesiastici*. The basic source material that Gallonio drew on consists of the acts of the martyrs, historical martyrologies and patristic writings. Pagan authors provided valuable practical information: Cicero, Plautus, Pliny, Vitruvius. Furthermore, Gallonio employed a range of visual and material sources. The ultimate goal was to facilitate devotion to the martyr saints.[18]

---

[14] Fiorelli P., *La tortura giudiziaria nel diritto comune*, 2 vols. (Varese: 1953–1954) I, 194.

[15] Gallonio, *Trattato* 134 "Di più altri modi, co' quali erano afflitti i nostri da gli Imperatori Gentili, e loro ministri. Cap. XI." ("On still other ways in which our men were afflicted by the Pagan Emperors. Chapter XI."); *De sanctorum* 183 "De aliis instrumentis, ac modis, quibus martyres cruciabantur. Cap. nonum" ("On other instruments for, and ways of, torturing martyrs. Ninth chapter").

[16] Gallonio closely supervised the production of the illustrations accompanying the test, as can be surmised from a letter of his to his fellow oratorian Antonio Talpa: 'un trattato nel principio diviso in quindici capitoli de gli instrumenti e modi di martirizzare usati da gli antichi contra i christiani con le loro figure in rame, che saranno quaranta di numero per lo meno, et al presente ne ho in ordine ventitré, le quali danno, per la gratia del Signore, grandissima divotione e soddisfattione ad ognuno che le vede' ('a treatise in principle divided into fifteen chapters of instruments and methods for martyring used by the ancients against the Christians with their figures in copper, which will amount to at least 40, and at present I have ready 23 of them, which, by the Grace of the Lord, give very great devotion and satisfaction to anyone who sees them'), cited in Cistellini A., *San Filippo Neri, l'Oratorio e la Congregazione oratoriana. Storia e spiritualità* (Brescia: 1989) I, 730–731 n. 17.

[17] Delehaye H., *Les passions des martyrs et les genres littéraires* (Brussels: 1966) 149–150.

[18] Mansour O., "Not Torments, but Delights: Antonio Gallonio's *Trattato de gli instrumenti di martirio* of 1591 and its Illustrations", in Hopkins A. – Wyke M. (eds.), *Roman*

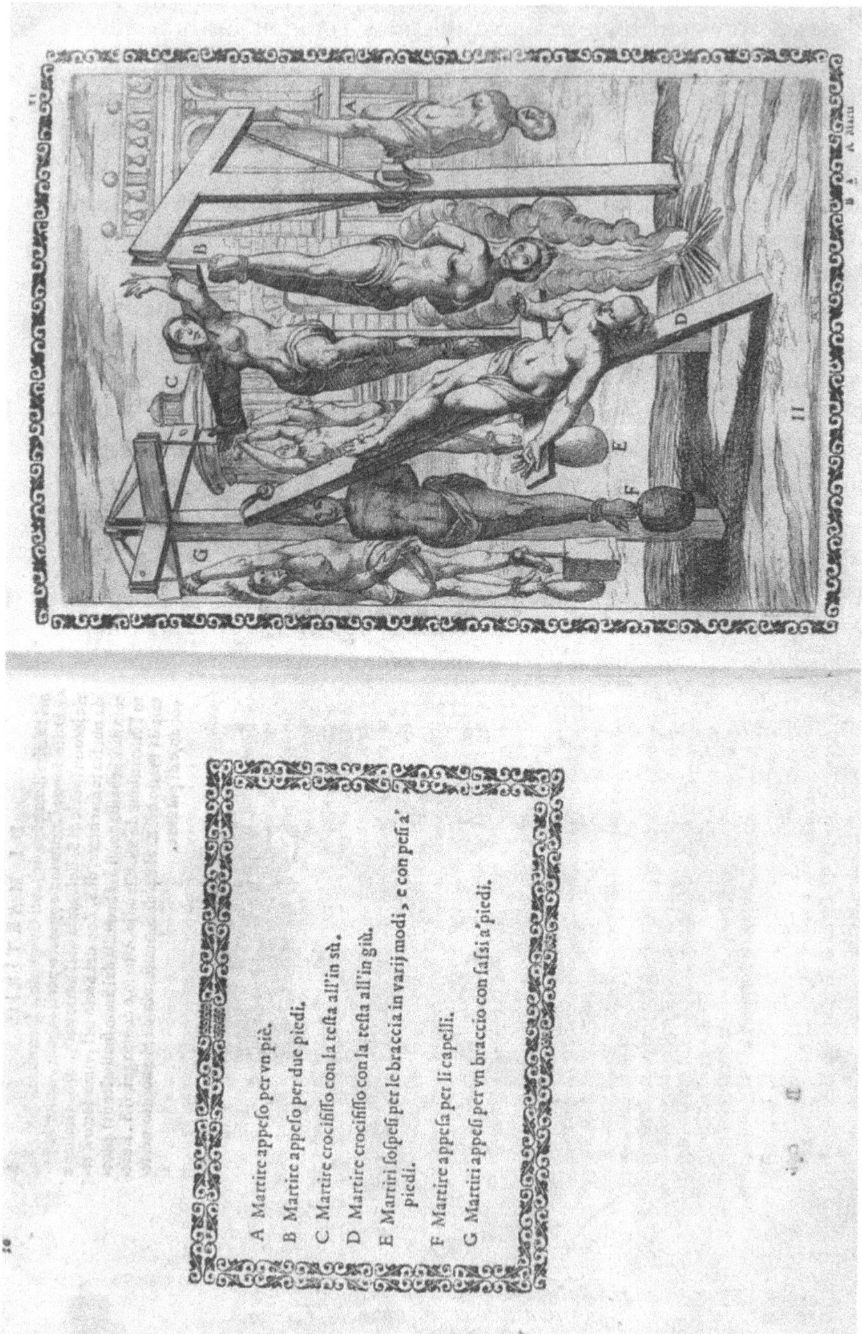

Fig. 1. An inventory of ways of crucifying. From Antonio Gallonio, *Trattato de gli instrumenti di martirio, e delle varie maniere di martoriare usate da'gentili contro christiani* (Rome, Ascanio and Girolamo Donangeli: 1591) 10–11, copper engraving. Biblioteca Vallicelliana.

More specifically, the treatise was designed to assist future missionaries in meditating on the fates of their predecessors.[19]

This leaves open the question of what exactly readers were supposed to admire and emulate in practice. Martyrology followed age-old traditions of endless reappropriation of the same hagiographical *topoi*.[20] Gallonio utilizes such genre-specific commonplaces when he introduces the martyrs as the subject matter of his treatise, and calls them the 'glorious warriors' and the 'unbeaten soldiers of Jesus Christ our Lord.'[21] However, in order to cope with the new confessional divide in Europe, the clerics of the Counter Reformation applied these conventions in creative ways.[22] The concern with current religious violence is evident in the treatise on martyrdom, at least in the Latin edition of 1594. In the preface to this edition, Gallonio announces that he has enriched it with references to recent events, taken from several contemporary publications authored mainly by English Catholics. Gallonio lists a variety of suffering that had recently been inflicted on Catholics in England and elsewhere, including incarceration, harassment, hanging,

Bodies. Antiquity to the Eighteenth Century (London: 2005) 167–183; Ditchfield S., "Text before Trowel: Antonio Bosio's *Roma sotterranea* Revisited", in Swanson R.N. (ed.), *The Church Retrospective: Papers Read at the 1995 Summer Meeting and the 1996 Winter Meeting of the Ecclesiastical History Society* (London: 1997) 343–360; Ditchfield, *Liturgy, Sanctity and History*, 85–90; Zuccari, "Politica culturale dell'Oratorio" 85–86; 90–91.

[19] Mansour, "Not Torments, but Delights" 171–172; 179–180; Piccirillo F., "VI.3 Fenomenologia del martirio", in Fagiolo M. – Madonna M.L. (eds.), *Roma, 1300–1875: l'arte degli anni santi*, exh. cat. (Milan: 1984) 282–291 Vannugli A., "Gli affreschi di Antonio Tempesta a S. Stefano Rotondo e l'emblematica nella cultura del Martirio presso la Compagnia di Gesù", *Storia dell'Arte* 48 (1983) 101–116.

[20] Aigrain R., *L'Hagiographie: ses sources, ses methodes, son histoire* (Brussels: 2000) 149; Goddard Elliott A., *Roads to Paradise: Reading the Lives of the Early Saints* (Hanover, NE – London: 1987) 1–10; Delehaye, *Les passions des martyrs* 133–169; Delehaye H., *Cinq leçons sur la méthode hagiographique* (Brussels: 1934) 18–41. The rhetorical conventions and historical particularities of hagiographical texts have long been studied by the Jesuits of the Société des Bollandistes, who were (and still are) devoted to the conservation of Latin and Greek hagiographical traditions, notably as editors of the *Acta Sanctorum*. De Gaiffier B., "Hagiographie et historiographie", *Settimane di studio del Centro Italiano di Studi sull'Alto Medioevo* 17 (1970) 139–166.

[21] 'I gloriosi combattenti' ('glorious warriors'); 'invicti Domini nostri Iesu Christi milites' ('invincible soldiers of our lord Jesus Christ'), see citations n. 10; for the image of the martyr as a victorious soldier, see Delehaye, *Les passions des martyrs* 152–154.

[22] Gregory, *Salvation at Stake* 255–272; 283–297. For the concept of the process of 'confessionalization' in the age of the Reformation, see MacCulloch, *Reformation* xxiv; Po-Chia Hsia R., *Social Discipline in the Reformation: Central Europe 1550–1750* (London – New York: 1989) 1–9.

drowning, and torture.[23] This suggests that studying the philology as well as the mechanics of torment contributed to the idea of martyrdom as a cohesive element of contemporary Catholic culture.

Torture in Society

To the modern reader, the endless cruelties listed and described in both editions of the treatise on martyrdom evoke associations with tremendous pain. Pain in pre-modern societies, however, is elusive. This is due partly to the nature of pain itself. In an important study of the human expression of pain, Elaine Scarry has pointed out that it is fundamentally impossible to share the concern with pain. One cannot communicate the exact nature or extent of the pain one feels

---

[23] Gallonio, *De sanctorum* fol. ++v: 'En tibi, lector, librum auctum tradimus, quem hoc tempore Latino sermone conscripsimus, non solum innumeris fere (si loqui sic licet) antiquorum martyrum tormentis, sed etiam nostrae aetatis Catholicorum, qui pro fide Catholica mortem constanti animo oppetivere: quorum si summam in cruciatibus perferendis patientiam, si invictum animi robur, si ingentem laetitiam, si numerum, si causum cognoscere tibi libeat; vide Sanderi libros de Schismate Anglicano, deq. visibili Ecclesiae Monarchia, item Concertationis Anglicanae volumen, simul etiam libellum de Persecutione Anglicana, Trophaea Ecclesiae Anglicanae, Theatrum insuper crudelitatum haereticorum nostri temporis, Suriique commentarium rerum in Orbe suo tempore gestarum et Thomae Bozii librum 11. ac 12. primi voluminis de Signis Ecclesiae Dei, et demum libellum Idibus Martii anno a partu Virginis MDXCII. impressum, cui est titulus, Exemplar litterarum missarum e Germania, in quo Anglus quidam Catholicus respondet Protestanti amico petenti ipsius sententiam de edicto quodam Regio Londini nuper promulgato, in quibus multa continentur scitu dignissima, quae ad praesentem persecutionem, Anglicaniq. Regni statum pertinet' ('Look, reader, we hand over to you the book, that this time we have written in Latin, enriched with (if it is allowed to put it this way) almost innumerable tortures of the ancient martyrs, but also of Catholics of our own age, who have faced death with a constant mind for the sake of the Catholic faith: if you would like to know about their great steadfastness in enduring torments, their invincible strength of soul, their immeasurable gladness, their number and the background, consult the books by Sander on the English schism, on the visible Monarchy of the Church and the book about the English Trial, and also the booklet about the English Persecution, the Trophies of the English Church, the Theatre of cruelties of the heretics of our time, the commentary by Surius on the deeds in the world of his days, and books 11 and 12 of the Signs of the Church by Tommaso Bozio, and finally the booklet printed 15 March 1592, with the title Example of the letters sent from Germany, in which a certain Catholic Englishman responds to his Protestant friend who wants to know his opinion about some edict recently decreed in the Royal Capital of London, in which much is mentioned that is worth knowing, pertaining to the current persecution and the state of the English Realm'). For the examples mentioned, see *De sanctorum* 76–94; 140: 176; 207; 223–224.

in his or her body.[24] In addition, pain in history eludes us also because of its relatively scarce occurrence in pre-modern sources. In the early modern period, pain was only beginning to be regarded as an occurrence worth of contemplation in its own right; one of the pioneers of this process was Michel Montaigne in his *Essais*. In general in the sixteenth, century pain as an integral part of the human condition was still only tentatively becoming the subject of reflection.[25] Christian theology and spirituality, however, formed an exception. Since late antiquity, pain had been perceived simultaneously as a consequence of the fall of mankind and as an element of human salvation.[26] As Mitchell Merback has shown, the rituals of late medieval and early modern criminal justice were effective ways of communicating the pain of biblical scenes involving violence, with the passion of Christ playing a central role.[27] In the same vein, the pain of the martyrs in the works of Antonio Gallonio can be assessed by tracing analogies with early modern judicial culture.

Physical cruelty in pre-modern societies has often been described in terms of display, rather than in terms of feeling. A number of historians have studied corporeal punishment inflicted by the state, especially in the early modern period. In the wake of one of the epoch-making studies by Michel Foucault, historians have approached public torture in early modern Europe as a ritual punishment.[28] The elaborate breaking, burning and maiming of the bodies of sentenced delinquents served as a collective vindication of the restored integrity of the social body. Corporeal punishment in judicial procedure could continue even after the deaths of the convicts. The cut-up body would be put on display, for example during a public dissection in the anatomical theatre, performed

[24] Scarry E., *The Body in Pain: The Making and Unmaking of the World* (New York: 1985) 3–11.

[25] Rey R., *The History of Pain*, trl. Wallace L.E. – Cadden J.A. – Cadden S.W. (Cambridge, MA: 1995) 10–70.

[26] Cohen E., "The Animated Pain of the Body", *American Historical Review* 105,1 (2006) 36–68.

[27] Merback M.B., *The Thief, the Cross and the Wheel: Pain and the Spectacle of Punishment in Medieval and Renaissance Europe* (London: 1999).

[28] The literature on corporal punishment in early modern Europe – my focus in this article – is vast. Some important studies: Muchembled R., *Le temps des supplices: de l'obéissance sous les rois absolus XVe–XVIIIe siècle* (Paris: 2006); Puppi L., *Lo splendore dei supplizi: liturgia delle esecuzioni capitali e iconografia del martirio nell'arte europea dal XII al XIX secolo* (Milan: 1990); Spierenburg P., *The Spectacle of Suffering: Executions and the Evolution of Repression: From a Preindustrial Metropolis to the European Experience* (Cambridge: 1984); Foucault M., *Surveiller et punir: naissance de la prison* (Paris: 1975).

by professors of medicine and their assistants. Such a spectacle obviously had nothing to do with pain, and has been interpreted as a form of humiliation through physical destruction.[29] It has become almost a commonplace to remark that the function of these executions was the public destruction of the body rather than the infliction of pain.

A less conspicuous strand of historical writing has studied judicial torture as a way of generating truth.[30] The study of this aspect of judicial practice has generally been restricted to legal history. Again, it was especially the early modern period, rather than the Middle Ages, that saw the structural application of torture in the law courts. The goal of torture was to have the defendant make a confession, and the means to reach this goal was pain. Although torture is nowadays widely considered cruel and ineffectual as a means of obtaining reliable testimony, in the period under scrutiny it seemed a sensible procedure. Because mankind in general was supposed to be sinful and unrepentant, always trying to evade punishment for its sins, the body with its involuntary reactions was deemed a more reliable witness than the devious mind. Significantly, interrogatory torment tended to take place behind closed doors, without spectators.[31]

The separation of these two aspects, inquisitive pain and punitive desintegration, might be the consequence of the divergent interests of modern historians, rather than early modern judicial practice itself. Though it is far beyond the scope of this article to address this question in general terms, the martyrological culture of Rome during the Catholic Reformation suggests that it is at least plausible that pain and disintegration were perceived as inseparable aspects of the process of generating true knowlegde. The trial of the martyr was in a sense an

---

[29] Egmond F., "Execution, Dissection, Pain and Infamy: A Morphological Investigation", in Egmond F. – Zwijnenberg R. (eds.), *Bodily Extremities: Preoccupations with the Human Body in Early Modern European Culture* (Aldershot – Burlington: 2003) 92–128; Scott P., "Some Perspectives on Execution and Martyrdom, during the Ancien Régime", in Dousteyssier-Khoze C. – Scott P. (eds.), *(Ab)Normalities* (Durham: 2001) 25–38; Sawday J., *The Body Emblazoned: Dissection and the Human Body in Renaissance Culture* (London – New York: 1995) 43–84; Lazzerini L., "Le radici folkloriche dell'Anatomia. Scienza e rituale all'inizio dell'età moderna", *Quaderni storici* 29 (1994) 193–233.

[30] Silverman L., *Tortured Subjects: Pain, Truth, and the Body in Early Modern France* (Chicago: 2001); Langbein J.H., *Torture and the Law of Proof: Europe and England in the Ancien Régime* (Chicago and London: 1977); Fiorelli, *La tortura giudiziaria*.

[31] Silverman, *Tortured Subjects* 62–68; Hanson E., "Torture and Truth in Renaissance England", *Representations* 34 (1991) 53–84, there 62–66; Von Dülmen R., *Theater des Schreckens. Gerichtspraxis und Strafrituale in der frühen Neuzeit* (Munich: 1985) 13–37.

inversion of the trial of the criminal or of the heretic. It is worthwhile to map the similarities and differences between accounts of Christian martyrdoms and the structure of judicial violence.[32]

Antonio Gallonio would have had ample opportunity to observe or learn about the functioning of both public execution and inquisitive torture. The highest frequency of public executions for heresy in Rome occurred during the pontificate of Pius V (1565–1572).[33] Penal executions took place on various squares around the city, were preceded by a defamatory tour on a cart and could be accompanied by various kinds of mutilations. In this period Gallonio was an adolescent, and he could easily have witnessed these ceremonies.[34] On the other hand, there were also occasions on which Gallonio could at least speak to victims of judicial torture. From 1580 onward the Oratorian fathers were engaged in comforting, confessing and educating prisoners of the Sant'Uffizio, the institution responsible for the Roman Inquisition. Gallonio was reported to be personally engaged in the assistance of detainees of the secular prisons of Campidoglio and Tor di Nona.[35] Far from being withdrawn in spiritual isolation, Gallonio had first-hand experience with suspected or convicted sinners and crooks.

---

[32] Lestringant F., *Lumière des martyrs: essai sur le martyre au siècle des Réformes* (Paris: 2004) 15–17; 137–138. Ditchfield has indicated the 'symbiosis' between those responsible for the canonisation of saints and those responsible for the persecution of heretics, pointing out that the curial judge Francisco Peña not only advised the commission that investigated the development of new cults around 1600, but also edited the fourteenth-century manual for inquisitors, *Directorium Inquisitorum*, by Nicolaus Eymericus (see n. 45). Ditchfield, "Il mondo della Riforma e della Controriforma" 288.

[33] Prosperi A., *Tribunali della coscienza: inquisitori, confessori, missionari* (Turin: 1996) 171–177. A chronological inventory of the public executions for heresy in Rome between 1567 and 1657, based on archival sources, is in Firpo L., "Esecuzioni capitali in Roma (1567–1671)", in Biondi A. (ed.), *Eresia e riforma nell'Italia del cinquecento* (Florence and Chicago: 1974) 307–342. An older publication, based on diplomatic correspondence, lists many more executions, but the criteria which the author employs for identifying 'free thinkers' are unclear, and it is not always certain that the death sentences were carried out: Bertolotti A., *Martiri del libero pensiero e vittime della Santa Inquisizione nei secoli XVI, XVII e XVIII* (Bologna: 1976).

[34] Calzolari M., "Delitti e castighi", in Calzolari M. – Di Sivo M. – Grantaliano E. (eds.), *Giustizia e criminalità nello stato pontificio. Ne delicta remaneant impunita* (Rome: 2002) 39–75.

[35] Cistellini A., *San Filippo Neri* I, 257 (with n. 38); Incisa della Rocchetta G. – Vian N. (eds.), *Il primo processo per San Filippo Neri nel Codice Vaticano Latino* 3798 *e in altri esemplari dell'archivio dell'Oratorio di Roma* I (Vatican City: 1957) 60 (testimony of Francesco Zazzara). For the application of torture to the accused in the prisons of Rome in the early modern period: Di Sivo M., "Per via di giustizia. Sul processo penale a Roma tra XVI e XIX secolo", in Calzolari – Di Sivo – Grantaliano, *Giustizia e criminalità* 13–35.

We might regard the treatment of martyrs described by Gallonio as executions. The destructive spectacle is very much present in his treatise, and the martyrdoms that he describes have a strongly theatrical element. Their effects could be spectacular, for example in the case of the bronze bull, a concept taken directly from ancient literature, and described by Ovid, for example, in his *Ars amatoria*.[36] The bull was a metal container; the martyr would be placed inside it, after which the object would be heated by a fire. The distorted screams of the victim coming from inside the bronze bull were likened to a bovine moo [Fig. 2].[37] This extravagant symbol of tyranny could hardly have been intended as a way of prying a confession from the defendant. Rather, it had an inherently dramatic dimension. Most of the illustrations in Gallonio's treatise show the martyrdoms takin place out in the open, as performances. The historian Adriano Prosperi has accordingly identified it as a public denouncement of the cruelties that Protestants inflicted on Catholics: a display of unjust executions.[38] One of the books Gallonio drew on for information about Protestant violence was aptly called the *Theatrum crudelitatum nostri temporis*, a combination of devotional and propagandistic literature written by a Catholic exile from England, Richard Verstegan.[39] Incidentally, 'theatre of cruelties' would also have been an appropriate title for the treatise of martyrdom.[40]

The martyrological writings of Gallonio also show a concern with inquisitive torment. The torture that the pagan judges in martyrology inflicted was usually closely bound up with extensive interrogation.[41]

---

[36] Ovidius, *Ars Amatoria* I, 653. For the literary tradition in classical antiquity concerning Phalaris, the Greek tyrant made famous by the bronze bull that was invented for him and in which he himself found a gruesome death, see Hinz V., *Nunc Phalaris doctum protulit ecce caput: Antike Phalarislegende und Nachleben der Phalarisbriefe* (Munich: 2001) 47–98.

[37] Gallonio, *Trattato* 80–81; Gallonio, *De sanctorum* 151–154.

[38] Prosperi A., "La mort de l'hérétique: normes juridiques et pratique concrète au temps de l'inquisition romaine", in Seidel Menchi S. (ed.), *Ketzerverfolgung im 16. und frühen 17. Jahrhundert* (Wiesbaden: 1992) 159–174.

[39] Richard Verstegan, *Theatrum Crudelitatum Haereticorum nostri temporis* (Antwerp, Adrianus Huberti: 1587); Arblaster P., *Antwerp & the World: Richard Verstegan and the International Culture of Catholic Reformation* (Louvain: 2004) 34–35, 40–42, 197–199; Lestringant F., *Lumière des martyrs* 137–176.

[40] For the metaphor of the theatre in the sixteenth and seventeenth centuries, see Lestringant F., *Lumière des martyrs* 140–142; Blair A., *The Theater of Nature: Jean Bodin and Renaissance Science* (Princeton: 1997) 153–179.

[41] For the importance of interrogation in inquisitorial procedure, see Romeo G., *L'inquisizione nell'Italia moderna* (Rome: 2002) 41–45; Prosperi, *Tribunali della coscienza* 199–202. Cf. Scarry, *The Body in Pain* 28–35, 57–59.

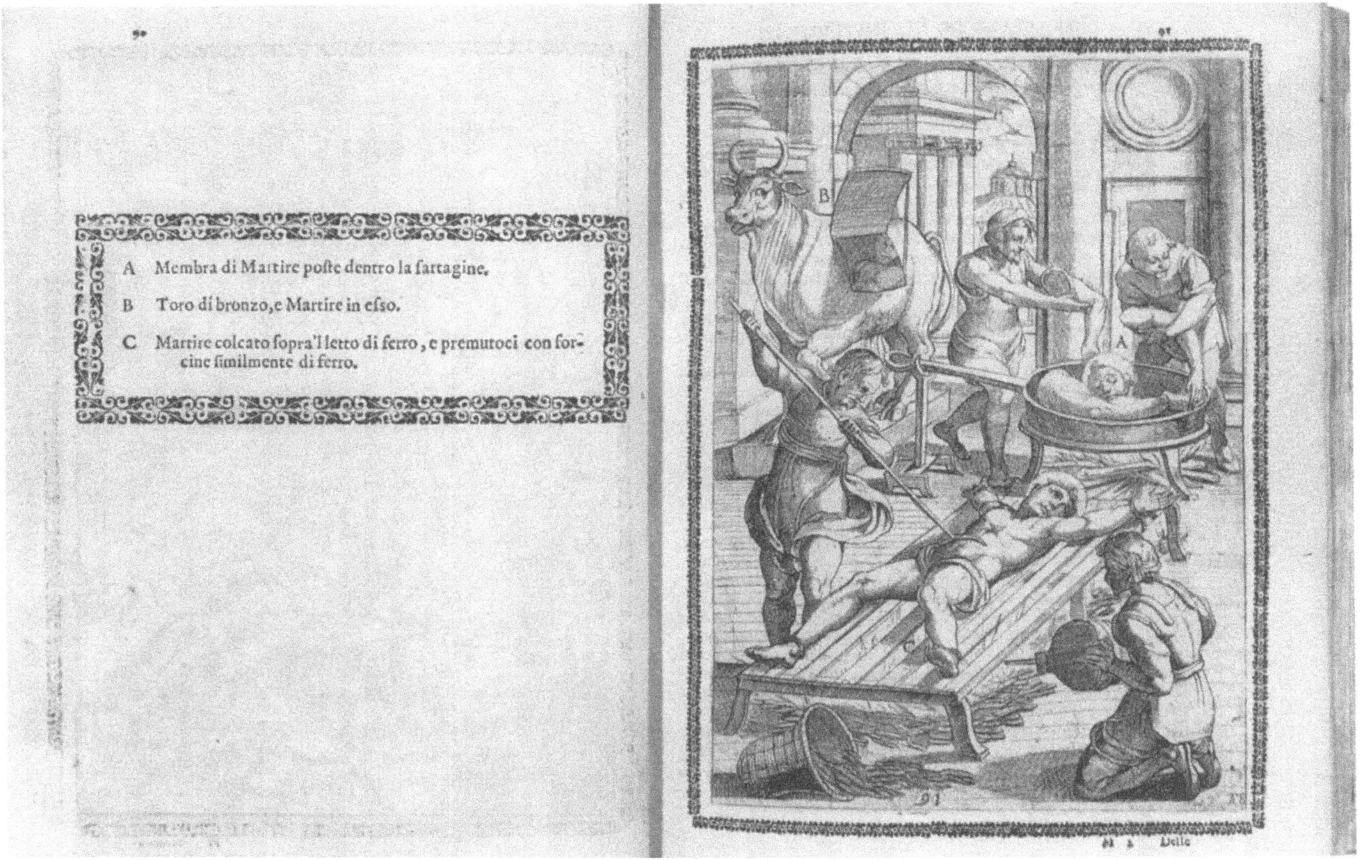

Fig. 2. The bronze bull, among a number of torture methods that involve fire. From Antonio Gallonio, *Trattato de gli instrumenti di martirio, e delle varie maniere di martoriare usate da'gentili contro christiani* (Rome, Ascanio and Girolamo Donangeli: 1591) 90–91, copper engraving. Biblioteca Vallicelliana.

The judges tried to undermine the resolution of the Christians on trial by socratically questioning them about the benefits they received from their god. Every round of questioning occasioned another torment. Instead of succumbing to the pressure of the judges, which would have amounted to a confession of error, the Christians continued to profess their faith until the end. Although the interrogation as such was not the subject of Gallonio's treatise, most if not all of the acts of the martyrs, the most fundamental group of sources for all martyrological writing, including Baronio's and Gallonio's, devoted a good deal of space to the dialogue between the judge and the Christian martyr.[42] Some of the *vitae* of the Roman virgin saints that Gallonio published together with the Italian edition of the treatise on martyrdom consisted of little else but questions by a Roman judge and pious answers by the virgin saint, alternating with violent torments.[43]

The treatise on martyrdom categorized the torments, but also presented them as successive stages in a more or less regular process. After a martyr had been pulled up (on the wooden horse or hanging from a rope tied to his hands behind his back), he would receive a beating first, then have his skin and flesh torn open, then be burnt with a fiery instrument of some sort.[44] Even though the extent of the torture to

---

[42] Delehaye, *Les passions des martyrs* 254–273.

[43] E.g. the *vita* of Saint Sothera, which begins as follows (Gallonio, *Historia delle sante vergini romane* 35–37): 'Fu questa Vergine nobilissima per sangue, e di tanto fervore, e spirito, che à tutte le grandezze, e vanità del mondo, diede con grandissimo ardir repulsa, e come cose basse, e vili, con altezza di cuore le dispreggiava. Avenne, che per esser'ella Christiana, fù fatta prigione: e commandandole il Giudice, che sacrificasse à gli Dei: rispose, che non voleva in modo alcuno farlo. All'hora pensando egli poter superare fortezza si grande, ordinò, che le fossero fate le guanciate [...]' ('This Virgin was of very noble blood, and of such fervor, and spirit, that she fiercely rejected all greatness and vanity of the world, and despised them virtuously as lowly and vile things. It so happened, that because she was Christian, she was made a prisoner: and the Judge ordered her to sacrifice to the Gods: she answered, that she would not do this in any way. Then, thinking he could overcome such great strength of will, he ordered her to be slapped'). The *vita* then continues with the torments Saint Sothera is subjected to, until she dies. In the same way the *vitae* of, for example, Saint Theodora, Saint Gliceria, Saint Cantiamilla and Saint Bonosa were hardly more than an exchange between the virgin in question and one or several adjudicating authorities (Gallonio, *Historia delle sante vergini romane* 45–46; 63–71; 106–108; 109–115).

[44] Gallonio, *Trattato* 42 (opening of chap. 4): 'Ho giudicato conveniente trattare doppo l'equuleo di quegli instrumenti, co'quali erano i Christiani battuti: imperoche solevano alle volte i Gentili, [...] stirati che havevano gli adoratori di Christo nell'equuleo, ivi ancor legati battergli, e dopo questo scarnificargli, come pure le historie nel cap. precedente riferite testimoniano, dar loro fuoco a'fianchi, overo à qualche altra parte del corpo' ('I have judged it to be convenient to treat after the wooden horse those

which the martyrs were subjected was excessive, the structure of the fixed sequence of torments is similar to what seems to have been common in torture in judicial courts.

According to early modern manuals, judges could put the defendant through a number of stages of torture during interrogation. The precise definition of these stages was contested by different sixteenth-century legal experts. According to the Spanish curial Francisco Peña, in a commentary to an influential thirteenth-century manual for inquisitors which he edited and published in 1578, the stages of torment were widely known and did not have to be discussed.[45] Of the secular legal experts that Peña refers to, Giulio Claro, in a 1568 collection of jurisprudence, advised the judge to limit torture to the rope (with the defendant pulled up by his hands tied behind his back). He identified the successive stages of torture on the basis of the moments that led up to its actual performance, first threatening the defendant with torture, then leading him to the place where it would be applied, then undressing him, then preparing him for the haul, and finally lifting him up.[46] Around 1545, Paolo Grillandi also limited torture to the rope, but he interpreted the five stages as five different degrees of painfulness, starting by threatening the defendant, then pulling him up for the duration of a *Pater Noster* or an *Ave Maria*, then for the duration of two *Miserere mei*, then for up to a full hour, and finally pulling him up with weights hanging from his legs. Grillandi expressed his admiration for another legal expert, Ippolito De'Marsili, who had listed as many as fourteen

---

instruments with which Christians were beaten: since now and then, having stretched the worshippers of Christ on the wooden horse, the Pagans used to go on beating them in that position, and after that tear off their flesh, as the histories mentioned in the previous chapter testify, put fire to their sides, or to some other part of their bodies'). Gallonio, *Trattato* 70 (opening of chap. 6): 'Non bastava alla fierezza de'Tiranni l'havere stracciate a'servi di Giesù Christo, legati nell'equuleo, ò a'pali [...], le carni, che ancora con diverse altre maniere di tormenti, così mal conci gli distratiavano' ('It did not satisfy the wickedness of the Tyrants to have torn open [...] the flesh of the servants of Jesus Christ while they were tied to the wooden horse or to poles, so, in their distress, they attacked them with still other kinds of torments'). In the Latin edition more or less the same indications of the regular sequence of torments in martyrdoms are given.

45 Nicolaus Eymericus, *Directorium Inquisitorum*, ed. Peña F. (Roma, in aedibus Populi Romani: 1578) 225.

46 I have used Giulio Claro, *Receptarum sententiarum opera omnia. His novissime accesserunt doctissimae additiones d. Hieronymi Giacharii; additae sunt denuo animadversiones Manfredi Goveani et Joannis Guiotii* (Frankfurt a.M., Wolfgang Richter: 1613) 230. The original edition: Giulio Claro, *Sententiarum receptarum liber quintus. Item practica criminalis* (Venezia, Giovanni Antonio Degli Antoni: 1570).

different kinds of torture, many of them derived from historical texts, but some of them invented by himself.[47] Ippolito De'Marsili description of possible techniques to be employed during torture, published in 1537, in fact bears the most resemblance to Gallonio's treatise on martyrdom. He distinguishes a number of sophisticated methods, which range from a kind of waterboarding (which he judges to be dangerous) to having a rodent eat through the defendant's stomach wall or having a goat lick the defendant's feet with his course tongue. His historical sources were medieval legal treatises rather than ancient literature, notably Azo's *Summa de questionibus* and Francesco Bruni's *Tractatus de indiciis et tortura.*[48]

This sample of ideas on the application of torture suggests a transformation from harsh physical violence (De'Marsili) to a more psychological approach (Claro). There clearly was a debate about the exact multi-stage procedure of torture, and both Claro and Peña admonish the reader not to apply creative new ways of torturing in the successive stages, in this way also implying that this was not entirely uncommon.[49] The reflections by early modern legal experts on the nature of the stages of judicial torture calls to mind Gallonio's categorization of the methods of torment, used in a more or less regular sequence in the torturing of early Christian martyrs. The painful extraction of truth from criminal suspects and the torments of martyrs were structured in similar ways.[50]

Gallonio's martyrological works thus approach torture partly as public execution, and partly as interrogatory torture. Like executions, the martyrdoms were spectacles of suffering, while at the same time involving a discursive exchange that was analogous to interrogation in judicial procedures. Gallonio's classification of torments into diverse categories has much in common with the instructions for inquisitive torture found in manuals written by legal experts. Instruments and methods of torture, therefore, appear to refer to destruction and pain at the same time. In one of the histories in Gallonio's *Historia delle sante vergini romane*, that of Saint Sothera, it is explicitly left undecided whether

[47] Paolo Grillandi, *Tractatus de hereticis et sortilegiis omnifariam coitu eorumque penis. De questionibus et tortura ac de relaxatione* (Lyon, Giunta: 1545) fols. 94v–100v.

[48] Ippolito De'Marsili, *Tractatus de questionibus nuperrime recognitus: in quo materie maleficiorum admodum diffuse subtiliterque pertractantum* (Lyon, Giunta: 1537) fols. 5v–6v.

[49] Claro, *Receptarum sententiarum opera omnia* 231; Eymericus, *Directorium Inquisitorum* 225–226.

[50] Silverman, *Tortured subjects* 46–48; Fiorelli, *La tortura giudiziaria* 192–214.

the torment of the virgin martyrs was a matter of disgrace or of pain. The anonymous judge who tries Saint Sothera has her face slapped, in order to persuade her 'out of shame or out of pain'.[51] The difference between inquisitive torture and executionary violence may well have been less clear-cut than modern historiography suggests.

The Execution of Gérard

The interest among oratorians in the sufferings of Catholics was not limited to the saintly models of antiquity. As I pointed out above, while Gallonio devoted the Italian edition of treatise on martyrdom exclusively to historical martyrs, he expanded the subsequent Latin edition with events that had recently taken place in north-west Europe. Especially English Catholics in exile on the European continent were actively publicising the persecution of their co-religionist in their home country.[52] The situation under Elisabeth I was precarious, since the English queen denounced Catholic loyalty to the pope as treason. While cardinal William Allen, Nicholas Sanders, Richard Verstegan, Robert Parsons and others, saw the violence they reported as a testing of (Catholic) Christian perseverance, according to the English authorities it was an instrument to suppress rebellion.[53] The authors of these books and pamphlets thus operated in the border zone between jurisprudence and martyrology. The oratorians owned many of these publications, and Gallonio himself possessed copies of books by Allen

---

[51] Gallonio, *Historia delle sante vergini romane* 35: '[...] ordinò, che le fossero fate le guanciate, affin che la tenera verginella, vinta dalla vergogna, ò dal dolore, se gli arrendesse: ma non gli successe, come s'era persuaso: [...]' ('he ordered her to be slapped, until the tender virgin, overcome by shame or by pain, would surrender: but it did not happen as he had convinced himself it would'); Gallonio cited his source faithfully: *De virginibus* by Saint Ambrosius of Milan.

[52] Dillon A., *The Construction of Martyrdom in the English Catholic Community, 1535–1603* (Aldershot: 2002) esp. 1–17; 72–113; Gregory, *Salvation at Stake* 268–272; 274–280; 283–297.

[53] William Allen, *Historia del glorioso martirio di sedici sacerdoti martirizzati in Inghilterra per la confessione, & difesa della fede catolica, l'anno 1581.1582. & 1583* (Macerata, Sebastiano Martellini: 1583) 3–6 (this work is a translation of William Allen, *A briefe historie of the glorious martyrdom of twelve reverend priests* (Reims, s.n.: 1582), with some additions); Verstegan, *Theatrum Crudelitatum* 8–14. The other publications mentioned are: Nicholas Sanders, *De visibili monarchia ecclesiae, libri 8* (Antwerp, John Fowler: 1578); Nicholas Sanders, *De origine ac progressu schismatis Anglicani libri tres* (Rome, Bartolomeo Bonfadini: 1586); Robert Parsons, *De persecutione Anglicana libellus* (Rome, Francesco Zanetti: 1582).

and Sanders.[54] Furthermore, he manually transcribed those parts of the *Theatrum crudelitatum* by Verstegan that contained the factual details of the torture and executions. He omitted the verses that accompanied the illustrations, and seems to have been interested only in the bare essentials of the tortures endured by Catholics.[55]

These excerpts from the *Theatrum crudelitatum* are part of a set of hagiographical writings, collected into a series of manuscript volumes by Gallonio.[56] In the same series, there is a volume with a section on another recent case of extreme judicial violence against a Catholic, the trial and execution of Balthasar Gérard. This Burgundian Catholic in 1584 answered the summons, issued by King Philip II of Spain, to kill Prince William the Silent, the leader of the protestant Dutch Revolt.[57] After he had shot the prince of Orange, Gérard was captured and subjected to a particularly gruesome sequence of torments during a number of days. The trial and death of Gérard were recorded in several written accounts, both by Protestants and Catholics. These narratives soon made their way around Europe.[58] Two of the accounts – obviously

[54] Sanders, *De origine ac progressu*, Biblioteca Vallicelliana S. Borr. F. V. 139, Gallonio's note of possession; Allen, *Historia del glorioso martirio di sedici sacerdoti*, Biblioteca Vallicelliana S. Borr. F. I. 145, Gallonio's note of possession.

[55] The transcription is in "Theatrum crudelitatum hereticorum nostri temporis", Biblioteca Vallicelliana, Ms. H. 5, fol. 118v–130v.

[56] Ditchfield, *Liturgy, Sanctity and History* 47–50. According to the preface to the "Index vetus nominum sanctorum et aliorum monumentorum quae sunt in codicibus manuscriptis collectis ab Antonio Gallonio", drawn up by a librarian of the Oratory in the eighteenth century, this series of nineteen volumes consisted of manuscript hagiographical texts collected by Gallonio: Biblioteca Vallicelliana Ms. H. 1, fol. IIr and IIIr. The fact that one of the volumes contains the holy office for the Lateran canons, printed in 1621, sixteen years after Gallonio had died, indicates that the present arrangement of sheets and quires cannot be assumed to be identical to the arrangement that Gallonio bequeathed to the oratorian library in 1605: *Officia canonicorum regularium Lateranensium S. Augustini* (Venice, Giunta: 1621) in: Biblioteca Vallicelliana, Ms. H. 2, fols. 226r–261r. Therefore, one should be cautious in attributing texts in this series to Gallonio's original collection. The appearance of the handwriting suggests that it was written some time in the last two decades of the sixteenth century, which increases the probability of it having belonged to Gallonio, even though he did not write it himself.

[57] For details see Jardine L., *The Awful End of Prince William the Silent: The First Assassination of a Head of State with a Handgun* (London: 2005), particularly 50–61.

[58] Pater Gerlach (Schümmer S.), *De verhalen over de dood van Balthasar Gérard* (Tilburg: 1949) 39–41; Fruin R.T., *Robert Fruin's verspreide geschriften*, part. VII, *Kritische studiën over geschiedbronnen*, vol. I, ed. Blok P.J. – Muller P.L. – Muller F.S. (The Hague: 1903) 247–266.

Catholic versions – ended up in the Roman Oratory, one of which is the document in the manuscript series of Gallonio.[59]

Gérard's first interrogation was accompanied by elaborate torture. He was beaten with rods; he was suspended from a rack with a weight of several pounds hanging from his toes; his armpits were burnt; boiling fat was poured over him. In the process, Gérard confessed that he had killed William of Orange. The authorities then passed a verdict and Gérard was to be put to death. The sentence involved another round of torments. The executioners tied Gérard up. They scorched his right hand between fiery hot plates; they burnt his limbs with a blazing grille; they cut off his genitals; they opened his body, emptying it of its entrails, and of the heart, which they threw into his face. His body was quartered and the different parts were exhibited over the gates of the town of Delft. The destruction of Gérard's body could hardly have been more complete. The embryonic state of the United Provinces, temporarily decapitated by the shooting of William the Silent, made a public show of its power over the body of the miscreant.

The reason for obtaining or receiving such a narrative was not the oratorians' predilection for gruesome prose, but because they were closely involved in the administrative procedures for determining who would be honoured in the Catholic liturgy.[60] After the death of Gérard, abortive attempts were made to have him venerated as a martyr of the Catholic church. The highest representative of the Catholic church in the United Provinces, apostolic vicar Sasbout Vosmeer, safeguarded relics of Gérard's body. He also wrote a holy office for the assassin, which he had sent to Rome for approval. It appears that the Oratory of Rome took part in the administrative deliberations concerning the veneration of Balthasar Gérard, which in the end faltered. In 1604 Cesare Baronio, by then a cardinal, informed Sasbout Vosmeer about the slow proceedings. He told Vosmeer that pope Clement VIII, rather

[59] Biblioteca Vallicelliana Ms. H. 6, fols. 157r–159v (in the collection attributed to Gallonio) and Biblioteca Vallicelliana Ms. N. 22, fols. 267r–268v.

[60] Gallonio himself occurred in a list of advisers to the Congregation of Sacred Rites, the department in the Curia Romana responsible for the inquiries that were part of canonisation procedure: Papa G., *Le cause di canonizzazione nel primo periodo della Congregazione dei Riti (1588–1634)* (Vatican City: 2001) 96–97; in general, the members of the Oratory were intensely engaged in hagiographical, liturgical en juridical aspects of canonisation procedure: Gotor M., *I beati del papa* 127–202.

than approve a holy office in honour of Gérard, preferred to have a single office composed in honour of a number of similar cases.[61]

Tommaso Bozio, another member of the Oratory, mentioned the trial of Gérard in an apologetic reference work, the *De signis ecclesiae Dei* (1591), a catalogue listing all the components of the one true Catholic church. These included theological doctrines, such as the intercession of saints on behalf of mortals and the soteriological necessity of all seven sacraments; historical principles, such as the continuous succession of popes since the death of Saint Peter and the validity of canon law; intellectual, moral and theological virtues; philosophical achievements; liberal and mechanical arts; spiritual and mystical accomplishments; and the efficacy and significance of miracles. For each hallmark of religious truth, Bozio ammassed historical examples to illustrate and prove that it found its main manifestation in the Catholic Church. One of the categories listed by Bozio is *patientia*, patience or endurance. Bozio presented the case of Gérard as illustrative of the strictness with which the Catholic church selected those worthy of veneration. Even though Gérard had shown incredible endurance, not showing any sense of pain, this was still not sufficient for the church to regard him as a holy marty.[62]

The clerics of the Counter Reformation appealed regularly to the authors of the second and third centuries, when the Christian church still struggled to survive and was persecuted by distrustful emperors and administrators. Especially Tertullian and Cyprian were cited often in relation to the merits of martyrdom. In both editions of the treatise on martyrdom, Gallonio referred to Cyprian in several passages.[63] Accord-

---

[61] Gerlach, *De verhalen over de dood* 37–42; another candidate for inclusion in such a collective holy office might have been Jacques Clémente, the dominican friar who had assassinated king Henry III of France: Gregory, *Salvation at Stake* 295–297.

[62] Gerlach, *De verhalen over de dood* 30–31; Tommaso Bozio, *De signis ecclesiae Dei libri XXIIII* (Cologne, Johann Gymnich: 1626) I, 425–426: 'Igitur aliquem nominemus, qui a nobis inter martyres haud recenseatur et crudelissima tamen tormenta sit constantissimè passus et patientissimè, nullum doloris sensum praeseferens' ('So I will mention one who is absolutely not counted by us among the martyrs, even though he suffered the most cruel torments with great constancy and endurance, showing no sense of pain'); the original edition is: Tommaso Bozio, *De signis ecclesiae Dei libri XXIIII*, 2 vols. (Rome, Giacomo Tornieri: 1591).

[63] E.g. Gallonio A., *Trattato* 34, with a reference to *De laude martyrii*; Gallonio, *Trattato* 38, with Gallonio citing *Epistula* IV; Gallonio, *Trattato* 70, where Gallonio mentions *De laude martyrii*; Gallonio, *De sanctorum* 59, where Gallonio cites the *Epistula ad Donatum, De lapsis* and *De laude martyrii*; Gallonio, *De sanctorum* 62, where reference is made to *Epistula* XXXIII; Gallonio, *De sanctorum* 139, where Gallonio refers to *De laude martyrii*.

ing to Gallonio, Gérard calmly spoke the words of Cyprian, 'Thank God', in response to his death sentence.[64] In the previous dialogue with his prosecutors, the magistrates expressed their admiration at how little Gérard seemed to have been moved by the tortures to which he was subjected. He replied that this was because of the mediation by the saints. In the intervals between the various tortures, he spoke clearly and without hesitation, 'which moved the spectators to tears'.[65] The account presents the interrogation already as a spectacle, with the pain of the torments determining the dynamics. In the narrative, Gérard is presented as possessing the constancy of the ideal martyr, as prescribed by Cyprian and his contemporaries. It was especially his response to pain that served as an indication of this firmness.

At first sight, the trial and execution of Gérard seem a typical example of interrogatory and punitive torment. Balthasar Gérard was made to tell the truth about his heinous crime by subjecting him to gruesome torture. Subsequently, the Delft authorities publicly demolished his body. As described in the account however, the torments were hardly separate stages. The painful torture of interrogation and the destructive torment of execution evolved in a continuous crescendo. From a Catholic viewpoint, Gérard's painful ordeal testified to the truth embodied by the Church. Torture and execution, hurting and shaming, together formed a process of literally wrenching the truth from

[64] Biblioteca Vallicelliana, Ms. H. 6, fol. 158v: 'ergo sepius auditus frequentissime et variis modis tortus, cum nihil diceret, quod illis arrideret, tandem decimatertia die prescripti mensis de ipsi imminenti morte certior factus, et sequenti die eius sententiam audiens, placide ac benigne cum sanctissimo Cipriano dixit: Deo gratias' ('Having been interrogated in this manner many times, and tortured in various ways, since he did not tell them anything that pleased them, in the end, on the thirteenth day of the aforesaid month (of July), he was informed of his own imminent death, and listening the following day to his sentence kindly and at ease, he said, as the most saintly Cyprian had done: "Thank God"').

[65] Biblioteca Vallicelliana, Ms. H. 6, fol. 158r: 'Quesitus, quomodo ad tantas paenas et tormenta non amplius moveretur. Beatorum, inquit, praeces id efficiunt. Consuli eius instantiam admiranti constantiam, inquit, morte intueri licebit. verum extra tempus torturae blandè, ac liberè cum singulis locutus, etiam tortoribus mirantibus, et spectatoribus ad lachrymas inclinatis, quibusdam eum hominem esse negantibus [...]' ('Asked how it could be that he was not affected more by such torture and torments, he said "The advocacy of the saints brings this about". To the magistrate, who admired his firmness, he said "constancy can be observed only in death". As a matter of fact, when not under torture he spoke freely and in a friendly manner to every single one, even to the torturers, who were very impressed, and to the spectators, who were moved to tears; some of whom even denied he was human [...]).

Gérard.[66] The martyrological value of Gérard's conduct was that he remained impassive. The fact that he did not express his pain is what proved him right.

The Instruments of Torture

After Gérard had been led to the scaffold, he was bound to a stake. The Latin report of the execution states that he was tied to a 'stake or a cross' ('Palo seu Cruci'), associating the stake with the universal Christian symbol of martyrdom. This link also runs parallel to the subject matter of the first chapter of Gallonio's treatise on martyrdom, in which he advances two reasons for placing 'stakes', and, more generally, 'ways of suspending Christians' in the same category as 'the cross'.[67] The first was a historical-linguistic argument: in antiquity, the word 'cross' had indicated stakes as well. The second argument drew on the mechanics of torture: crosses and stakes were both methods of suspending people.[68] In this way, Gallonio created a rational foundation for associating stakes with the cross.

---

[66] Asad T., "Notes on Body Pain and Truth in Medieval Christian ritual", *Economy and Society* 12,3 (1983) 287–327. A similar dual perspective, in which both the inquisitor and the victim make a claim to have generated truth in the process of the tortures, has been described in relation to the persecution of English catholics under Elizabeth I, by Hanson, "Torture and Truth" 61.

[67] Biblioteca Vallicelliana, ms. H. 6, fol. 158v: 'in Theatrum processit, Palo seu Cruci se alligari passus [...]' ('he went forth to the scaffold, allowing himself to be tied to the Stake or Cross [...]'); see the titles of the first chapters of the Italian and the Latin edition, as cited in n. 11.

[68] Gallonio, *De sanctorum* 1: 'Quoniam vero stipites erecti sub hoc eodem crucis nomine ab antiquis comprehendebantur, ideo et de his erit nobis ibidem agendum, sicuti et de modis, quibus sancti martyres pro Christi fide defendenda suspendebantur: nam, tam cruci affixi, quam palis alligati, erant aliquo modo pendentes' ('Because upright poles were in fact included under this same name of the cross since antiquity, and therefore I will need to write about them in this same place, as well as about the ways in which martyr saints were suspended on account of their defence of the Christian faith, both those nailed to the cross and those tied to stakes were in a sense suspended people'). For the same passage in the Italian edition see Gallonio, *Trattato* 1: 'e perche i pali dritti vengono da gli antichi con questo medesimo nome chiamati, Croce; però di questi ancora quì scriveremo, come similmente de'modi di sospendere, essendo che e nella croce, e ne'pali stavano i condannati pendenti' ('and because upright stakes are called by the ancients by this same name "Cross", therefore we will write also about them, as well as about ways of suspending, since on crosses as well as on poles convicts were suspended').

This is one of several coincidences between Gallonio's treatise on martyrdom and the account of the Gérard's execution. In the latter source, the executioners are said to squeeze his arms between 'fiery plates' ('candentes laminas'), while Gallonio devotes an entire section to 'burning plates' ('de laminis ardentibus').[69] Gérard's entrails were pulled out, and the same torment appears in the treatise on martyrdom. Moreover, the description of this atrocious torment in the Latin edition of Gallonio's treatise is similar to its depiction by his contemporary Frans Hogenland in his illustration of the execution of Gérard [Fig. 3, 4].

Gallonio's treatise and the anonymous account of Balthasar Gérard's execution not only have a set of themes in common, but also a vocabulary for discussing them. One last example will show that the painstaking accuracy of their formulations presuppose a continuum of pain and destruction. The account of Gérard's execution in Gallonio's manuscript collection claims that the assassin is tied to the *eculeus* or 'wooden horse'.[70] The exact appearance and workings of this antique torture instruments were the subject of some scholarly debate during these decades.[71] Gallonio discusses the *equuleus* extensively in chapter 3 of the treatise on martyrdom, and declares his indebtedness to his fellow oratorian, Tommaso Bozio, in the reconstruction of the device. Indeed, Bozio left a handwritten description of the device that accords with Gallonio's account. According to Gallonio, the *equuleus* consisted of a traverse beam on four legs. The victim would be placed on the beam and stretched out.[72] The stretching could continue until the

[69] Gerlach, *De verhalen over de dood* 51–54; Gallonio *Trattato* 6–7; 70; Gallonio, *De sanctorum* 7; 9; 139–140.

[70] Biblioteca Vallicelliana, ms. H. 6, fol. 157r: 'tortus horribiliter in eculeo suspensus [...]' ('tortured horribly, put up on the wooden horse [...]'). In the other known versions of the account, different words have been used instead of *eculeus*.

[71] See for this debate the publications by Sigonio and Gallonio mentioned below, and Girolamo Maggi, *De equuleo hactenus incognito liber*, ed. Jungermann G. (Hanau, Claude Marne: 1609). The book by Maggi was included in a later edition of the treatise on martyrdom: Antonio Gallonio, *De sanctorum martyrum cruciatibus liber*, ed. Trichet du Fresne R. (Paris, Claude Cramoisy: 1660). Maggi, who died in 1572, explained that *eculeus* is the orthography commonly accepted, whereas *equuleus* would be more correct: Gallonio, *De sanctorum martyrum*, ed. Trichet du Fresne, 273.

[72] Gallonio, *Trattato* 35: 'Disconvengono poi in assegnargli la forma: intorno à che, per fuggire troppa lungezza, mi sono risoluto riferire l'opinione del P. Thomaso Bozzi, la quale tra tutte le altre mi è parsa più conforme al vero, narrata da lui nell'historia che ha scritta de'nostri santi Papia, e Mauro, non ancor data in luce; dicendovi, esser esso un'instrumento antico di legno, ritrovato per martoriare, fatto à foggia di un cavalletto con quattro piedi, e con alcune girelle dalle parti, accomodate nel modo che hora s'esplicarà' ('Then they disagree on which form to attribute to it: regarding

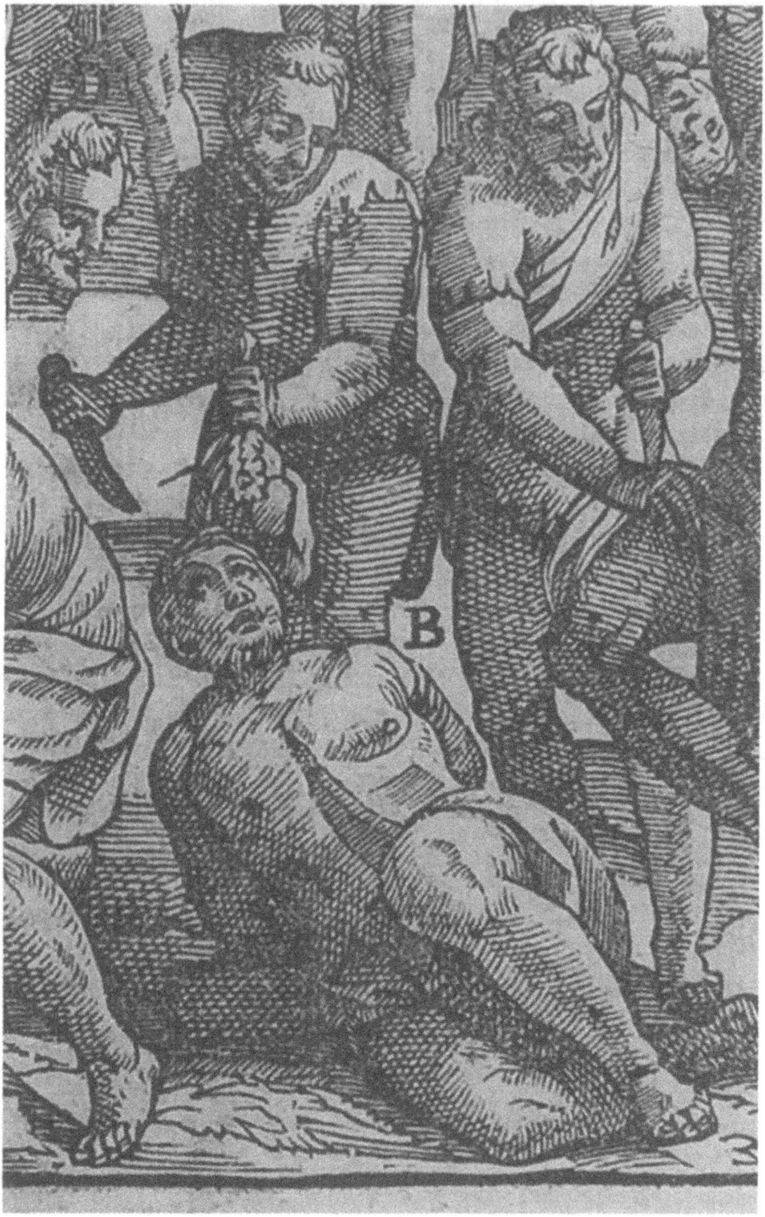

Fig. 3. A martyr's entrails are cut out. Detail of an engraving depicting various forms of torture. From Antonio Gallonio, *De sanctorum martyrum cruciatibus liber quo potissimum instrumenta et modi, quibus iidem Christi martyres olim torquebantur, accuratissime tabellis expressa describuntur* (Rome, Typographia Congregationis Oratorii: 1594) 253, woodcut. Biblioteca Vallicelliana.

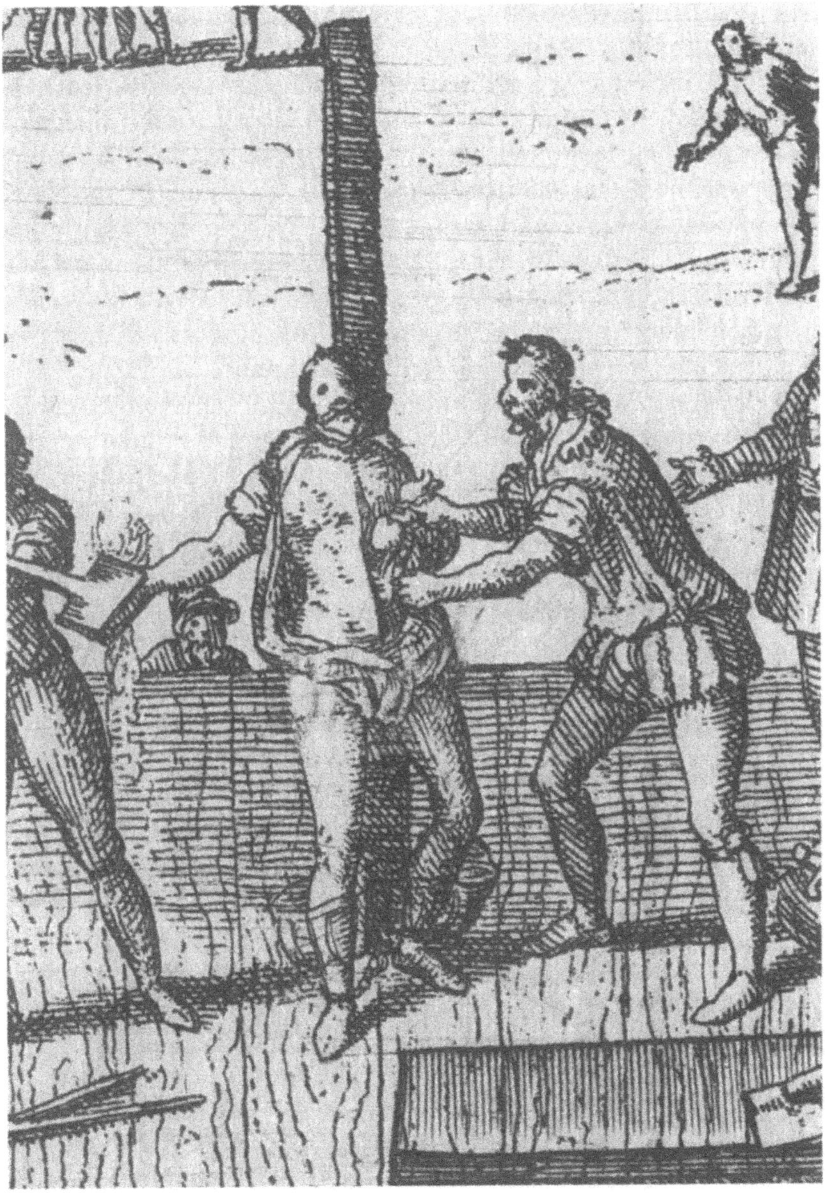

Fig. 4. Gérard's heart and entrails are taken out. Detail of an engraving depicting the execution of Balthasar Gérard. From Frans Hogenberg, *Kroniek van de opstand in de Lage Landen, 1555–1609: actuele oorlogsverslaggeving uit de zestiende eeuw met 228 gravures van Frans Hogenberg*, ed. K. Kinds (Wenum – Wiesel: 1999) vol. II, 57.

joints of the victim would snap. Several arguments serve to support this reconstruction. On a philological level, the word *equuleus*, meaning 'little horse', suggested that the machine should have four legs. On a level of mechanics, ancient texts claim that once the ropes were relaxed, the victim would hang underneath the *equuleus*. According to Gallonio, this implied that the victim was bound on the *equuleus* in a horizontal position; once the ropes were relaxed, the victim would fall down and dangle underneath the crossbeam. Gallonio repeatedly stressed this point, emphasizing that falling underneath the *equuleus* would continue the painful dislocation of the victim's joints, causing excruciating pain – in this way, disintegration and pain merge.[73] The description of Balthasar Gérard as having been tortured on the *equuleus* not only suggested the continuity between the ancient and the early modern *Ecclesia Militans*, but also implied the continuity between pain and the destruction of Gérard's body.

Elaine Scarry has argued that in violent interrogations, the instruments of torture come to embody the pain inflicted. Showing the instruments to the victim is an element of the process of torture, inseparable from the actual application of the instruments. Although Scarry is concerned with twentieth-century political torture, the situation she

---

which, to avoid too much prolixity, I have decided to render the opinion of father Tommaso Bozio, which among all the others seemed most in accordance with the truth, expounded by him in the history that he has written of our saints Papias and Maurus, as yet unpublished; as I was saying to you, this was an ancient wooden instrument, invented for torturing, made in the guise of a little horse with four legs, and with some pulleys on the sides, mounted as will be explained next' (the discussion of the *equuleus* takes up the whole of chapter 3, ibid. 34–41).

Gallonio, *De sanctorum* 49 (the discussion of the *equuleus* takes up half of chapter 3; Gallonio, *De sanctorum* 47–63): 'Alii postremo, machinam ligneam fuisse ad equi similitudinem (veluti infra diffuse explicabitur) fabricatam, cum duabus striatis rotulis in extremis excavatisque eius partibus positis, quae quidem per axiculos ductoriis funiculis traiectis versabantur; unde fiebat, ut rei illis alligati varie excruciarentur atque distenderentur. Fuit huius opinionis P. Thomas Bozius nostrae Congregationis sacerdos, in historia, quam de sanctis martyribus Papia et Mauro descripsit, nondum excusa' ('Still others, at last, that it was a wooden machine made in the likeness of a horse (as will be explained in detail below), with two little wheels with grooves at the far ends, positioned in the cut-out sides, which were turned by windlasses with cords reeled around them; which cause the criminals tied upon them to be tormented as well as stretched. Father Tommaso Bozio, priest of our Congregation, held this view, in the history that he has written of the martyr saints Papias and Maurus, as yet unpublished').

[73] Gallonio, *De sanctorum* 51: 'vel, Iudice annuente, funiculos relaxantes, incurvum ac pendulum sub equuleo cadere, non sine maximo dolore faciebant' ('or, at a nudge of the Judge, they made (the martyr) fall under the wooden horse, stooped and swinging, not without the greatest pain').

describes is that of secluded interrogatory torture. The importance of watching the instruments as part of judicial torture is also suggested by sixteenth-century manuals for magistrates.[74] Rosalyne Rey has shown that for early modern Catholics, it was hurting the body, not breaking it, that facilitated contrition and thus salvation. The sinner who castigated himself allowed his body to ache, to speak, so as to come to terms with it.[75] Combining these two observations, it follows that displaying – and theorising about – instruments of torture evoked the pain of torture, and this in turn evoked reflection on the superiority of divinely inspired spirituality to physical comfort. The elaborate and meticulous reconstruction of the *equuleus*, the rack on which the victim's limbs were gradually torn apart, was a meditation on the evangelical message that the application of the instrument conveyed. This applied to late antique and early modern Christian martyrs. The instrument of pain evoked the truth to which the martyr testified. Both the instrument that generated truth and the martyr that uttered it required an audience that would be edified by the spectacle.

Conclusion

Gallonio's treatise on martyrdom is a surgical analysis of the infliction of pain and the destruction of the body. The essence of martyrdom implied renouncing the carnal shell in which the pure Christian soul resided, yet in order to clarify the nature of what exactly happened when martyrs renounced their bodies, ecclesiastical writers occupied themselves with the more physical aspects of martyrdom. With respect to torture, Gallonio shows a great interest in the mechanical workings of the human body in relation to pain. If the painful demolition the victim's body in torture was supposed to produce truth, this occasioned academic reflection on the instruments used to lay bare this truth.

Ecclesiastical scholars engaged with current experiences, as well as with past traditions. Moreover, in Gallonio's analysis of martyrdom,

---

[74] Scarry, *The Body in Pain* 15–19; 27–59; see also the publications cited in nn. 39–40. Cardinal Gabriele Paleotti implicitly associated the torments of the martyrs, and the instruments that inflicted it, with the experience of pain. In *De sacris imaginibus* he argued for depicting the instruments of martyrdom in painting, in order to remind the onlooker that our personal weaknesses and pains were relatively mild. Mansour, "Not Torments, but Delights" 169–171.

[75] Rey, *The History of Pain* 54–55.

interrogatory torture merged with punitive torment, both current in theory and practice of criminal justice in his own days. The accounts of trials and executions in the religious upheavals of Europe reveal how strongly legal conflicts and martyrdom were interconnected. The account of the ordeal endured by Balthasar Gérard, the assassin of William the Silent, contains elements that recurred in martyrological literature. The adaptation of this account by Tommaso Bozio shows how such an ordeal acquired martyrological meaning in terms of *patientia*, or endurance of pain. The infliction of pain in order to gain truthful knowledge and the infliction of destructive pain in order to stage the spectacle of salvation were both part of a continuous process.

Gallonio and Bozio both paid particular attention to the mechanics of the instruments of judicial violence; a philologically and logically correct language to write and talk about instruments of torture was vital to a proper reading of martyrdom. Gallonio's treatise is a systematic reflection on the instruments of torture, and this amounts to a reflection on pain itself. Since martyrs testified to the truth of salvation, articulating their physical suffering was a way of mediating this truth.

Selective Bibliography

Manuscripts

Biblioteca Vallicelliana, Rome:

Ms. H. 1, fol. Ir–IVr; 1r–27v, "Index vetus nominum sanctorum et aliorum monumentorum quae sunt in codicibus manuscriptis collectis ab Antonio Gallonio".

Ms. H. 2, fol. 226r–261r, *Officia canonicorum regularium Lateranensium S. Augustini* (Venice, Giunta, 1621).

Ms. H. 5, fol. 118v–130v, "Theatrum crudelitatum hereticorum nostri temporis".

Ms. H. 6, fol. 157r–159v.

Ms. N. 22, fol. 267r–268v.

Old Printed Books

Allen William, *Historia del glorioso martirio di sedici sacerdoti martirizzati in Inghilterra per la confessione, & difesa della fede catolica, l'anno 1581.1582. & 1583.* (Macerata, Sebastiano Martellini: 1583).

Bozio Tommaso, *De signis ecclesiae Dei libri* XXIIII, 2 vols. (Cologne, Johann Gymnich: 1626).

Claro Giulio, *Receptarum sententiarum opera omnia. His novissime accesserunt doctissimæ additiones d. Hieronymi Giacharii; additae sunt denuo animadversiones Manfredi Goveani et Joannis Guiotii* (Frankfurt a.M., Wolfgang Richter: 1613).

De' Marsili Ippolito, *Tractatus de questionibus nuperrime recognitus, in quo materie maleficiorum admodum diffuse subtiliterque pertractantum* (Lyon, Giunta: 1537).

Eymericus Nicolaus, *Directorium Inquisitorum*, ed. Francisco Peña (Rome, in aedibus Populi Romani: 1578).

Gallonio Antonio, *Historia delle sante vergini romane con varie annotationi e con alcune vite breui de' santi parenti loro, e de' gloriosi martiri Papia e Mauro soldati romani* (Rome, Ascanio and Girolamo Donangeli: 1591).

——, *Trattato de gli instrumenti di martirio, e delle varie maniere di martoriare usate da'gentili contro christiani* (Rome, Ascanio and Girolamo Donangeli: 1591).

——, *De sanctorum martyrum cruciatibus liber quo potissimum instrumenta et modi, quibus iidem Christi martyres olim torquebantur, accuratissime tabellis expressa describuntur* (Rome, Typographia Congregationis Oratorii: 1594).

Grillandi, Paolo, *Tractatus de hereticis et sortilegijs omnifariam coitu eorumque penis. De questionibus et tortura ac de relaxatione* (Lyon, Giunta: 1545).

Maggi, Girolamo, *De equuleo hactenus incognito liber*, ed. Gottfried Jungermann (Hanau, Claude Marne: 1609).

Scholarly Literature

Aigrain R., *L'Hagiographie: ses sources, ses methodes, son histoire* (Brussels: 2000).

Bonadonna Russo M.T., "La cultura storica nella Congregazione dell'Oratorio", in Bonadonna Russo M.T. – Del Re N. (eds.), *San Filippo Neri nella realtà romana del XVI secolo* (Rome: 2000) 69–88.

Bynum Walker C., *The Resurrection of the Body in Western Christianity, 200–1336* (New York: 1995).

Calzolari M., "Delitti e castighi", in Calzolari M. – Di Sivo M. – Grantaliano E. (eds.), *Giustizia e criminalità nello stato pontificio. Ne delicta remaneant impunita* (Rome: 2002) 39–75.

Cohen E., "The Animated Pain of the Body", *American Historical Review* 105,1 (2006) 36–68.
Delehaye H., *Les passions des martyrs et les genres littéraires* (Brussels: 1966).
——, *Cinq leçons sur la méthode hagiographique* (Brussels: 1934).
Di Sivo M., "Per via di giustizia. Sul processo penale a Roma tra XVI e XIX secolo", in Calzolari M. – Di Sivo M. – Grantaliano E. (eds.), *Giustizia e criminalità nello stato pontificio. Ne delicta remaneant impunita* (Rome: 2002) 13–35.
Ditchfield S., "Il mondo della Riforma e della Controriforma", in Benvenuti A. *et al.* (eds.), *Storia della santità nel cristianesimo occidentale* (Rome: 2005) 261–329.
——, "Text before Trowel: Antonio Bosio's *Roma sotterranea* Revisited", in Swanson R.N. (ed.), *The Church Retrospective: Papers Read at the 1995 Summer Meeting and the 1996 Winter Meeting of the Ecclesiastical History Society* (London: 1997) 343–360.
——, *Liturgy, Sanctity and History in Tridentine Italy: Pietro Maria Campi and the Preservation of the Particular* (Cambridge: 1995).
Egmond F., "Execution, Dissection, Pain and Infamy: A Morphological Investigation", in Egmond F. – Zwijnenberg R. (eds.), *Bodily Extremities: Preoccupations with the Human Body in Early Modern European Culture* (Aldershot – Burlington: 2003) 92–128.
Fiorelli P., *La tortura giudiziaria nel diritto comune*, 2 vols. (Varese: 1953–1954).
Firpo L., "Esecuzioni capitali in Roma (1567–1671)", in Biondi A. (ed.), *Eresia e riforma nell'Italia del cinquecento* (Florence – Chicago: 1974) 307–342.
Foucault M., *Surveiller et punir: naissance de la prison* (Paris: 1975).
Gotor M., *I beati del papa. Santità, Inquisizione e obbedienza in età moderna* (Florence: 2002).
Gregory B., *Salvation at Stake: Christian Martyrdom in Early Modern Europe* (Cambridge, MA: 1999).
Guazzelli G.A., "Cesare Baronio e il *Martyrologium Romanum*: problemi interpretativi e linee evolutive di un rapporto diacronico", in Firpo M. (ed.), *Nunc alia tempora, alii mores. Storici e storia in età postridentina. Atti del Convegno internazionale Torino, 24–27 settembre 2003* (Florence: 2005) 47–89.
Hanson E., "Torture and truth in Renaissance England", *Representations* 34 (1991) 53–84.
Jardine L., *The Awful End of Prince William the Silent: The First Assassination of a Head of State with a Handgun* (London: 2005).
Langbein J.H., *Torture and the Law of Proof: Europe and England in the Ancien Régime* (Chicago – London: 1977).
Lestringant F., *Lumière des martyrs: essai sur le martyre au siècle des Réformes* (Paris: 2004).
Mansour O., "Not Torments, but Delights: Antonio Gallonio's *Trattato de gli instrumenti di martirio* of 1591 and its Illustrations", in Hopkins A. – Wyke M. (eds.), *Roman Bodies. Antiquity to the Eighteenth Century* (London: 2005) 167–183.
Merback M.B., *The Thief, the Cross and the Wheel: Pain and the Spectacle of Punishment in Medieval and Renaissance Europe* (London: 1999).
Prosperi A., *Tribunali della coscienza: inquisitori, confessori, missionari* (Turin: 1996).
Rey R., *The History of Pain*, trl. Wallace L.E. – Cadden J.A. – Cadden S.W. (Cambridge, MA: 1995).
Romeo G., *L'inquisizione nell'Italia moderna* (Rome: 2002).
Scarry E., *The Body in Pain: The Making and Unmaking of the World* (New York: 1985).
Scott P., "Some Perspectives on Execution and Martyrdom, during the Ancien Régime", in Dousteyssier-Khoze C. – Scott P. (eds.), *(Ab)Normalities* (Durham: 2001) 25–38.
Silverman L., *Tortured Subjects: Pain, Truth, and the Body in Early Modern France* (Chicago: 2001).
Simoncini S., "Tendenze e figure della cultura", in Pinelli A. (ed.), *Storia di Roma dall'antichità a oggi. Roma del Rinascimento* (Rome: 2001) 199–266.

Spierenburg P., *The Spectacle of Suffering: Executions and the Evolution of Repression: From a Preindustrial Metropolis to the European Experience* (Cambridge: 1984).
Zen S., *Baronio storico: Controriforma e crisi del metodo umanistico* (Naples: 1994).
Zuccari A., "Politica culturale dell'Oratorio romano nella seconda metà del Cinquecento", *Storia dell'Arte* 41 (1981) 77–112.

PAIN AS PERSUASION: THE PETRARCH MASTER INTERPRETING PETRARCH'S *DE REMEDIIS*

Karl A.E. Enenkel

Petrarch's *De remediis utriusque fortune* was certainly one of the most influential books of the early modern period. From its publication in 1366 on, it was disseminated all over Latin-speaking Europe, and found its way in the libraries of a range of intellectuals, clerics and laymen.[1] Much ahead of its time, it represents a very early example of Renaissance Neo-Stoicism (which is generally associated with sixteenth-century intellectuals such as Du Vair and Lipsius), and offers a manual of more than 250 meditative exercises that teach its reader how to master as many different situations in life. As the huge number of manuscripts, printed editions and translations demonstrates, the influence of *De remedies* even grew in the fifteenth and sixteenth centuries. In the sixteenth century, part of its tremendous success was due to the large set of illustrations (261 woodcuts), made in 1519–1520 by an anonymous artist from Augsburg in Southern Germany, the so-called Petrarch Master.[2] The German *De remediis* editions with the Petrarch

---

[1] The Latin text was disseminated in an enormous number of manuscripts, of which more than 245 have been preserved, and a considerable number of printed editions. Cf. Mann N., "Manuscripts of Petrarch's *De remediis*. A Checklist", *Italia medioevale e umanistica* 14 (1971) 57–90 and Trapp J.B., "Illustrated Manuscripts of Petrarch's *De Remediis Utriusque Fortunae*", in idem, *Studies of Petrarch and his Influence* (London: 2003) 118–170. Moreover, the work was translated into French, German, Italian, Spanish and other languages. The translations were circulated in manuscripts and printed editions alike.

[2] The illustrations of the Petrarch Master normally accompany the German translations of *De remediis* and are found for instance in the printed editions Augsburg, Heinrich Steyner: 1532; 1539; Frankfurt, Christoph Egenolff: 1551; 1559; 1572; 1583; 1584; 1596; Frankfurt: 1604; 1620; 1672; Lüneburg: 1637. For the illustrations of the Petrarch Master cf. Scheidig W., *Die Holzschnitte des Petrarca-Meisters* (Berlin: 1955); Enenkel K.A.E., "Der Petrarca des Petrarca-Meisters: Zum Text-Bild-Verhältnis in illustrierten *De-Remediis*-Ausgaben", in Enenkel K.A.E. – Papy J. (eds.), *Petrarch and his Readers in the Renaissance*, in *Intersections. Yearbook for Early Modern Studies* 6 (2006) 91–169.

Master's illustrations figure among the most intriguing bi-medial book productions of the early modern era.[3]

The woodcuts have often been interpreted as being essentially in line with Petrarch's text. For example, Fraenger and Scheidig see them as realistic genre scenes or *Schaubilder* that are meant to express Petrarch's humanist and Renaissance world view. More recent interpretations by Raupp, Knape and Wohlfeil-Wohlfeil argue that they should be read as *didactic images* or *Lehrbilder* that are intended to express Petrarch's Neo-Stoic and humanistic doctrines.[4] Detailed recent analysis, however, has cast doubt on these interpretations. Some two years ago, I made a first attempt to offer a new interpretation of the relationship between word and image. In the *Glücksbuch*, the *Von der Artzney baider Glück, des guten und des widerwertigen*, illustrated by the Petrarch Master, word and image operate within remarkably dissimilar discourses. While Petrarch's text is situated in Christian Stoicism, the images participate in the discourses of the house book, moral satire (the *Narrenschiff*), of collections of proverbs and of political and religious polemics.[5]

---

[3] For the relationship between word and image, see especially Enenkel, "Der Petrarca des Petrarca-Meisters" and R. Falkenburg, "Speculative Imagery in Petrarch's *Von der Artzney bayder Glueck*", in Enenkel – Papy (eds.), *Petrarch and his Readers* 171–189.

[4] Scheidig, *Die Holzschnitte des Petrarca-Meisters*, passim; Fraenger W., *Altdeutsches Bilderbuch. Hans Weiditz und Sebastian Brant* (Leipzig: 1930); Raupp H.-J., "Die Illustrationen zu Francesco Petrarca ,Von der Artzney bayder Glueck des guten und des widerwertigen' (Augsburg 1532)", in *Wallraf-Richartz-Jahrbuch* 45 (1984) 59–112; Knape J., *Dichtung, Recht und Freiheit. Studien zu Leben und Werk Sebastian Brants 1457–1521* (Baden-Baden: 1992) 271–317; Wohlfeil R. – Wohlfeil T., "Verbildlichung ständischer Gesellschaft. Bartholomäus Bruyn d.Ä. – Petrarcameister (mit Exkursen von Marlies Minuth und Heike Talkenberger)", in Schulze W. (ed.), *Ständische Gesellschaft und soziale Mobilität* (Munich: 1988) 269–331, esp. 308–319. According to Raupp and Knape the woodcuts partly summarize 'die Lehraussage' (didactic message); partly they depict the examples mentioned in Petrarch's text; partly they provide examples that are not mentioned in the text but that reinforce the '*Lehre des Textes*'; cf. Raupp, "Die Illustrationen zu Francesco Petrarca", 100; Knape, *Dichtung, Recht und Freiheit*, 298. Wohlfeil and Wohlfeil, "Verbildlichung ständischer Gesellschaft", 314 agree with this view: 'Nicht selten löste der Künstler meisterhaft die Schwierigkeiten, humanistische Gedanken in eine Form zu kleiden, wie sie Lehr- und Lesebilder erforderten'. P. Michel, in an unpublished article on the Petrarch Master "Transformation und Augmentation bei Petrarca und seinem Meister" (www.enzyklopaedie.ch/dokumente/Petrarcameister.pdf), also believes in the contingency of word and image. Despite 'transformations' that cause major difficulties with understanding the relationship between word and image, it is the Petrarch Master's goal to 'teach' Petrarch's thoughts.

[5] Enenkel, "Der Petrarca des Petrarca-Meisters".

Physical Pain, Stoicism and the Illustrations

The object of this volume offers an excellent opportunity to analyse more closely a striking feature of the relationship between word and image in the illustrated *Remedies against Foul and Fortune*, the *Von der Artzney baider Glück, des guten und des widerwertigen*: the function and meaning of physical pain. This paper is not meant to single out a somewhat marginal aspect of the *Glücksbuch*, but touches on the very core of the book, since in a large number of illustrations the Petrarch Master focuses on physical pain, for example in the illustrations to chapters II, 7; 19; 27–29; 36; 38–39; 43; 46; 49; 55; 59–60; 65–67; 70–71; 73–74; 77; 81–82; 84–85; 90; 94–98; 100; 102–105; 113; 116–118; 120–124, and 131. Interestingly enough, in these cases the Petrarch Master does not simply amplify the message of Petrarch's text. In marked contrast with the illustrations, Petrarch's philosophical argument mostly downplays or even excludes physical pain, and focuses on the realm of the mind, especially the emotions, the passions (*passiones animi; pathe*).

In his tendency to marginalize physical pain, Petrarch closely follows the discourse of antique Stoicism (as presented by Cicero and Seneca).The Stoics did their best largely to ignore physical pain, and emphasized the power of reason over bodily affects. While they did not deny that the wise man could feel physical pain as a bodily sensation they ascribed to *Ratio* the fundamental ability not to 'assent' to this sensation, that is to say not to let it through to the soul or the mind.[6] They classified bodily sensations among the essentially meaningless and 'indifferent' aspects of human life. Also, they did their best to live in accordance with their theoretical views and provide others with their living example. Thus, Stoics liked to cultivate an attitude of bravery. Posidonius, for instance, who in old age suffered so heavily from gout that he could not leave his bed anymore, did not stop receiving visitors and lecturing. He was visited by Scipio the Younger, for whom he lectured on the 'summum bonum'. When, during his lecture, he was almost overwhelmed by physical pain that was 'burning like fire', he said: 'You will not achieve anything, pain. Although you are annoying, I will never admit that you are an evil'.[7]

---

[6] Cf. e.g. Weinkauf W., *Die Stoa. Kommentierte Werkausgabe* 58–62 ("Affektenlehre"); Rist J.M., *Stoic Philosophy* (Cambridge: 1980, 3rd ed.) 37–53.

[7] Cicero, *Tusculanae disputationes* II, 61: 'nihil agis, dolor. Quamvis sis molestum, numquam te esse confitebor malum'.

To modern readers, Posidonius' attitude may seem exaggerated. The crucial issue, however, was that of *autarkeia*: the individual's independence, which could only be safeguarded if the philosopher was able to downplay all kinds of physical sensations or 'outward' influences.

Petrarch, who knew the source of the story, Cicero's *Tusculanae disputationes* (in itself a kind of manual on Greek philosophy), almost by heart, was not only familiar with Posidonius' example but above all with the Stoic's contempt of bodily pain. Although he did not strive to appear as a Stoic hero like Posidonius, he adopted the Stoic principle of ignoring physical pain. He also successfully combined Stoic meditative practice with Christian dualism, which departs from the clear-cut division between body and mind, and between earthly and spiritual things. Physical pain is not considered as a serious danger, since it does not hinder man's salvation. On the contrary, pain may help us to understand the vanity of all earthly things, and, therefore, it may even contribute to salvation. Thus, in his meditations, Petrarch powerfully organizes the human mind on the basis of both Christian and Stoic models. In the case of the illustrated *De remediis*, we are confronted with the puzzling fact that we have a Neo-Stoic and Christian treatise, in which physical pain holds at best a marginal position, while a considerable number of the large images[8] precisely focus on or emphasize physical pain. This points to a clash between two paradigms: the visual artist and the writer seem to have interpreted physical pain in radically different ways. In what follows I will examine the two paradigms more closely, starting with a form of pain that seems difficult to ignore, namely toothache.

Toothache

Petrarch deals with rotten teeth in *De remediis*, chapter II, 94 ("De dentium egritudine").[9] Somewhat surprisingly, he is not at all concerned with the mental suppression of a bodily sensation that must have been acute, since especially in the late Middle Ages, efficient pain-killers

[8] Mostly 14.5 × 9.8 cm.

[9] A critical edition of the Latin text of Petrarch's *De remediis* is still a desideratum. For this study, I have used the edition by Joannes le Preux (second edition, Bern: 1600) ('editio secunda, priore longe castigatior'), which goes back to Joannes Paganinus' edition dedicated to Pope Leo X from 1515. This edition offers a much better text than the commonly quoted edition in the *Opera omnia*, vol. I (Basel: 1554). In Le Preux's editio secunda, chapter II, 94 is on pp. 574–576.

against toothache were hardly available.[10] Instead, Petrarch exclusively focuses on the emotions, particularly on grief. Most remarkably, in Petrarch's philosophical argument, grief is *not* caused by physical pain, but by the consequences of bad teeth: the loss of teeth, for example, brings about a loss of beauty of the face ('decus oris'), and difficulties with daily matters such as eating, drinking and speech.

Petrarch unfolds his consolatory argument on two levels. First he argues, in the vein of antique Stoicism, that teeth should not be regarded as man's property, but as a temporary gift of Nature/God. Man should be grateful for what he has received from God instead of complaining about the loss of what he wrongly considers as his property. If it is only in old age that he loses his teeth he should 'give thanks to Nature for permitting him to keep until senility this gift of hers, which she demands back from many when they are still young'.[11] The second level is that of the Christian *contemptus mundi*: Petrarch argues that the loss of teeth is in fact desirable since it helps us to prevent deadly sins such as gluttony, lust and vanity. He who has lost his teeth, will eat less ('minus comedes'), refrain from gossiping or offending others,[12] and from voluptuous kisses,[13] which he regards as a manifestation of forbidden lust (*luxuria*). Furthermore, the loss of teeth will remind man strongly of the weakness, transience and frailty of his body: If even 'solid' parts of the body cease to function, what can one expect from 'soft' parts such as muscles and skin?[14] Also, the loss of teeth prevents man from being too cheerful, and especially from committing the sin of (loud) laughter ('parcius ridebis', 'you will laugh less'). According to (medieval) clerical and monastic values, man should avoid laughter, especially loud laughter (*multus risus et excussus*).[15] In fact, as RATIO argues, the loss of teeth brings

---

[10] This is not to say that medicine in the late Middle Ages was not interested in alleviating pain. Cf. Schmitz R. – Kuhlen F.-J., "Schmerz- und Betäubungsmittel vor 1600", *Pharmazie in unserer Zeit* 18 (1989) 10–19.

[11] *Petrarchs Remedies for Fortune Fair and Foul*, transl. by C.H. Rawski, Indiana U.P. 1991, vol. III, 231. Le Preux 575. The idea that man receives health, strength and physical beauty not as property, but only 'on loan' occurs very frequently in Seneca's Letters and philosophical dialogues.

[12] *Petrarchs Remedies*, transl. Rawski, vol. III, 231: 'You bite less mordantly when you chew up another's reputation. The broken row of your teeth will curb your ready tongue [...]'.

[13] Le Preux 575: 'ab illicitis osculis [...] cohibebit'.

[14] Le Preux 575.

[15] Cf. St. Benedictus, *Regula* IV, 54: 'Risum multum aut excussum non amare'. Cf. ibidem VI, 8 and VII, 59.

man closer to his desired future existence in heaven: instead of eating, drinking and talking immoderately, it teaches man to concentrate on spiritual food (*cibus animae*).[16] Thus, in Petrarch's philosophical argument, physical pain is largely ignored, while physical decay is presented as an important means of spiritual progress.

How did the Petrarch Master illustrate these thoughts? First of all, he rendered a scene focused on the sensation of physical pain that early modern users of the book would have recognized immediately. It presents an early modern dentist, or rather a strolling practitioner or surgeon, 'curing' a woman by pulling a tooth [Fig. 1]. Strolling practitioners wandered from village to village and offered their service especially on market places. The Petrarch Master's image resembles a certain type of genre scene, that of the "charlatan" ("kwakzalver"; "tandentrekker"; "Zahnbrecher"), a practitioner who frequently figures in Dutch and Flemish paintings, drawings and etches a century later. Maria Elisabeth Wasserfuhr, in her monograph on this genre scene in Dutch art, collected some forty examples of the "Zahnbrecher" ("tooth-puller"), and there are more.[17] Somewhat surprisingly, Wasserfuhr does not mention the image of the Petrarch Master as a possible forerunner of the Dutch genres scenes, although its pictorial invention is much closer to them than that of Lucas van Leyden, whom she presents as a 'Wegbereiter' of the genre [Fig. 9].[18]

It is, of course, not my intention to limit my interpretation of the Petrarch Master's image by linking it exclusively to Dutch and Flemish renderings of the scene. There are, however, several aspects which the Petrarch Master's illustration and the Dutch examples have in common. First, the scene, which represents an experience shared by many (it usually took place on markets), is characterized by a satirical tendency, sometimes connected with fraud and deceit. Second, although the image depicts a medical cure, it concentrates precisely on pain *caused by the cure*. For example on the painting by the Utrecht Caravaggist Gerard

[16] 'Reason: '[...] If you do not fool yourself, you will think about the road you must walk upon, which leads to the place where one does not eat material food, but where one lives exclusively from joy and spiritual food.' ('[...] nisi dissimulans cogitandum eo tibi iter instare ubi nil editor, atque ubi solo gaudio cibisque aimae vivitur', Le Preux 576).

[17] *Der Zahnarzt in der Niederländischen Malerei des 17. Jahrhunderts* (Cologne: 1977) (Kölner medizinhistorische Beiträge 1); Maar F.E.R. de, *Vijf eeuwen tandheelkunde in de Nederlandse en Vlaamse kunst* (Nieuwegein: 1993).

[18] Wasserfuhr, *Der Zahnarzt* 25–28.

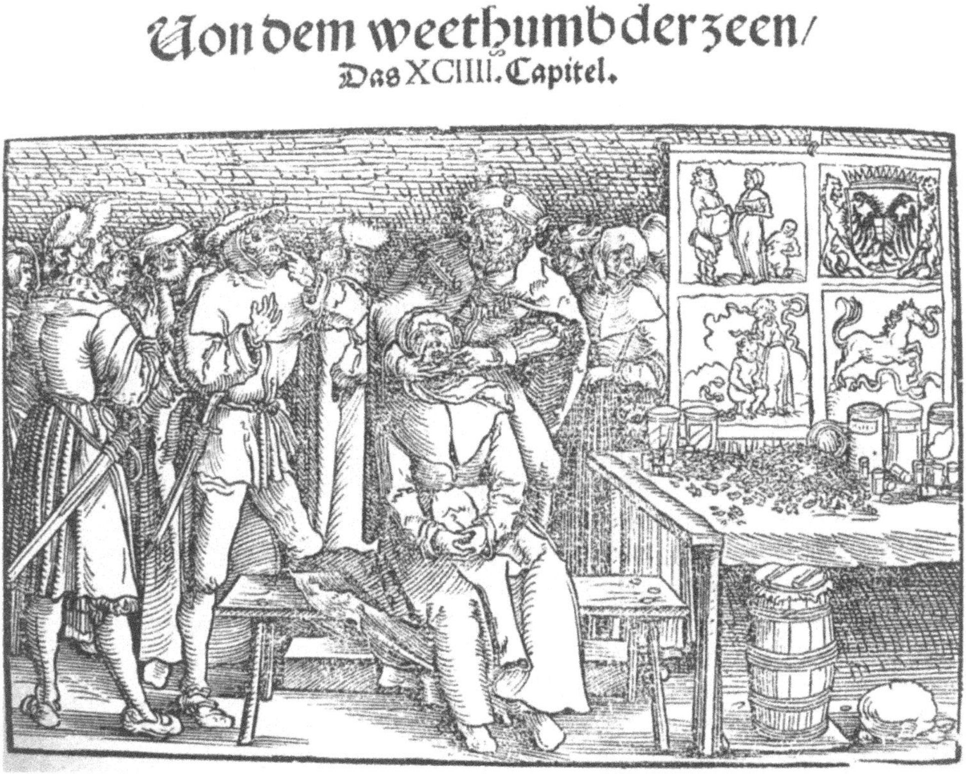

Fig. 1. The Petrarch Master, Woodcut illustration to Petrarch's *Von der Artzney baider Glueck* [...] (Augsburg: 1532), book II, chapter 94, fol. CXIXv.

van Honthorst (1628) the patient flails his arms in response to the pain, while his eyes are wide open as a sign of the stress he is undergoing [Fig. 2]. Three visitors of the market look with great compassion at the poor man in such intense pain. Jan Victors expresses the pain the young patient suffers from by depicting him with crossed legs, clenched fists and closed eyes [Fig. 3]. The Leiden specialist in humorous scenes Jan Steen depicts the physical pain of the patient by having him stamp his feet and clench his fists [Fig. 4].[19] The young client in a scene by the Flemish painter Theodoor Rombout flails his left arm [Fig. 5],[20] a gesture similar to that of the peasant in the woodcut of the Petrarch Master. Lucas van Leyden, a contemporary of the Petrarch Master, also emphasizes the patient's pain by his hand gestures [Fig. 9].

The expression of *physical* pain plays an important role in the pictorial rhetoric of the Petrarch Master [Fig. 1]. The persons who have come to visit the surgeon obviously suffer from severe pain. This is expressed, for example, in the flailing arms of the second and fifth figures from the left (respectively a patrician and a peasant). Moreover, the peasant is pointing his finger in the direction of his mouth, obviously the source of the intense pain he is suffering from. As is the case with the Dutch and Flemish images, the Petrarch Master emphasizes that the remedial operation, the pulling of teeth, in fact causes severe pain: the face of the female client in the centre, is contorted with pain, while her cramped hands express the same sensation.

How should one 'read' this pictorial invention? Scheidig considers it a perfect example of his 'Schaubilder' interpretation – realistic scenes taken from daily life bearing a moral message which he identifies with Petrarch's humanist outlook. According to Scheidig the moral message of the image is that '*vor dem Schmerz sind alle Stände gleich*; Bauern, Landsknechte, Patrizier und ihre Frauen suchen einträchtig Hilfe bei dem Zahnbrecher' (italics mine).[21] Interestingly enough, this moral message fits in extremely well with the socialist morals of the German Democratic Republic, the context in which Scheidig worked; the Petrarch Master and Petrarch himself appear as the venerable forefathers of

---

[19] Cf. Brown Ch., *Holländische Genremalerei im 17. Jahrhundert* (Amsterdam – Munich: 1984) 67–70; 98–99.

[20] Cf. de Jong E. – Luijten G., *Spiegel van alledag. Nederlandse genreprenten 1550–1700* (Gent: 1997) 221–225; Maar, *Vijf eeuwen tandheelkunde in de Vlaamse en de Nederlandse kunst* 197–223.

[21] Scheidig, *Die Holzschnitte des Petrarca-Meisters* 297.

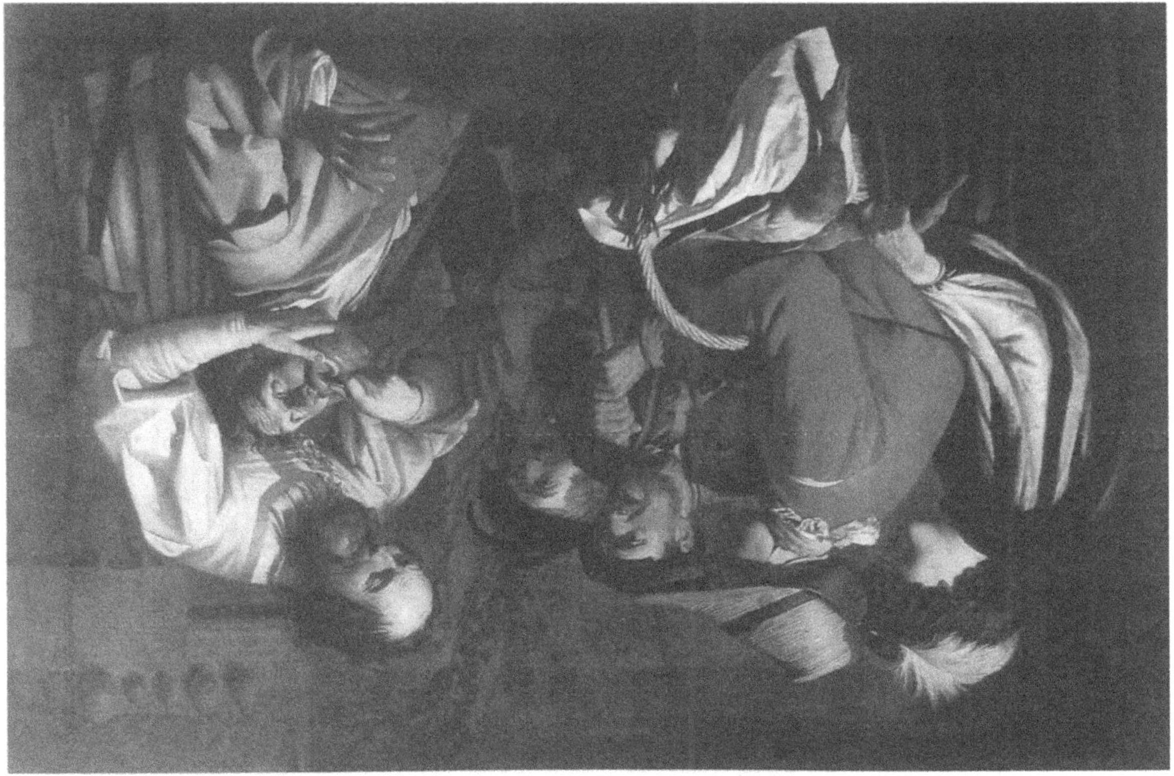

Fig. 2 [Col. pl. II]. Gerard van Honthorst, *The Tooth-puller* (1628). Oil on canvas, 137 × 200 cm. Paris, Musée du Louvre.

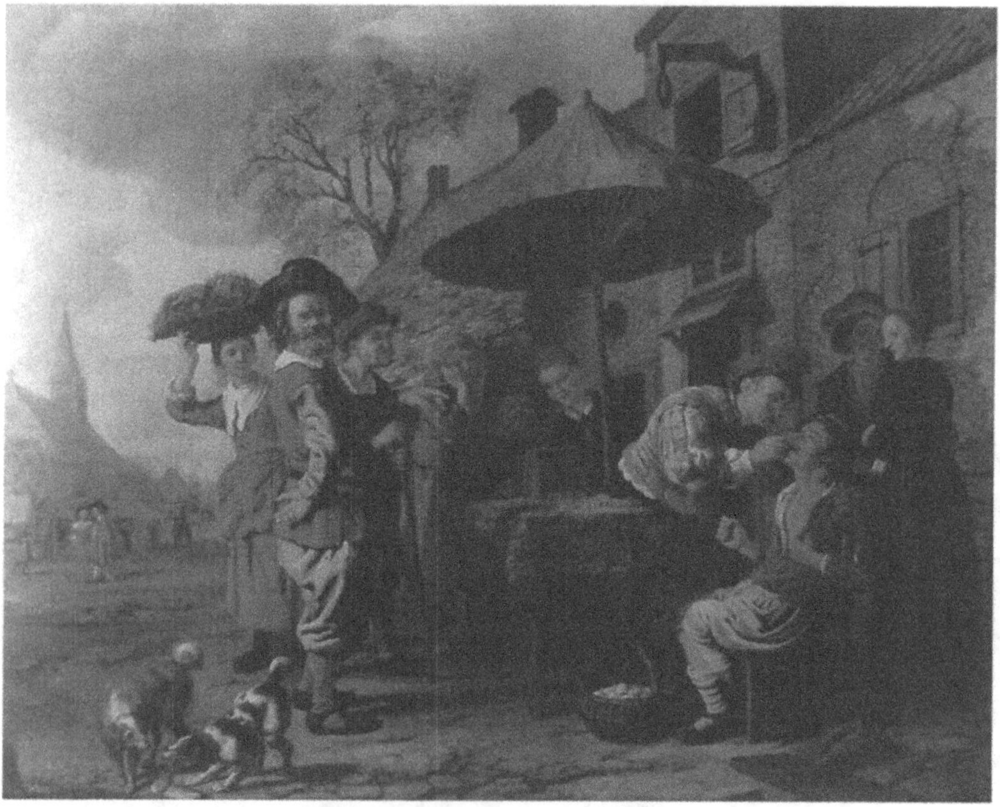

Fig. 3 [Col. pl. III]. Jan Victors, *The Tooth-puller* (1654). Oil on canvas, 76 × 94.5 cm. Amsterdam, Rijksmuseum.

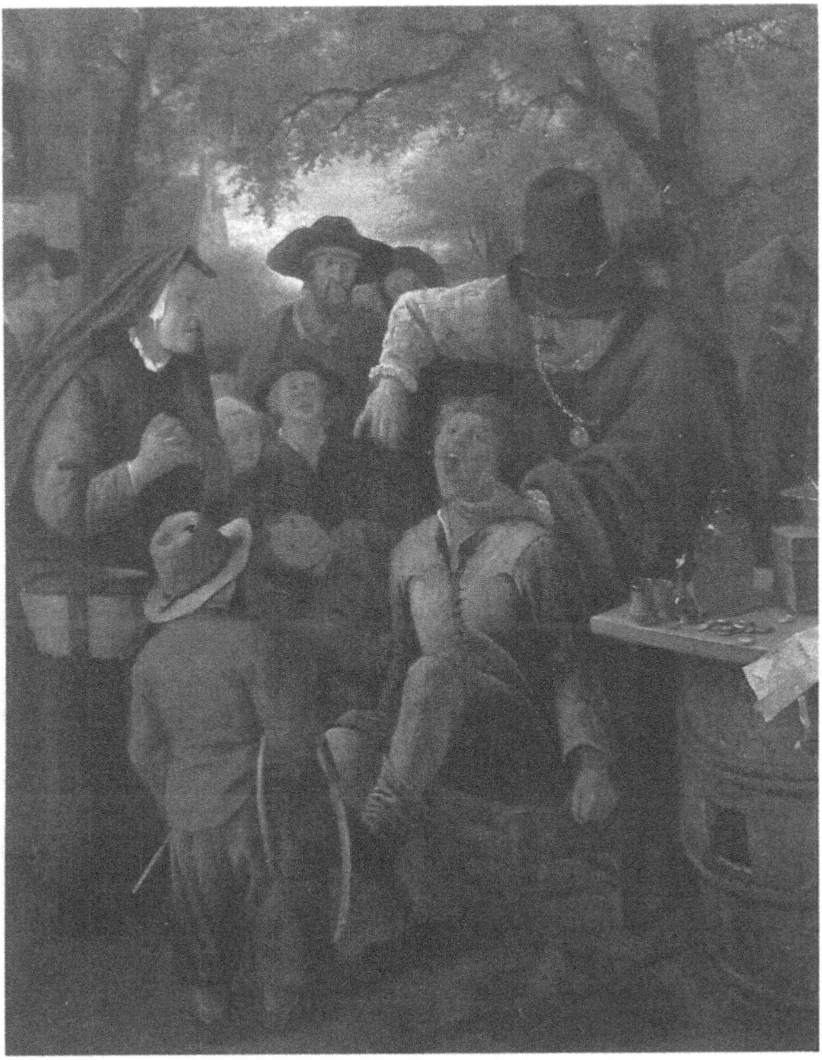

Fig. 4 [Col. pl. IV]. Jan Steen, *The Tooth-Puller* (1651). Oil on canvas, 32.5 × 26.7 cm. The Hague, Mauritshuis.

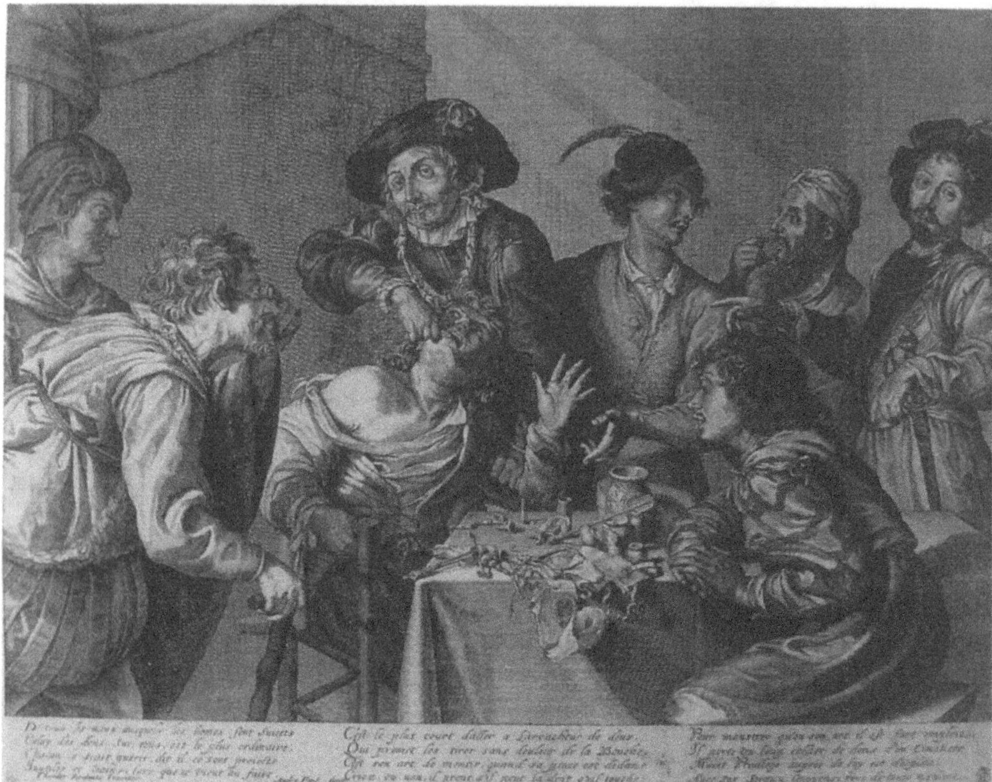

Fig. 5. Andries Pauli, etching after Theodoor Rombouts, *The Tooth-Puller*, 29.6 × 38.2 cm.

Marxist philosophy. As we have seen already, Petrarch's argument unfortunately has nothing to do with that type of message.

But what about the Petrarch Master? In my view, his pictorial invention is far from Scheidig's naïve, simple, and politically correct message. Consider, for example, the enormous number of teeth on the surgeon's table, on the right of the image. If these were pulled out the same day, this early modern dentist must already have treated, or perhaps rather maltreated, some 100 clients. One can imagine how careful and precise his diagnosis must have been. Such an enormous number of teeth, however, was neither a 'realistic' detail nor a standard element of pictorial images of the tooth-puller. The image on the "Augsburger Monatsbild" ("Winter"), which shows a tooth-puller at work at the market place of Augsburg in the year 1532, has nothing similar [Fig. 6].[22] From the exaggerated number of pulled teeth, the viewer may deduce that the 'dentist's' treatment may be questionable, and that he may in fact be a charlatan.[23] The clients on the image, however, are obviously unaware of this, and fall into the trap. Probably, by drawing on common social and gender prejudices, the Petrarch Master wanted to emphasize this by the fact that peasants and women are first in line to be cheated. There are even more disturbing elements in the picture, such as the strange decoration on the dentist's cloak, which resembles the decorations worn by noblemen. The pendants on the decoration, however, are not made of gold or silver, but represent teeth [Fig. 1].

The Petrarch Master's woodcut, then, is certainly neither a neutral rendering of a scene from "daily life", or merely a realistic description of early modern dentistry, but clearly has a satirical dimension. As a dentist, I would be reluctant to hang this image in my office. The

---

[22] Cf. Grüber P.M. (ed.), *"Kurzweil viel ohn' Maß und Ziel". Alltag und Festtag auf den Augsburger Monatsbildern der Renaissance* (Munich: 1994) 192–193.

[23] This is not meant as a teleological judgement from the point of view of modern medical standards. Late medieval and early modern readers may have come to the same conclusions on the basis of personal or collective experience. Cf. Wasserfuhr's brief but convincing description of the practice (*Der Zahnarzt* 6): 'Neben den von der Zunft her ausgewiesenen Zahnärzten spielten bis an die Neuzeit heran die Zahnbrecher oder Zahnreißer eine große Rolle, "Doktoren der Landstrasse", die wie Starstecher und Steinschneider von Ort zu Ort zogen. Zu dieser Kategorie gehörten sowohl ehrliche Praktiker als auch bloße Marktschreier und Scharlatane, die lediglich Zähne herausbrachen und wertlose, wenn nicht gar gefährliche Wundarzneien feilboten, nach der "Behandlung" sofort verschwanden und ihre "Patienten" ohne jede Kontrolle oder Nachbehandlung ihrem weiteren Schicksal überließen'. Cf. also Andel M.A. van, *Chirurgyns Vrye Meesters, Beunhazen en Kwakzalvers* (The Hague: 1981, second edition).

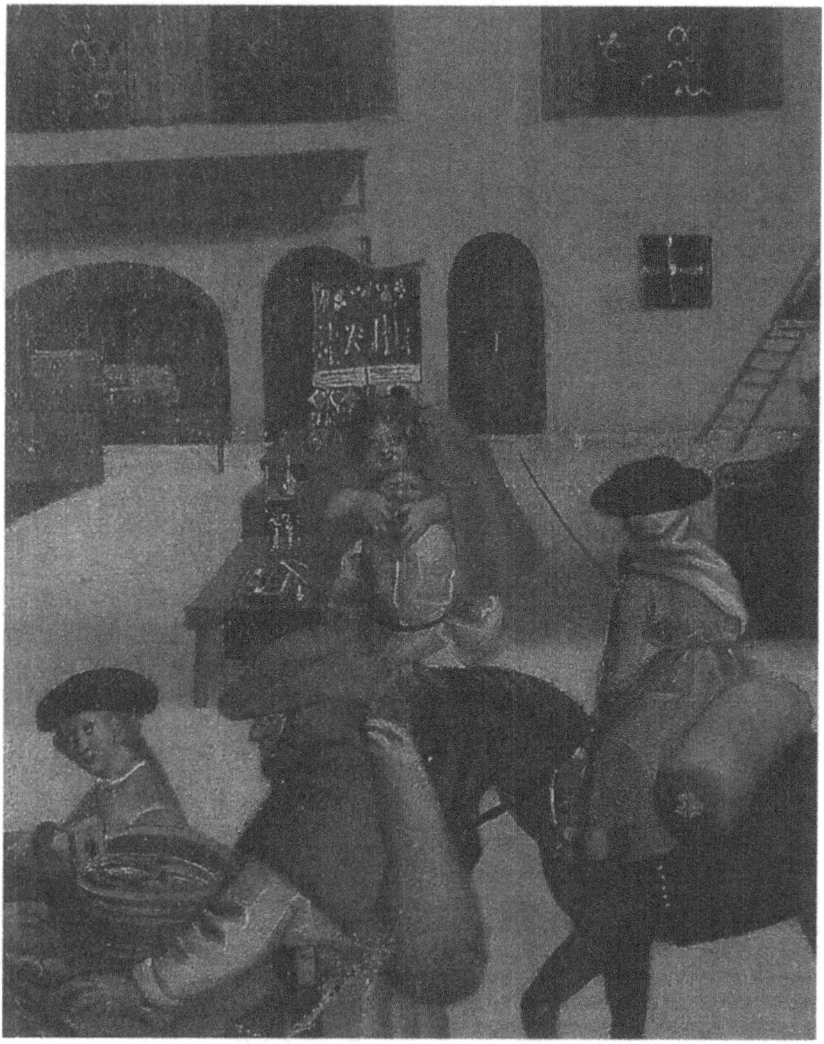

Fig. 6 [Col. pl. V]. "Augsburger Monatsbild", "Winter", detail with tooth-puller. Oil on canvas. Augsburg, Städtische Kunstsammlungen, Maximiliansmuseum.

image is in fact characterized by a mordant and aggressive rhetoric of *unmasking* of both the dentist and his clients. It unmasks the dentist as a dangerous charlatan and the behaviour of his patients as utterly foolish. Indeed, it transforms Petrarch's Stoic meditation into an argument in the vein of the *Ship of Fools*, the *Narrenschiff*. This kind of satire is one of the more important elements of the pictorial rhetoric on which the Petrarch Master's inventions are based.[24] As can be demonstrated by several images, the Petrarch Master was very well acquainted with Sebastian Brant's *Narrenschiff*. Interimaginality shows that he sometimes imitated Dürer's famous illustrations of Brant's work [Figs. 7 and 8]. For example, in his pictorial invention for the illustration belonging to chapter II, 107 of the *Glücksbuch*, he imitated Dürer's illustration of chapter 35 of the *Narrenschiff* (depicting the proverb 'den Esel reiten' or 'sich auf den Esel setzen lassen', which literally means 'to ride the donkey' and refers proverbially to an attack of anger).[25]

In his illustrations of Petrarch's *De remediis*, the Petrarch Master used the discourse of the *Ship of Fools* for various purposes and types of arguments.[26] In the case of chapter II, 94, he might have invited the viewer to construe the message as a kind of practical advice or warning: 'if you suffer from toothache, avoid visiting practitioners. They are untrustworthy, only interested in your money, and they won't properly cure you'. The illustration may be usefully compared to the "Augsburger Monatsbild" ("Winter") from 1532: it represents the tooth-puller as a fat and cruel man with bad eyesight [Fig. 6]. That blood is spouting from the victim's mouth [Fig. 6] suggests that one should not trust the technical skills of the tooth-puller. In fact, in 1532 complaints were issued in Augsburg against unauthorized practitioners.[27]

An even more ugent warning against the "Zahnbrecher" can be found in an etching by Lucas van Leyden, which was made only a few years after the Petrarch Master's image [Fig. 9]. While the foolish

[24] See Enenkel, "Der Petrarca des Petrarca-Meisters" 131–147 (chapter "*De remediis* in den Narrenschiffdiskurs").

[25] Röhrich L., *Lexikon der sprichwörtlichen Redensarten* (5th edition, Freiburg – Basel – Vienna: 2001) 398, s.v. "Esel". Interestingly enough, Röhrich presents the Petrarch Master's illustration chapter II, 107 as a comprehensive pictorial rendering of the proverb.

[26] Cf. Enenkel, "Der Petrarca des Petrarca-Meisters" 131–147.

[27] Gensthaler G., *Das Medizinalwesen der freien Reichsstadt Augsburg bis zum 16. Jahrhundert* (Augsburg: 1973) 78–79. The complaints, however, came from four medical doctors who had, of course, a financiel interest in measurements against practitioners.

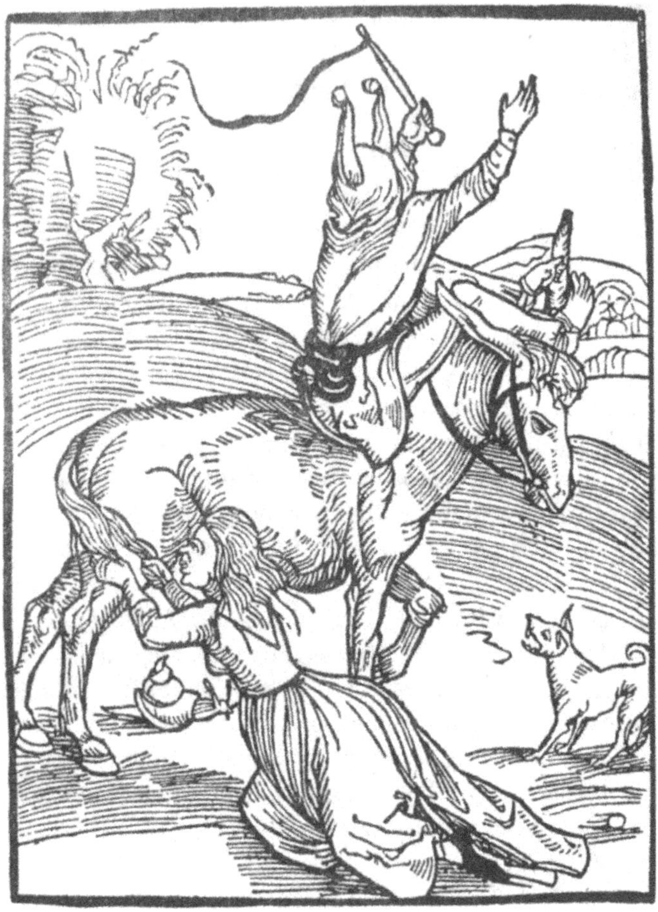

Fig. 7. Albrecht Dürer, woodcut illustration to Sebastian Brant, *Narrenschiff*, chapter 35.

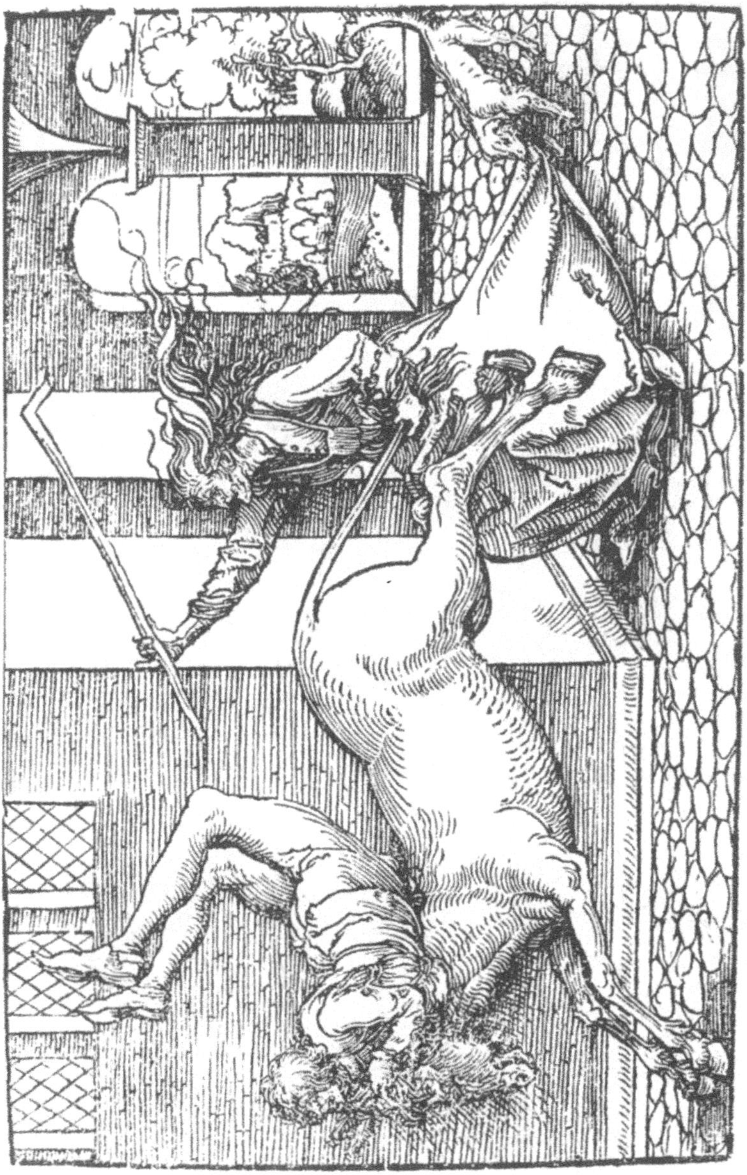

Fig. 8. The Petrarch Master, Woodcut illustration to Petrarch's *Von der Artzney baider Glueck* [. . .] (Augsburg: 1532), book II, chapter 107 (erroneously 112), fol. CXXXXIIIIv.

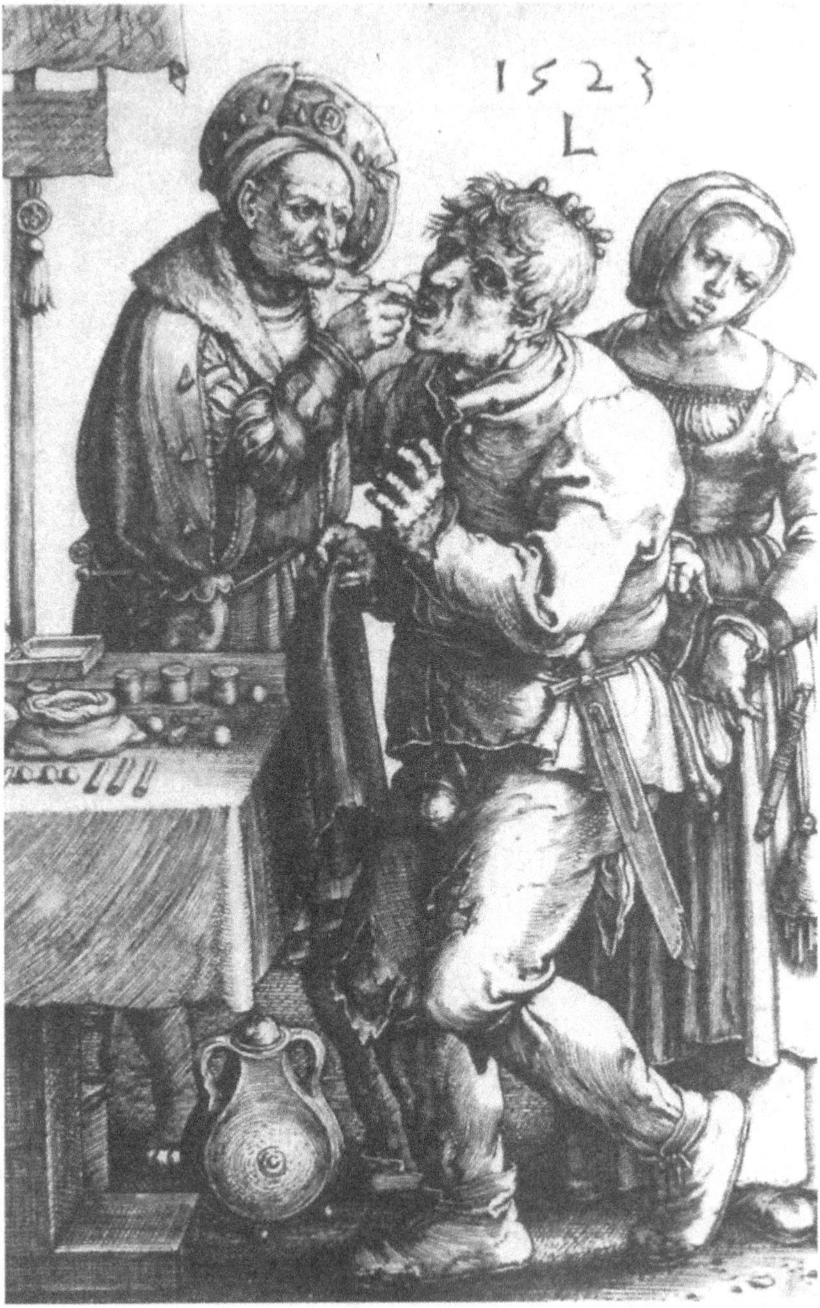

Fig. 9. Lucas van Leyden, *The Tooth-Puller*. Engraving (1523), 11.6 × 7.5 cm.

patient is treated, a woman coming from behind steals his money.[28] Its practical orientation brings Lucas van Leyden's message close to house book wisdom. Its satirical elements, however, suggest that the image's message is more sophisticated. Physical pain seems to be presented as something ridiculous and even humiliating. The social position of the patient, together with his ragged clothes and untidy hair seems to point in that direction: he is an uncouth peasant, an uneducated person whom one cannot take seriously. That he lets himself be cheated by the woman on the right underscores his stupidity. All these elements together made it difficult for the early modern viewer to identify with the person undergoing physical pain.

The same is true for quite a number of Dutch representations of the 'tandentrekker'. The clients are ignorant boys, as on the paintings by Jan Victors [Fig. 3] and Jan Steen [Fig. 4], peasants, or peasant women, as on an etching ascribed to Pieter van den Borcht.[29] This etching characterizes everyone involved as dim-witted peasants. They let themselves be cheated by an extremely untrustworthy "tandentrekker", a sordid tramp with a ragged hat who even remains seated on his donkey when he is pulling teeth. Similar satirical elements expressing social alterity can be detected in the image by the Petrarch Master, for example the peasant pointing at his open mouth [Fig. 1]. Nevertheless, they do not produce the same overall effect as on the etching ascribed to Pieter van den Borcht. Most of the clients depicted by the Petrarch Master are not peasants. This means that the Petrarch Master made a "Leseangebot" which invited the early modern users of the *Gluecksbuch* to identify with the clients of the dentist. In this "Leseangebot", the Petrarch Master used pain as a means of persuasion with respect to the practicalities of everyday life.

In the case of chapter II, 94, the pictorial rhetoric by the Petrarch Master is even more sophisticated and complex, in the sense that it transcends the level of literal interpretation, and adds to the satire on early modern dentistry a political or even propagandistic dimension.

---

[28] Vos R., *Lucas van Leyden* (Maarssen: 1978) 103, considers Lucas van Leyden's etch as a warning, as 'een ernstige boodschap' presented in a 'vrolijke verpakking'. His moralistic interpretation of the scene is shared by Filedt-Kok J.P., *Lucas van Leyden* [...] (Amsterdam: 1978) 72 and Reys K., *De grafiek van Lucas van Leyden, een beschrijving en vergelijking met tijdgenoten* (unpublished MA thesis, Leiden: 2004) 292 ('een waarschuwing tegen "varende luyden"').

[29] New York, Metropolitan Museum of Art. Cf. de Jong – Luijten, *Spiegel van alledag* 222.

A number of hints point in this direction. On a kind of advertising poster hanging above the table of the surgeon, a shield of arms with the double-headed eagle of the German Emperor can be seen, held by heraldic lions [Fig. 10; detail of Fig. 1]. At the top of the shield a crown is depicted. On a smaller shield, the double-headed eagle bears the arms of Austria (left) and Old Burgundy (right). In this way, the Petrarch Master conspicuously connects the seducing charlatan with the Roman Emperor. At first sight, this may have been interpreted by contemporary viewers as implying that the charlatan sells his doubtful services under the protection or authorization of the Emperor. Advertizing posters were used by surgeons in order to attract clients and to persuade them of their trustfulness.[30] Such posters would celebrate the practitioner's medical successes by showing operated body parts or kidney stones, for example in a drawing by Lambert Doomer [Fig. 11] or in the etching ascribed to Pieter van den Borcht (kidney stones).[31] In addition, surgeons could present letters of authorization, as in Jan Steen's painting in the Mauritshuis [Fig. 12; detail of Fig. 4],[32] in the 1523 etching by Lucas of Leyden [Fig. 9] or in Jost Amman's "Zanbrecher" in his *Ständebuch* [Fig. 13].[33]

It was not normal practice of surgeons, however, to present themselves with the most venerable coat of arms, that of the Roman Emperor. Moreover, in the Petrarch Master's image the coat of arms of the Emperor is not put on a letter of authorization or something similar, but is painted directly on his advertizing panel. One must bear in mind that it was of course strictly forbidden for ordinary people to bear the coat of arms of the Roman Emperor. Thus, for early modern viewers, the strange association of the charlatan with the Holy Roman Emperor must have been a remarkable detail that required some specific explanation. It invites the user of the book to identify the charlatan with the Roman Emperor. The chain which the dentist wears, and the strange decoration on his cloak may have reinforced this identification. On a

---

[30] Cf. Andel M.A. van, "Kwakzalver-reclames in vroeger eeuwen", in *Nederlands tijdschrift voor geneeskunde* 5 (1912) 297–310.

[31] Brown, *Holländische Genremalerei* 99 (Oxford, Ashmolean Museum).

[32] Ibidem 70.

[33] *Eygentliche Beschreibung Aller Staende auff Erden/Hoher und Nidriger* [...] (Frankfurt a.M.: 1568), nr. 52. Wasserfuhr, *Der Zahnarzt* 26: 'Ähnliche Schriftstücke, die sehr häufig abgebildet wurden, waren entweder Meisterbriefe einer Gilde oder Ehrenurkunden, die den Zahnbrechern von kirchlichen und weltlichen Fürsten für erwiesene Dienste verliehen wurden'.

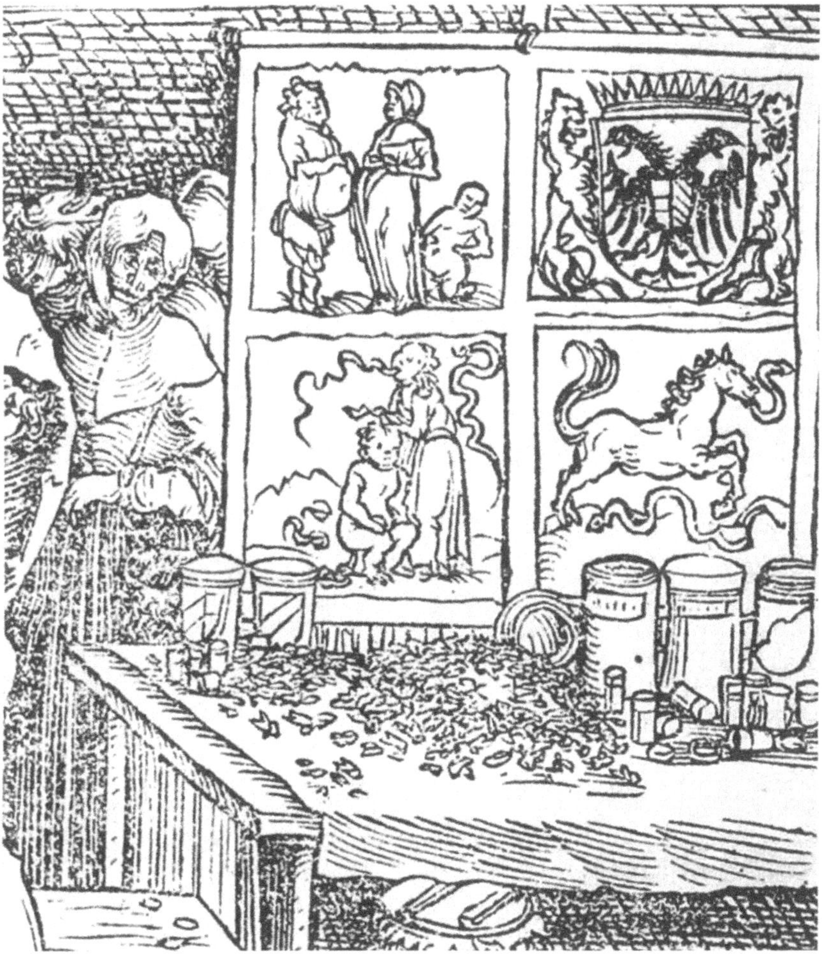

Fig. 10. The Petrarch Master, Woodcut illustration to Petrarch's *Von der Artzney baider Glueck* [...] (Augsburg: 1532), book II, chapter 94, fol. CXIXv. Detail.

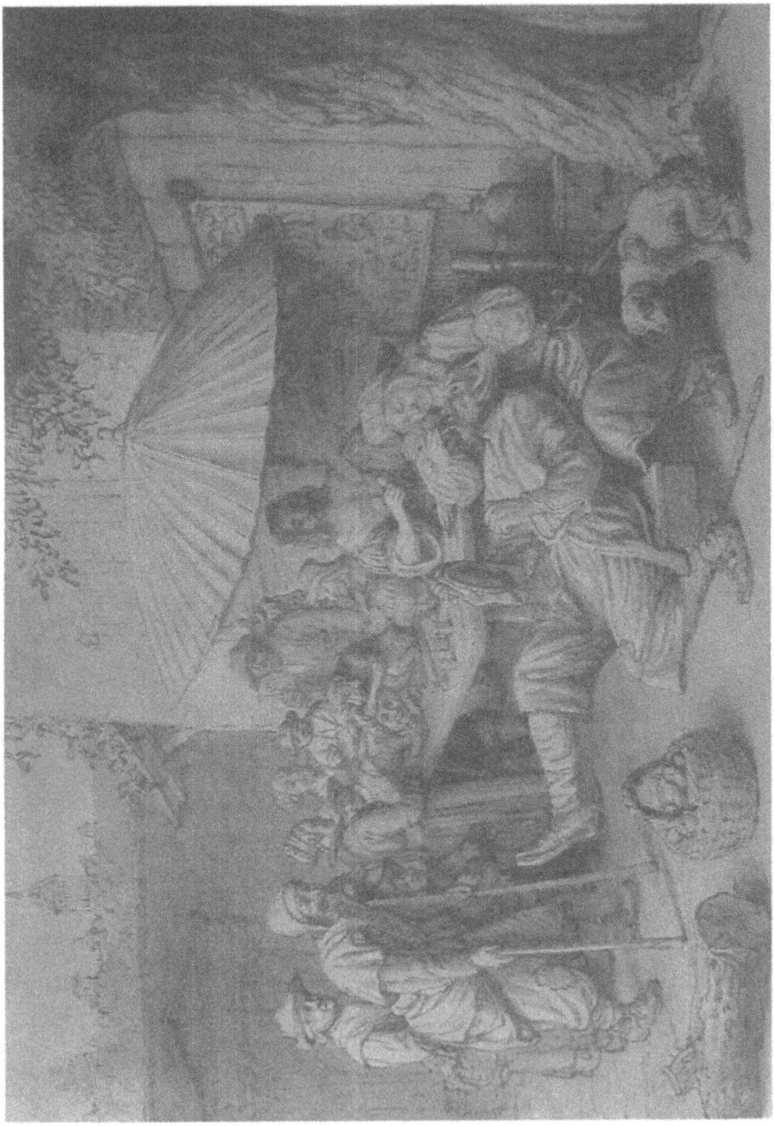

Fig. 11. Lambert Doomer, *The Tooth-Puller*. Drawing, 28.7 × 40.2. Oxford, Ashmolean Museum.

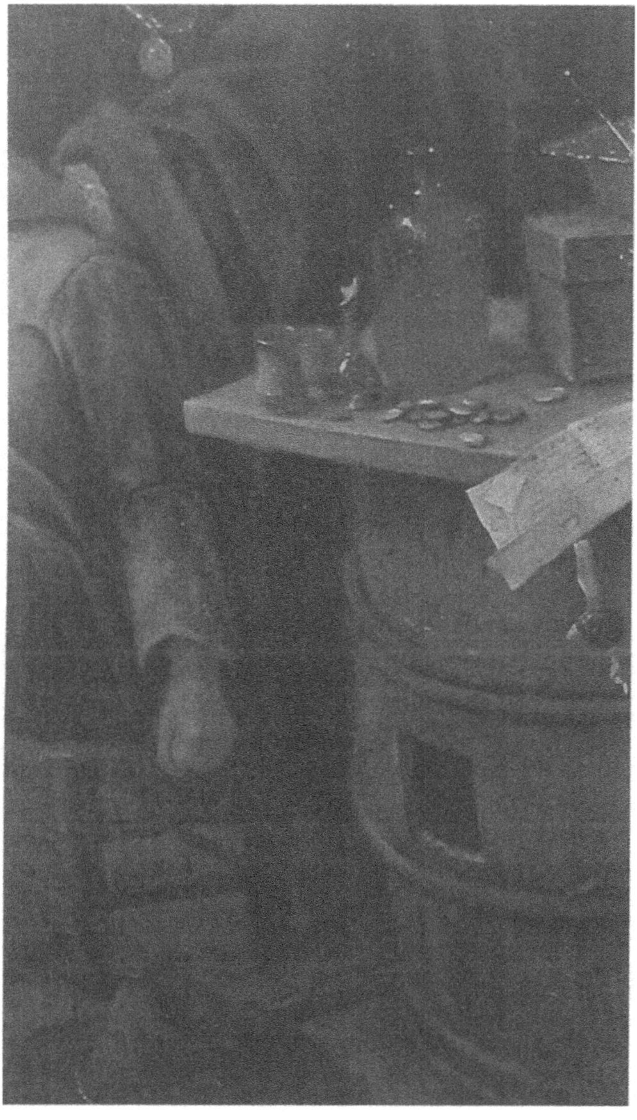

Fig. 12. Jan Steen, *The Tooth-Puller* (1651). Oil on canvas, 32.5 × 26.7 cm. The Hague, Mauritshuis. Detail.

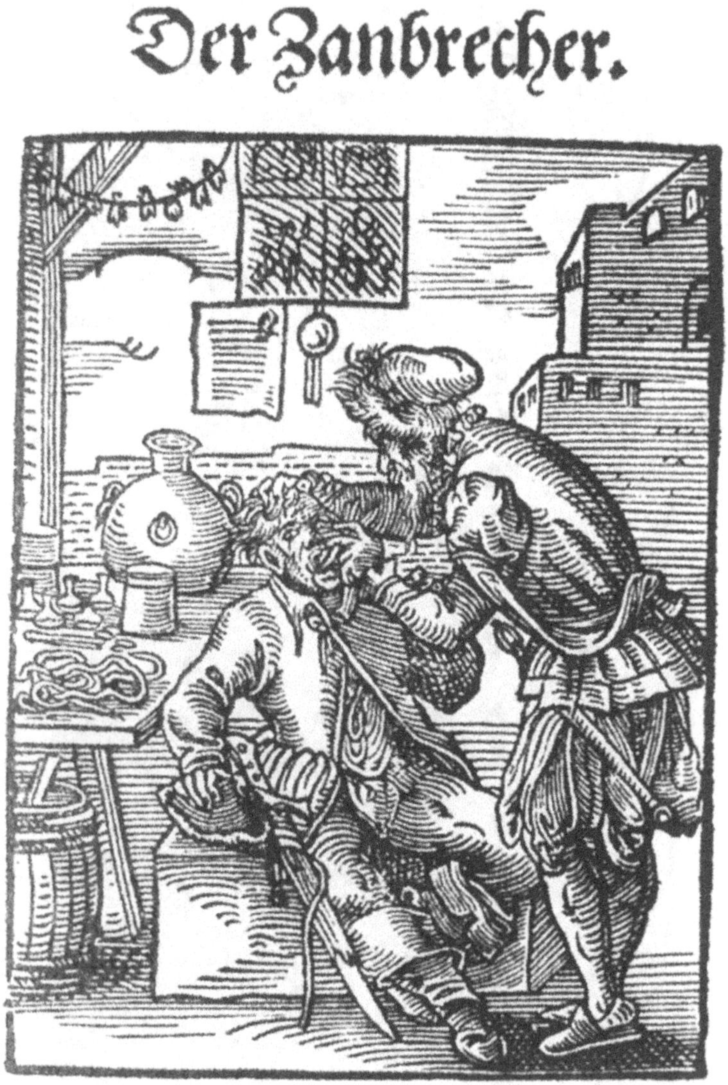

Fig. 13. Jost Amman, The "Zanbrecher". From Hans Sach's *Eygentliche Beschreibung Aller Staende auff Erden* [...] (Frankfurt a. M.: 1568), no. 52.

literal 'reading' of the image, of course, the pendants on the decoration and the chain represent teeth. In visual representations, early modern dentists sometimes wear chains of teeth, as on the painting by Theodoor Rombouts [Fig. 5]. These may have been meant as a caricature of the charlatans' advertising practices.[34] In connection with the Emperor's coat of arms, however, the pendants on the Petrarch Master's image display a remarkable resemblance to one of the Emperor's main markers of identity, the Golden Fleece. Since Maximilian I [Fig. 14], Charles' V predecessor, the Roman Emperor had been the president of the Order of the Golden Fleece. As on Lucas van Leyden's etching, the Petrarch Master's dentist wears the robe of a nobleman, for example the beret. This is a satirical element introduced to express the charlatan's pretensions. In the Petrarch Master's image however, the dentist wears on his beret the weapon of Austria.

In the visual rhetoric by which he presented his statement, the Petrarch Master – as in many cases – makes use of proverbial expressions. In this specific case, he refers on the one hand to the German proverb 'die Zähne ziehen', which means something like 'to harm someone' or, more specifically, 'to get money out of someone'.[35] If the Emperor pulls the people's teeth ('zieht dem Volk die Zähne'), it means he will harm them and try to get money out of them. On the other hand, the Petrarch Master alludes to the popular expression 'wie ein Zahnbrecher lügen' ('to lie like a practitioner').[36] Thus, in referring to the German Emperor, the image suggests that he is a liar and a fraud.

The context of this satirical attack is the German political situation of 1519–1520, the period in which the woodcuts were made, specifically the election of the new Emperor after the death of Maximilian I (1519). The town of Augsburg – the very place where the Petrarch Master worked – financed the election of Maximilian's grandson Charles by huge sums of money from the famous Augsburg bankers Fugger (543.585 guilders) and Welser (143.333 guilders).[37] Conrad Peutinger, the councillor of Augsburg, argued in favour of Charles, in order to

[34] Jost Amman's "Zanbrecher" has a chain of teeth fixed to his advertising poster [Fig. 13].

[35] Röhrich, *Lexikon der sprichwörtlichen Redensarten* V, 1756, s.v. "Zahn".

[36] Ibidem V, 1757, s.v. "Zahnbrecher". For the Dutch version of the proverb ('Hij liegt als een tandentrekker'), cf. de Jong – Luijten, *Spiegel van alledag* 222; also the French poem which accompanies Andries Pauli's etching of Theodoor Rombout's "De tandentrekker" refers to this notion: 'C'est son art de mentir [...]' (ibidem).

[37] Cf. the manuscript Augsburg, Staats- und Stadtbibliothek, 2o Cod. Aug. 126.

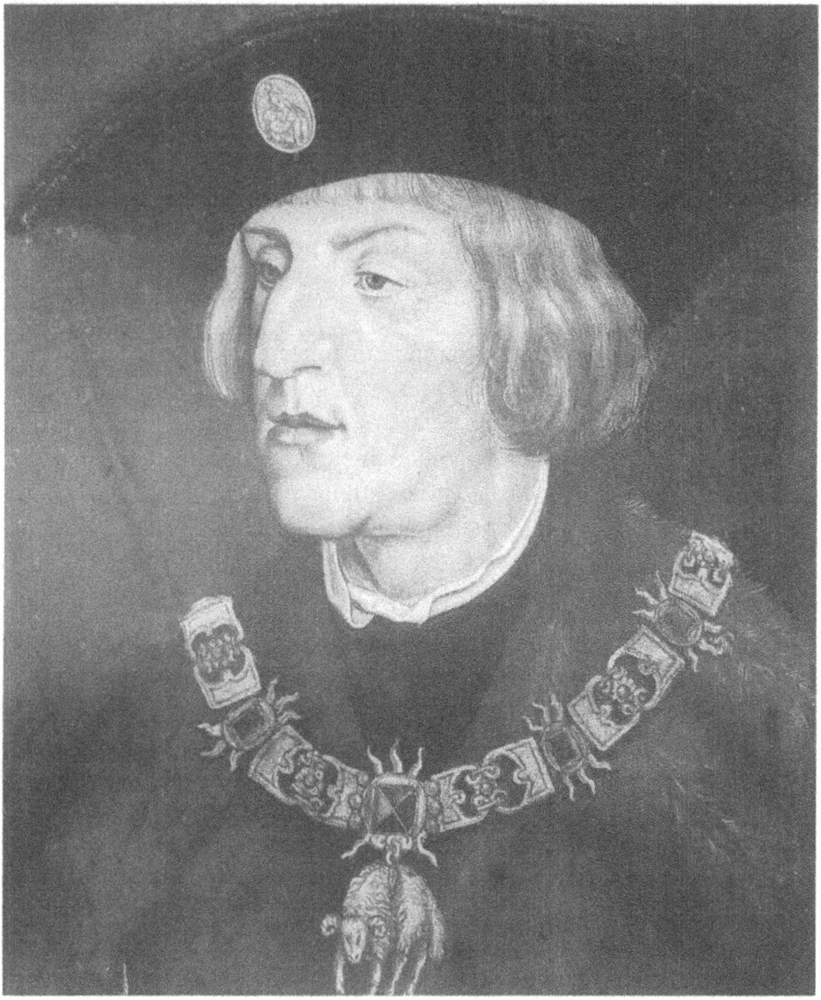

Fig. 14. German Painter, Portrait of the Emperor Maximilian I, after Albrecht Dürer. Oil on wooden panel, 40 × 31 cm. Vienna, Kunsthistorisches Museum.

bring about an alliance between the new Emperor and the Pope. He was eager to have Charles elected in order to destroy the Lutheran heresy. In the end Peutinger's wish was fulfilled, and in the summer of 1520 he was sent to the Low Countries to welcome Charles as he prepared for his coronation.[38] His speech was published by Erasmus' friend Peter Gillis (Petrus Aegidius). As the analysis of a number of images has shown, the Petrarch Master was an ardent Lutheran. Time and again he attacks the Pope, the Catholic Church, clerics, Catholic rites,[39] as well as the Roman Emperor. His opposition to the election of Charles V has already been observed by Ulrich Steinmann.[40] It is this context that helps us to understand the aggressive polemic in the image accompanying Petrarch's *De remediis*, chapter II, 94.

What, then, is the function of physical pain in this image? Why does it play such an important part? It is, of course, most remarkable that the Petrarch Master's image has so little to do with Petrarch's argument. In his chapter, Petrarch does not offer any practical advice concerning visits to a dentist, and does not engage in political polemic, nor does he discuss physical pain. So why did the Petrarch Master focus so strongly on pain? It could very well be that he almost automatically associated dental problems with toothache. Yet the association had also already been made by the German translator, who rendered 'illness of the teeth' as 'toothache': "Von dem weehtumb der zeen", as becomes clear already in the title of the chapter (fol. CXIXv).[41] In other words, the German translator already changed the tone of Petrarch's argument by giving physical pain a prominent place. We could interpret this as a feature of vernacular discourse which was somewhat alien to the humanist's Stoic way of thinking. In vernacular discourse, the mental 'dolor', the Stoic *pathe*, was probably difficult to understand or, at least, hard to grasp as a phenomenon fundamentally different from physical pain. Since it better fitted the vernacular discourse, the translator introduced physical pain where Petrarch exclusively talked about mental suffering.

[38] Cf. Lutz H., *Conrad Peutinger. Beiträge zu einer politischen Biographie* (Augsburg: 1958) 160–163.

[39] Enenkel, "Der Petrarca des Petrarca-Meisters". Cf. Lanckoronska M., "Der Petrarcameister und die Reformation", *Imprimatur* 11 (1952/53) 162–174.

[40] "Die politische Tendenz des Petrarca-Meisters. Seine Stellungnahme gegen die Wahl Karls V. und sein Verhalten zu den Ereignissen in Württemberg", *Staatliche Museen zu Berlin. Forschungen und Berichte* 6 (1964) 40–90.

[41] Scheidig adopts the questionable old German translation (297: "Von dem Wehtum der Zähne").

This suggests that physical pain played different roles within learned Latin and vernacular discourses.

The function and meaning of pain becomes even more interesting if one considers the political and propagandistic dimension of the Petrarch Master's rhetoric of pain. Here, physical pain functions as an important means for conveying a political statement. 1520 Germany was full of political tensions in which aggressive advertisement strategies and powerful propaganda were required. Especially the rise of the Reformation brought about a new use of printed media. Luther was one of the first to use the printed pamphlet and the printed images as means of propaganda.[42] In II, 94 and in a number of other chapters, the Petrarch Master used physical pain in a comparable propagandistic manner.

In terms of propaganda, pain serves first of all to attract the viewer's attention by emotionalizing the viewer. This is possible because physical sensations are extremely powerful identifiers. Furthermore, the physical sensation of pain causes emotional reactions such as fear, distress, grief, panic, shame and embarrassment. These reactions may be used for rhetorical means as well, for example in order to make the audience receptive to various messages, and to advices and warnings. Moreover, images of physical pain may also cause identification by compassion. The viewer may feel compassion for the pain-sufferers, which again may serve as an effective means to convey a range of messages. Compassion may also serve as a means to incite hatred in the viewer against the people who cause physical pain, and hurt or even torture others. The production of negative feelings, of course, is an important propagandistic device. Last but not least, images of physical pain are especially useful for political and religious propaganda since they can express relationships in terms of power and hierarchy. The persons who cause physical pain are the powerful; those on whom pain is inflicted are their subjects.

In the case of II, 94, the image of physical pain will immediately attract the viewer's attention. His gaze is drawn directly to the open mouth and the contorted face of the woman in the centre of the wood-

---

[42] Edwards M.U., *Printing, Propaganda, and Martin Luther* (Berkeley: 1994); Faulstich W., *Medien zwischen Herrschaft und Revolte. Die Medienkultur der Frühen Neuzeit (1400–1700)* (Göttingen: 1998); Hamm B., "Die Reformation als Medienereignis", *Jahrbuch für Biblische Theologie* 11 (1996) 138–166.

cut. The image may activate the viewer's own memories of toothache, as well as unpleasant or even humiliating situations when he had a tooth pulled in the marketplace, in front of a crowd of spectators. The viewer will identify with the image of pain, and in this way he will become receptive to the warning which the Petrarch Master's image seeks to put across. As a consequence, he will rethink his response to the pain depicted in the image. Ashamed of having surrendered to physical pain, he will be inclined to be more cautious henceforth. He will understand that it is dangerous to be driven into the hands of a charlatan by a toothache. Thus, the image arouses feelings of fear from practitioners in the viewer. Yet once the viewer has also discovered the political dimension of the image, he will transfer his fear of the charlatan to the Roman Emperor. As a consequence, he will feel hatred against this powerful fraud and torturer, and he will be embarrassed at having been cheated by him. He will come to distrust and feel anger against the Emperor. In this way, he will easily accept the image's message: 'avoid being hurt by Charles. Don't be so foolish as trust or support him. If you do so, you will end up paying for your naive attitude, just like the foolish people who trust practitioners'.

Eye-Piercing

Spectacular differences in attitude towards pain between word and image also occur in chapter II, 96 "De cecitate" ("On Blindness"). In his argument, Petrarch does not discuss physical pain, but is concerned with grief about loss of vision. As with chapter II, 94, the humanist's argument is shaped partly by antique Stoic statements, partly by Christian patterns of thought in the *contemptus mundi* tradition. The *contemptus mundi* patterns of thought are very similar to those presented in chapter II, 94. Loss of eyesight means freedom from sensual temptations, for example beautiful women and exquisite food:

> DOLOR: I have lost my vision.
>
> RATIO: And the view of women's faces. Hence rejoice! Closed are the windows through which normally death enters, and the way is barred to many vices; greed (*avaritia*), gluttony (gula), lust (*luxuria*), and other pests have lost their helpmeets and accomplices. As much as these friends took away from your soul, that much, you should understand, have you now regained.
>
> DOLOR: I have lost my eyes.

> Ratio: You have lost evil guides (*duces malos*), who were used to lead you to ruin (*qui in precipitium te ducebant*). It is amazing how often the most lucid part of the body (*lucidissima pars corporis*) casts mind and soul into darkness. Begin now to follow the spirit that calls you to better things, and listen to the truth which shouts into your ears. Seek not for 'the things which are seen, but the things which are not seen. For the things which are seen are temporal: but the things which are not seen, are eternal' (*Nolite querere que videntur. Que enim videntur, temporalia sunt. Que autem non videntur, eterna*).[43]

In the last two lines Petrarch quotes Paul's Letter to the *Corinthians* II, 4,18, in which the apostle persuades his audience to put aside earthly things in search of the heavenly kingdom. The Christian argument culminates in the paradox that whoever who has lost his vision has begun to see the light, the light of God and spiritual truth: 'When Saint Anthony came to see the old man (Didymus), he told him not to worry about the loss of the eyes one has in common with flies, mice, and lizards but to exult that those eyes he had in common with the angels were safe and sound. Words worthy of Anthony, the pupil of the heavenly Schoolmaster'.[44] Petrarch quotes the Latin version of the famous *Life of Anthony*, one of the key texts of medieval monastic spirituality.[45] Thus, he who has lost his physical eyes has the advantage of having (re)gained his inner sight, which enables him to perceive the true light.

The Stoic line of argument concentrates on examples of antique heroes who either ignored blindness or were not prevented by blindness from extreme forms of bravery. The first in line are of course Homer who despite his blindness was able to deliver no less than 48 books of epic poetry, and the philosopher Democritus, who was said to have deliberately deprived himself of his eyesight in order to better perceive philosophical truth.[46] As is the case with Homer, the Stoic philosopher Diodotus, Cicero's house philosopher, refused to be prevented by his blindness from pursuing demanding intellectual activities. He continued to study books incessantly, which he had read to him by slaves. As a

---

[43] Trsl. Rawski, III, 235–236; Le Preux 579 (additions of the Latin text in italics mine).

[44] Rawski III, 237; Le Preux 580–581.

[45] Athanasius, *Vita Antonii* (*Life of Anthony*), translated into Latin by Hieronymus' friend Euagrius bishop of Antiochia, in Migne, *Patrologia Latina* vol. LXXIII, 158.

[46] Cf. Cicero, *Tusculanae disputationes* V, 114; Gellius, *Noctes Atticae* X, 17; Valerius Maximus, *Factorum et dictorum memorabilium* libri VIII, 7 ext. 4.

telling detail, he managed even to construct geometrical drawings by meticulously describing the figures to Cicero's servants.[47] As an example of a military hero, Petrarch refers to the otherwise unknown soldier Tyrrhenus (taken from the Stoic poet Lucan) who fought in the battle of Massilia.[48] This example is especially interesting in relation to the role of pain in Petrarch's text, since it is connected with an extreme form of violence and pain. Lucan tells us that a lead bullet crushed the bones of Tyrrhenus' temples, causing his eyeballs to jump from their sockets and blood to gush from his head. This dramatic accident did not prevent the brave soldier from continuing his fighting. Petrarch, however, does not give any of these bloody details, but only briefly mentions Thyrrenus' name. In other words, Petrarch did not consider physical pain important enough to discuss it when dealing with the loss of functions of the body. Whenever possible – or even impossible – in his argument, the state of mind (grief, sorrow, fear et cetera) prevails over the physical sensation.

In marked difference, the Petrarch Master illustrated the chapter with an image that precisely exaggerates physical pain and violence [Fig. 15]. In the centre of the woodcut a patient lying on a bench is being operated upon by a wild-looking surgeon in primitive dress, who is into his eyes with a sharp instrument. Obviously the operation causes so much pain that the patient is tied to a bench. This is done in such a strange and exaggerated way – the patient is tied at the feet, knees, hands, arms, body and head – that the patient resembles more a victim of judicial torture. Behind the bench, a bird scratches out the eyes of a queen. Moreover, the queen is about to commit suicide in a painful way, by stabbing a dagger into her breast. Modern viewers are likely to be puzzled by this extraordinarily cruel image. It is difficult to understand how the Petrarch Master came to his pictorial invention. Even Scheidig, who thinks that the Petrarch Master closely followed Petrarch's text, admits that 'Petrarca nennt kein Beispiel einer Herrscherin, die so ihrem Leben ein Ende bereitet hätte'.[49]

With this illustration as with others, it is not plausible to argue that the Petrarch Master was dependent on images of physical pain *because he had to translate a philosophical text into visual objects*. Petrarch's text offers

[47] Cicero, *Tusculanae disputationes* V, 113.
[48] Lucan, *Bellum civile* III, 709–722.
[49] Scheidig, *Die Holzschnitte des Petrarca-Meisters* 299.

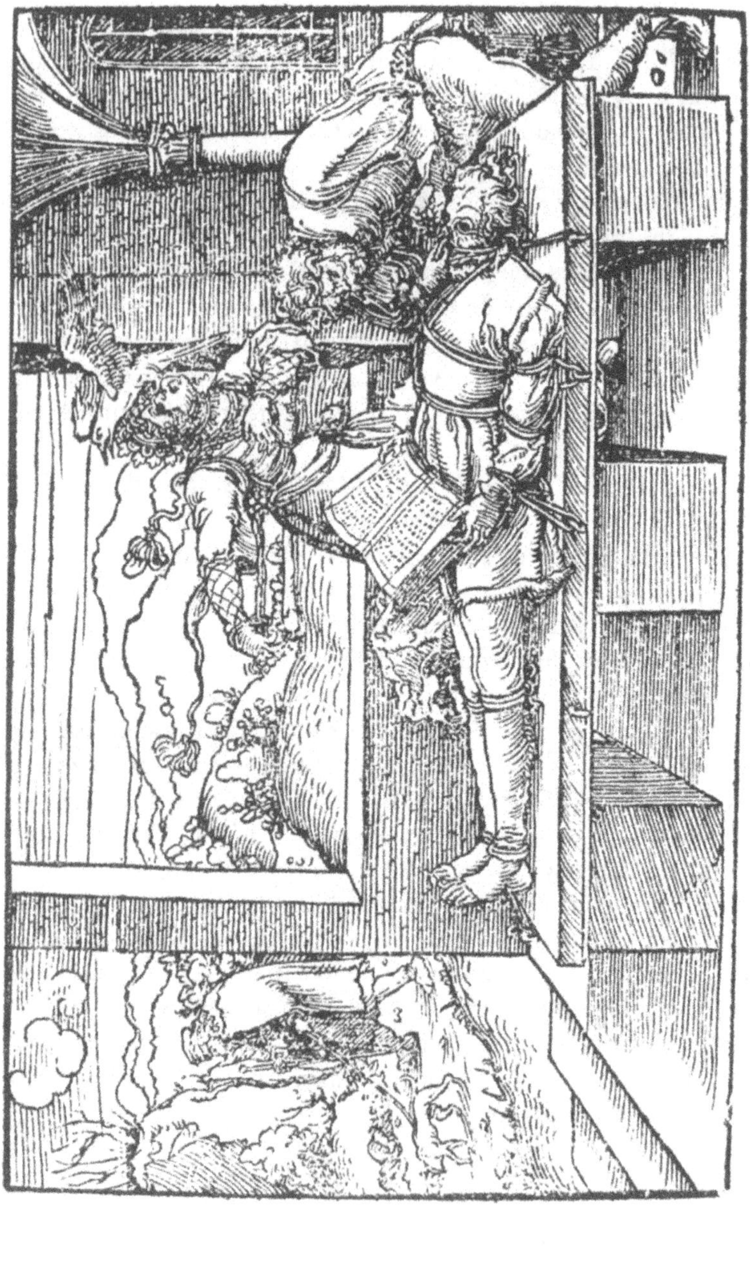

Fig. 15. The Petrarch Master, Woodcut illustration to Petrarch's *Von der Artzney baider Glueck* [...] (Augsburg: 1532), book II, chapter 96, fol. CXXIv.

generally a considerable amount of topics which could easily have been visualized. In the chapter on blindness, for example, the Petrach Master could have depicted the blind seer Tyresias, the blind poet Homer, the blind philosopher Democritus, Saint Anthony visiting the blind man Didymus (including the mice and lizards of Anthony's argument), the blind philosopher Diodotus constructing geometrical figures with the help of Cicero's servants, the blind jurist Gaius Drusus receiving a crowd of visitors, the famous censor Appius Claudius Caecus presiding over the venerable Roman senate, the biblical hero Simson who, for his love of Delilah, had forsaken his duties and had been punished by God with blindness,[50] the brave soldier Tyrrenus heavily wounded in the battle of Massilia, and not in the last place the emotional story of blind King John of Bohemia who sacrificed himself in the battle of Crécy (1346), which could have been an especially impressive image with a large battle scène. Moreover, the Petrarch Master could have depicted just the pictorial type of the blind man in its various manifestations, such as the blind man in despair and distress, the blind man who has lost his orientation, or the blind man who became a beggar (as often was the case in the late Middle Ages). For images of the blind man the Petrach Master easily could have drawn on the rich iconographical tradition from the Middle Ages ('the blind man'),[51] with which he was very well acquainted, as is demonstrated by the background figure of the blind man on the left (blind man's stick, hat of tramp, 'Augenbinde'; additionally guide dog).

How, then, is the strange pictorial invention of the Petrarch Master, in which he focuses on physical pain in such an exaggerating way, to be explained? First of all, the Petrarch Master associates the topic of the chapter, blindness, with yet another wide-spread medical technique of the late medieval and early modern period, the so-called "Starstich" (literally 'piercing of the cataract'). Cataract ("grauer Star"), especially during old age, was at least as frequent in the late Middle Ages as it is nowadays. It implies a deterioration of the lens that progressively robs patients of clear eyesight and, in the end, leads to blindness. The cure that was applied for this illness was to remove the cataract by piercing

[50] *Book of Judges* 13–16.
[51] Cf. *Lexikon des Mittelalters*, vol. II (Zurich: 1999) col. 279, s.v. "Blindheit" (W. Jaeger).

the lens push it back into the eyeball.[52] If the patient was lucky and the operation was done properly, he would regain his eyesight, yet since the lens had been displaced or partially destroyed, the patient would be unable to see sharply. As this short description already suggests, there was no guarantee that the operation would be successful, and even if the operation was done well, its success was limited. Moreover, the very poor hygienic circumstances in the late middle Ages frequently caused inflammations in operated parts of the body, which was all the more dangerous, of course, in the case of a delicate organ like the eye. It was no exception that patients died some time even after "successful" surgery. The problems were increased by the fact that there was no official or officially controlled ophthalmology.[53] As was the case with dentistry, eye surgery was done by strolling practitioners. They traveled from town to town, from village to village, were paid for their dubious skills and disappeared as quickly as they had appeared on the market place. There was no cure after the treatments and when inflammations or other complications occurred, the strolling practitioner was gone with the wind. Yet for late medieval patients of cataract who wanted to regain vision again, there were hardly any alternatives to visiting "Starstecher" ("cataract piercers").

There is, then, a puzzling discontinuity between word and image. Whereas Petrarch deals with the mental consequences of blindness, the Petrarch Master discusses a medical cure for blindness which – painful as it was – did offer some hope of regaining eyesight. It seems unconvincing to construe the image as a kind of practical advice: if you lose your vision, visit a surgeon and have a cataract operation. The figure in the background (the blind man with guide dog) points exactly in the opposite direction, showing the deplorable results of the operation: it has failed completely, and the man became blind. Thus, the Petrarch Master in fact dissuades people from visiting cataract piercers. The figure in the centre (the woman about to commit suicide) probably reinforces this: if you trust a "Starstecher" you are in fact as mad as a

[52] The "Starstecher's" instruments (needles etcetera) are exhibited for example in the Pathologisch-anatomisches Bundesmuseum Narrenturm in Vienna. The piercing of cataracts was already practiced in antiquity, cf. Künzl E., "Der Starstich [...]", in *Antike Welt. Zeitschrift für Archäologie und Urgeschichte* 35 (2004) 45–50.

[53] Cf. Hirschberg J., *The History of Ophthalmology*, vol. II *The Middle Ages, the 16th and 17th centuries* (1985); *Lexikon des Mittelalters*, vol. II (Zurich: 1999) col. 1845–1859, s.v. "Chirurg".

person trying to commit suicide.[54] Suicide was, of course, condemned by Christian religion, and punished as a crime by the confiscation of the suicide's possessions.[55] The bird scratching out the woman's eyes may hint at the madness or 'furor' ('Verblendung') of suicide. Yet the bird may also connect the *exemplum historicum* more closely with the client of the "Starstecher". The bird probably represents a starling, German 'Star' – a homonym of the illness from which the operated person suffers (Star, i.e. cataract).[56] The viewer discovers the terrible fact that the starling bird does exactly the same as the practitioner: it renders the "cured" person forever blind.

As is the case with II, 94, the Petrarch Master's pictorial emphasis on pain has a polemical and satirical dimension, and is connected with the discourses of the *Ship of Fools* and the house book. The satirical polemic is directed against patients and practitioners alike. It accuses the strolling surgeons/practitioners of charlatanry and their patients of foolishness. Instead of curing patients, the untrustworthy surgeons will make them definitively blind. Instead of helping patients, they *torture* them. As the pictorial devices used by the Petrarch Master show, this last accusation is to be taken literally. The Petrarch Master represents

[54] I cannot exclude the possibility that the iconographical archetype of the woman committing suicide by stabbing a dagger in her breast was the Roman heroine Lucretia who was raped by Tarquinius Superbus (Livy, *Ab urbe condita* I, 57,6–59,6). But there is another, more plausible iconological tradition, that of Dido who stabbed a sword into her breast (Virgil, *Aeneis* IV, 642 ff.). The Petrarch Master was familiar with the pictorial representation of Dido's suicide. Compare his illustration to *De remediis* chapter II, 120 [Fig. 16]. For his image of Dido committing suicide, he imitated the woodcut illustration of the Virgil edition, Straßburg 1502 [Fig. 17]. As is the case with chapter II, 96, Petrarch does not mention the historical example depicted by the Petrarch Master. Two pictorial elements, the long hair and the crown [Fig. 18; detail of Fig. 15], strongly suggest that the historical example of the Petrarch Master's image of chapter II, 96 is Dido. Dido was a queen (wheras Lucretia was not) and Virgil describes her as wearing long hair (which was cut off by Iris; last lines of *Aeneid*, book IV). According to Virgil Dido committed suicide in an attack of madness ('effera', IV, 642; 'furibunda', IV, 646), a mental blackout so to say. Thus, her suicide has especially negative connotations. If the woman committing suicide in illustration II, 96 is Dido, winged Iris is replaced by the starling bird scratching out her eyes. It does not bring relief by death, as Iris did, but permanent blindness, i.e. long suffering on earth. This suffering may be expressed by the image of the strolling blind man on the left part of the woodcut.

[55] Cf. Wacke A., "Selbsttötung, – mord", in *Lexikon des Mittelalters*, vol. VII, col. 1727.

[56] That the illness 'Star' has different etymological roots (old German 'starablint', i.e. 'mit offenen, starren Augen blind', cf. Pfeifer W. [ed.], *Etymologisches Wörterbuch des Deutschen*, [Munich: 2005, 8th edition] 1344) from the bird 'Star' (cf. ibidem), is of course less relevant for the Petrarch Master's pun.

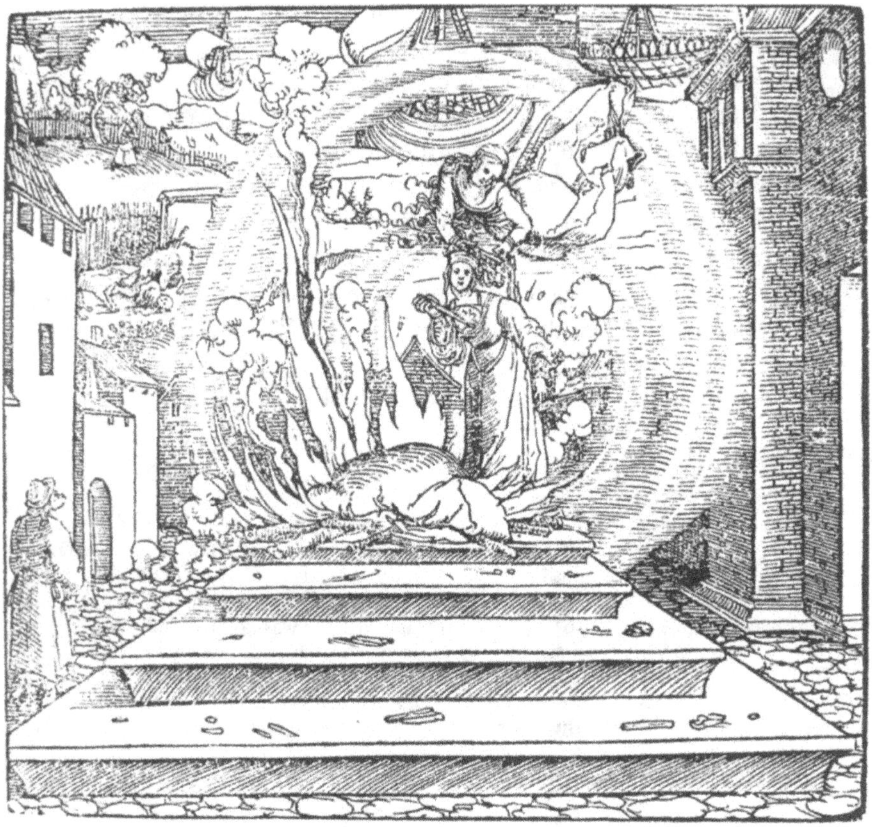

Fig. 16. The Petrarch Master, Woodcut illustration to Petrarch's *Von der Artzney baider Glueck* [...] (Augsburg: 1532), book II, chapter 120, fol. CLVIIIr.

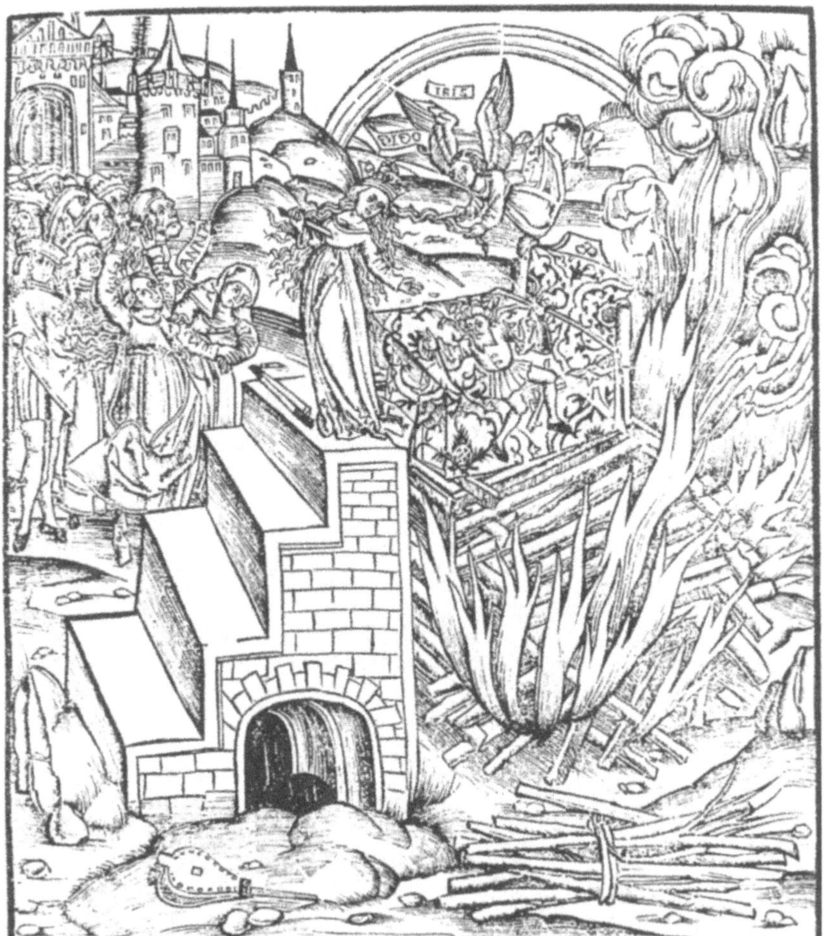

Fig. 17. Dido committing suicide. Woodcut illustration in Sebastian Brant's edition of Virgil (Straßburg: 1502), at the end of book IV.

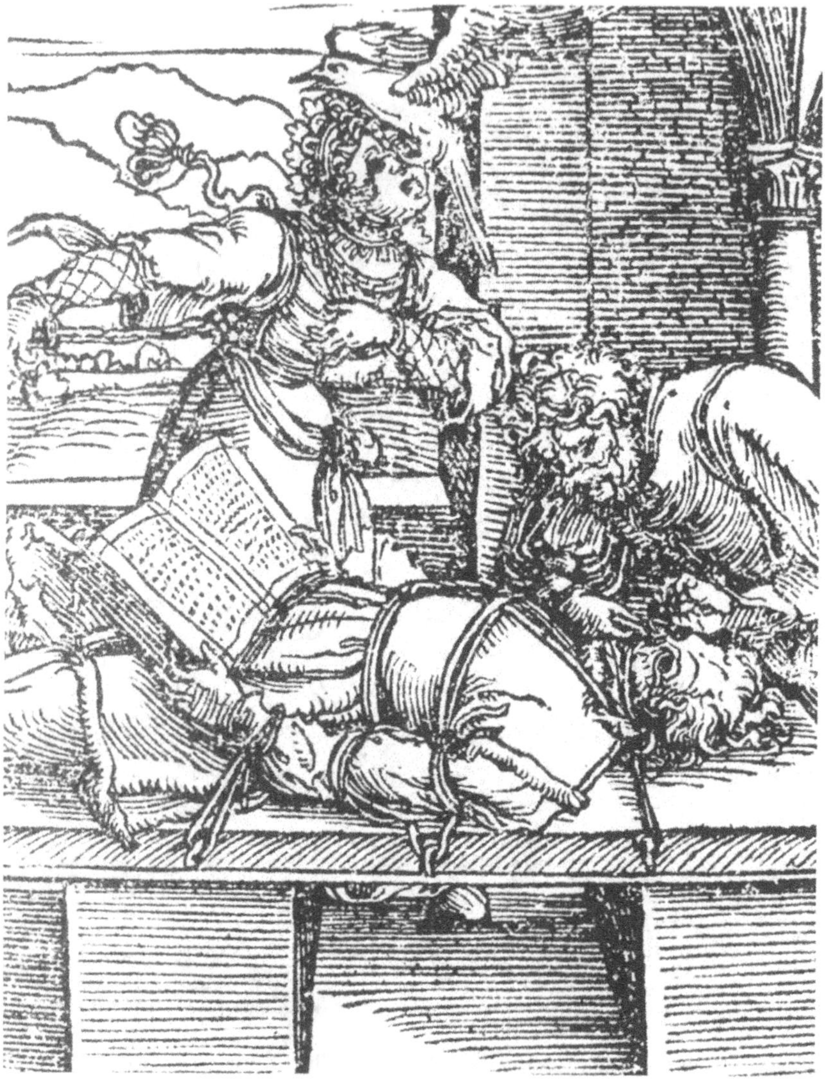

Fig. 18. The Petrarch Master, Woodcut illustration to Petrarch's *Von der Artzney baider Glueck* [...] (Augsburg: 1532), book II, chapter 96, fol. CXXIv. Detail.

the patient lying *tied to a bench.* This is a curious distortion of the normal practice. The operations were normally done with both patient and surgeon sitting opposite each other. The patient was held from behind by an assistant, so that he could not move. When the Petrarch Master renders the patient lying tied to a bench he is referring to the widespread and well-known medieval instrument of torture, the rack. That the Petrarch Master knew about the rack is also suggested by his illustration of chapter II, 65, in which the victim in the foreground is stretched on the rack while water is being poured into its mouth [Fig. 19].

Patients who undergo torture out of their own free will are of course fools. The same is true for patients who believe that they will be able to read again after a cataract operation, as the book in the hands of the tortured person shows [Fig. 15]. Instead of being able to read again he will become blind forever, as the blind man in the background (of the left part of the image) suggests. That people who commit suicide are fools was already indicated above. It is even more foolish to choose the dagger or the sword as a means of suicide. This will certainly be very painful whereas it is uncertain whether the attempt will succeed. The woman committing suicide may well be modeled on Dido – the long, flying plaits point in that direction – and it is worth noting that Dido's attempt was not successful, and she was only relieved by Juno who, out of pity, sent winged Iris to her, in order to cut off the queen's long blond hair, the symbol of her life force.[57]

Thus, in chapter II, 96 again, the Petrarch Master uses pain as a powerful means to drive his point home: to make his audience refrain from undergoing the cataract operation that was so widespread and popular. The painful torture of the violent eye operation on the rack and the painful suicide by stabbing a dagger into one's breast are meant to emotionalize the viewer and to make him receptive to the Petrarch Master's practical warning.

Whipping, Scourging, Torturing

The view that in his pictorial inventions the Petrarch Master tried to stir up the emotions of the reader is reinforced by the fact that he time

[57] Virgil, *Aeneid* IV, 693–705.

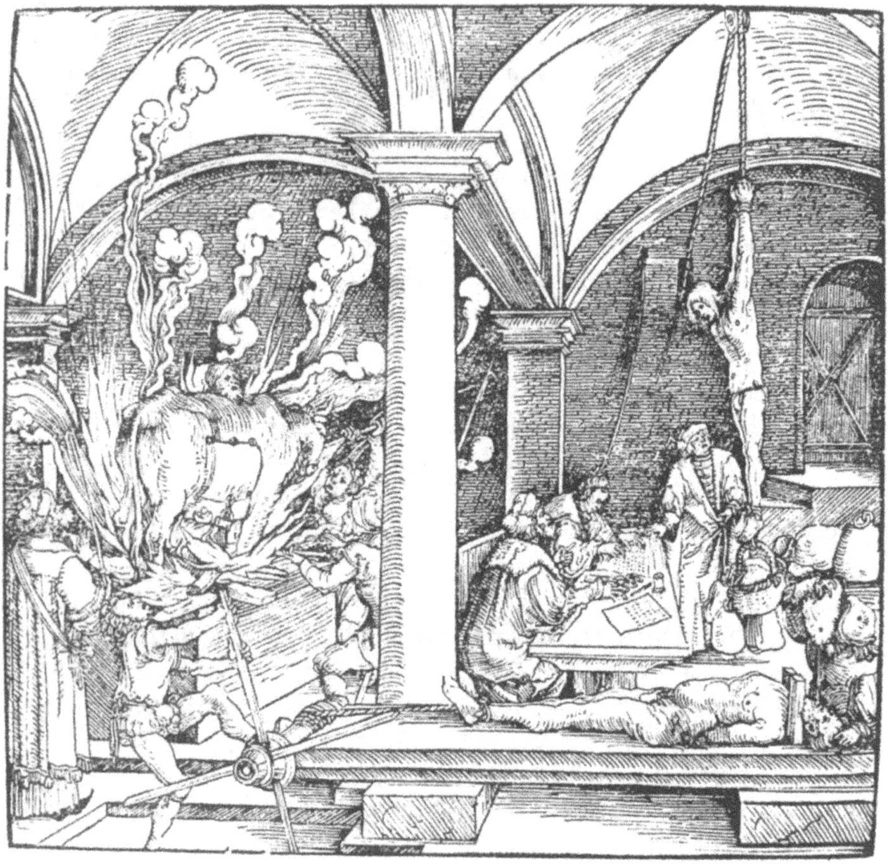

Fig. 19. The Petrarch Master, Woodcut illustration to Petrarch's *Von der Artzney baider Glueck* [...] (Augsburg: 1532), book II, chapter 65, fol. LXXVIv.

and again represents *extreme forms of pain and violence*. In his woodcuts he repeatedly present the human body naked, that is in as vulnerable a state as possible (for example in chapters II, 7; 27; 28; 29; 46; 65; 67; 100; 105; 122; 124). The naked body is scourged or whipped (II, 7 [Fig. 20]; 29 [Fig. 21]; 67 [Fig. 22]; 100; 122), scratched (II, 27); pierced by arrows, swords or daggers (for example in II, 29; 46 [Fig. 23]); literally roasted (II, 65 [Fig. 19]), tortured by means of the strappado technique, the rack (II, 65 [Fig. 19]), the wheel or the cross (II, 122 [Fig. 24]), it will be torn into pieces by wild animals (II, 7), crucified, hanged or burnt alive (II, 122 [Fig. 24]). Several times tongues are cut off (Fig. II, 29 [Fig. 21] (left part of the image)); II, 103 [Fig. 25] (right part of the image)), eyes are gouged out (II, 60 [Fig. 26] (detail, left part of the image)), ears are cut off (II, 97) as well as heads (II, 102).

The pictorial inventions by the Petrarch Master are all the more remarkable since in most cases the text does not speak about those specific forms of physical pain or violence. In chapter II, 67 ("De exilio") Petrarch discusses the grief caused by exile, which, from Antiquity to the early modern period, was considered one of the most severe punishments. The Petrarch Masters illustration, however, focuses on the scourging of a man with a naked back and his hands tied [Fig. 22]. The scourged man is represented with his mouth open, which suggests that he is screaming with pain. His bending forward, moreover, suggests that he is attempting to escape from the pain. Interestingly enough, there is no obvious juridical connection between the punishments of exile and scourging.

In II, 7 ("De servitudine") Petrarch discusses the deplorable state mind caused by the loss of freedom and offers Stoic arguments against it. One can only free oneself if one deals with philosophy. Thus, the most important argument is derived from the Stoic paradox that 'only the wise man is free' ('solus sapiens liber est'). The Petrarch Master, however, presents the physical punishment of a servant by severe scourging. The servant is represented as a naked victim bound to a pillar and relentlessly whipped by two men, one behind the pillar with a 'flagellum' in his left hand, and by another man in the centre of the woodcut. The face of the victim shows the effects of physical pain. His mouth is open, which probably suggests that he is groaning from pain. His eyes are opened wide, which suggests fear of receiving yet another blow. His body is contorted as if he is trying to escape the intense physical pain afflicted on him. The cruelty of the scene is enlarged by the fact that the man

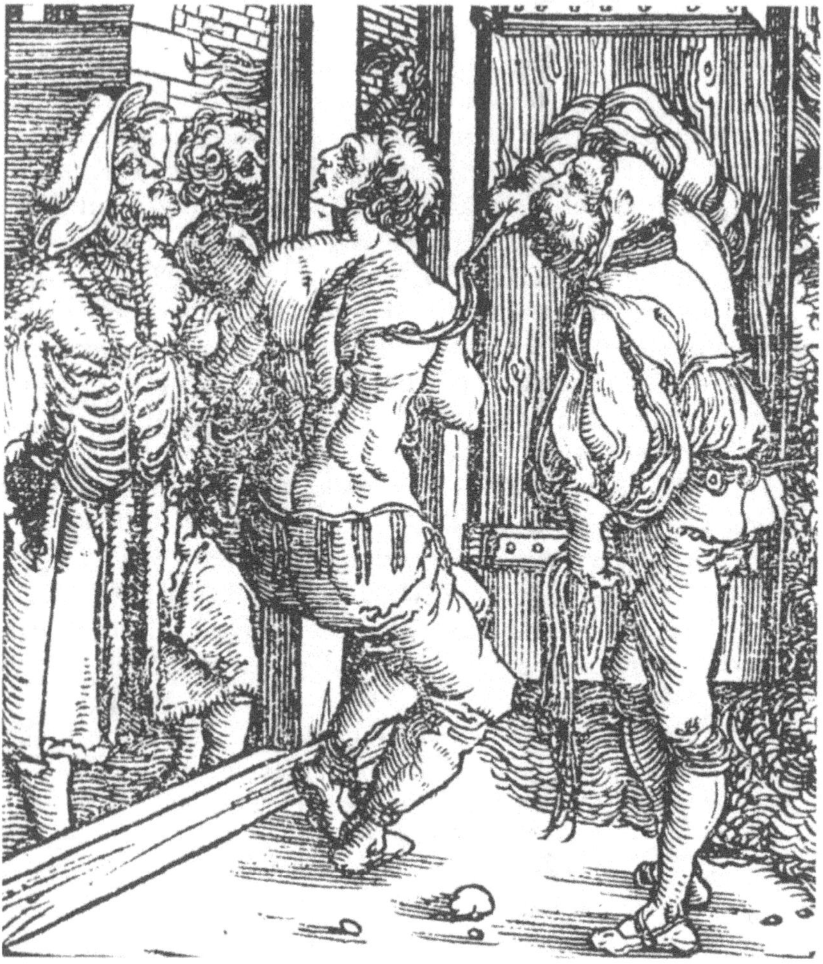

Fig. 20. The Petrarch Master, Woodcut illustration to Petrarch's *Von der Artzney baider Glueck* [...] (Augsburg: 1532), book II, chapter 7, fol. VIIIv. Detail, left part of the image.

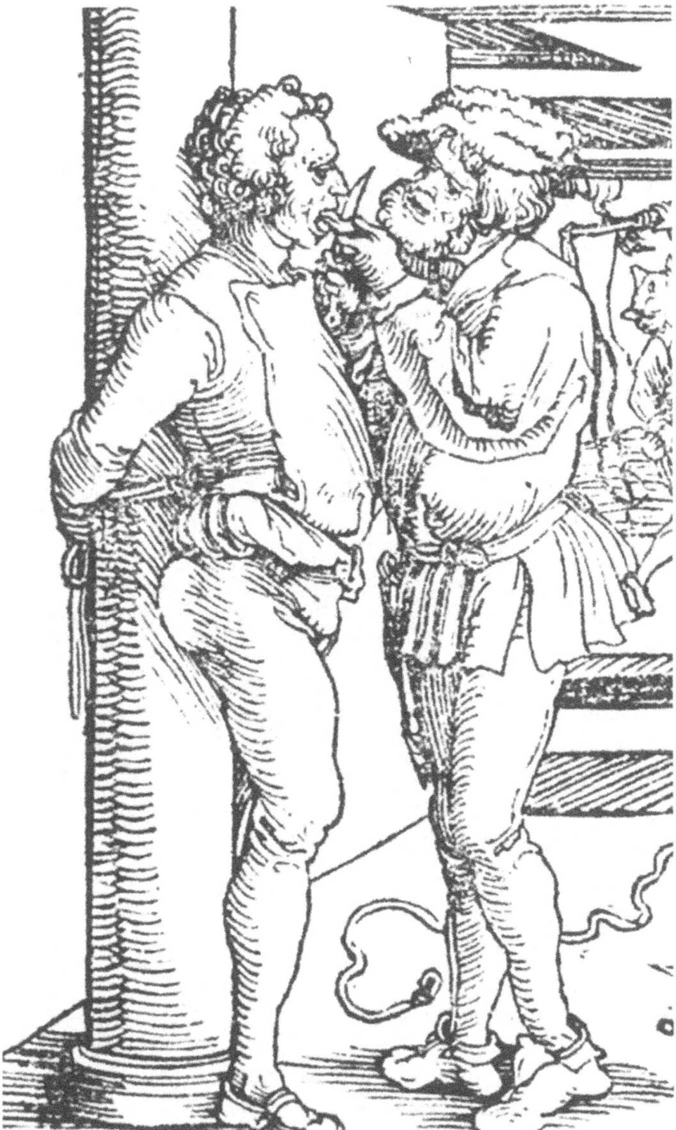

Fig. 21. The Petrarch Master, Woodcut illustration to Petrarch's *Von der Artzney baider Glueck* [...] (Augsburg: 1532), book II, chapter 29, fol. XXXVIIIr. Detail, left part of the image.

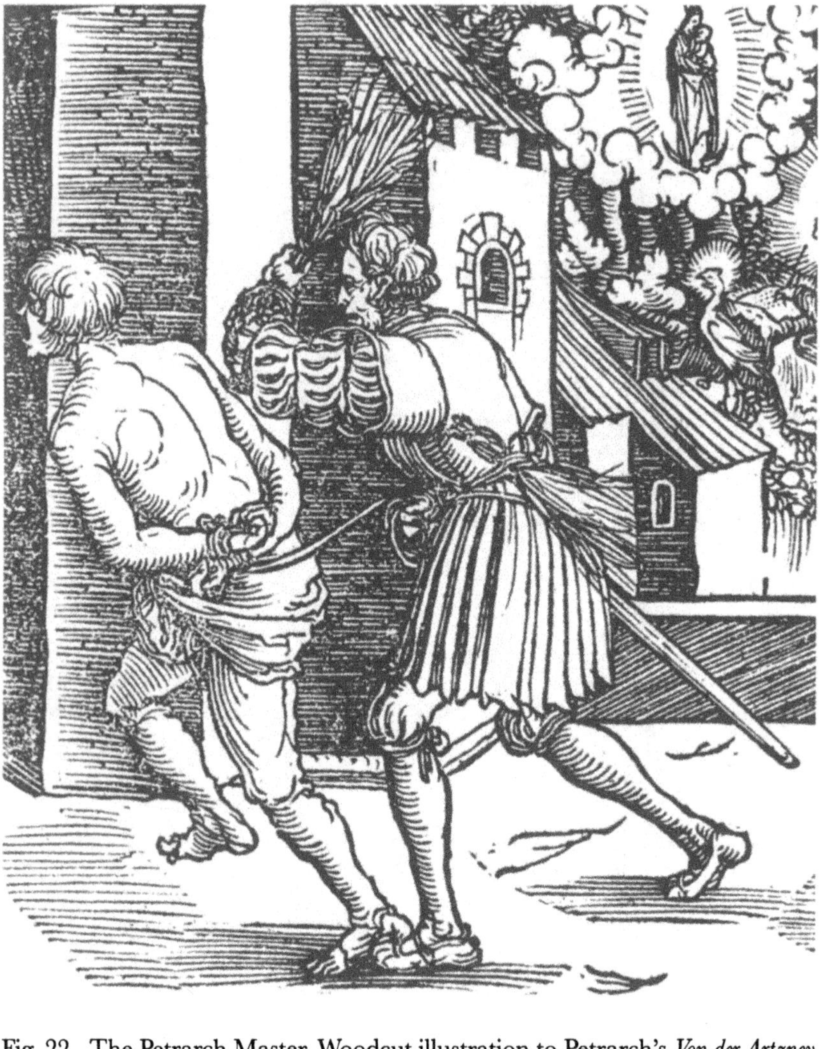

Fig. 22. The Petrarch Master, Woodcut illustration to Petrarch's *Von der Artzney baider Glueck* [...] (Augsburg: 1532), book II, chapter 67, fol. LXXIXr. Detail, left part of the image.

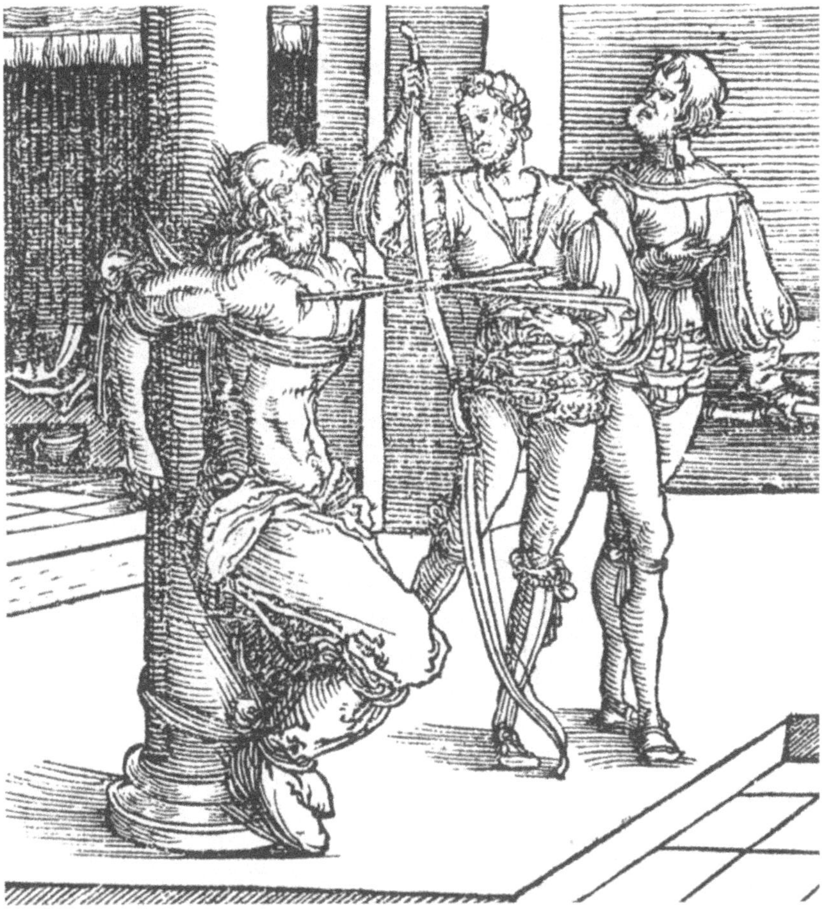

Fig. 23. The Petrarch Master, Woodcut illustration to Petrarch's *Von der Artzney baider Glueck* [...] (Augsburg: 1532), book II, chapter 46, fol. LVv. Detail, left part of the image.

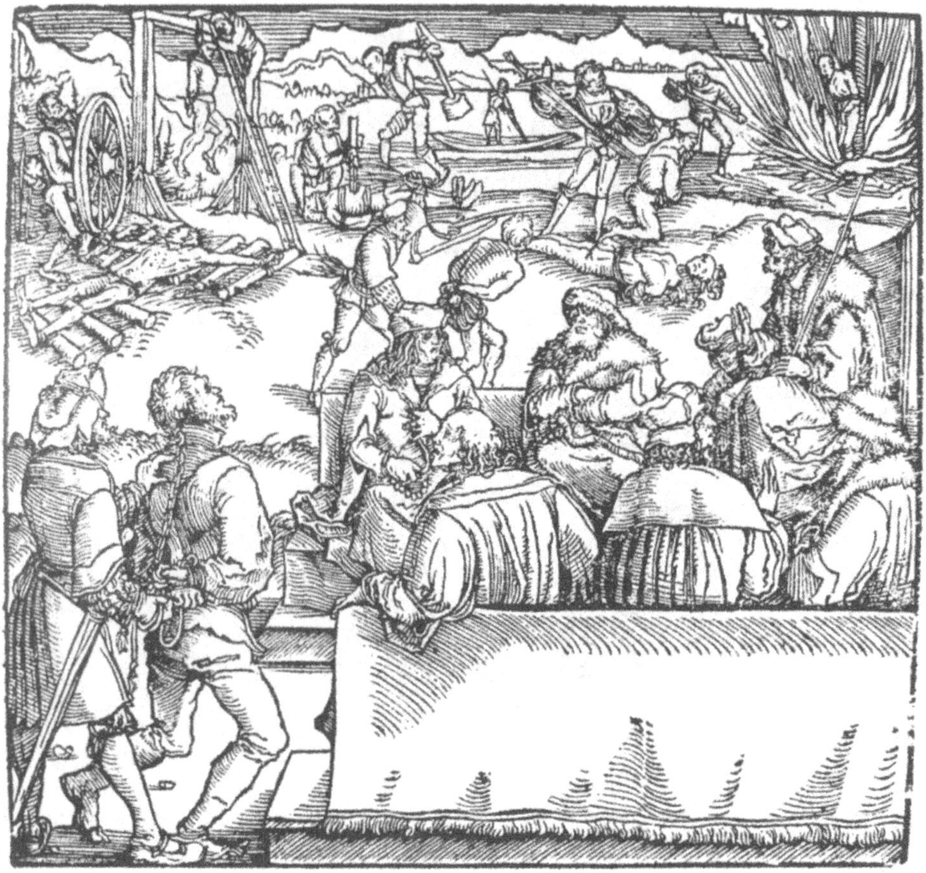

Fig. 24. The Petrarch Master, Woodcut illustration to Petrarch's *Von der Artzney baider Glueck* [...] (Augsburg: 1532), book II, chapter 122, fol. CLXIIr.

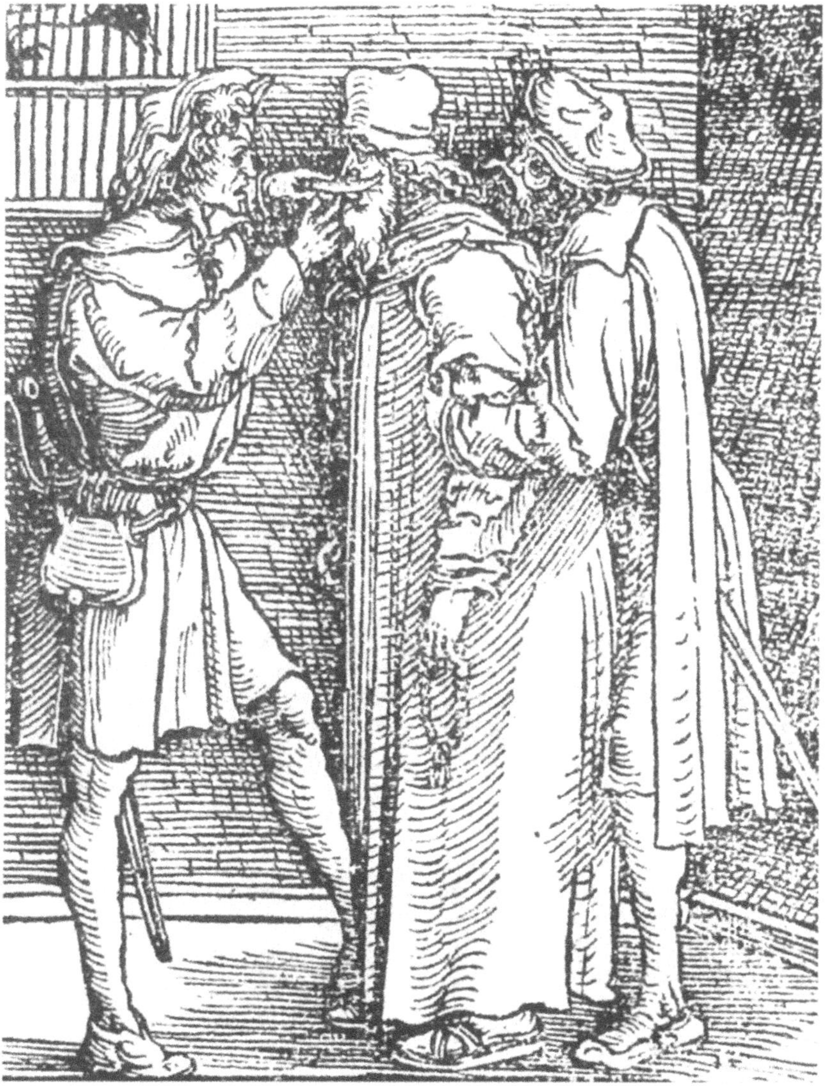

Fig. 25. The Petrarch Master, Woodcut illustration to Petrarch's *Von der Artzney baider Glueck* [...] (Augsburg: 1532), book II, chapter 103, fol. CXXXr. Detail, right part of the image.

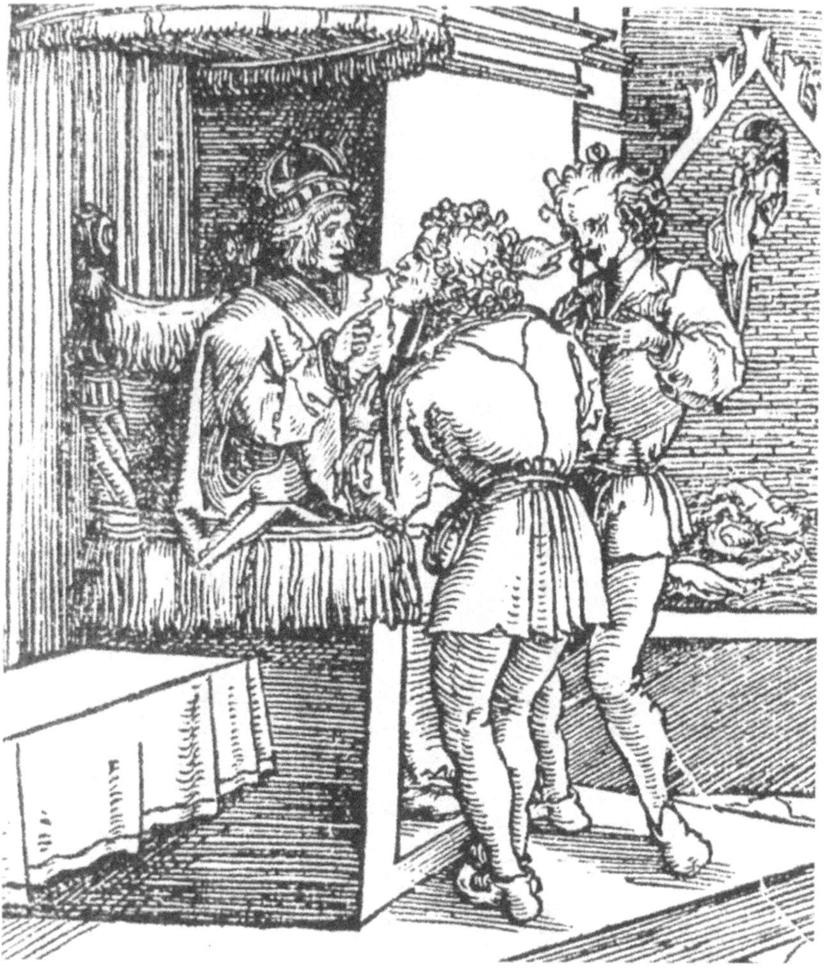

Fig. 26. The Petrarch Master, Woodcut illustration to Petrarch's *Von der Artzney baider Glueck* [...] (Augsburg: 1532), book II, chapter 60, fol. LXXIIr. Detail, left part of the image.

in the centre is so eager to scourge his victim that he uses even two whips, one in his right and one in his left hand [Fig. 20].

By constructing the image in this way, the Petrarch Master aimed at associating the punishment of the servant with the well known pictorial type of the flagellation of Christ, frequently depicted in late medieval painting from the fourteenth to the sixteenth century. The pillar reminds the viewer of the column to which Christ was tied (see below). The two man scourging Christ are standard elements of the 'flagellation'. For these elements compare for example Duccio's "Flagellation of Christ" on the *Maestà* painted for the cathedral of Siena (1308–1311) [Fig. 28] or the Master of the Osservanza's *Flagellation of Christ* in the Vatican Museum's (ca. 1425–1450 [Fig. 29]). The late medieval "Flagellations of Christ" have a clearly religious meaning: they are part of the passion of Christ and thus, they belong to the summit of late medieval religious experience, the so called 'Leidensmystik'. In the 'Leidensmystik' the believer is meant to identify with Christ and to re-experience the 'unsägliche' pain which He had to endure.

One wonders whether the Petrarch Master who was a Lutheran did participate in the late medieval 'Leidensmystik'. Luther, in fact, had outspoken views on the way in which one should meditate on the passion of Christ. Quite a number of contemporary habits he considered as wrong or even dangerous. He certainly did *not* approve of far-reaching identifications with the pains of Christ. In his 1519 treatise *A Sermon Concerning Meditation on the Holy Sufferings of Christ* (*Sermon von der Betrachtung des heiligen Leidens Christi*), he wants the believer above all to identify with the torturers. The believer should focus on the thought that it is *he* who tortured Him, *he* who crucified Him: 'Deeply believe and never doubt the least, that you are the one who thus martyred Christ. For your sins most surely did it. Therefore, when you view the nails piercing through his hands, firmly believe it is *your* work. Do you behold his crown of thorns, believe the thorns are your wicked thoughts'. Occupied with this thought, we will 'view Christ' and be 'terror-stricken in heart at the sight, and [our] conscience at once sinks in despair. This terror-stricken feeling should spring forth, so that [we] see the severe wrath and the unchangeable earnestness of God in regard to sin and sinners'.[58]

[58] For this article I have made use of an online translation, entitled "Christ's Holy Sufferings", published by the Christian Classics Ethereal Library, www.ccel.org/ccel/luther/sermons.iv.html, accessed 20 May 2008, italics mine.

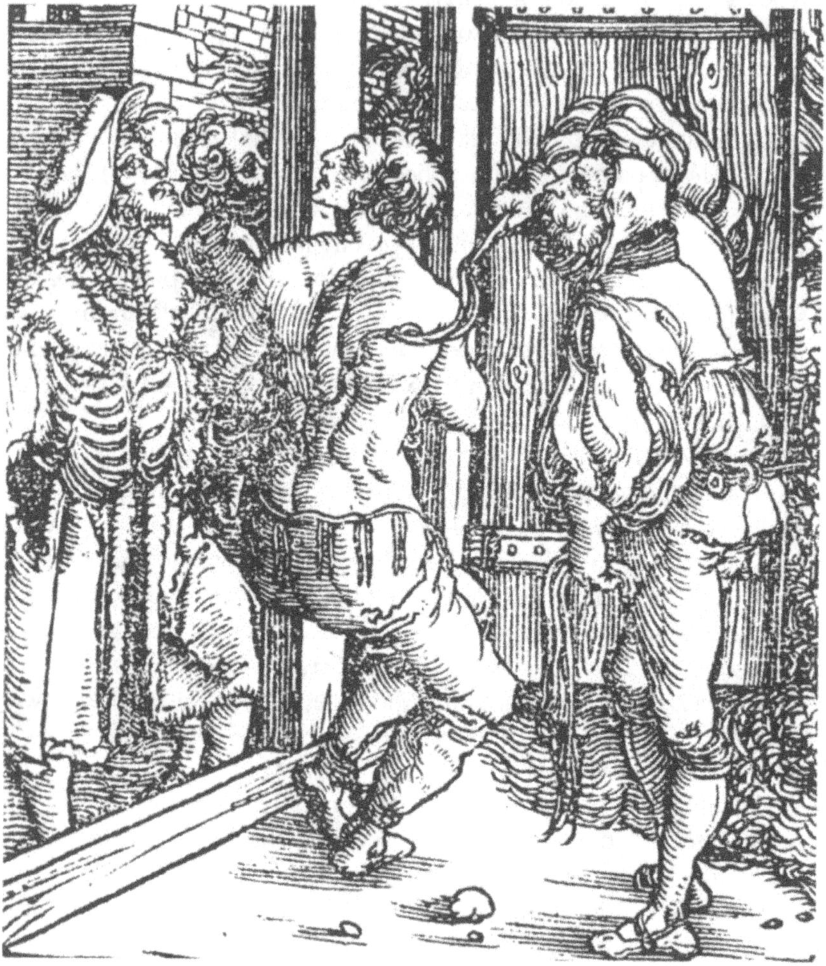

Fig. 27. Fig. 20. The Petrarch Master, Woodcut illustration to Petrarch's *Von der Artzney baider Glueck* [...] (Augsburg: 1532), book II, chapter 7, fol. VIIIv. Detail, left part of the image.

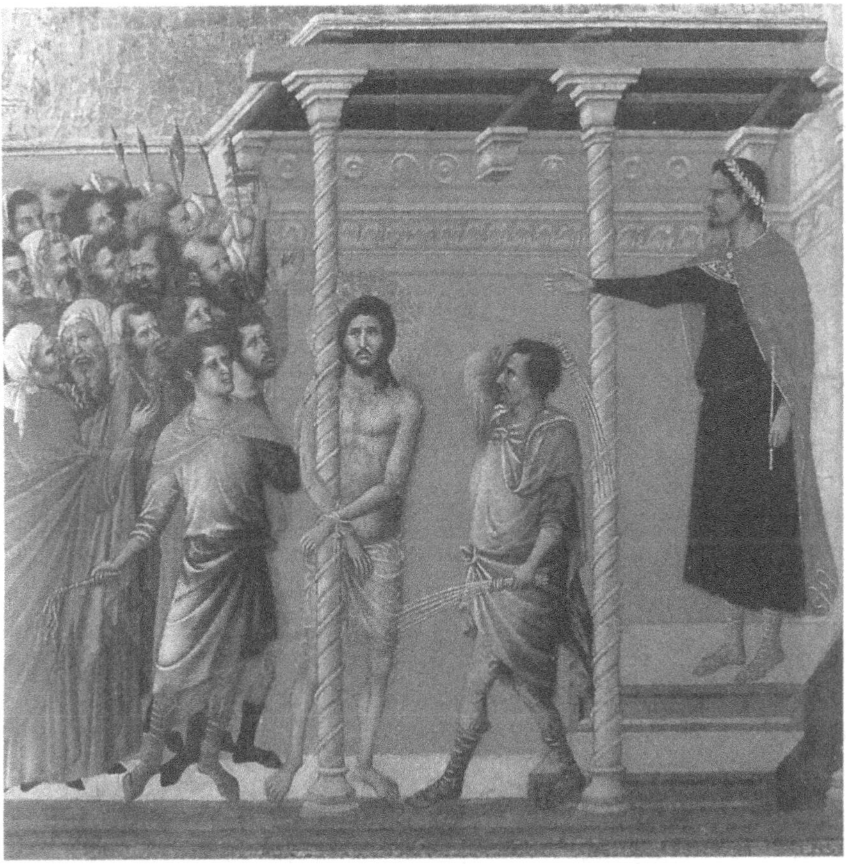

Fig. 28 [Col. pl. VI]. Duccio, "Flagellation of Christ", part of his *Maestà* painted for the cathedral of Siena (1308–1311). Tempera on wood, 99.6 × 53.2 cm. Siena, Museo dell' Opera di Duomo.

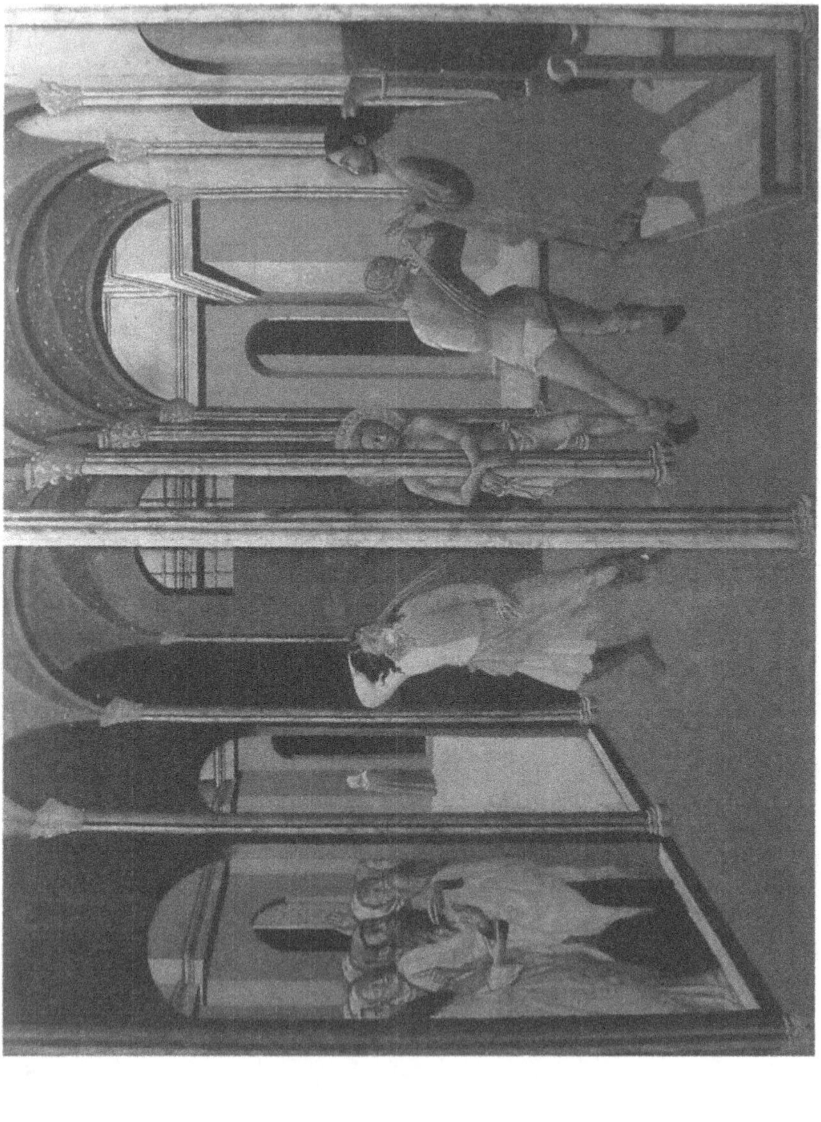

Fig. 29 [Col. pl. VII]. Master of the Osservanza, "Flagellation of Christ" (ca. 1425–1450). Tempera and gold on wood, 36.5 × 45.7 cm. Vatican, Musei Vaticani.

It is not clear, of course, if, and to what degree, the Petrarch Master was acquainted with Luther's thoughts on the meditation on the Passion of Christ. In the case of image II, 7 it is clear, however, that the Petrarch Master did not aim at making the viewer identify profoundly with the victim, since he glorifies neither the victim nor pain. As is the case with the other images by the Petrarch Master, pain does not have any transcendent or positive meaning. It is something exclusively negative, inflicted by people who display morally questionable behaviour. Most probably, the Petrarch Master wanted the viewer to see the cruel master as a reflection of himself. Interestingly enough, it is indeed the master who watches the scene, standing in the door. By making the viewer identify with the cruel master, the artist puts forward a moralistic critique of the outrageous punishments inflicted by early modern servant keepers. The viewer who watches the flagellation of the servant should understand that he is not any better than the Roman hypocrite governor Pontius Pilatus, who ordered the flagellation of Christ. In this ingenious construction of the image, physical pain serves as a means of simultaneously moral, social, religious and political commentary.

An interesting and to a certain degree related example is chapter II, 29 "On bad servants" ("De servis malis"). In this chapter, Petrarch deals with the troubles that are caused by bad servants, who may turn out to be disobedient, to steal and to cheat. Petrarch's perspective clearly is that of the early modern master who suffers from the presence of this seemingly inevitable household staff. As an exception, Petrarch, in this chapter, does not so much engage in mental therapy, but offers practical advice. This may be due to the fact that in this case, he largely identifies with the position of Dolor, i.e. the grief of the servant keeper. As a scholar, dedicated to *otium*, study and silence, he considered servants annoying and noisy. If one keeps many servants, as he puts it, one will house as many enemies. They will do their best to turn the scholar's life into hell. Thus, he dissuades the reader from keeping a large number of servants and advises him not to choose handsome, but rather ordinary and trustworthy servants: 'protect yourself by keeping only a few servants of the most ordinary sort. Throw out the handsome ones, throw out the refined and cunning ones, and throw out those who take pride in a pretty face, a sly wit, or their sophistication. Among a few servants – and the stupid and rude ones – you live safer, not because they are better, but because they dare less, like snakes in the winter, hampered by their congealed venom and vile torpor of their numbness'.[59]

As the last comparison shows, Petrarch was inclined to regard his servants as a kind of dangerous *domestic enemies*. Scheidig misses the point when he identifies Petrarch's view on the matter as follows: 'Man soll mit den Knechten freundlich, glimpflich und gütig umgehen, leben und handeln [...]. Man soll nicht gebrauchen der Strafe, nicht der Schläge, sondern der Worte'. These are in fact Seneca's words,[60] with which Petrarch vehemently disagrees. It is no coincidence that Petrarch's concept of 'domestic enemies' ('hostes domestici', 'hostes familiares') occurs in the first lines of chapter II, 29 ('non familiari solum exercitu, sed hostili'). A letter which Petrarch wrote to Sennucio of Florence makes the autobiographical vein of this chapter of *De Remediis* visible:

> I have with me at home some three pairs of servants, or, to speak more modestly, of lower-class friends, or, to speak more truthfully, of *domestic enemies*. Of the first pair, one is tremendously doltish, the other dangerously sly. Of the second, one is rendered useless by his extreme youth, the other by old age. Of the third pair, one is shockingly mad, the other shockingly lazy [...]. Amidst such contrasts I used to be the overseer with the whip, but now, I just sit and observe them. Nor can I wonder enough about the purpose of those who consider throngs of servants as something glorious, and enjoy being forever besieged by those they feed, that is, their domestic plotters [...].[61]

Thus, in II, 29, Ratio surprisingly enough reinforces Dolor's complaints about bad slaves and states that the best thing is in this case to reduce the evil somewhat, according to the lines quoted above.

The Petrarch Master, by contrast, presents a much different argument, in which he emphasizes rather the extreme cruelty of early modern masters towards their servants; the same thing he has already done in his illustration to chapter II, 7. *It is, in fact, the master who turns the servant's life into hell.* In the left part of the image [Fig. 30] a master in person cuts off the tongue of a servant who is tied to a column; on the right part, another master beats a servant so violently on his buttocks that the instrument of punishment, a birch, falls into pieces. The broken twigs of the birch are scattered all over the floor. By his focus on physical pain the Petrarch Master suggests that the punishments are morally

[59] Trsl. Rawski, vol. III, 85.
[60] Seneca, *Epistulae ad Lucilium* 47.
[61] *Familiares* IV, 14 (ed. Rossi); trsl. by Rawski, vol. IV, 140 (italics mine).

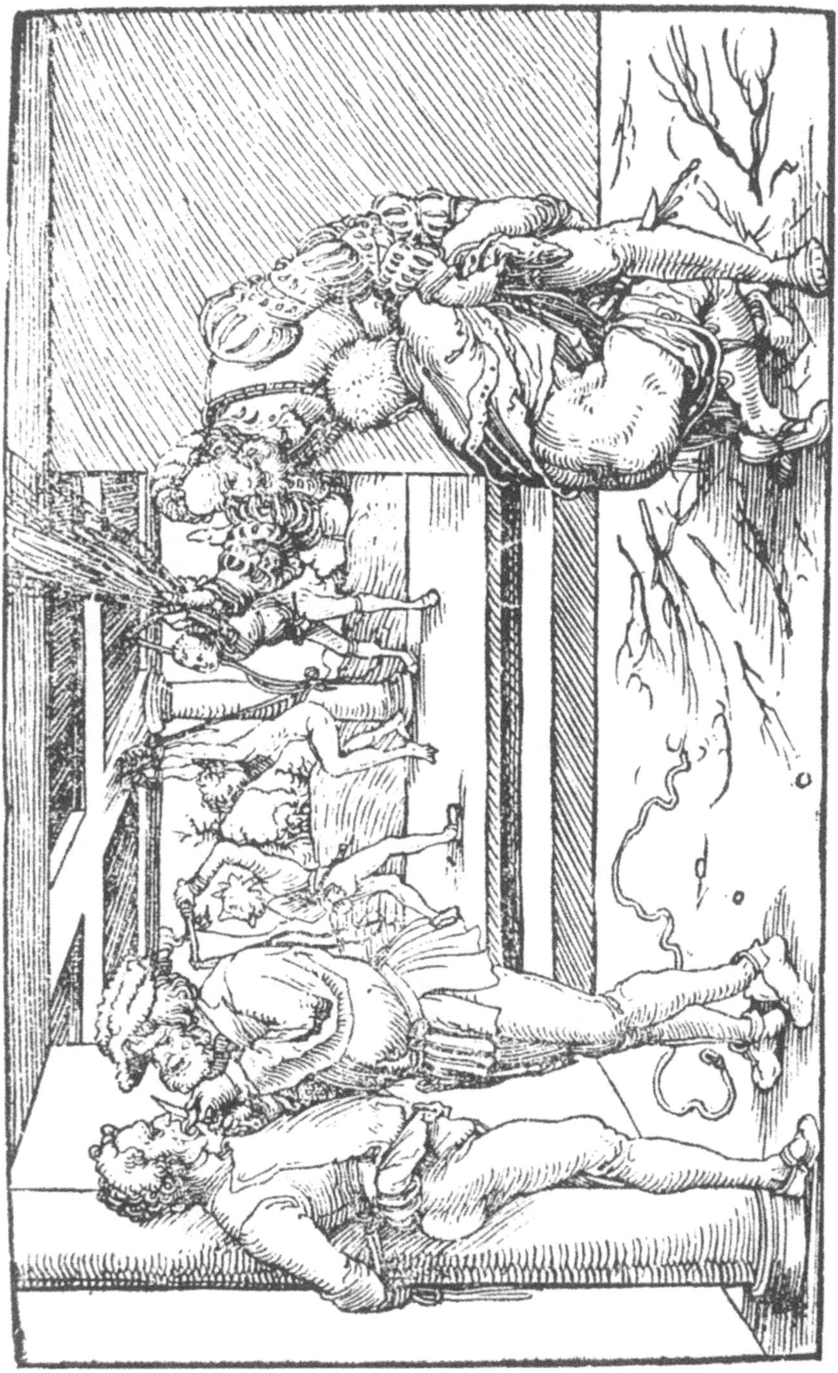

Fig. 30. The Petrarch Master, Woodcut illustration to Petrarch's *Von der Artzney baider Glueck* [...] (Augsburg: 1532), book II, chapter 29, fol. XXXVIIIr.

wrong, and that they are in fact tantamount to torture. The result of this spectacular rhetoric of pain is that the emotionalized viewer will feel compassion with the poor servants. This is meant to make the viewer embark on a moral meditation in which he will reconsider his behaviour towards his servants.

As is the case with II, 7, the meditative process activated by the Petrarch Master is essentially steered by the powerful religious image of the flagellation of Christ. The background scene shows a man, bound to and lifted up on a pillar, who is cruelly whipped by two tormenters. Here we have the standard elements of the traditional image: the column (the 'Geisselsäule' or 'flogging column'), the naked Christ, two (or more) tormenters with whips or flagella.[62] In the late Middle Ages, this scene was also singled out for panels meant for private devotion ('Andachtsbilder'), for example in Piero della Francesca's "Flagellation of Christ" in the Palazzo Ducale in Urbino. The Petrarch Master who was, of course, well acquainted with the iconography of the flagellation of Christ,[63] drew on it in order to put forward a Christian moral similar to II, 7: 'Do not treat your servants in a cruel way. If you do so, you are not any better than the tormenters of Christ'. In II, 29, the Petrarch Master ingeniously connects the "Flagellation of Christ" of the background scene to the scenes in the foreground: the servant in the left corner whose tongue is cut out is tied to a pillar like Christ, whereas the servant on the right is flogged like Christ.

Generally speaking, the Petrarch Master's Christian moral may fit in with the discourse of a house book as well as that of the Christian meditative treatise. In both cases the viewer is made to ponder Christian values such as mildness, compassion and forgiveness. In a meditative treatise, this may be a stepping stone towards a more profound contemplation of the relationship of the individual towards other human beings, or of Christian living as such. In the discourse of a house book, the statement may have practical implications as well: if one treats one's servants well, they will repay with good behaviour. If one treats them cruelly, they might take revenge. That the Petrarch Master wanted

[62] Kirschbaum E. S.J., *Lexikon der christlichen Ikonographie* (Rome – Freiburg – Basel – Vienna: 1994), vol. II, 126–130, s.v. "Geisselsäule, Christus an der" and "Geisselung Christi".

[63] The fact that he adds the strappado technique to his "Flagellation of Christ" does not prove his lack of knowledge. On the contrary, the strappado serves as a means to surpass his iconographic forerunners by increasing the cruelty of the torture.

the viewer to consider this possibility is suggested by the fact that the servant on the right, who is beaten by a birch, stabs his master in his left leg with a knife. The cruelty of the revenge is emphasized by the blood splashing out of the wound [Fig. 30].

How is the Petrarch Master's use of the flagellation of Christ related to late medieval 'Leidensmystik'? Did the Petrarch Master use physical pain as a means to make the viewer identify with the passion of Christ? This question is difficult to answer. While it is true that the servants are tortured like Christ, the servant to the right does not display anything like Christ's endurance. Instead of suffering willingly, he stabs his master in the leg. Similarly, the boorish-looking servant on the left hardly seems a glorification of martyrdom. It seems more likely, therefore, that also in II, 29 the Petrarch Master wanted the viewer to identify with the cruel masters. In emphasizing physical pain, he aims to persuade his viewer to adopt a milder and more compassionate behaviour towards his servants. Thus, moral, religious and political commentaries are interwoven.

Cutting off Ears

In the illustration to chapter II, 97 "On the Loss of Hearing" ("De auditu perdito") the Petrarch Master once more presents an image of extreme physical pain, while Petrarch's treatment of the topic is similar to his discussion of blindness in II, 96 or the loss of teeth in II, 94. Chapter II, 97, however, is especially remote from the discussion of physical pain, since Petrarch, in fact, treats the loss of hearing as a blessing. In doing so, he closely associates the physiological defect with the most positive aspects of human life, namely study, silence and contemplation. The deaf person is not distracted anymore by people who ly, cheat, gossip, quarrel and shout, but is able to dedicate his life to contemplation, inner dialogue, reading books, writing, prayer and religious meditation. As RATIO puts it,

> If one cannot converse with others, one can converse with himself, mindful of the Ciceronian maxim: 'Who can converse with himself does not need the conversations of another'.[64] Of course, even a deaf person can enter into discourse by reading and writing, for when we read we talk

[64] Cicero, *Tusculanae disputationes* VI, 117.

> with the ancients, and when we write we talk to posterity. But when we read the books of sacred philosophy, we hear the Lord God, and when we pray we talk to Him. For these we need neither tongue nor ears – only eyes and fingers, and a devout heart. [...] Therefore, since you cannot hear the voices of your fellow men, you should read the books written by them and write books for them to read. And contemplate in silence the heavens, the earth, the sea – and the Creator of it all.[65]

Thus, "On the Loss of Hearing" is one of the most peaceful chapters of *De remediis*. In marked difference, the Petrarch Master once and again perceives the loss of hearing in the first place as an illness, and focuses on medical treatment and on pain. On the left part of the image, an officially recognized medical doctor treats the ear of a patient with an ointment. Most eye-catching, however, is the violent scene in the centre of the woodcut, which shows St Peter cutting off the ear of the high priest's servant Malchus [Fig. 31]. The story is mentioned in all four Gospels (*Matth.* 26, 51; *Marc.* 14, 47; *Luc.* 22, 50), but most explicitly by John, who is the only one to give the servant's name (18, 10). When the soldiers of the high priest came to Gethsemane, as John tells us, 'Simon Peter, who had a sword drew it and smote the high priest's servant, and cut off his right ear. The name of the servant was Malchus'. It is a telling detail that the gospels of Matthew, Mark and Luke do not specify that it was Peter who struck off the servant's ear. They understood very well that this was a crime and refrained from accusing Peter of it. Luke even tries to undo the act of violence by telling a miracle: He claims that Christ healed the ear by putting it back on the servant's head.[66]

The story of St Peter and Malchus is not only absent from Petrarch's text; it is, in fact, irrelevant to the topic "On the Loss of Hearing" ("De auditu perdito").[67] If an ear is cut off, this does of course not necessarily mean that one becomes deaf. The image by the Petrarch Master engages in totally different arguments, which are situated in two discourses. The first argument regards practical life: it connects the image of Peter's sword cutting off the servant's ear with the German proverbial expression 'jemanden übers Ohr hauen', which means to cheat someone in a

[65] Trsl. Rawski, vol. III, 240–241.

[66] *Luc.* 22, 51: 'et cum tetigisset (sc. Iesus) auriculam eius, sanavit eum'.

[67] Scheidig, *Die Holzschnitte des Petrarca-Meisters* 300, admits: 'Dieses Beispiel ist nicht gut gewählt, denn mit dem Abhauen des Ohres geht das Gehör nicht verloren'.

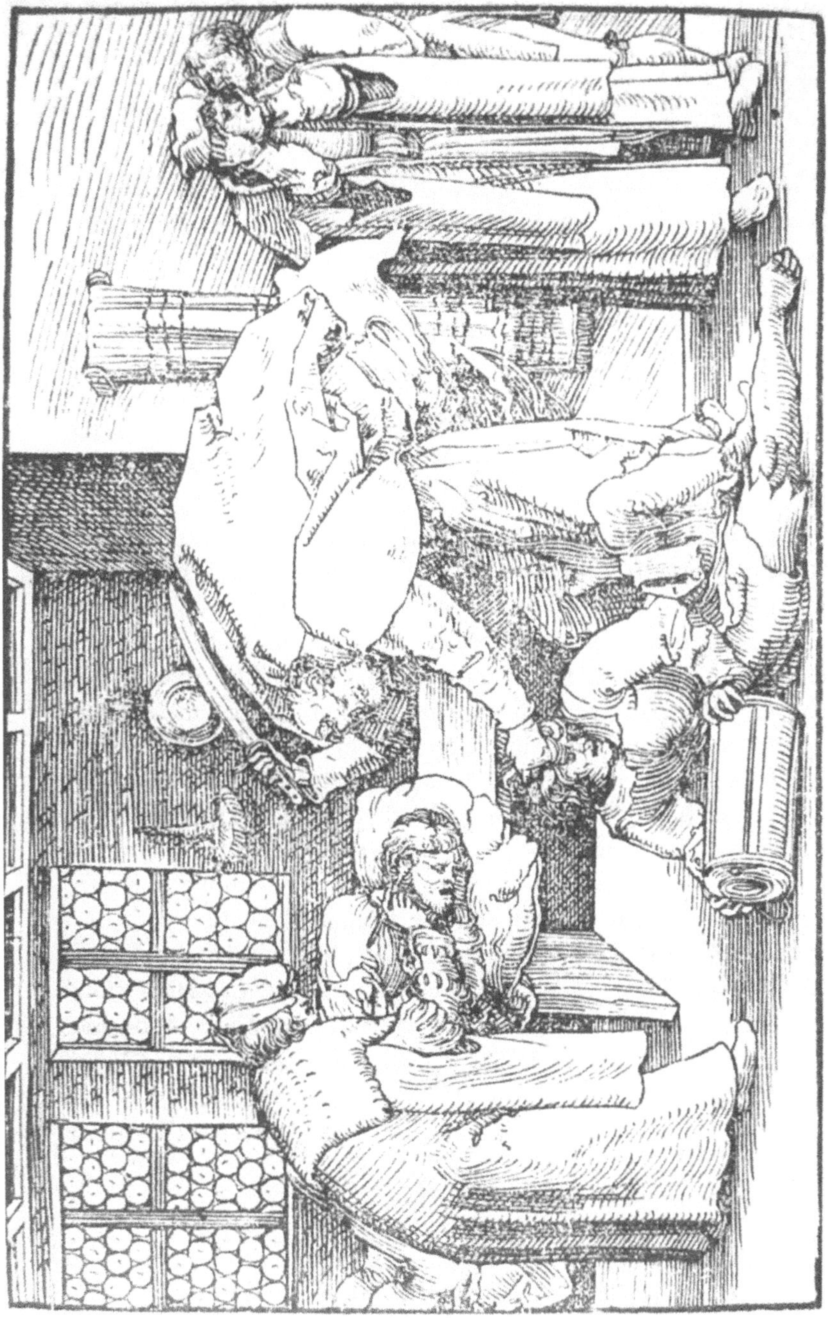

Fig. 31. The Petrarch Master, Woodcut illustration to Petrarch's *Von der Artzney baider Glueck* [...] (Augsburg: 1532), book II, chapter 97, fol. CXXIIIIr.

material or economic sense ('jemanden übervorteilen').[68] The proverbial expression is indeed derived from sword-fighting, and literally means 'to strike someone a blow on the ear' [Fig. 32]. In its proverbial, metaphorical sense the expression is akin to 'jemandem die Zähne ziehen', i.e. to harm someone, to get out money of him (cf. above). Thus, the Petrarch Master again launches an attack against contemporary medical doctors by warning their patients: if they hand themselves over to doctors in order to be treated for their loss of hearing, they will be cheated. The doctors will take their money, but the poor patients will stay as deaf as they were before.

On a second level, the polemic against doctors is superseded by an aggressive religious argument focusing on St Peter: it is Peter who will cut off the people's ear, i.e. who will cheat them. This argument was certainly relevant in 1520, the year in which the woodcut was probably made. It was in 1520 that the struggle between Peter's successor, Pope Leo X and Luther escalated. The papal ban against Luther which Leo X issued in the same year was published accompanied by an additional expression of support from the bishop of Augsburg, Christoph von Stadion.[69] It was also in 1520 that Luther himself published his pamphlet *Von dem Papsttum zu Rom*, in which he questioned the authority of the Pope, and argued against the financial exploitation of Germany by the Roman Church. As appears from a number of images, the Petrarch Master was an ardent Lutheran.[70] In several images, he attacks Peter as the first Pope and questions his legitimacy, for example in his illustration of *De remediis*, chapter I, 13.[71] Thus, the rhetoric of the image conveys a satirical warning against the Pope, Luther's archenemy.

In fact, the story, as told by St John, provides a beautiful and effective argument against St Peter and the Roman Pope, first because it proves that the first Pope was not infallible, as the Catholic Church claimed, but capable of unchristian behaviour. A true Christian should not physically harm his fellow humans, even less wound them. Second, St John's text demonstrates that Christ disagreed with the first Pope's behaviour. Christ in fact reproached Peter by telling him: 'Put back your sword'.[72] It is no coincidence that the Petrarch Master's rendering

[68] Röhrich, *Lexikon der sprichwörtlichen Redensarten*, IV, 1113, s.v. "Ohr".
[69] *Bulla contra errores Martini Luther et sequacium, cum mandato Reverendissimi domini Episcopi* Augustensis (Ingolstadt, Andreas Lutz: 1520).
[70] Cf. Enenkel, "Der Petrarca des Petrarca-Meisters" 95–115.
[71] For a discussion of this image see ibidem 95–104.
[72] John 18, 11: 'dixit ergo Iesus Petro: mitte gladium in vaginam'.

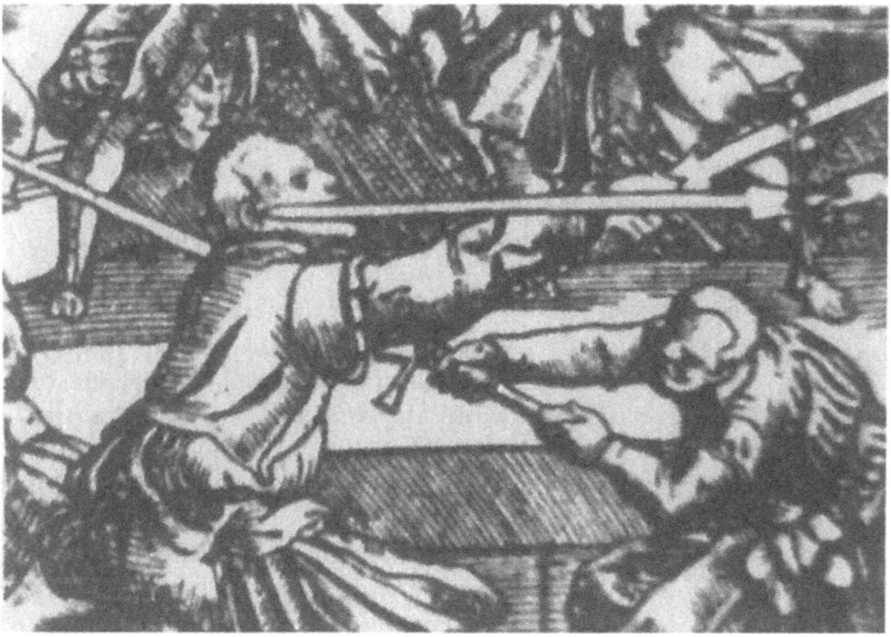

Fig. 32. "Übers Ohr hauen". Illustration from Röhrich, *Lexikon der sprichwörtlichen Redensarten*, 1113.

of the scene goes back to the gospel of John, whereas it deliberately leaves out Christ's healing that is included in Luke's version.

In his composition, the Petrarch Master focuses on Peter's unchristian behaviour and even enlarges it by his sophisticated use of the iconography of the scene. Scheidig has criticized the Petrarch Master's composition: 'So steht denn auch diese Gruppe (i.e. St Peter with Malchus) mit dem unmotiviert fliegenden Mantel des Jüngers fast wie ein Fremdkörper in der Komposition'.[73] Far from being 'unmotivated', Peter's floating cloak is in fact linked to the core of the Petrarch Master's interpretation. Moreover, the very fact that the scene looks unmotivated at first glance, is part of the Petrarch Master's pictorial rhetoric. For the construction of his image, the Petrarch Master could draw on a rich iconographic tradition, since the "Arrest of Christ", like all scenes of Christ's Passion, was depicted many times, especially in the Late Middle Ages. The scene was generally known, not in the last place because it was shown on many altar pieces in medieval churches. It is beyond doubt that contemporary users of the *Glücksbuch* would have immediately recognized it.

It should be noted that the scene of Peter cutting off Malchus' ear was always part of a larger composition in which Christ, the soldiers of the high priest (many a times in aggressive poses), and the kiss of Judas are to be seen. In many cases the emphasis is put on Judas' kiss, and hence on the betrayal of Christ. The very fact that the Petrarch Master singled out the scene with Peter and Malchus is vital to his iconographic construction and therefore to his argument, since the immediate result is that Peter's act of violence appears entirely unmotivated. There is no Christ anymore to be defended by his follower. There is no betrayal and there are no soldiers threatening Peter's master. Thus, in the Petrarch Master's image, it is Peter, not the high priest's henchman, who appears as the aggressor.

A second important device is that Peter strikes Malchus' ear while the poor servant lies on the ground, and does not struggle against Peter, nor bear any weapon. His hands hold a larger object which is not easy to identify at first glance, but, as other representations of the scene show, e.g. by Jan Joest of Kalkar, must be a lantern [Fig. 33]. The fact that Peter is bending over to strike Malchus as hard as possible emphasizes Peter's cruelty. By means of the floating cloak, the Petrarch Master

[73] Scheidig, *Die Holzschnitte des Petrarca-Meisters* 300.

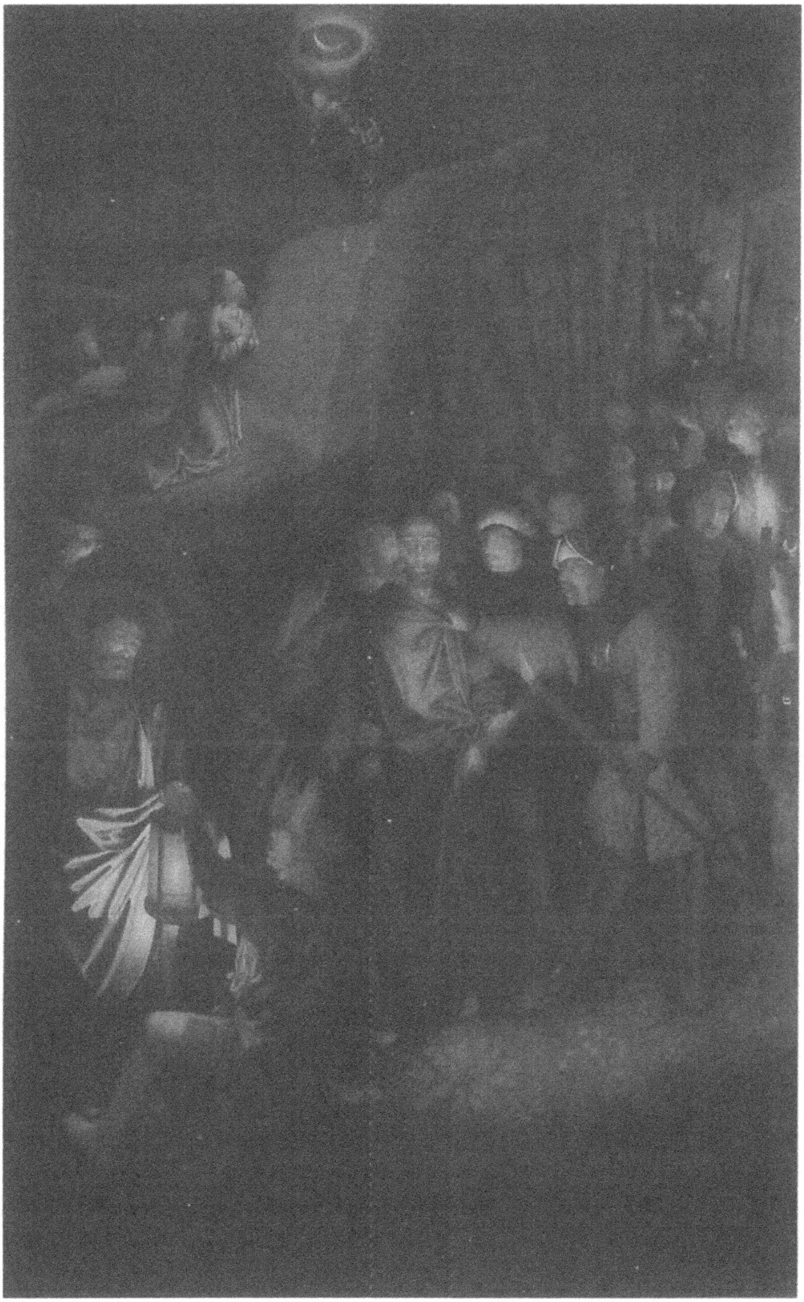

Fig. 33 [Col. pl. VIII]. Ascribed to Jan Joest of Kalkar, "Arrest of Christ" (ca. 1500). Altar table, 173 × 111 cm. Wittenberg, Schloßkirche.

succeeds in focusing attention on Peter's violent movement. It looks as if Peter is about to chop off Malchus' head. This is also suggested by the fact that Peter has seized the victim Malchus by the hair with his left hand. In fact, the scene comes close to an execution by sword. Malchus not only is lying helplessly on the ground, but also does not show any sign of resistance, defence or emotion (fear, surprise, pain). It looks as if he has patiently agreed to be beheaded.

Only if one compares the Petrarch Master's image with its iconographic forerunners do the subtlety, argumentative force and uniqueness of his visual construction become clear. There is not a single work of art that renders the scene in the same way. Indeed, the Petrarch Master makes idiosyncratic use of certain elements in the iconographic tradition of the scene to build up his argument. Malchus lying on the ground, for example, was part of the iconography as early as in the tenth century (Codex Egberti). Yet this was normally presented *as the result* of Peter's blow. It is never suggested that Peter was about to chop off the poor servant's head. If Malchus is depicted as lying on the ground, (from the thirteenth century on) he normally shows signs of defence, pain or emotional behaviour. Also, Peter is mostly depicted in an upright position, as for example in the painting of Duccio on the *Maestà* [Fig. 34],[74] on a Dutch altar table from Roermond (1435) now in the Rijksmuseum in Amsterdam,[75] on the altar of monastery Tempzin in Mecklenburg (1411) [Fig. 35][76] or Jan Joost of Kalkar's "Arrest of Christ" (ca. 1500) [Fig. 33].

There is one iconographic forerunner, however, on whom the Petrarch Master drew in particular: Dürer's woodcut with the "Arrest of Christ" of 1510 [Fig. 36]. The Petrarch Master is likely to have known this woodcut, since Dürer's passion cycle was published in 1511 (by Benedikt Schwalbe). In my view, the Petrarch Master's Peter is an imitation and further development of Dürer's Peter. He copied Dürer's depiction of Peter's movement, but enlarged the figure of the apostle, especially by adding the floating cloak in order to increase the violence of the movement [Fig. 37 Dürer versus Fig. 38 Petrarch Master]. In Dürer's woodcut, however, Peter's act of violence is motivated by the fact that Christ is surrounded by aggressive and fierce-looking soldiers. Dürer

---

[74] Cf. Weber A., *Duccio di Buoninsegna, um 1255–1319* (Cologne: 1997) 78.
[75] Depicted in Kirschbaum, *Lexikon der christlichen Ikonographie*, vol. III, 82.
[76] Krüger R., *Altdeutsche Tafelmalerei* (Berlin: 1974) no. 5.

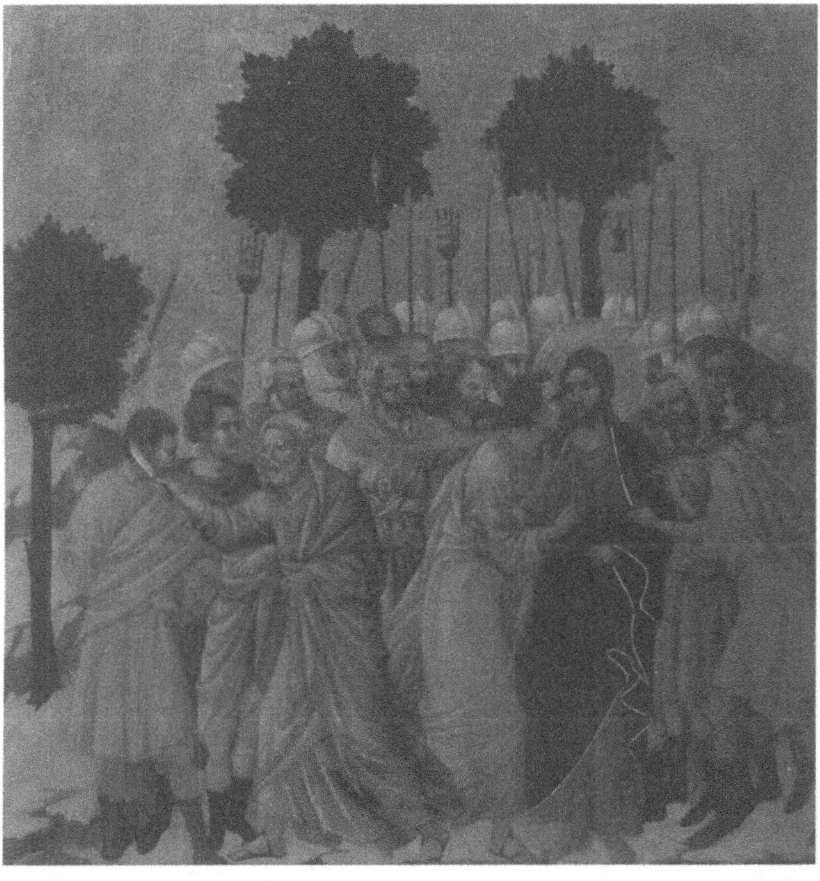

Fig. 34 [Col. pl. IX]. Duccio, "Imprisonment of Christ", part of his *Maestà* painted for the cathedral of Siena (1308–1311). Tempera on wood, 102 × 76 cm. Siena, Museo dell' Opera di Duomo. Detail, left part of the painting.

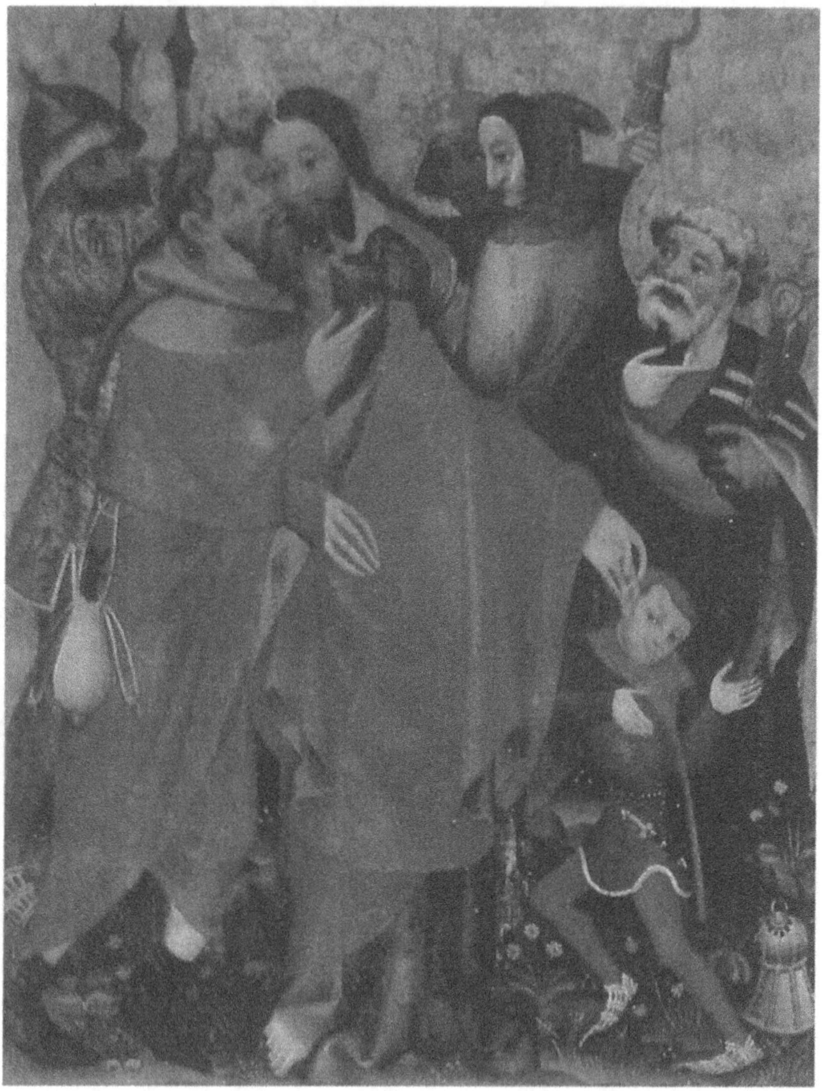

Fig. 35 [Col. pl. X]. Anonymous, Altar of monastery Tempzin (Mecklenburg, 1411). Tempera on wood, 180 × 204 cm. Schwerin, Staatliches Museum. Detail.

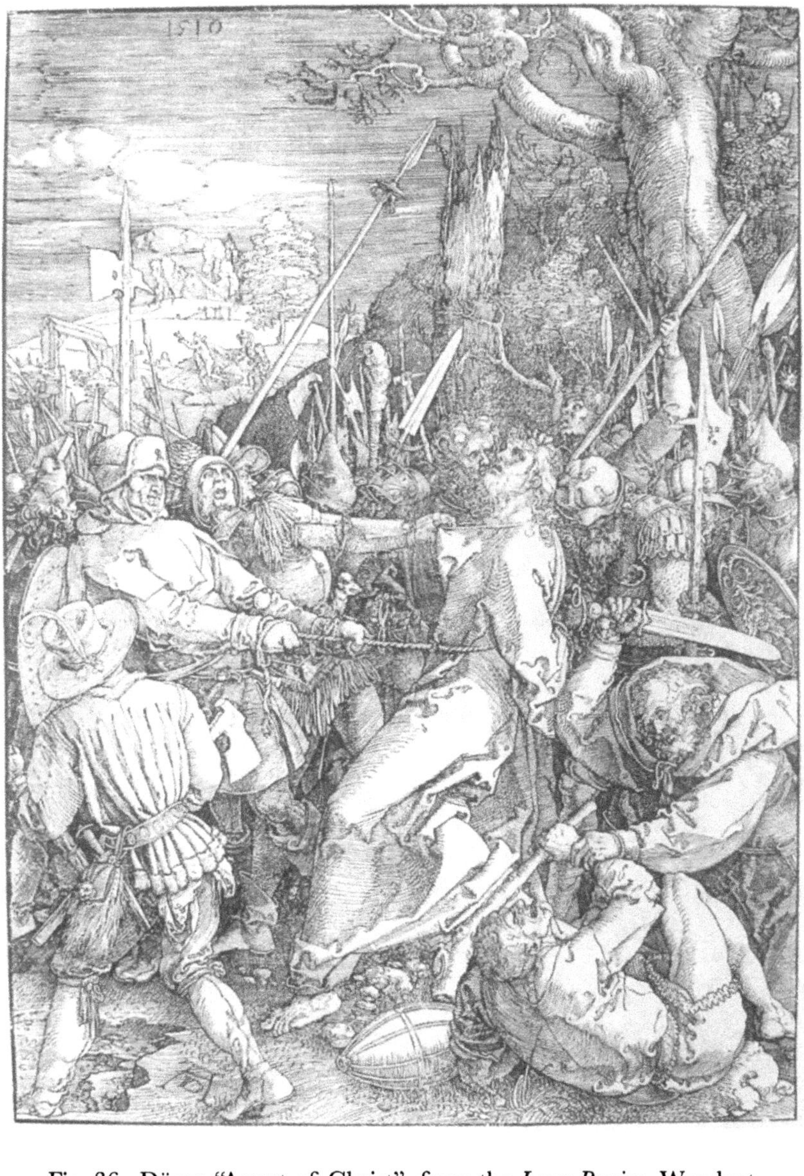

Fig. 36. Dürer, "Arrest of Christ", from the *Large Passion*. Woodcut, 39.1 × 27.7 cm.

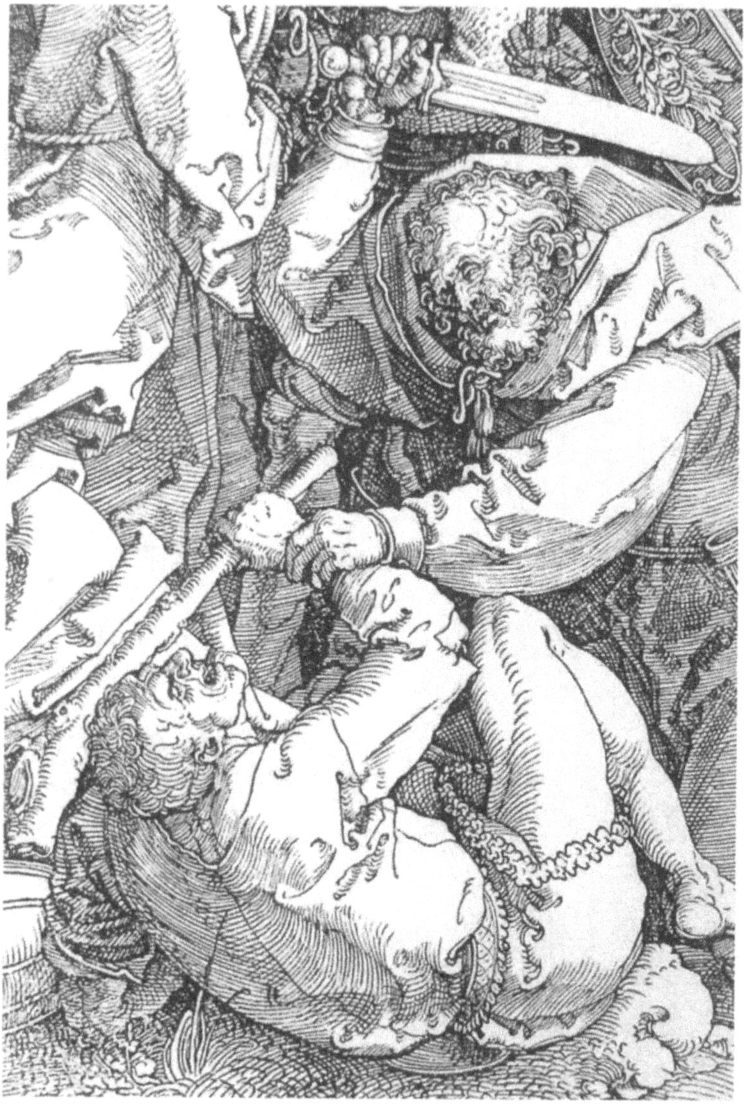

Fig. 37. Dürer, "Arrest of Christ", from the *Large Passion*. Woodcut, 39.1 × 27.7 cm. Detail.

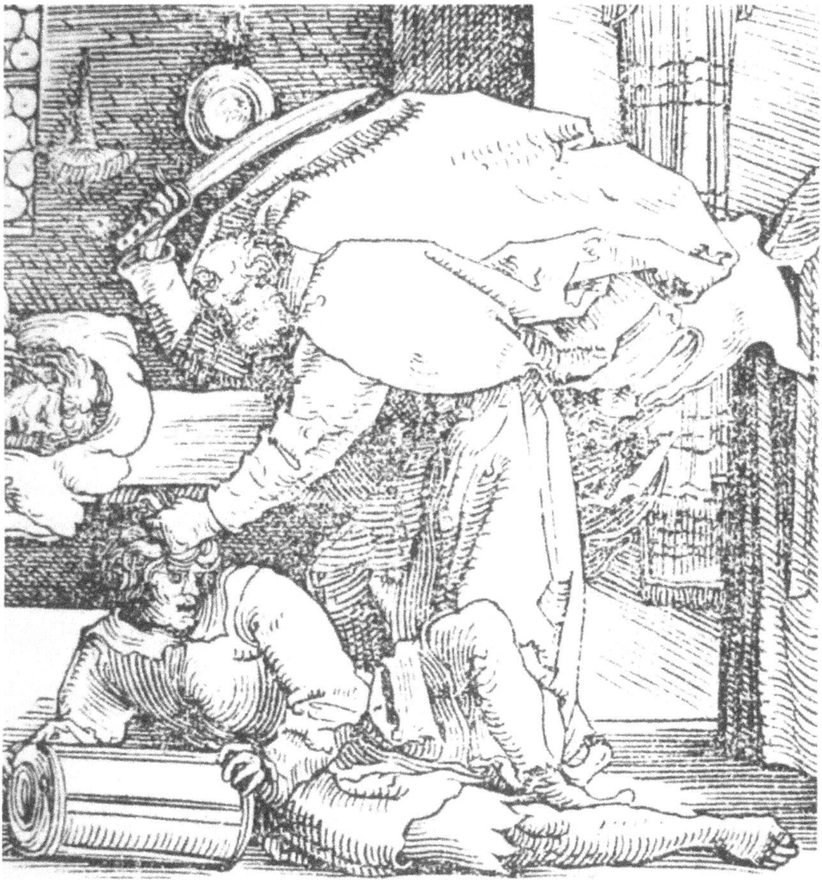

Fig. 38. The Petrarch Master, Woodcut illustration to Petrarch's *Von der Artzney baider Glueck* [...] (Augsburg: 1532), book II, chapter 97, fol. CXXIIIIr. Detail, central part of the image.

emphasized the threat of the soldiers by depicting a large number of weapons, more than 40 (!), halberds, spears, pikes, axes, swords, daggers, stars, clubs and so on [Fig. 36]. It is a telling detail that Malchus, too, has a weapon in his right hand: a large club, which he apparently had lifted up with the intention of hitting Peter. It seems only logical that Peter seizes Malchus' right hand to prevent him from doing so. Furthermore, Malchus' face shows a blend of fear and aggression. Thus, Dürer's scene depicts a fierce physical struggle, rather than the slaughtering of a helpless victim. The Petrarch Master, however, reinterpreted the gesture of Peter's left hand, which now seizes Malchus' hair. Since his Malchus does not show any signs of aggression, resistance or defence, the result is, of course, the opposite: his scene does not portray a fight, but *a cruel execution.*

By means of his intriguing play with the iconographic forerunners of the scene, the Petrarch Master launches a fierce polemical attack on the Roman Pope, suggesting that he is a violent aggressor, a ruthless slaughterer, a pitiless executioner, or in short: the Anti-Christ whom true Christians should fear, as Luther argued. If they erroneously support the Anti-Christ, they will be cruelly hurt by him, just like the poor victim lying on the ground. In his rhetoric of physical pain, the Petrarch Master makes the viewer identify with Malchus, not with Peter. He emotionalizes the viewer, so as to make him fear and hate Peter and the Roman Pope. Thus, in this image, physical pain functions as a trigger for religious polemic. In this sense, the image accompanying chapter II, 97 looks like a Lutheran pamphlet against the pope.

Conclusion

The Petrarch Master attributed to physical pain meanings and functions that differ markedly from Petrarch's text. This may be due partly to the vernacular context in which the artist worked, partly to the various discourses in which his pictorial inventions are situated (the Ship of Fools, and a range of proverbial expressions), and partly to the historical context of confessional strife in the crucial year of 1520, which caused an increased interest in political and religious propaganda. Petrarch's Christian Neo-Stoicism, however, conveyed a message that uneducated people would have found difficult to understand. In his images, the Petrarch Master did not try to illustrate Petrarch's thought, or to explain it to the uneducated, but showed a remarkable independence by conveying radically different ideas. For this, he invented a powerful rhetoric of physical pain which functioned as a means to achieve various goals. Through the Petrarch Master's intensive use of physical pain, the Stoic striving against the emotions, the *passiones animi*, is superseded by other discourses, such as practical advice for daily life in the manner of a house book, social and religious criticism, political satire and aggressive Lutheran religious polemic. In his pictorial inventions, the Petrarch Master sometimes uses pain in order to make the viewer identify with those who suffer from it. Sometimes he wanted the viewers to identify with those who inflict pain, in order to make them change their behaviour. By emphasizing physical pain, he stirs up emotional reactions such as fear, distress or grief, by which he makes his audience receptive to his advice and to his warnings. In his political and religious polemics he uses physical pain to incite hatred against the most powerful, among others the Emperor and the Pope. The Petrarch Master makes the viewer feel the violation, and indeed the humiliation of the human body, partly in order to make him question existing structures of power. In this sense, the remarkable focus on physical pain to be seen in the Petrarch Master's images is connected with the increased tension of political, religious and social life around 1520, a crucial year in the history of the Protestant Reformation.

Selective Bibliography

Buchner E., "Der Petrarka-Meister als Maler, Miniator und Zeichner", in *Festschrift für H. Wölfflin* (Munich: 1924) 209–232.
Bynum Walker C., *The Resurrection of the Body in Western Christianity, 200–1336* (New York: 1995).
Cohen E., "The Animated Pain of the Body", *American Historical Review* 105,1 (2006) 36–68.
Edwards M.U., *Printing, Propaganda, and Martin Luther* (Berkeley: 1994).
Constable G., *Attitudes towards Self-Inflicted Suffering in the Middle Ages* (Brookline, MA: 1982).
Enenkel K.A.E., "Der Petrarca des Petrarca-Meisters: Zum Text-Bild-Verhältnis in illustrierten *De-Remediis*-Ausgaben", in Enenkel K.A.E. – Papy J. (eds.), *Petrarch and his Readers in the Renaissance*, in *Intersections. Yearbook for Early Modern Studies* 6 (2006) 91–169.
——, *Die Erfindung des Menschen. Die Autobiographik des frühneuzeitlichen Humanismus von Petrarca bis Lipsius* (Berlin: 2008).
——, "Das Unglück des körperlichen Schmerzes: zur Leistung von Text und Bild in der Augsburger Ausgabe von Petrarcas Glücksbuch", Vortrag am Max-Plank-Institut für Kunstgeschichte (Florence: 2007).
——, "Der Zusammenprall frühneuzeitlicher Weisheitssysteme in Wort und Bild: Die Augsburger Ausgabe von Petrarcas Glücksbuch (*De remediis utriusque fortune*)", in *Östliche und Westliche Weisheitssysteme*. Vortraggsreihe der Universität Trier (Trier: 2008).
——, *Francesco Petrarca, De vita solitaria, Buch 1. Kritische Textausgabe und ideengeschichtlicher Kommentar* (Leiden – New York – Cologne – Kopenhagen: 1990).
Faulstich W., *Medien zwischen Herrschaft und Revolte. Die Medienkultur der Frühen Neuzeit* (1400–1700) (Göttingen: 1998).
Fraenger W., *Altdeutsches Bilderbuch. Hans Weiditz und Sebastian Brant* (Leipzig: 1930).
Geiss, J., "Herausgeber, Korrektor, Verlagslektor. Sebastian Brant und die Petrarca-Ausgabe von 1496", in Wilhelmi Th. (ed.), *Sebastian Brant. Forschungsbeiträge zu seinem Leben, zum Narrenschiff und zum übrigen Werk* (Basel: 2002) 83–102.
Gregory B., *Salvation at Stake: Christian Martyrdom in Early Modern Europe* (Cambridge, MA: 1999).
Hamm B., "Die Reformation als Medienereignis", *Jahrbuch für Biblische Theologie* 11 (1996) 138–166.
Heitmann K., *Fortuna und Virtus. Eine Studie zu Petrarcas Lebensweisheit* (Cologne: 1958).
Hess G., *Deutsch-Lateinische Narrenzunft. Studien zum Verhältnis von Volkssprache und Latinität in der satirischen Literatur des 16. Jahrhunderts* (Munich: 1971).
Hoffmann K., "Wort und Bild im *Narrenschiff*", in Grenzmann L. – Stackmann K. (eds.), *Literatur und Laienbildung im Spätmittelalter und in der Reformationszeit*. Symposion Wolfenbüttel 1981 (Stuttgart: 1984) 392–426.
Iserloh E., *Geschichte und Theologie der Reformation im Grundriß* (Paderborn: 1985, 3rd. ed.).
Knape J., *Die ältesten deutschen Übersetzungen von Petrarcas 'Glücksbuch'. Texte und Untersuchungen* (Bamberg: 1986) (Gratia. Bamberger Schriften zur Renaissanceforschung 15).
Lanckoronska M. Gräfin, "Der Petrarcameister. Eine vorläufige Mitteilung", *Gutenberg-Jahrbuch* 27 (1952) 111–120.
——, "Der Petrarcameister und die Reformation", *Imprimatur* 11 (1952–1953) 162–174.
——, "Weiteres zur Identifizierung des Petrarcameisters", *Stultifera navis* 11 (1954) 35–43.
——, "Die Burgkmair-Werkstatt und der Petrarcameister", *Gutenberg-Jahrbuch* 29 (1954) 171–180.
Lemmer M., "Nachwort", in Petrarca, Francesco, *Von der Artzney* [...] 181–209.
——, *Die Holzschnitte zu Sebastian Brants 'Narrenschiff'* (Leipzig: 1964).

MANGER K., *Das 'Narrenschiff'. Entstehung, Wirkung und Deutung* (Darmstadt: 1983) (Erträge der Forschung 186).

MANN N., "Manuscripts of Petrarch's *De remediis*. A Checklist", *Italia medioevale e umanistica* 14 (1971) 57–90.

MARXER E.M., *Text und Illustration bei Sebastian Brant und Konrad Celtis*, Diss. Ms. (Vienna: 1960).

MERBACK M.B., *The Thief, the Cross and the Wheel: Pain and the Spectacle of Punishment in Medieval and Renaissance Europe* (London: 1999).

MORRIS D.B., *The Culture of Pain* (Berkeley – Los Angeles: 1993).

MÜLLER J.-D., "Poet, Prophet, Politiker: Sebastian Brant als Publizist und die Rolle der laikalen Intelligenz um 1500", *Zeitschrift für Literaturwissenschaft und Linguistik* 10 (1980) 102–127.

MUSPER Th., *Die Holzschnitte des Petrarca-Meisters. Ein kritisches Verzeichnis mit Einleitung und 28 Abbildungen* (Munich: 1927).

PERKINS J., *The Suffering Self: Pain and Narrative Representation in the Early Christian Era* (London: 1995).

PETRARCA FRANCESCO, *De remediis utriusque fortune* s. idem, *Opera latina*, ed. J. Herold (Basel: 1981) 1–254 (reprint Ridgewood, New Jersey: 1965).

—— (Pétrarque), *Les Remèdes aus deux fortunes. De remediis utriusque fortune*, vol. I, Texte et traduction par Ch. Carraud; vol. II, Commentaires, notes et index (Grenoble: 2002).

——, *Von der Artzney bayder Glueck, des guten und widerwertigen* (Augsburg, H. Steyner: 1532), Facsimile-Edition, *herausgegeben und kommentiert von* M. Lemmer (Leipzig: 1984).

——, *Remedies for Fortune Fair and Foul. A Modern English Translation of* De remedies utriusque fortunae, *with a Commentary by* C.H. Rawski, 5 vols. (Bloomington – Indianapolis: 1991).

RAUPP H.-J., "Die Illustrationen zu Francesco Petrarca 'Von der Artzney bayder Glueck des guten und des widerwertigen' (Augsburg 1532)", *Wallraf-Richartz-Jahrbuch* 45 (1984) 59–112.

REDGRAVE G.R., *The Illustrated Books of Sebastian Brant* (London: 1896).

RÖHRICH L., *Lexikon der sprichwörtlichen Redensarten* (Munich: 2001).

ROSENFELD H., "Sebastian Brant und Albrecht Dürer. Zum Verhältnis von Bild und Text im Narrenschiff", *Gutenberg-Jahrbuch* 47 (1972) 328–336.

——, "Sebastian Brants Narrenschiff und die Tradition der Ständesatire, Narrenbilderbogen und Flugblätter des 15. Jahrhunderts", *Gutenberg-Jahrbuch* 40 (1965) 242–248.

RÖTTINGER H., *Hans Weiditz, der Petrarca-Meister* (Straßburg: 1904).

SCARRY E., *The Body in Pain: The Making and Unmaking of the World* (Oxford: 1985).

SCHEIDIG W., *Die Holzschnitte des Petrarca-Meisters* (Berlin: 1955).

SCHNEIDER B., "Virgilius pictus – Sebastian Brants illustrierte Vergilausgabe von 1502 und ihre Nachwirkung", *Wolfenbüttler Beiträge* 6 (1983) 202–262.

SCHOTTENLOHER K., "Der Augsburger Verleger Sigmund Grimm und sein Geschäftszusammenbruch im Oktober 1927", *Der Sammler* 11 (1921) 344–345.

SILVERMAN L., *Tortured Subjects: Pain, Truth, and the Body in Early Modern France* (Chicago: 2001).

SPIERENBURG P., *The Spectacle of Suffering: Executions and the Evolution of Repression: From a Preindustrial Metropolis to the European Experience* (Cambridge: 1984).

STEINMANN U., "Die politische Tendenz des Petrarca-Meisters. Seine Stellungnahme gegen die Wahl Karls V. und sein Verhalten zu den Ereignissen in Württemberg", *Staatliche Museen zu Berlin. Forschungen und Berichte* 6 (1964) 40–90.

——, "Der Ständebaum des Petrarkameisters. Ein Hinweis auf seine Beziehungen zu den 'Böhmischen Brüdern'", *Letopis. Jahresschrift des Instituts für serbische Volksforschung. Festschrift für Paul Neto. Reihe C – Volkskunde* 11/12 (Bautzen: 1968–1969) 251–263.

TRAPP J.B., *Studies of Petrarch and his Influence* (London: 2003).

——, "Illustrated Manuscripts of Petrarch's De Remediis Utriusque Fortunae", in idem, *Studies of Petrarch and his Influence* 118–170.
Welt im Umbruch. Augsburg zwischen Renaissance und Barock (Augsburg: 1980).
Winkler F., *Dürer und die Illustrationen zum Narrenschiff* (Berlin: 1951).
Wohlfeil R. – Wohlfeil T., "Verbildlichung ständischer Gesellschaft. Bartholomäus Bruyn d.Ä. – Petrarcameister (mit Exkursen von Marlies Minuth und Heike Talkenberger)", in Schulze W. (ed.), *Ständische Gesellschaft und soziale Mobilität* (Munich: 1988) 269–331.

GREEN WOUNDS: PAIN, ANGER AND REVENGE IN EARLY MODERN CULTURE

Kristine Steenbergh

Recent research argues that, in early modern culture, the passions were experienced as bodily phenomena. The emotions were produced by the humours. These four fluids should not be seen as metaphorical concepts; rather, choler, melancholy, blood and phlegm are material substances that literally travel through the body.[1] As a consequence, the emotions in this psychological materialism are physically felt: a passion is a bodily sensation. In the words of Robert Burton's *Anatomy of Melancholy*, the passions 'are drowned in corporeal organs of sense'.[2] One sensation that the passions could be experienced as, is the feeling of pain.[3]

Richard Strier recently argued that this material approach to the emotions, which studies the bodily processes associated with the passions in early modern texts, will not render any insights into actual experience. Emotions may be described as physical phenomena in medical texts of the period, but that does not mean that early modern subjects also *felt* the emotions as such. 'When an early modern person got angry', he writes, 'he or she did not say to her/himself: "Oh dear, my liver is heating up; my choleric humour is being activated, etc." [...] Instead, then, as now, people said, "That makes me mad, and I'm going to retaliate, or remember", or something along those lines'.[4] A proper historical phenomenology, in Strier's view, should not concentrate on the operations of the body, but on the mental processes of anger. Research ought to focus on the reasons that made people angry as well as on the decisions that result from the passion: 'To make a phenomenology historical, one needs to reconstruct the kinds of things that

[1] See Paster G.K., *Humoring the Body: Emotions and the Shakespearean Stage* (Chicago: 2004).

[2] Burton R, *The Anatomy of Melancholy* (Oxford, John Lichfield: 1621) fol. H8v.

[3] Babb L., *The Elizabethan Malady: A Study of Melancholia in English Literature from 1580 to 1642* (East Lansing: 1951) 13.

[4] Strier R. – Mazzio C., "Two Responses to 'Shakespeare and Embodiment: An E-Conversation'", *Literature Compass* 3,1 (2005) 17.

made persons at some time react (anger, in both men and women, to continue the instance, was often tied to ideas about honor)'.[5] In Strier's view, a history of ideas would bring us closer to past experiences of anger than a reconstruction of early modern ideas about the bodily operations of passion.

This article is not a defence of historical phenomenologies based on bodily experience, simply because they do not need defending.[6] Many characters in early modern literature do precisely what Strier denies: they remark on the heat in their liver or the boiling of their blood. Other characters do in turn proclaim that they will remember or retaliate. The distinction Strier makes between bodily experience and what we could call intentionality ('I am going to retaliate') should not lead to an exclusive choice between these two approaches to the experience of the emotions. In fact, I would argue that the distinction is one that was made in the early modern period itself, and it was a distinction that functioned politically. Rather than argue for either approach to the role of anger, it interests me to see how these two perspectives on anger operated in early modern culture, and in which institutional and political circumstances the choice between these two views was made. In what follows, I will explore representations of the role of pain in the anger of the avenger to trace the ways in which this distinction between the bodily experience and the goal-orientedness of anger is used politically in different discourses. As I will argue, the conflicts between these discourses in their outlook on anger centre in part around their understandings of pain.

Pain in Aristotelian and Senecan Views of Anger

The division that Strier makes between anger as a purely physical experience and as a means unto a goal is inherent in two conflicting views of anger from antiquity current in the early modern period. Whereas

[5] Strier – Mazzio, "Two Responses" 16–17.

[6] Recent works on the passions from a material perspective include Schoenfeldt M., *Bodies and Selves in Early Modern England: Physiology and Inwardness in Spenser, Shakespeare, Herbert and Milton* (Cambridge: 1999); Paster G.K. – Rowe K. – Floyd-Wilson M. (eds.), *Reading the Early Modern Passions* (Philadelphia: 2004); Paster G.K., *Humoring the Body*, and Floyd-Wilson M. – Sullivan G.A. Jr. (eds.), *Environment and Embodiment in Early Modern England* (Houndmills, Basingstoke: 2007). The introduction to the latter work includes a longer list of recent works on the 'ecology of the emotions' in note 5.

Aristotle's philosophical works allow for a view of anger as contributing to virtue, Senecan Stoicism views anger as an irrational emotion that needs to be suppressed by reason at all cost. The experience of pain plays an important role in both these philosophers' thinking on anger.

Aristotle defines anger as 'a longing, accompanied by pain, for a real or apparent revenge for a real and apparent slight'.[7] He acknowledges that the emotions have a physical basis, but he does not view the emotions solely in terms of their material states, such as the temperature of the blood or the workings of bile. Instead, he stresses the rational and cognitive aspects of emotion. Anger in Aristotle's view is not a bodily reflex, but depends on a subtle set of judgements.[8] Therefore, anger does not need to be suppressed in all cases. When it is felt for the right reasons, anger can be morally right. Indeed, Aristotle distinguishes a type of martial anger, which 'is more like a universal drive toward the particular goods of honour and freedom from tyranny'.[9] This type of martial anger is oriented towards a goal; it is a rational type of anger. When the bodily experience, the feeling of pain, comes into play however, Aristotle's position on anger becomes more ambiguous. Although he defends martial anger, he does not unequivocally approve of courage that is sparked by the pain of anger:

> [H]uman beings also feel pain when angry, and take pleasure in revenge. But those who fight for these motives, though valiant fighters, are not courageous; for the motive of their confidence is not honor, nor is it guided by principle, but it springs from feeling. However, they show some affinity to true Courage.[10]

Aristotle's ambiguous view of anger and courage is rooted in the opposition between the senses and moral principles. If a warrior is spurred to courage by a bodily sensation, a 'feeling' of pain and the consequent desire for revenge, then he is not as courageous as a valiant fighter who is motivated rather by honour or principle.

Whereas Aristotle acknowledges that valiant warriors spurred by the pain of anger at least display some signs of courage, Seneca disapproves

---

[7] *Aristotle, The Art of Rhetoric*, trl. Freese J.H. (Cambridge: 1924) 2.84, 1378a.

[8] Konstan D., "Aristotle on Anger and the Emotions," in Braund S. – Most G.W. (eds.), *Ancient Anger: Perspectives from Homer to Galen* (Cambridge: 2003) 105–107.

[9] Koziak B., *Thumos, Aristotle, and Gender* (University Park, PA: 2000) 86.

[10] Aristotle, *Nicomachean Ethics*, trl. Rackham H., *Aristotle in 23 Volumes*, vol. 19 (Cambridge, MA – London: 1934) Book 3, 1117A.

of the emotion altogether. Anger is a complicated emotion in Stoic philosophy, because it combines two of the primal emotions: pain and desire. Anger is characterized by a desire for revenge, but that desire arises from the impression of an injustice in the present, and not from something desirable in the future. This double motor behind anger is made explicit in the first sentence of Seneca's treatise on anger, *De Ira*, where anger is characterized by pain (*dolor*), and the desire (*cupiditas*) for revenge.[11] From the perspective of Stoicism, reactions to an injury should be based on rational deliberation rather than on emotion. In the seventeenth-century English translation of Seneca's *De Ira*, Thomas Lodge phrases it as follows: 'Reuenge is a confession of paine. The minde is not great which is animated by iniurie'.[12] As a confession of pain, the passion of anger in Seneca's philosophical writing causes more pain. Even though it is aimed at hurting another person, anger eventually wounds the choleric persons themselves. *De Ira* describes anger as 'neglecting oneself so one may hurt another' (510). This neglect of the self has a tendency to backfire, and Seneca warns of the consequences: 'we ought to consider [...] how many men wrath hath armed to wound themselues. Some thorow too much rage haue burst their veines, and by force of crying haue vomited blood' (550–551). He draws a picture of anger that stresses this danger of self-inflicted wounds:

> In such manner should we picture out anger, that hath fierie furie in her eyes, [...] shaking in both her handes her dierful weapons *without care of couering her bodie*, frowning, *couered with bloud and wounds: yea mortified with strokes which shee hath giuen her selfe*, [...] *and aboue al things wishing her owne death*. [...] Or if a man will behold her in such sort as our Poets describe her: She in her hand shaketh a bloudie whip (550) [italics mine].

Whereas Aristotle argued that the painful feeling of anger can spur a man to a kind of courage, Seneca sees anger as an inherently excessive emotion that is incapable of being directed at a higher goal. Instead, it turns in upon itself. Aristotle's angry person channels his anger to inflict pain on another, but Seneca's angry person is so lost in the emotion that he can do nothing but inflict pain on his own body. These two views on anger, which also reverberate in Strier's opposition between

---

[11] See Vogt K.M., "Anger, Present Injustice and Future Revenge in Seneca's *De Ira*", in Volk K. – Williams G.D. (eds.), *Seeing Seneca Whole: Perspectives on Philosophy, Poetry and Politics* (Leiden – Boston: 2006) 57–74.

[12] Thomas Lodge, *The Workes of Lucius Annaeus Seneca* (London, William Stansby: 1614) 55–57.

bodily experience and intentionality, also circulated in early modern culture. They were not neutral views, but connected to networks of political discourses.

The Politics of Anger

Norbert Elias in his *Civilizing Process* described how the centralization of power in the early modern period led to a state monopoly of physical violence, and to what he called a 'civilizing process': a restraint and moderation of the emotions. With the feuds of the Wars of the Roses well in mind, the Tudor state was especially aware of the dangers of a strong nobility. Queen Elizabeth in her royal proclamations objected to the scale of some aristocratic households, which 'plainly hinder justice and disorder the good policy of the realm [...] by stirring up and nourishing of factions [and] riots'.[13] The state adapted socio-legal systems to replace forms of aristocratic self-government with a centralized system of power. One of the key rights to be appropriated from the nobility by the state was the right to execute legitimate violence. By means of a growing number of Justices of the Peace, the state sought to replace private practices of retribution with a national legal system.[14] Lawrence Stone described how the Tudors not only tried to control the amount of weapons and the size of retainers' armies that aristocrats attached to themselves, but also approached matters from a moral angle:

> they sought to change men's attitudes of mind, to persuade the nobility themselves that resort to violence was not merely illegal and impolitic but also dishonourable and morally wrong; and to persuade the dependants and tenants of the nobility that loyalty to their lord should not extend to support of private quarrels by force of arms, much less to the taking up of arms against the sovereign.[15]

These strategies resulted in changes in conceptions of heroism in the period. The figure of the independent, aristocratic warrior became anachronistic: 'his status became ever more residual, like the chivalric

[13] Hughes P.L. – Larkin J.F., *Tudor Royal Proclamations*, vol. II: The Later Tudors (New Haven – London: 1969) 495–497.

[14] Smith A.G.R., *The Emergence of a Nation State: The Commonwealth of England 1529–1660* (London – New York: 1984) 134.

[15] Stone L., *The Crisis of the Aristocracy 1558–1641* (Oxford: 1965) 201.

imagery that adorns the Elizabethan court'.[16] In the place of the chivalric heroics of action came a heroic of endurance, a private heroic of patient suffering, humility, loyalty and obedience. These processes also affected the role of anger in early modern society. The emotion had been part of aristocratic patterns of behaviour, but was now starting to go out of favour. Gail Kern Paster has examined the role of Galenic humoralism in the social tropes of early modern urbanization and elite socialization.[17] She opens her analysis with a quotation from Thomas Wright's *The Passions of the Minde in General*, in which he complains of the proverbial anger of the English nobleman: 'how vngratefull must his company seeme, whose passions ouer-rule him? and a man had need of an Astrolabe alwayes, to see in what height or eleuation his affections are, lest, by casting forth a sparke of fire, his gun-powdred minde of a sudden bee inflamed'.[18] The passions were thus enlisted in a critique of the nobility's behaviour in this shift from chivalric codes to a new set of social conventions.

Although these notions of residual and emerging ideas elucidate long term processes of change, they tend to obfuscate the conflicts that took place between different discourses during these changes. The chivalric discourse had by no means lost its power in the early modern period. Richard McCoy has shown how the nobility resisted the centralization of power, and how figureheads such as Essex and Leicester, but also authors such as Spenser, Sidney, and Daniel employed chivalric discourse as a way to protect the position of the aristocracy while at the same time avoiding conflicts with the monarch.[19] The passion of anger and its connection with pain play a role in these conflicts, as will appear from an analysis of the Elizabethan translations of Seneca's tragedies, and the representation of anger in Sir Philip Sidney's chivalric romance *The Countess of Pembroke's Arcadia*.

---

[16] Rose M.B., *Gender and Heroism in Early Modern English Literature* (Chicago: 2002) xiii.

[17] Paster G.K., *Humoring the Body* 194. See also Bryson B., *From Courtesy to Civility: Changing Codes of Conduct in Early Modern England* (Oxford: 1998).

[18] Paster, *Humoring the Body* 191.

[19] McCoy R., *Rites of Knighthood: The Literature and Politics of Elizabethan Chivalry* (Berkeley – Los Angeles: 1989).

Anger and Pain in Seneca's Revenge Tragedies

Seneca's tragedies were first translated into English in the 1560s, by a group of students and writers associated with the Inns of Court, the London schools of law. The translations are usually studied as precursors of the genre of revenge tragedy that was to flourish later in the period. Just recently, Jessica Winston was the first to examine them against the background of the social and political culture of the Inns of Court in the 1560s. She concluded that the work on the tragedies facilitated the translators' Latin learning, personal interactions, and political thinking and involvement.[20] If we consider not only the personal politics of the translators, but also the pivotal position of the Inns of Court in the expanding nation state, these translations can be seen to intervene in the conflict over the politics of anger. They take up Seneca's view of anger as a dangerous emotion. By feeding this view into early modern society, the translators can be said to intervene in aristocratic discourses that represented anger as a more positive emotion, following Aristotle.[21]

In comparison to the Latin original, the early modern translations of Seneca's tragedies emphasize the pain of anger. If the nurse in Seneca's text tells us that she 'recognize[s] the marks of [Medea's] old-time rage' (*irae novimus veteris notas*), then John Studley translates that phrase as

[20] Winston J., "Seneca in Early Elizabethan England", *Renaissance Quarterly* 59 (2006) 29–58.

[21] Jonathan Bate writes that 'the Elizabethans did not doubt that the stoic philosopher Seneca who put forward these views in works such as his *Epistles* was the same man as the dramatist whose *Tenne Tragedies* were collected in English translation in 1581' (Bate J. [ed.], *Titus Andronicus* [London: 1995] 30). If *De Ira* warns against the effects of passion, the tragedies enact the effects of anger on a person. Berthe Marti argued that Seneca's characterizations of Medea and Phaedra, when viewed in connection with *De Ira*, display concrete examples of one of the harmful passions deplored by the Stoic philosophers. She writes that these two plays 'illustrate the most significant contribution of the Stoics to psychology, the analysis of the effect of emotional impulses upon the struggle between vice and virtue. They provide exempla for a Treatise of the Passions' (Marti B., "Seneca's Tragedies: A New Interpretation", *Transactions of the American Philological Association* 76 [1945] 220). More recently, Anne Pippin Burnett suggested that Seneca's plays are in accordance with his philosophy, since the reception of a play is an exercise in the control of the emotions. A member of the audience 'can rehearse himself in not surrendering, and learn to view horror and injustice with no more than an agreeable thrill because his mind has chosen not to be affected' (*Revenge in Attic and Later Tragedy* [Berkeley: 1998] 10).

'The token olde of pinching ire full well ere this know I'.[22] The added adjective describes Medea's rage as causing physical or emotional pain, especially associated with pressing or biting.[23] The Latin *furore ore signa lymphati gerens* ('[bearing] marks of distracted passion in here face') is translated as 'The signes pronouncing proofe of pangues her frensy Face doth show'.[24] The painful experience of anger is here conveyed by the word pang – 'a sudden sharp spasm of pain which grips the body or a part of it; a shooting pain' also used in a more figurative sense to refer to an intense emotional pain or a sharp feeling.[25]

In the translations of Seneca's tragedies, the pain of anger is seen as a necessary step towards revenge. Medea, for example, feels that she cannot take revenge on her husband without first having been tormented by the Furies herself. Those who brood on revenge in early modern English revenge tragedy often invoke the Furies. With this dramatic convention, they invite the goddesses of revenge to take possession of their body, in order to infuse it with anger.[26] The three Furies come armed with instruments of torture: 'Alecto with her brand and bloudie torch,/ Megaera with her whip and snakie haire,/ Tysiphone with her fatall murthering yron'.[27] With their torches, whips and knives, these goddesses carry out acts of retribution, but in these tragedies they also paradoxically use their instruments of torture to inflict pain on the prospective avengers themselves. In a deviation from the Latin original, Medea asks the goddesses of revenge: 'in plunge of passing payne/Torment yee mee, that on my spouse do wishe this woe to raygne'.[28] To be able to enact the murder of her own children, Medea needs to be

[22] The first translation is from Frank Justus Miller in *Seneca's Tragedies*, Loeb Classical Library (London – New York: 1961), vol. I, 261; the second translation by John Studley, in Eliot T.S. (ed.), *Seneca His Tenne Tragedies Translated into English* (Bloomington – London: 1964), *Medea* Act III, 73. This is Eliot's edition of the ten tragedies originally edited by Thomas Newton in 1581, who brought together translations of Seneca's tragedies written during the 1560s. All quotations from early modern English translations of Seneca's plays are taken from this edition.

[23] *Oxford English Dictionary*, s.v. "pinching" *adj.* 2a.

[24] The Latin and modern English translation derive from the Loeb edition (see footnote above); the line is on page 72 of Eliot's edition of the *Tenne Tragedies*.

[25] *Oxford English Dictionary*, s.v. "pang" *n.* 1a and 2.

[26] On the invocation to the Furies as a set speech in early modern English tragedy, see Clemen W., *English Tragedy Before Shakespeare: The Development of Dramatic Speech* (London: 1961) 243–246.

[27] George Peele, *The Battle of Alcazar* (London, Edward Allde: 1594) fol. B3.

[28] *Medea* Act I, 56. The Latin reads: 'Mihi pelius aliquid, quod precer sponso', which the Loeb edition translates as 'I have yet curse more dire to call down on my husband' (229).

thrown into a state of fury that gives her the force to enact such a horrific deed. She asks to be immersed in a pool of extreme pain ('plunge of passing pain') in order to reach this level of fury. Elsewhere in the play, the torments of the Furies are described in more detail: 'flap thou fearce the fierbrandes full dasshed in myne Eyes,/ Dig, rent, scrape, burne and squeas them out, loe ope my breast it lyes,/ To fighting furies bobbing strokes'.[29]

The experience of the pain inflicted by the Furies is all-absorbing. When they are thus tormented, angry characters explain in detail what they feel is happening to their bodies. They seem unable to describe anything else than the very physical and painful emotion they are experiencing. In Seneca's *Agamemnon*, translated by John Studley, Clytemnestra describes her anger as follows:

> So grievous is my careful case which plungeth me so sore
> That deale I cannot with delay, nor linger any more.
> The flashing flames and furious force of fiery fervent heate,
> Outraging in my boyling breast, my burning bones doth beate:
> It suckes the sappy marrow out the juice it doth convay,
> It frets, it teares, it rents, it gnaws, my guttes and gall away.[30]

The words Clytemnestra uses in the first two lines of this quotation to describe her case refer metaphorically to the experience of pain, but could also be read in a literal sense. The word 'grievous' generally means 'pressing heavily upon a person', and is also used to describe a wound or pain that causes great suffering.[31] The verb plunge is here used in the sense of 'overpower, overwhelm, oppress'; the *OED* cites as and example of this use the line 'This womans harte is plungid with payn' from a 1520 play.[32] 'Sore' can similarly refer to mental pain, but can also refer to 'considerable physical pain or bodily injury'.[33] More elaborate than Seneca's original text, the last four lines of the quotation emphasize this physical aspect of her anger, and describe

---

[29] *Medea* Act V, 96. The Latin original reads 'fige luminibus faces, lania, perure, pectus en Furiis patet'. Loeb edition, vol. I, 308. The translation there: 'Plunge your brands into my eyes, tear, burn; see, my breast is open to the Furies'.

[30] *Agamemnon* Act II, 107. *Agamemnon* was translated by John Studley in 1566. The Latin reads: 'Maiora cruciant quam ut moras possim pati;/ flammae medullas et cor exurunt meum' (Loeb edition, vol. II, 13), translated there as 'Passions rack me too strong to endure delay; flames are burning my very marrow and my heart'.

[31] *Oxford English Dictionary*, s.v. "grievous" a. 1a and 3.

[32] *Oxford English Dictionary*, s.v. "plunge" v. 8.

[33] *Oxford English Dictionary*, s.v. "sore" adv. 1.

how the heat of fury eats at her inner organs. The alliteration and the metre enact on a level of poetic form the painful throbbing sensation of Clytemnestra's boiling breast and burning bones. Her physical pain seems to inhibit her from taking vengeful action at this point: even though she claims that she cannot 'linger any more', she is unable to do anything else than attempt to communicate the pain of the fury that rages within her.

It is not only women who invite the anger of the furies into their bodies. In *Thyestes*, translated by Jasper Heywood, Atreus longs to take revenge on his brother. He calls upon the Furies in order to bring his body into a state of great anger:

> And now let all the flock of furies dire,
> And full of strife Erinnys come, and double brands of fire
> Megaera shaking! For not yet enough with fury great
> And rage doth burn my boiling breast; it ought to be repleat
> With monster more.[34]

The Furies are once more depicted with their instruments of torture, in this case Megaera's burning pieces of wood. Like Clytemnestra, Atreus describes the experience of anger in bodily terms: 'a tumbling tumult quakes within my bosom, lo,/ And round it rolls. I moved am, and wot not whereunto,/ But drawn I am'. He feels a plan for revenge 'begins to swell' and tells his servant 'what thing it is I cannot tell/But great it is'.[35] As in the other examples, the furious anger of the avenger is represented as a purely bodily process caused by the Furies, which lies outside the agency of the angry persons themselves.

In a fascinating transmigration of forms, Jasper Heywood employs this model of a painful, bodily inspiration to revenge in the preface to his translation of the play. The conventional invocation of the Muses in this preface merges with the invocation of the Furies. Heywood sees himself faced with a writer's block. He paces the room, curses and cries. He depicts his persona as a 'wight that waxed wood' (furiously insane) and uses the traditional, feminine, Senecan image of an angry 'panther of her prey depriv'd, or tiger of her brood'. In this troubled state, the poet decides to call upon the Furies:

---

[34] *Thyestes* Act II, 63: 'dira Furiarum cohors/ discorsque Erinys veniat et geminas faces/ Megaera quatiens; non satis magno meum/ ardet furore pectus; impleri iuvat maiore monstro' (Loeb, vol. II, 110).

[35] *Thyestes* 63–64: 'tumultus pectora attonitus quatit/ penitusque volvit; rapior et quo nescio, sed rapior' (Loeb, vol. II, 112).

'O thou, Megaera', then I said, 'if might of thine it be
Wherewith thou Tantal drov'st from hell, that thus disturbeth me,
Inspire my pen; with pensiveness this Tragedy t'indite,
And, as so dreadful thing beseems, with doleful style to write'.
My hair stood up, I waxed wood, my sinews all did shake,
And as the Fury had me vexed my teeth began to ache.
And thus enflam'd with force of her, I said it should be done,
And down I sat with pen in hand, and thus my verse begun.[36]

The possession by this Fury-as-Muse is again described as a painful experience, which here causes not only the familiar symptom of shaking sinews, but also an agonizing Elizabethan ailment, the toothache. John Kerrigan writes that it is hard to explain 'the clash between this prologue and what the Fury represents in the translation proper: a destructive spirit of ire which drives Thyestes and Atreus to disaster'.[37] I think the awkward conflation of a Muse with a Fury could be explained in terms of bodily experience and intentionality. Both the muses and the Furies represent external forces of inspiration that need to be invoked and allowed to take possession of the body in order to inspire ideas and action. The pain that is foregrounded in these passages draws attention to the bodily nature of the process. Descriptions of the experience in terms of bodily pain emphasize a loss of control over their body. The speakers can only hope that their fury will inspire them to create, whether that creation is a translation or a deed of revenge. In the case of Atreus, for example, his vindictive plan is described as growing, or swelling within him. However, the danger that Seneca's tragedies point to time and again, is that the birth-pains of anger do not lead to creation, as in the case of Heywood, but to self-destruction. The invocation to the Furies can lead a loss of self in anger, since all rational capacities need to submit to violent passion.[38] Then, the engendered violent passion may direct itself inward instead of outward. Indeed, avengers in Seneca's tragedies often kill what is closest to themselves: Atreus makes his own brother eat his nephews, Clytemnestra kills her husband, Medea her children.

---

[36] Jasper Heywood, *Thyestes*, ed. Joost Daalder (New York: 1982), Preface ll. 333–342.

[37] Kerrigan eventually reads this 'conceptual awkwardness' as deriving from a divergence between classical and Christian ideas of the role of anger. Kerrigan J., *Revenge Tragedy: Aeschylus to Armageddon* (Oxford: 1996) 112–113.

[38] See also Hallett C.A. – Hallet S., *The Revenger's Madness: A Study of Revenge Tragedy Motifs* (Lincoln – London: 1980) 45.

The dangers of uncontrolled fury are brought to the fore most clearly in the play that opens the collection of ten tragedies published by Thomas Newton in 1581, *Hercules Furens*, also translated by Jasper Heywood. In this play, the hero of classical antiquity returns from the twelve works set him by the goddess Juno. She is furious at Hercules' successful completion of the works, and broods on revenge. Deciding that the only way to defeat the half-god is to use his own strength against him, she plans to possess him with a fury that will lead to his own destruction:

> Seekes thou a match t'Alcides yet?
> Thers none, except hymselfe: let him agaynst himselfe rebell.
> Let present be from bottome deepe upraysd of lowest hell
> Th'Eumenides, let flaming lockes of theyrs the fires out flinge,
> And furious hands bestowe aboute the stroakes of vipers sting.
> [...]
> Let hateful hurt now come in anger wood,
> And fierce impyety imbrew himselfe with his owne bloud,
> And errour eke, and fury arm'd agaynst it selfe to fight.[39]

The Furies are here once more depicted as torturers, whose flaming hair and furious hands instil an anger that hurts like the viper's sting. As in Seneca's *De Ira*, this anger will turn against Hercules, and smear his body with his own blood: his fury is armed to fight against itself. The half-god suddenly sees 'fearce Tisyphone with head and ugly heare' and 'Erynnis bringing flames', who throws burning firebrands in his face. When the Furies have thus incited his painful anger, Hercules in his blind rage thinks his wife and son are the children of his enemy, the tyrant Lycus, and kills them with his bow and club. As he wakes from his madness and sees his family dead, his first instinct is to take revenge for their murders. His father, knowing who the killer was, advises against this, and captures the essence of the play in a phrase: 'Revenge oft hurtful was'.[40]

---

[39] *Hercules Furens* Act I, 11–12. After checking the 1561 original, I have silently emended T.S. Eliot's 'vipers fling' in the fifth line of the quotation to 'vipers sting'. The Latin reads: 'quaeris Alcidae parem?/ nemo est nisi ipse; bella iam secum gerat./ absint ab imo Tartari fundo excitae/ Eumenides, ignem flammeae spargant comae,/ viperea saevae verbera incutiant manus [...] veniet invisum Scelus/ suumque lambens sanguinem Impietas ferox/ Errorque et in se semper armatus Furor (Loeb edition, vol. I, 10).

[40] *Hercules Furens* Act V, 47. In *The Second Maiden's Tragedy*, Govianus shows himself aware of this danger of vindictive fury, when he asks the heavens for patience: 'Give me a sober fury, I beseech thee,/ A rage that may not overcharge my blood/ And do myself most hurt!' (V, 2.50–53).

Although Juno is aware of the self-destructive qualities of anger, she invites the Furies to take possession of her own breast first, before she lets them drive Hercules mad: 'Wherfore doth Juno yet not into raging fall?/ Mee, me, ye Furye, systers three throwne quite out of my wit,/ Tosse fyrst, if anything to do'.[41] This invocation of the Furies shows the double bind of the avenger: Juno knows that anger can turn against itself, and it is her very plan to make use of the pain that anger can inflict on an angry person. Yet, to be able to take revenge on Hercules, she too needs to be possessed by the Furies. Although Juno here does not literally state that the experience will be painful, it can by implication be assumed that the methods the Furies use to 'tosse' her, involve pain.

In the translations of Seneca's tragedies, then, anger is represented as a primarily bodily experience that is intensely painful. Aspiring avengers call upon the Furies to inflict this pain on them, in order to reach a state of fury that is so painful they can no longer delay their act of revenge. The risk inherent in this painful method of revenge, however, is that the pain of fury turns against itself, and inflicts the most painful wounds on the avenger. In Seneca's tragedies, this is often the case. The pain of anger in his tragedies is not a means to an end. With their translations of Seneca's tragedies, in which they enforce the association between anger and pain already present in the plays, the Inns of Court men introduce a discourse into early modern English culture in which anger is depicted as an uncontrollable, bodily process that leads to destruction and even self-destruction.

Memory, Pain and Revenge

One of the instruments to counter this loss of reason in fury and its subsequent wounding of the self, is the use of memory. Strier mentions it as one of the possible responses resulting from anger: 'I'm going to retaliate, or remember'.[42] Seventeenth-century philosophers who looked for ways to discipline passion also turned to memory as a solution. Their techniques were concerned with organizing and ordering the past

[41] *Hercules Furens*, Act I, 12.
[42] Strier – Mazzio, "Two Responses" 16–17.

in an attempt to control the unruly emotions.[43] Katherine Rowe has recently stressed the importance of this function of memory in early modern revenge tragedies. Referring to Vindice's remembrance of the past in *The Revenger's Tragedy* as well as Hamlet's resolve to remember the words of the ghost, she writes that '[t]he strenuous, even strained claims for memory in these plots suggest how much energy is required to maintain a backward accounting of the self against the entropy of humoral affection'.[44]

Memory can indeed be a method to guard the self against being engulfed in humoral affection, but paradoxically there are also discourses in which it is represented as a painful, bodily process that can lead to a loss of self-control. Francis Bacon, a member of the Inns of Court and author of various edicts against the duel, views the role of memory in revenge as a bodily process, and thinks of it in terms of pain. 'This is certain' he writes, 'that a man that studieth *Reuenge* keepes his owne Wounds greene, which otherwise would heale, and doe well'.[45] The word green in this quotation could refer to the rawness of the wounds, implying that thinking of the injury and its revenge keeps the wounds open and bleeding, and therefore painful. Bruce Smith has recently traced the association between the word green and the senses in early modern culture. He found that hearing or seeing green is a way of perceiving associated with the body, a combined sensory experience, and with the passions. 'To hear green would mean attending to sounds that spiral away from denotative meaning toward wordless sensation', he writes.[46] Perhaps the green wounds in this quotation also evoked in an early modern reader this association of memory and revenge with the body and the passions: a green feeling of wounds that is not rational, but spirals away into the passions.

One could argue that the wounds in this quotation are not literal gashes, but metaphors for the mental state of a person who broods

[43] See Sutton J., "Controlling the Passions: Passion, Memory and the Moral Physiology of Self in Seventeenth-century Neurophilosophy", in Gaukroger S. (ed.), *The Soft Underbelly of Reason: The Passions in the Seventeenth Century* (London – New York: 1998) 115–146.

[44] Rowe K., "Inconstancy: Changeable Affections in Stuart Dramas of Contract", in Floyd-Wilson – Sullivan, *Environment and Embodiment in Early Modern England* 93.

[45] Francis Bacon, "Of Revenge", in *The essayes or counsels, ciuill and morall, of Francis Lo. Verulam, Viscount St. Alban* (London, John Haviland: 1625) fol. D3.

[46] Smith, "Hearing Green", in Paster – Rowe – Floyd-Wilson, *Reading the Early Modern Passions* 161.

over revenge. The distinction between literal and metaphorical is not so easy to make for the early modern period, however. This is not only the case for the operations of the humours, but also for the workings of memory and the mind. John Sutton describes how excessive emotions were thought to wreak havoc in the brain. His description shows that in early modern physiology, the fixation of Bacon's man who studies revenge would be explained with reference to literal wounds in the brain:

> If one is not defended against violent passions, error inevitably follows through the confusions of brain traces. Fixations and obsessions can result. If one passion dominates, then as some animal spirits 'violently descend' in unnatural motions to the periphery of the body, others, 'swirling irregularly in the brain, stir up so many traces' that the soul, which is 'continually constrained to have the thoughts tied to these traces', 'becomes, as it were, enslaved to them'. [...] Once the dispositions of confusion are in place in a set of superposed traces, it is hard to displace them, for 'wounds received by the brain heal with greater difficulty than those in other parts of the body'.[47]

The wounds to the brain caused by animal spirits swirled irregularly into the brain by excessive passion are literal, not metaphorical wounds. Animal spirits physically trace ideas into the surface of that part of the brain that houses memory, leaving 'structural alterations to the brain pores', according to Descartes.[48] The process of remembering is therefore a bodily process that leaves wounds in the brain.[49]

In Thomas Nashe's *The Unfortunate Traveller* (1594), this process of remembering is explicitly expressed in terms of pain. An avenger called Cutwolfe has travelled years to find the murderer of his brother. During his travels, he has devoted all his energy to the pursuit of revenge. In the process his body has become a revenge machine:

> Looke how my feete are blistered with following thee from place to place. I haue riuen my throat with ouerstraining it to curse thee. I haue ground my teeth to pouder with grating & grinding them together for anger when any hath namde thee. My tongue with vaine threates is bolne, and

[47] Sutton, "Controlling the Passions" 130; 132. The quotations are from Malebranche's *De la recherche de la vérité.*

[48] Sutton, "Controlling the Passions" 122–123.

[49] In her contribution to this volume, Anita Traninger quotes Jörg Jochen Berns' description of memory as 'the art of carefully calculated self-harm'. Her article describes the crucial connection between memory and pain in the teaching of Latin to young boys.

> waxen too big for my mouth: my eyes haue broken their strings with their staring and looking ghastly, as I stood deuising how to frame or set my countenance when I met thee. I haue neer spent my strength in imaginarie acting on stone wals, what I determined to execute on thee: intreate not, a miracle may not repriue thee: villaine, thus march I with my blade into thy bowels.[50]

Cutwolfe's body has become trained in the execution of revenge. He has cracked the strings of his eyes in practising the harrowing look he will use to confront his brother's murderer. He has practised his revenge 'in imaginarie acting on stone wals', wearing down his body in trying out on walls the stab that he now intends to deal to his enemy. In the process, Cutwolfe has become a body – he thinks of himself in terms of body parts, and uses his body as a material repository of his memory. The phenomenon of bodily memory was not unknown in the early modern period. Descartes noticed that a lute player 'has a part of his memory in his hands; for the ease of bending and positioning his fingers in various ways, which he has acquired by practice, helps him to remember the passages which need these positions when they are played'.[51] In a similar way, Cutwolfe has lodged his memory in his eyes, teeth, tongue and hands. This corporeal, material memory is represented as a painful affair that leads the avenger to wound himself in the pursuit of revenge. Even if memory was seen as a safeguard against the painful and overwhelming bodily operations of the passions, then, it was at the same time also conceived of as susceptible to passion, and could be a painful experience.

Objectified Pain in Chivalric Discourse

Pain's effect of directing a person's attention inward, cutting them off from all other sensations, is central to Elaine Scarry's theory in *The Body in Pain*. There, she argues that what sets pain apart from other human physical experiences such as hearing, touching, or desiring, is the fact that pain has no object in the external world: 'it is not *of* or *for*

[50] Thomas Nashe, *The Unfortunate Traveller or the Life of Jacke Wilton* (1594), ed. Brett-Smith H.F.B. (Oxford: 1920) 119.

[51] Descartes in a letter to the French mathematician Marin Mersenne, quoted in Roodenburg H., *The Eloquence of the Body: Perspectives on Gesture in the Dutch Republic* (Zwolle: 2004) 13.

anything'.[52] As a result, pain resists objectification in language. Interestingly, other human experiences can come to be expressed in terms of pain when they, too, are characterized by this lack of an object. 'Often', writes Scarry, 'a state of consciousness other than pain will, if deprived of its object, begin to approach the neighborhood of physical pain; conversely, when physical pain is transformed into an objectified state, it (or at least some of its aversiveness) is eliminated'.[53] We encountered an example of the first case in the translations of Seneca's tragedies, where anger is deprived of its object. When vengeful characters in these plays experience the emotion of anger, they tend to forget that they had an object of revenge in mind. They are fully occupied by the bodily experience of anger, and, as Scarry states, their anger indeed approaches physical pain.

This is not the only view on anger to be found in early modern culture, however. In a counter discourse, anger is an emotion that does serve a greater purpose: it enables courage and valiant behaviour in warlike circumstances. Anger in these cases has an object, and in this objectified state it is not a painful experience. Rather, the state in which anger can serve a purpose is a state in which a warrior is able to forget his wounds. These two discourses of anger and pain are not neutral, but function in specific political contexts.

Robin Headlam Wells has demonstrated how such concepts as masculine virtue or noble manly courage function politically in early modern England. They play a significant role in the political discourse of members of the Sidney-Essex faction and of later admirers of the young Henry Prince of Wales, expressing a commitment to the ideals of militant Protestantism.[54] The notion of choler as conducive to courage is associated in early modern culture with this aristocratic tradition. An example of this more positive view of anger can also be found in an emblem representing the humour of choler in Henry Peacham's *Minerva Brittanna* (1612) [Fig. 1]. Peacham, an admirer of the young and militant Prince Henry, produces works that take part in this aristocratic discourse. Mervyn James in his influential study of concepts of honour in early modern England affirms that Peacham

[52] Scarry E., *The Body in Pain: The Making and Unmaking of the World* (New York – Oxford: 1985) 5.

[53] Scarry, *The Body in Pain* 6.

[54] Headlam Wells R., *Shakespeare on Masculinity* (Cambridge: 2000) 7–19.

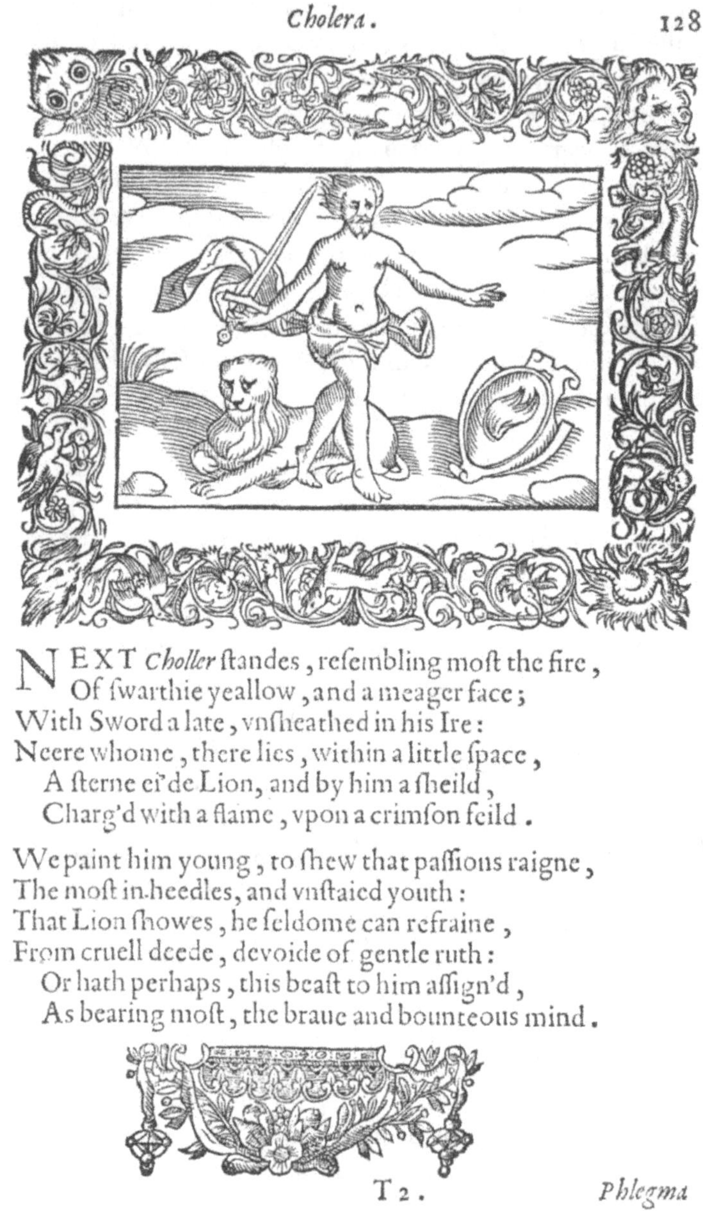

Cholera. 128

NEXT *Choller* ſtandes, reſembling moſt the fire,
Of ſwarthie yeallow, and a meager face;
With Sword a late, vnſheathed in his Ire:
Neere whome, there lies, within a little ſpace,
A ſterne ey'de Lion, and by him a ſheild,
Charg'd with a flame, vpon a crimſon feild.

We paint him young, to ſhew that paſſions raigne,
The moſt in.heedles, and vnſtaied youth:
That Lion ſhowes, he ſeldome can refraine,
From cruell deede, devoide of gentle ruth:
Or hath perhaps, this beaſt to him aſſign'd,
As bearing moſt, the braue and bounteous mind.

T 2. *Phlegma*

Fig. 1. Henry Peacham, "Cholera". From idem, *Minerva Britanna* (London, Walter Dight: 1612) 128. Copy of Leiden University Library.

tends to defend the more aggressive and military aspects of honour.[55] The emblem features a young man speeding towards us, his hair blowing in the wind, his sword drawn. The wild shape of the man's hair is mirrored in the picture of a flame, emblazoned on what the epigram tells us is a 'crimson' shield. The flame, the red colour, the desert-like surroundings of the young man, the lion that is couched behind him, as well as his unsheathed sword, combine to refer to the hot and passionate nature of the choleric temperament, 'resembling most the fire'.[56] The epigram tells us that the choleric man depicted is a young man, 'to shew that passions raigne,/ The most in heedless, and unstaied youth'. If Peacham's emblem seems to imply that choler is not compatible with adult masculinity, there is a sting in the tail of the epigram. The young man is depicted with a lion, whose presence is initially explained by the epigram as signifying the cruelty that results from choler. The final two lines challenge this interpretation of anger, however: 'Or hath perhaps', the poem wonders, 'this beast to him assign'd/As bearing most, the braue and bounteous mind'? Instead of constructing choler as unbridled and cruel, as the Senecan tragedies do, the closing couplet presents its readers with a counter-discourse that suggests the lion might also signify choler's contribution to courage. In his later collection of essays, Peacham compares the lion to the nobility – 'man of greater perfection, of nobler form'.[57] Also, the adjective 'bounteous' in a chivalric context carried the now obsolete meaning of prowess; it was a synonym for the adjective 'valiant'.[58] The emblem in Peacham's *Minerva Britanna*, dedicated to the young 'and hopefull' Prince Henry, openly questions the humanist view on anger by suggesting that this passion might be of use to the aristocratic male.

This view of anger also affects the representation of the relation between anger and pain. An example of this can be found in Sir Philip Sidney's chivalric romance *The Countess of Pembroke's Arcadia*. The genre of the chivalric romance had been mocked for its 'open manslaughter' by humanists such as Roger Ascham, but Sidney turned to the genre

[55] James M., "English Politics and the Concept of Honour 1485–1642", in *Society, Politics and Culture: Studies in Early Modern England* (Cambridge: 1986) 406–407.

[56] Henry Peacham, *Minerva Britanna* (1612) (Amsterdam-New York: 1971) 128.

[57] Henry Peacham, *The Complete Gentleman* (1632), ed. Virgil B. Hetzel (Ithaca, NY: 1962) 11–12.

[58] *Oxford English Dictionary*, s.v. "bounteous" *a.* 1b.

to give it a new political significance.[59] Fulke Greville, who edited the *Arcadia* for publication after Sidney's death, connected the romance with a prominent faction of nobles concerned with these rights of the nobility, the Essex circle.[60] In the *Arcadia*, Sidney underscores the need to limit royal power, and preserve the ancient rights of the aristocracy. Alan Sinfield writes that 'we may understand this text as a continuation of his concern with the rights of the nobility and gentry as against any absolutist tendency'.[61]

Within this political context, the *Arcadia* stresses the positive value of martial anger. The concluding couplet of a dialogue between passion and anger in the Second Eclogues, in which Reason and Passion after their 'skirmish' join hands and decide to give way to 'heavenly rules' is often seen as emblematic for the attitude to passion in the *Arcadia* as a whole.[62] The chivalric romance portrays the rational faculties as equal to the passions; indeed, the two are in constant need of each other. Fear is said to breed wit, for example, joy to strengthen the heart, and sorrow leads one to look inward and correct the self.[63] Anger is shown to have positive effects as well. Instead of representing it as a destructive emotion that needs to be avoided at all times, the *Arcadia* brings to the fore anger's positive contribution to honour and virtue: 'anger is the cradle of courage' (133). Martial anger is not portrayed as an uncontrolled rage that wounds the warrior himself, rather, the choler

---

[59] Roger Ascham refers to *Morte D'Arthur*'s 'open manslaughter and bold bawdry' in *The Schoolmaster* (1570), ed. Ryan L.V., *Folger Documents of Tudor and Stuart Civilization* (Charlottesville: 1967) 68–69.

[60] See Wood R., "'The Representing of so Strange a Power in Love': Philip Sidney's Legacy of Anti-factionalism", *Early Modern Literary Studies* Special Issue 16 (2007) 4.1 www.chass.utoronto.ca/emls/si-16/woodsidn.htm>, accessed 17 June 2008.

[61] Sinfield A., "Power and Ideology: An Outline Theory and Sidney's *Arcadia*", *English Literary History* 52,2 (1985) 265. For various interpretations of the role of chivalry in the new *Arcadia*, see (among others) Montrose L.A., "Celebration and Insinuation: Sir Philip Sidney and the Motives of Elizabethan Courtship", *Renaissance Drama* 8 (1977) 3–35, McCoy R., *The Rites of Knighthood: the Literature and Politics of Elizabethan Chivalry* (Berkeley: 1989), chapter 3; Norbrook D., *Poetry and Politics in the English Renaissance* (London: 1984) 106–107; Kinney C.R., "Chivalry Unmasked: Courtly Spectacle and the Abuses of Romance in Sidney's *New Arcadia*", *Studies in English Literature, 1500–1900* 35,1 (1995) 35–52.

[62] See also Maurice Evans' endnote to this line in his edition of the *Arcadia*. Philip Sidney, *The Countess of Pembroke's Arcadia*, ed. Maurice Evans (London – New York, etc.: 1977) 859. n. 1.

[63] Philip Sidney, *The Countess of Pembroke's Arcadia*, ed. Evans M. (London – New York: 1977) 133.

is firmly controlled by virtue and honour. This element of control is essential since true valour is only achieved if the passion of anger is moderate: 'people who show indeed in themselves the right nature of valour, which, as it leaves no violence unattempted while the choler is nourished with resistance, so, when the subject of their wrath doth of itself unlooked-for offer itself into their hands, it makes them at least take a pause before they determine cruelty' (382). Choler is shown to be essential to valour, but when the object of danger is defenceless, it needs to be controllable.

This martial kind of anger is not represented as a painful experience, but as a force that leads the warrior to ignore his pain to reach the higher goal of glory. The third book of the new *Arcadia* is the most chivalric in nature, and tells of many knightly combats. In the descriptions of these fights, anger is not represented as painful:

> These thoughts indeed not staying, but whetting their angry swords, which now had put on the apparel of cruelty: they bleeding so abundantly, that everybody that saw them fainted for them; and yet they fainted not in themselves: their smart being more sensible to others' eyes than to their own feeling. Wrath and courage barring the common sense from bringing any message of their case to the mind: paine, weariness, and weakness not daring to make known their case (though already in the limits of death) in the presence of so violent fury; which filling the veins with rage instead of blood, and making the mind minister spirits to the body, a great while held out their fight (541).

The violent fury of these knights keeps them from experiencing their pain at all. As Sidney puts it: 'pain rather seemed to increase life than to weaken life in these champions' (542). The passage provides a physiological explanation for the phenomenon: wrath and courage interfere with the operations of common sense, the faculty that collects sense data such as pain and presents them to the reason.

This idea occurs more than once in the *Arcadia*'s descriptions of chivalric encounters. When Phalantus has been hit on the head in single combat 'in such sort that his feeling sense did both dazzle his sight and astonish his hearing' it is his anger that allows him to continue the fight: 'choler took away either the bruise or the feeling of the bruise, so as he entered afresh into the combat' (498–499). In a combat between Amphialus and the forsaken knight, the anger of the two adversaries is stimulated both by the fighting itself, as well as by the hurt they incur: 'choler no less rising of the doing than of the suffering'. While it originates in their suffering, choler also enables the knights to ignore their pain, as if their bodies were senseless: 'Their very armour by piecemeal fell away from them; and yet their flesh abode the wounds constantly, as though it were less sensible of smart than the senseless armour' (538). In this chivalric context, anger is aimed at an outward object, and is no longer experienced as painful. Instead, it makes the angry person forget his pain in his fury. In the words of Elaine Scarry, 'when physical pain is transformed into an objectified state, it (or at least some of its aversiveness) is eliminated'.

Bodily Experience and Intentionality in Political Context

To return to Richard Strier's words, there are indeed angry characters in early modern culture who say 'That makes me mad, and I'm going to retaliate, or remember'. I found such characters in Sir Philip Sidney's *Arcadia*. In this specific literary genre, written in negotiation with a specific political context, characters use their anger to reach the goal of revenge. Interestingly, these characters do not experience their anger as a painful passion. Their fury enables them to ignore their wounds in combat. In the genre of Senecan revenge tragedy, produced in a different political context, characters express their anger in terms that approach quite closely Strier's mock-rendition of a humoral phenomenology: 'Oh dear, my liver is heating up; my choleric humour is being activated, etc'. In these tragedies, anger is a painful emotion that eats at a inner organs and burns in bones. It is an emotion without an object that wounds the self, rather than the other. The connection between pain and anger, then, is construed differently in these two discourses. The tragedies of the Inns of Court portray anger as an excessive, destructive emotion that is better avoided. The translators draw on the language of the psychophysiology of the humours to render anger as explicitly bodily in nature. The pain of anger underscores this purely bodily nature of the emotion. On the other hand, militant aristocrats who attach great value to martial anger and masculine aggression, follow Aristotle in his perception of anger as a positive force that can enable courage. In their counter discourse, anger is not a painful emotion: it can make a valiant fighter forget his pain during combat. Representations of anger as either a bodily process or a matter of intentions and action, then, both figure in Renaissance culture. The choice between the two manners of representation is political: militant members of the aristocracy sought to preserve their privileges of anger, while a pivotal institution in the fast-growing legal system of Elizabethan England appropriated a classical genre in which anger's raging and burning serves no purpose but painful, uncontrollable self-destruction.

Selective Bibliography

ARISTOTLE, *Nicomachean Ethics*, trl. H. Rackham, in *Aristotle in 23 Volumes*, vol. 19 (Cambridge, MA – London: 1934).

——, *The Art of Rhetoric*, trl. Freese J.H. (Cambridge: 1924).

ELIOT T.S. (ed.), *Seneca His Tenne Tragedies Translated into English* (Bloomington – London: [1927] 1964).

HEYWOOD JASPER, *Thyestes*, ed. Daalder J. (New York: 1982).

KERRIGAN J., *Revenge Tragedy: Aeschylus to Armageddon* (Oxford: 1996).

LODGE THOMAS, *The Workes of Lucius Annaeus Seneca* (1614), STC 22213.

MCCOY R., *Rites of Knighthood: The Literature and Politics of Elizabethan Chivalry* (Berkeley – Los Angeles: 1989).

PASTER G. KERN, *Humoring the Body: Emotions and the Shakespearean Stage* (Chicago: 2004).

PASTER G. KERN – ROWE K. – FLOYD-WILSON M. (eds.), *Reading the Early Modern Passions* (Philadelphia: 2004).

ROSE M.B., *Gender and Heroism in Early Modern English Literature* (Chicago: 2002).

SCARRY E., *The Body in Pain: The Making and Unmaking of the World* (New York – Oxford: 1985).

SCHOENFELDT M., *Bodies and Selves in Early Modern England: Physiology and Inwardness in Spenser, Shakespeare, Herbert and Milton* (Cambridge: 1999).

SIDNEY PHILIP, *The Countess of Pembroke's Arcadia*, ed. Evans M. (London – New York: 1977).

SMITH B., "Hearing Green", in Paster – Rowe – Floyd-Wilson (eds.), *Reading the Early Modern Passions* 147–168.

STRIER R. – MAZZIO C., "Two Responses to 'Shakespeare and Embodiment: An E-Conversation'", *Literature Compass* 3,1 (2005) 15–31.

SUTTON J., "Controlling the Passions: Passion, Memory and the Moral Physiology of Self in Seventeenth-century Neurophilosophy", in Gaukroger S. (ed.), *The Soft Underbelly of Reason: The Passions in the Seventeenth Century* (London – New York: 1998) 115–146.

WELLS R. HEADLAM, *Shakespeare on Masculinity* (Cambridge: 2000).

PARTAKERS OF PAIN: RELIGIOUS MEANINGS OF PAIN IN EARLY MODERN ENGLAND

Jan Frans van Dijkhuizen

In the *Meditations on First Philosophy* (1641), René Descartes analysed pain as a way of investigating the philosophical conundrum of the relation between mind and body.[1] He saw the experience of pain as simultaneously psychological and physical, and it was for this reason that it undermined the clear-cut distinction between the two that he attempted to set up in much of the *Meditations*. For Descartes, pain showed that the mind cannot succesfully purge itself of the epistemological uncertainties engendered by the body. In addition, Descartes approached pain from a purely utilitarian perspective; it serves as a potentially unreliable yet ultimately useful warning system that helps to maintain bodily health.

In effectively locating the religious dimension of pain solely in its god-given medical usefulness, Descartes departed radically from pain discourses that had long been central to Christianity, and significantly narrowed the spiritual significance that pain possessed within these discourses. As I will discuss in more detail below, the meaning and experience of pain had been inextricably bound up with issues of salvation and spiritual self-transformation since the beginnings of Christianity. This link between pain and religious experience became especially pronounced in late medieval culture, which helped to create a discourse of physical suffering that was very much alive during Descartes' own lifetime, and had been a subject of theological concern throughout the sixteenth century. It is precisely on early modern religious conceptions of pain that the following analysis will concentrate. As we will see, one central idea that was upheld and attacked in equal measure by religious writers was that suffering pain, and experiencing it in all its physical intensity, is theologically and spiritually meaningful and efficacious, and is therefore even something to be actively sought.

[1] For a more detailed discussion of Descartes comments on pain in the *Meditations*, see the introduction to this volume, and Stephen Pender's article on pain in the early modern imagination.

There is also an unexpected parallel between Descartes' understanding of pain and early modern religious pain discourses, however: in both cases, the question of pain is intimately linked to the relation between mind and body. Pain spoke to Descartes because it posed the question of mind and body in a particularly stark form. Pain spoke to religious writers of the early modern period because it posed in equally stark form a number of analogous theological questions: is religious experience located in the mind or in the body? What is the theological role of the body? Can justification be obtained via the body, or is it a matter exclusively of the inner life? As we shall see, sixteenth- and early seventeenth-century theological controversies about the meaning of pain revolved in part around these questions.

My main focus will be on the interplay between two competing religious understandings of physical suffering that can be broadly characterized as Catholic and Reformed. I will look at early modern English translations and adaptations of works by three Spanish writers of the Catholic Reformation – Teresa of Avila (1515–1582), Ignatius of Loyola (1491–1556) and Louis of Granada (1505–1588) – and at the first English translation of the final version of John Calvin's *Institutes of the Christian Religion*, published in 1561, only two years after the Latin original. It is one of my contentions that the religious upheavals of the early modern period also affected perceptions of physical pain, and formed a watershed moment in what we might call 'the history of pain'. The Protestant Reformation, in its preoccupation with the theological role of the human body, and of the physical world in general, did much to forge what was in some respects a radical revision of Catholic conceptions of bodily anguish, while the Catholic Reformation was in part an attempt to re-assert some of the Catholic attitudes towards pain that reformers were at pains to discredit. Both movements drew on the long-standing centrality of physical suffering in the Christian tradition. Judith Perkins has persuasively argued that pain was at the heart of new Christian views of the self that emerged in the early Roman empire. Part of the triumph of Christian discourse, she notes, lay in the fact that it constructed a notion of the self as 'a mind/soul joined to a body liable to pain and suffering', as opposed to the more traditional Graeco-Roman representation of the self as 'a soul/mind *controlling* the body'.[2] Early Christianity not only presented itself as a

[2] Perkins J., *The Suffering Self: Pain and Narrative Representation in the Early Christian Era* (London: 1995) 3, my italics.

succesful healing cult, but also created a discourse 'for understanding suffering if healing should fail'. Suffering, in the early Christian understanding, could be 'profitable in itself' and could serve as a form of empowerment, analogous to the way in which Christ's pain had led to a triumph over death.[3] In this sense, early Christian conceptions of bodily suffering entailed a rejection, and even an inversion of prevailing notions of power and prestige – pain gave power to the marginalized. It is this heritage which both the Protestant and Catholic Reformations had to grapple with; rethinking some of the fundamentals of Christian culture was impossible without also addressing the meaning of pain and suffering.

In *The Body in Pain*, Elaine Scarry has argued, somewhat notoriously, that bodily pain is ineffable. If language and, for example, the creating of artefacts can be seen as forms of communication and self-extension, as ways of making the contents of consciousness sharable and tangible, pain represents a state of extreme isolation in which human beings are cut off from the world: 'pain comes unsharably into our midst as at once that which cannot be denied and that which cannot be confirmed. [...] Its resistance to language is not simply one of its incidental or accidental attributes but it essential to what it is'.[4] Scarry's view has been criticized for being reductive and even 'wrong' by Lucy Bending, in a study of representations of pain in nineteenth-century England.[5] The question of whether pain can be accurately 'captured' in language may ultimately be metaphysical. At the very least, the myriad nineteenth-century attempts to interpret physical suffering that Bending traces in her study testify to an overwhelming human need to make sense of pain, as well as to the large reservoirs of cultural meaning that enable them to do so, and this article will investigate similar processes of meaning-giving. Yet Scarry's argument does alert us to the problematic nature of what Roy and Dorothy Porter have called 'the

---

[3] Perkins, *The Suffering Self* 129.

[4] Scarry E., *The Body in Pain: The Making and Unmaking of the World* (Oxford: 1985) 4–5. It should be emphasized that this is of necessity an extremely brief account of Scarry's sophisticated argument, and it would be difficult to do full justice to the complexity of her ideas, even in a much more extended treatment.

[5] Bending L., *The Representation of Bodily Pain in Late Nineteenth-Century English Culture* (Oxford: 2000), 86. For another critique of Scarry, see Silverman L., *Tortured Subjects: Pain, Truth, and the Body in Early Modern France* (Chicago: 2001) 20–22.

annals of pain'.[6] The experience of pain tends to elude the historical gaze, and some forms of pain are more easily recorded than others:

> The most acute fevers have left the fewest records. *De profundis*, people have neither strength, time, nor wish to pen their pains. [...] Likewise, those most susceptible to life-endangering diseases, the very young, left no eyewitness records. The same goes for the mentally ill. [...] Innumeral mothers died in childbed; all had better things to do than document their own demise. [...] Chronic complaints leave more record than acute, those attacking visible parts are described in greater detail than those of the internal organs. Thus gout is richly recorded [since it] produced precisely the kind of pain sufferers could readily write about: tedious enough to be capable of description (what can be said about instantaneous spasms?), severe enough to command attention, yet not so deranging as to preclude writing.[7]

Of the writers discussed in this article, only Teresa of Avila writes about personal pain experiences, and only her work can legitimately be thought of as the record of a sufferer attempting to understand her pain. Louis of Granada, Ignatius and Calvin write *about* pain, not *from* pain. The works by Ignatius and Louis de Granada, moreover, are instructional works that clearly attempt to engender in their readers a certain attitude towards physical suffering, while Teresa's *Flaming Hart*, as an autobiography, is more experiential and less interested in the doctrinal meaning of pain. Yet there is a remarkable overlap in the categories in which these writers discuss pain, and it is clear that they all operate within a shared discourse of bodily suffering. The meanings of pain are not created only by those who suffer, or have suffered, from it; pain sufferers both draw on and help to create the pain discourses by which they are surrounded.

I have so far used the term 'pain' to refer to *physical* suffering, not to mental trauma. Having said this, it is precisely the distinction between the two that has been called into question by recent medical thinking.[8] David Morris has dismissed dualist conceptions of bodily suffering as the 'Myth of Two Pains' and stresses that pain is always simultaneously physical and cultural or psychological.[9] My discussion in this article will proceed from pain that has a recognizably physical dimension, but it is

---

[6] Porter R. – Porter D., *In Sicknesss and in Health: The British Experience, 1650–1850* (London: 1988) 102.

[7] Porter – Porter, *In Sicknesss and in Health* 102–103.

[8] Wall P., *Pain: The Science of Suffering* (London: 1999) 32–39.

[9] Morris D.B., *The Culture of Pain* (Berkeley – Los Angeles: 1993) 9.

also alert to the extent to which the language of bodily pain can shade into that of emotional pain, or serve as a way of discussing emotional pain. Indeed, as we shall see, it was partly the extent to which bodily and mental pain were intertwined in Catholic understandings of the matter that disturbed Calvin, and his comments on the meaning of suffering in the *Institutes* are in part an attempt to disentangle the two. In a sense, therefore, modern dualist notions of pain as either physical or mental can be traced to early Protestant attempts to make a distinction between the two, rather than to the Cartesian *cogito*.

While the changes in early modern religious notions of pain clearly had a wider European resonance, this article will zoom in on the question of how this broader debate was received and conducted in England. The English debate forms a specifically useful case study since, as has been pointed out by a number of historians, the English Reformation was in many ways an incomplete process: even after the Elizabethan Settlement of 1560, English attitudes both towards the recent English Catholic past and towards post-Tridentine Catholicism remained volatile and ambivalent.[10] Moreover, in spite of its officially avowed Protestantism, the identity of the English Church continued to be the object of intense scrutiny and debate until well into the second half of the seventeenth century.

The relatively undecided character of post-Settlement English religion is also borne out by the lively culture of translating continental Catholic devotional works into English (indeed, printed works have been said to serve to some extent as substitutes for the real presence of priests), and this article will look at a small selection of them. The first is the *Libro de la oración y meditación* by the Spanish Dominican theologian and devotional writer Louis of Granada, which was translated into English by the Catholic exile Richard Hopkins (ca. 1546–1596[?]), under the title *Of Prayer and Meditation* (1582). Hopkins' translation, published in

[10] See for example Lake P., "Religious Identities in Shakespeare's England", in Kastan D.S. (ed.), *A Companion to Shakespeare* (Oxford: 1999) 57–85; Duffy E., *The Stripping of the Altars: Traditional Religion in England, c. 1400–c. 1580* (New Haven: 1992); Duffy E., *The Voices of Morebath: Reformation and Rebellion in an English Village* (New Haven: 2001); Jones M., "Choosing Reformations", in idem, *The English Reformation: Religion and Cultural Adaptation* (Oxford: 2002) 7–33; Walsham A., *Church Papists: Catholicism, Conformity and Confessional Polemic in Early Modern England* (London: 1993).

no less than eleven editions between 1582 and 1634,[11] contains only the first, most practically oriented book of the *Libro*, which consists mostly of a two-week programme of morning and evening meditations. The second work which I will discuss is a translation of Teresa of Avila's autobiography, entitled *The Flaming Hart, or the Life of the Glorious S. Teresa* (1642) by Sir Toby Matthew (1577–1655), a lifelong friend of Francis Bacon.[12] Matthew's turbulent career can be said to embody the religious vicissitudes of England during this period. He was an MP from 1601 until 1604 but travelled to the continent the following year and converted to Catholicism in Florence in 1607.[13] On his return to England, Matthew refused the oath of allegiance, and was forced to leave the country. He was ordained priest in 1614 and during his time abroad translated the work of Catholic writers such as the Jesuit Francisco Arias (1533–1605) and the preacher and mystic Juan of Avila (1500–1569). He was eventually allowed to return to England in 1621 and, following diplomatic missions in Spain, was knighted by James I in 1623. His ties with the royal court became closer during the reign of Charles I but he left England for good in 1641, after he had been accused of taking part in a conspiracy to murder Charles and Archbishop Laud. The dedicatory letter to *The Flaming Hart* suggests that in 1642, on the eve of the English Civil War, Matthew was still attempting to regain favour with the court. In it he claims that Henrietta Maria 'carr[ies]

---

[11] Murphy G.M., "Hopkins, Richard (*b. c.* 1546, *d.* in or before 1596)", *Oxford Dictionary of National Biography*, Oxford University Press, 2004 <www.oxforddnb.com/view/article/13752>, accessed 3 Oct 2007. For this article, I have relied mainly on the 1611 edition. Granada's treatise was first published in Salamanca in 1554. Various revised versions appeared between 1554 and 1579. For an overview of the, see the textual commentary in Fray Luis de Granada, *Obras Completa, Tomo 1: Libro de la Oración y Meditación*, ed. Huerga A. (Madrid: 1994) 581–653, esp. 592, 648–53. Hopkins' translation is based on an edition published in Antwerp by Plantin in 1572. For a useful overview of the first English translations of the *Libro*, see Hagedorn M., *Reformation und Spanische Andachtsliteratur. Luis de Granada in England* (Leipzig: 1934) 25–48.

[12] The first translation of Teresa's autobiography was *The lyf of the mother Teresa of Iesus, foundresse of the monasteries of the descalced or bare-footed Carmelite nunnes and fryers, of the first rule* (Antwerp, Henry Jaye: 1611), translated by the Jesuit Michael Walpole (1570–1625). For biographical information about Walpole, see Jessopp A., "Walpole, Michael (bap. 1570, d. 1625)", rev. Milward P., *Oxford Dictionary of National Biography* (Oxford U.P.: 2004); <www.oxforddnb.com/view/article/28597>, accessed 3 Oct 2007.

[13] For biographical details about Matthew, see also Loomie A.J., "Matthew, Sir Toby (1577–1655)", *Oxford Dictionary of National Biography* (Oxford U.P.: 2004), <www.oxforddnb.com/view/article/18343>, accessed 3 Oct 2007; and Mathew A.H. – Calthrop A., *The Life of Tobie Matthew (1577–1655): Bacon's Alter Ego* (London: 1907).

an extraordinary devotion' to Teresa, and to 'the holy Religious woemen of her Angelicall Order; whereof, the English Nation [...] hath a Monastery at Antwerpe'.[14] He invites the Queen to

> march at the very head of that whole Troope, which may addresse it selfe, to the imitation of [Teresa's] Heroicall actions, and to the admiration of those incomparable Graces, and Favours, which the God of Heaven, and Earth, thought fitt to infuse, with his enamoured hart, and omnipotent hand, into that most happy Soule (fol. 3r).

Ignatius' *Spiritual Exercises* was not directly translated into English until 1736, but Henry More (ca. 1587–1661), another seventeenth-century English Catholic with an erratic public career, translated an adaptation of Ignatius' work by Tomas de Villacastin that was printed in 1618 at the Jesuit press in St Omer as *A Manuall of Devout Meditations and Exercises*.[15] The *Manuall* is loosely modeled on the basic thematic structure of the *Spiritual Exercises*, with its division into the 'purgative way', the 'illuminative way', and the final 'unitive' or 'perfective' way.[16] Unlike Ignatius, it does not divide these three stages on the basis of a four-week time-schedule, nor does it specify a time-frame for the process of the exercitant's spiritual growth. Like Granada's *Of Prayer and Meditation* (especially in its abbreviated English translation), De Villacastin's *Manuall* is a practical guidebook presenting a range of meditation exercises. A small duodecimo volume, it was intended to be carried around by the exercitant; De Villacastin describes it as 'my little Manuall, desiring to have that portable in our bosome, which ought ever to be fixed in our soule & hart.'[17]

---

[14] St Teresa of Avila, *The flaming hart, or, The life of the glorious S. Teresa*, trl. Toby Matthew (Antwerp, Johannes Meursius: 1642) fol. 2v.

[15] The Spanish title of De Villacastin's adaptation is *Manual de ejercicios espirituales para tener oracion mental* (first published in 1612; for this article I have consulted an edition from 1618 [Valladolid: Geronymo Murillo]). Both Henry More and De Villacastin were Jesuits. The 1736 translation of the *Spiritual Exercises*, also printed at the Jesuit press in St Omer, is entitled *The spiritual exercises of S. Ignatius of Loyola. Founder of the Society of Jesus*. The identity of the translator is unknown. More's translation follows the Spanish original closely.

[16] For a brief account of these four stages, see Ignatius of Loyola , *The Spiritual Exercises and Selected Works*, ed. Ganss G.E., S.J. (New York: 1991) 51–54. De Villacastin explains the nature of the three ways at the beginning of each of the three books of his manual.

[17] Tomas de Villacastin, *A manuall of devout meditations and exercises instructing how to pray mentally*, trl. Henry More (Saint Omer, English College Press: 1618) fol. 5.

The *Manuall* reads primarily as an extended commentary on Ignatius' *Exercises* that enlarges on the latter's often terse directions, teasing out their implications. For example, if Ignatius' fifth exercise, a meditation on hell, takes up merely a single page of short, one-sentence comments, De Villacastin extends this to a detailed, seven-page description of the pains of hell. Similarly, De Villacastin turns Ignatius' brief pointers for a meditation on the conversion of Mary Magdalen into a six-page meditation in which the significance of Mary's conversion is clarified. Although De Villacastin reads Mary's conversion in generalized spiritual rather than denominational terms, his exhortations to follow her example must have had a seditious resonance in the politico-religious context of late Jacobean England: 'Purpose not to deferre thy conversion when God shall call thee; learne of this holy penitent to reject and abhorre those things which were instruments of offending him' (295). Indeed, More was imprisoned in 1628, along with six other Jesuits. He had worked in London during most of the 1620s, and his English translation of De Villacastin had been reprinted in 1623 and 1624.[18] By the time of More's release in 1633, conditions for Jesuits had changed greatly, with Queen Henrietta both openly Catholic and openly sympathetic towards Catholic priests, and the Laudian establishment seeking rapprochement with the Catholic church. From 1635 until 1639, More was provincial for the English province of the Society of Jesus, and when Charles I disapproved of his appointed successor, Edward Knott, he continued to act as vice-provincial until 1642.

All three texts share a central concern with the meaning of physical suffering – Teresa of Avila's autobiography is easily one of the most extended meditations on pain of the period. Moreover, as we shall see, they offer religious conceptions of pain that are in some respects radically at odds with the Reformed models of suffering that were forged in the course of the sixteenth century, represented in this article by Thomas Norton's influential translation of Calvin's *Institutes*. Yet they also share a number of central preoccupations with these models.

[18] McCoog Th.M., "More , Henry (c. 1587–1661)", *Oxford Dictionary of National Biography* (Oxford University Press: 2004), <www.oxforddnb.com/view/article/19180>, accessed 15 May 2008.

The Flaming Hart, A Manuall of Devout Meditations and Exercises, and *Of Prayer and Meditation* share an overwhelming concern with the meaning of the physical suffering of Christ. Relating the spiritual struggles of her early adult life, Teresa describes her own emotional response to seeing an image of the suffering Christ. It is Christ's bodily agony that fills her with a sense of spiritual inadequacy:

> I saw a Picture [...] of Christ our Lord, full of wounds, & soares; and it was so devoutly made, that when I looked up on, it moved me much, for it represented very well, what he had endured for us. And the sense of the little gratitude to our Lord, which I had conceaved, and expressed, for those wounds of his, was such, that me thought, my verie hart, did even splitt. And I cast my self earnestly downe, near the Picture, with a great shower of teares (98).

The image of Christ also fosters a desire in her to be mentally present at the scene of Christ's lonesome suffering in the Garden of Gethsemane, and to wipe the bloody sweat off his forehead. She is kept from doing so by her own sense of sinfulness: 'I never durst resolve, to presume to doe it; so grievously, did my Sinnes represent themselves to me' (100). The reader of Henry More's translation of De Villacastin is urged to ponder and visualize Christ's pain in a similar manner: 'Ecce homo, behold o my soule this man: [...] so wounded with stripes, so defiled with spittle, so bruized with buffets, crowned with thornes' (412). De Villacastin makes Christ's suffering vividly present to the mind by dwelling on visual details such as the garments that stick to the dried-up wounds on Christ's body: 'Ponder how Christ our Lord, to carry his Crosse, layd aside the garments which others had put on him in Herods, and Pilats house, & cloathed himselfe with his owne, not without extreme great payne, for they cleaved fast to his sacred wounds & were dryed into them, they being now cold' (416–417). Louis of Granada also incites his reader to concentrate mentally on the Agony in the Garden as a prelude to the Passion, in which Christ becomes mentally aware of the bodily pains he will have to undergo: 'Consider now attentively, in what a dolorous case our Saviour was, and how there were presented unto him, all the cruell paines and torments he had to suffer, even as though they had beene then presently in doing before his eyes'.[19] The

[19] Louis of Granada, *Of prayer and meditation contayning foureteene meditations, for the seaven dayes of the weeke, both for mornings and evenings*, trl. Richard Hopkins (London, Edward White: 1611) 429.

intensity with which Christ grasps the horror of his own impending agonies serves as a model for the focused meditation that Granada seeks to cultivate in his reader.

The centrality of Christ's suffering leads these writers to the question of how Christ's divine pain relates to human suffering. Does Christ's Passion exist in a realm of its own that cannot be approximated by human beings, or are humans able to share in the pain undergone by Christ? Louis of Granada stresses that the sufferings of Christ can never be *fully* shared. It is impossibe to undergo sufficient pain to atone for one's sins, and Christ's self-sacrifice is always needed: 'although I alone should suffer all the paines & torments, that both the Devils, and damned persons doe suffer in Hell, yet should I not be able with all this, to make a sufficient satisfaction for all that which my sinnes have deservd. Wherefore, I beseech thee (O Lorde) to cast the cloake of thy mercy uppon mee' (40–41). At the same time, Granada urges his reader to 'heape paines and despightes against [him] selfe' (42), and presents these pains as a technique for getting closer to, and even becoming, Christ: 'so that by them I may be brought to my most sweet & mercifull Lord' (43). Meditating on Christ's pain, moreover, can be enhanced by thinking of Christ's pain not as a distant historical event 'but as a thing present', and by mentally placing oneself in Christ's place, imagining his pain to be one's own: 'thinking with thy selfe what a terrible paine it would be unto thee, if in so sensible and tender a part as the head is, men should fasten a number of thornes, yea and those so sharpe, that they should pierce into thy skull' (486). Similarly, De Villacastin sees a sharing in Christ's suffering as a prerequisite for salvation:

> [G]ather [...] a great desire to suffer persecution in imitation of Christ: [...] if it was necessary that Christ our Lord shold passe through innumerable tribulations and afflictions, and so enter into his owne glory; it is evident that neither thou nor any other shal enter into the glory which is not thine, but only by this way of persecution (282).[20]

[20] In the *Spiritual Exercises*, Ignatius advises the exercitant to inflict pain on himself as a form of penance for his sins. It is worth noting that this is a carefully calibrated pain, and the bodily damage it causes carefully controlled: '[t]he best and safest form of penance seems to be that which produces physical pain but does not penetrate to the bones, so that it brings pain but no illness. Therefore the most suitable form of penance is to hurt oneself with light cords that inflict the pain on the surface, rather than some other manner which might cause noteworthy illness inside' (Ignatius of Loyola, *Spiritual Exercises and Selected Works* 144.).

We have seen that Teresa wishes to be present at the scene of Christ's suffering, but that her awareness of her sins makes her realize the gap between herself and Christ. Yet the idea that human pain and disease can be a way of participating in Christ's self-sacrifice is repeatedly voiced in *The Flaming Hart*, both as a source of comfort in suffering, and as an element in Teresa's struggle to become one with Christ. Teresa describes the debilitating and inexplicable pains from which she suffered during her adolescence – 'the sharp, and bitter paine, which neuer gaue me ouer, but vexed me, euen all alike, from head to foot' – and early in her autobiography she wonders whether 'our Lord may be, peradventure, served, in some sort' by her agony (43; 72). When her father begins to suffer from the pains from which he will eventually die, she comforts him by reminding him that 'his Divine Majestie had been pleased to give him a feeling, of some part of that, which himselfe had undergone' (76). It is this rationale which leads her to the notion that pain can serve as 'the way of the Crosse' (262), an avenue to the mystical union with Christ for which she longs.

Conversely, the language of pain provides Teresa with a vocabulary for discussing the sense of alienation from the world, and the disintegration of the self, which the turning towards God brings with it. Teresa's mystical experiences bring about in her 'a kind of totall untying, and loosning [...] from all things' and lead to 'such a new kind of shynesse, and mislike, in order to the things of this world, that it makes even our verie life much the more painefull to us' (254). Moreover, Teresa's soul is 'alienated even from her self' and it seems that 'she, and [God], were one, and the self-same thing, without division, or distinction' (515). The sense of becoming dead to the world is also painful in that it intensifies Teresa's desire for a full mystical union with Christ that is as yet beyond her reach – she is in an inbetween state, both cut loose from the world and not yet at one with Christ. It is partly in this sense that Teresa's pain is both agonizing and uplifting:

> that which comes to [the soul] from Heaven, [...] doth but serve for her greater torment, because it multiplyes the same desire, in such sort, that the excessive paine therof, doth put her, in my opinion, even past her senses [...]. Now this condition of mind, seemes to be no lesse, then even the verie agonie, and passage of death it self; yet withall, there is so very great a contentment taken in this suffering, that I know not, to what, in fine, I may possible be able to compare it. It is a feirce, and yet a savourie, and delightfull kind of Martyrdome (258–259).

It is worth noting that the *Oxford English Dictionary* lists 'torment, agony; extreme or severe pain or suffering, esp. when protracted or prolonged' as one of the meanings of 'martyrdom'.[21] Teresa's mysticism makes her a martyr, not so much in a political sense, but in that it leads to the pain of rejecting the world and of shedding the self.

If the process of becoming divorced from the world is initially painful, eventually it is the world *itself* that becomes a source of pain in that it draws attention away from God: 'all things are wont to afflict; all things to wearie, & tyre; and all things doe even torment [the soul], unlesse it be only God, or for God' (359). Teresa also describes her isolation from God in terms of bodily pain; she speaks, for example, of 'the wound, which growes to be made in her, by the absence of our Lord' (417). Yet, like the anguish of self-loss, it is a sweet pain in that she knows it is inflicted upon her by God, not primarily as punishment, but as a necessary stage in her spiritual progress: 'the Soule was purifyed by this paine; and for that it was burnished, & refined heer, as gold might be in the Chrysuble' (263). For Teresa, as for De Villacastin, there is also a manifest soteriological dimension to pain. Whatever anguish she suffers during her earthly life she will not have to undergo as a punishment after death: 'that was to be wiped away, which would otherwise have made worke for Purgatorie' (263).

The Flaming Hart forms an apt illustration of Ariel Glucklich's observation that in mystical discourse, pain can become 'an alchemical force, like the forger's fire, which magically transforms its victim from one state of existence to a higher, purer state'.[22] In a sophisticated attempt to interpret religious pain from a combined cultural and biological perspective, Glucklich claims that 'pain weakens the individual's feeling of being a discrete agent; it makes the "body-self" transparant and facilitates the emergence of a new identity'.[23] Yet for Teresa, the idea that pain can serve as an agent of mystical self-transformation is not always self-evident, or easily grasped. It takes a deliberate effort on her part to remain aware of this meaning of pain, since it can easily slide into its opposite. Pain can also be inflicted by the devil in an attempt to lead her into religious despair: '[the devil] was some five howers togeather, tormenting me, with very terrible paine, and both exteriour,

---

[21] *OED*, s.v. "martyrdom" 3.
[22] Glucklich A., *Sacred Pain: Hurting the Body for the Sake of the Soul* (Oxford: 2001) 25.
[23] Glucklich, *Sacred Pain* 207.

and interiour disquiet; in such sort, that it was even past enduring' (447). This demonically inflicted pain is void of the paradoxical dimension of joy that characterizes Teresa's mystical pain; she describes it as 'past enduring'. Moreover, rather than fostering a form of spiritual self-transformation, it leads only to 'an inward kind of restlesnes, and disquiet' (446). Teresa is even initially unsure whether this pain is indeed demonic or whether it comes from God, and it is only after she has prayed for patience, and after she has considered whether she may serve God even in suffering this unbearable pain, that 'our Lord was pleased [...] that I should clearly understand it, to be the Divel' (447).

Teresa is similarly ambivalent about the question of where her pain is located. She wonders whether it is primarily physical or spiritual and concludes hesitantly that it cannot be categorized in dualist terms: 'that Paine seemes to be such, as that, although the Soule doe feele it, yet it feeles it, togeather, with the Bodie; and so, both of them, participate therin' (255).[24] She later writes that her spiritual pain also 'peirces the whole body, through, and through' (419). This commingling of the physical and the spiritual is especially evident in what is arguably the most celebrated passage in Teresa's autobiography. An angel appears to her in a vision, with

> a long Dart of gold in his hand; and at the end of the iron below, me thought, there was a little fire, and I conceaved, that he thrust it, some severall times, through my verie Hart, after such a manner, as that it passed the verie inwards of my Bowells; and when he drew it back, me thought, it carried away, as much, as it had touched within me; and left all that, which remained, wholy inflamed with a great love of Almightie God. The pain of it, was so excessive, that it formed me to utter those groanes, and the suavitie, which that extremitie of pain gave, was also so very excessive, that there was no desiring at all, to be ridd of it; nor can the Soule then, receave anie contentment at all, in lesse then God Almightie himself.
>
> This is no Corporall, but a Spirituall paine; though yet the Bodie doe not faile, to participate some part thereof; yea and that, not a little. And it is such a deare, delightfull kind of entercourse, which passes heer, between the Soule, and Almightie God, as I beseech him of his infinite goodnes, that he will give some touch, or tast of it, to whosoever shall

[24] It is worth noting that, as Giles Constable writes, 'dualism as a philosophical or metaphysical doctrine [...] has always been rejected by Christians, [...] in opposition to the beliefs of the Manicheans. [...] As a religious temper, however, dualism has played an important part in the history of Christian ascetiscism and apolypticism' (see his *Attitudes towards Self-Inflicted Suffering in the Middle Ages* [Brookline, MA: 1982] 9.

> believe, that I lye. During the time, when I was in this state [I cared not], either to see anie thing, or to speake; but contented my self to consume with burning-up in my paine, which was to be the greatest glorie for me, that this whole world could affoard (420–421).

In the second paragraph of this passage, Teresa has hardly claimed that her pain is spiritual before she goes on to stress the extent to which it is physical, and the diction of the first paragraph leaves little doubt about the overwhelmingly bodily nature of her experience. The passage also underlines that Teresa's pain alienates her from the world, yet also transforms her sense of self, and even creates it anew *ex nihilo*. She is literally emptied out by pain – the dart 'carried away, as much, as it had touched within me', and what is left of her is only a 'great love of Almightie God'. Indeed, this is where part of pain's potential for mystical self-transformation is located, and from which it derives its double nature as both agonizing and pleasurable. As David Morris notes, 'it is impossible to say where pain leaves off and ecstasy or vision begins'.[25]

In De Villacastin, the languages of bodily and mental suffering also flow into each other. Drawing on the long *christus medicus* tradition in which Christ heals both body and soul, he explains to his reader that it is both Christ's 'sorrowes & pains' that serve as a form of 'medicine' to cure 'the swellings of thy pride' and the 'soares rancled and putrifyed by the inveterate and continuall custome of sinning' (534–535) – sin is presented as a physical disease and as a form of bodily corruption. Louis of Granada especially sees the Agony in the Garden as evidence of the mixed nature of Christ's suffering. It is because of Christ's 'remembrance & imagination of that which was yet to come' that his 'flesh suffered such grievous paines', while his soul 'suffered those paines even dyrectly in it selfe?' (430). Christ's imagination is presented as capable of producing physically experienced pain.

If the boundaries between the physical and the spiritual in these texts are sometimes hazy, Louis of Granada's *Of Prayer and Meditation* leaves no doubt that the body is a source of moral corruption – 'a sack of earth, a continuall flowing water of all filth and stench' (71) – that needs to be tamed by means of mortification. De Villacastin urges his reader to cultivate a contempt of the body: '[beseech] our Lord to open the eyes of thy soule, that from this day forward, thou cease to

[25] Morris, *The Culture of Pain* 132.

seeke delights and contentments for thy body, which is so unworthy of them; chastising it with rigorous pennance' (72–73). Yet it should be emphasized that the human body is just as much of an overwhelming presence in Granada and De Villacastin as it is in *The Flaming Hart*, and that it forms an important part of the material from which they construct their theology. In Louis of Granada, pain is presented as a defining characteristic of human existence – 'it be indeed very short for all good thinges, yet in one thing I find it long, that is, in bearing of paine and misery' (98) – and he meditates at great length on the frailty and mortality of the human body. If De Villacastin's Ignatian exercises are designed to subject the body by causing it discomfort and pain, the human body also forms his most important locus of religious experience, and it is primarily via the body that his readers can reach spiritual insight. Not only do the techniques for prayer which De Villacastin offers include advice about 'the composition of body in Prayer' (22), but the human body serves as a reference point to which he returns time and again. He meditates at length on the minutiae of Christ's Passion, elaborating on them in detailed visual tableaux, and finds evidence for the centrality of physical suffering in Christ's life even in Christ's circumcision, which points to his willingness to embark on his pre-ordained suffering for humankind almost immediately after his birth, and should create in human beings a similar acceptance and even active seeking of hardship, in a range of metaphorical circumcisions:

> it is Gods will & pleasure, that thou circumcise thy selfe spiritually (that is) that thou cut off all superfluityes in pampering thy flesh, in honour and commodityes of this world, circumcising and mortifying thyne eyes, not suffering them to behold that which is not lawfull to desire; circumcising thy tongue, making it to keep silence, from vaine and idle words; circumcising thy tast, that it feed not it selfe with gluttonies and delicacies (203).

De Villacastin's repeated insistence on the importance on mortifying the body, moreover, keeps it at the centre of his attention, and continuously offers the body up as a tool for spiritual enlightenment. It is precisely the attempt to overcome the body that requires a sustained preoccupation with it.

If the concern with physical suffering is related to a wish to identify with and participate in Christ's suffering, and a desire to subdue the body, it has also to do with the compelling nature of bodily sensations, with the ability of physical experiences to lend authority to otherwise abstract concepts. This is most evident in *The Flaming Hart*. If for Teresa, the union with God implies a form of self-loss, bodily pain forms a tangible illustration of this spiritual 'untying': 'our Lord is pleased, that even the Body also it self, shall put this point in practice' (254). Indeed, physical pain sensations possess a reality by which the authenticity of spiritual pain can be gauged; spiritual pain is real insofar as it can take on the intensity of a sensory experience. After a vision of hell, Teresa writes that 'in this other present Vision, our Lord was pleased, that I should really feele those torments, and afflictions in Spirit, even as if my verie Bodie, has been suffering them there' (474). The vision derives its truth value, its reality, from its almost bodily intensity; it leaves a lasting impression on Teresa because it makes her 'really feele', on a physical level, the torments of hell. Similarly, the psychological distress that a 'wicked man' feels when he has to part with the things of the world at the moment of death is presented by means of an arresting dental metaphor that implies that worldliness is located in the body itself: 'The deeper roote the tooth hath in the Jaw, the greater griefe it causeth at what time it is plucked out. Now the heart of a wicked man, being so fast rooted in the love of thinges of this life, it cannot, but that it must needes bee a very great griefe unto him, when he seeth the houre is now come, wherein he must depart from them all' (146).

In a similar vein, for Louis of Granada the multitude of marks that pain leaves on Christ's body captures the overwhelming nature of the evidence for his divinity: 'if the testimonies be so many, as the stripes were that thou sufferedst for my sake, who can then put any doubt in the proofe, being as it is, so plainelie avouched and prooved, by so many witnesses?' (475). The reality of Christ's scarred body serves as the measure of the truth of his divinity. Moreover, Granada repeatedly urges his reader to try and grasp the meaning of eternal damnation by pondering a form of earthly physical pain, and extrapolating its aversiveness to the scale of divine punishment:

> When a man hath by reason of some great fall, put his arme out of joynt, the more griefe and paine must hee afterwardes abide, before it can bee set in joynt againe, and brought to his due proper place. Now whereas the wicked have disordered al things in this World, and set them out of joynt, and wrenched them out of their naturall placed, when that heavenly reformer shall come to restore the world, by punishment of so many disorders; howe great shall the punishment be, where so many and so great disorders have beene? (213–214).

Although Granada, in this passage, concludes that earthly pain is almost negligible compared to the pains of eternal punishment, it still serves to make those eternal pains, abstract and remote in themselves, vivid and graspable.

De Villacastin claims that after his death Christ descended into purgatory to carry the souls of 'those holy fathers that were there' (446) up to heaven. In order to make the reality of their salvation unambiguously clear to them, Christ took them to the sepulchre and

> Discover[ed] unto them the lamentable shape of his sacred body, that they might understand how deere their ransome had cost him: and when they beheld that holy body all blacke and blew, out of ioynt, and so bruized & mangled on evry side, they yeilded againe unto their deliverer infinite thankes for having redeemed them with so great labours and paynes (449).

In all three texts, the abstract concept of salvation is made tangible and concrete by equating it with Christ's bodily suffering: salvation is not only the result of, but effectively *consists in* Christ's passion. The meditation on Christ's pain in which the readers of Granada and Ignatius are urged to take part, therefore, is an exercise in the internalizing, and becoming fully conscious, of the reality of salvation. In this respect, Edward Howell's description of Teresa's mysticism as 'the more bodily approach found in Bernard of Clairvaux and various other late medieval mystics, which regards the *bodily* senses as capable of mediating spiritual benefits [...] through the union of spirit and flesh in the incarnation,' is applicable also to De Villacastin and Granada.[26]

We have seen that for Teresa of Avila pain both assists her in cutting herself loose from the world and provides an idiom for expressing the anguish which this process of alienation brings with it. Physical suffering also plays a crucial part in preparing the ground for the mystical disembodiment that *The Flaming Hart* works towards. Teresa is eventually granted visions that are marked by an absence of pain, and by an escape from the physical body itself. In these visions, 'our B.Ladie' clothes Teresa's formerly suffering body 'in a Garment of much whitenes, and clearnes', and this moment signifies that 'I was now growne, to be cleansed, from my Sinnes' (503). Mary herself is also 'apparrelled in white, with excesse of splendour' (504), and she has been restored to an 'extraordinarily young' version of herself (505). The human body, which has so far been characterised by its suffering, has now become

[26] Howells E., *John of the Cross and Teresa of Avila: Mystical Knowing and Selfhood* (New York: 2002) 135.

diaphanous and has shed it physical particularities, and it seems that this is the precondition of its newly acquired beauty: 'The beautie also, which I saw in our B. Ladie, was excessive, though yet I could not determine the forme, or figure of anie particular part, which I might assigne her, but only the frame, and ayre of the whole face togeather' (504–505). If Teresa is now 'wholy, as it were, out of [her]self' (505), this self-loss is no longer accompanied by pain or distress.

This sense of disembodiment is even more pronounced in De Villacastin, who emphasizes that Mary's exemplarity lies partly in the fact that she 'lived in continuall payne and griefe' (169). In this way, she became like Christ, 'crucifyed in his paynes and Passion', and this is what ultimately enabled her to 'rise as he did, to a new life of glory' (454). If Christ's resurrected body is no longer 'disfigured as he was at his death but replendent & beautifull' (454), Mary is similarly rewarded in heaven by means of a glorification of her body, in which it becomes impervious to pain, and semi-weightless:

> [T]he third day after the death of our Blessed Lady, Christ Jesus her Sonne, came downe from heaven, attended on by innumerable Angells, with the soule of his most B. Mother, & infused it into her body, and made it a thousand tymes more beautiful then the Sunne it selfe, and restoring it to life, invested it with immortality, & with a beauty and grace so divine, as neither can be explicated by wordes, nor comprehended by humane understanding.
>
> Ponder how glorious the body of this pure Virgin was, raysed out of the sepulcher, with those foure dowries of glory, which the glorified bodies have, of impassibility, agility, subtility, and clarity. And beholding her selfe in this manner, what thanks would she render unto her most B. Sonne, for having dealt so liberally with her, not permitting her body (albeit she dyed a naturall death, as other children of Adam) to be dissolved and turned to dust, conserving it with the same integrity and purity, it had in life.[27]

Louis of Granada presents both heaven and hell first and foremost as physical states. The damned in hell undergo a comprehensive array of highly specialized pains, and the etymological link between 'pain' and 'punishment' in the Latin *poena* becomes literalized in Granada's account of hell. Not only are all the senses targeted by means of specific pains,

[27] 509–510. The meaning of 'subtility' in this passage is best captured by one of the definitions of 'subtlety' given by the *Oxford English Dictionary*: 'Thinness, tenuity, exility; penetrativeness arising from lack of density' (*OED*, s.v. "subtlety" 8). None of the definitions listed under 'subtility' are apposite in the present context.

but the damned are also made to suffer pains linked to their particular sins. The ears are targeted by 'the confusion of such terrible cries and lamentations, as shall there be heard' the nose by the 'intollerable stench of that filthy & lothsom place', the taste 'with a most ravenous hunger and thirst' (251), while the touch is tormented simultaneously by extreme heat and cold. In addition, 'there shall be one kind of paine for the proud man, another for the envious; one for the covetous, and another for the lecherous' (253). Moreover, once the bodily torments of hell reach a certain intensity, the distinction between physical and mental pain will blur in that consciousness is effectively taken over by the awareness of pain: 'the griefe it selfe occupieth the imagination so vehemently, that is cannot think upon any other thing' (271).[28] The result of this is that a condemned soul will come to hate his own body as the 'beginning and ende of [his] paynes and sorrowes' (229).

The treatment of the body in heaven is symmetrical to the punishments of hell. In heaven, each of the senses will 'have his owne proper delight and glory' (331), yet at the same time, the body will shed its materiality, and become not only impervious to decay but will also be characterised by 'subtilty, swiftnesse, imp[a]ssibility, and clearenesse. And this clearenesse shall bee so great, that everie one of the Saints bodies shal shine like the Sun in the kingdom of their father' (302).[29] If all three texts present the heavenly body as 'unbodied', defined first and foremost by its translucent immateriality, their concern with the state of the human body in heaven once again underlines their broader preoccupation with the body as a key site of religious experience.

In presenting pain as a useful spiritual tool, as a form of *imitatio Christi*, a key ingredient of Christian identity, and a source of mystical insight and self-transformation, the texts that I have discussed operate within a long tradition of Christian conceptions of pain, and re-assert some of its central assumptions. Earlier in this essay, I referred to Judith Perkins' analysis of the crucial role of pain in early Christian understandings of the self. This concern with physical suffering also characterised later medieval Christianity. Giles Constable notes the emergence of a range of devotional exercises, around the turn of the millennium, that were

[28] It should be noted that in early modern English, 'grief' also referred to physical pain (see *OED*, s.v. 'pain' 6).

[29] The text itself reads 'impossibility'; I have emended this to the more plausible 'impassibility'.

to become 'standard aspects of spiritual life in the late Middle Ages'.[30] Among these exercises were 'breast-beating, and whipping, [...] the wearing of hairshirts, chain-mail and plates of metal; flagellation' and 'praying with outstretched arms and in other painful positions'.[31] Diarmaid MacCulloch has described how late medieval Christianity was characterised by a new 'emphasis on the suffering Christ' who 'endured the worst possible physical and emotional pains to atone for human sin'.[32] This focus on Christ's suffering was 'part of a new exploration of his true humanity' that played an especially powerful role in Franciscan Christology:

> From the time of its foundation in the thirteenth century, the Franciscan Order of Friars emphasized this humanness of Jesus when they preached about him. St Bonaventure, one of their most celebrated early theologians, preachers and mystics, wrote passionately about his vision of sleeping beside the crucified Christ: the image of divine empathy with human suffering much comforted the generation traumatized by the Black Death and left a lasting impression on late medieval spirituality.[33]

Similarly, Esther Cohen has argued that late medieval religious culture was characterised by what she describes as an attitude of 'philopassianism' – a valorization, as well as an active seeking, of pain as spiritually meaningful and productive.[34] Physical anguish could serve as a source of spiritual enlightenment partly because it was a way of imitating Christ, and so offered an avenue to salvation, or to mystical union with Him. While the most extreme manifestations of philopassianism may have been confined to a small group of mystics and monks and nuns, its underlying attitude towards pain was 'was clearly grounded in a widespread popular form of piety'.[35]

John Calvin's *Institutes of the Christian Religion* (1536), first translated into English by Thomas Norton in 1561, is in part an engagement with this legacy. Calvin addresses the notions of physical suffering we

---

[30] Constable, *Attitudes towards Self-Inflicted Suffering* 15.

[31] Constable, *Attitudes towards Self-Inflicted Suffering* 15.

[32] MacCulloch D., *Reformation: Europe's House Divided 1490–1700* (London: 2003) 20.

[33] MacCulloch, *Reformation* 20.

[34] Cohen E., "Towards a History of European Physical Sensibility: Pain in the Later Middle Ages", *Science in Context* 8 (1995) 47–74.

[35] Cohen, "Towards a History of European Physical Sensibility" 59. For suffering as *imitatio Christi* in late medieval culture, see also Bynum C.W., *Holy Feast and Holy Fast: The Religious Significance of Food to Medieval Women* (Berkeley: 1987). Walker writes that late medieval fasting female mystics strove 'to merge their own humiliating and painful flesh with that flesh whose agony, espoused by choice, was salvation' (246).

have encountered and seeks to formulate a new model that continues to reserve a central role for suffering, and operates within the same parameters as medieval Catholic views, yet redefines these views in key areas. Calvin addresses the question of Christ's suffering most elaborately in Book 2 of the *Institutes*. Like his Catholic counterparts, he stresses the physical dimension of Christ's humanity, and he repeatedly condemns the views of 'Manichees' who, in the words of Norton's translation, 'framed Christ a body of ayre' (2.xiii.2; fol. 85v).[36] For Calvin, Christ's dual nature as both God and man includes a fully incarnate humanity: 'Christ toke upon him the true substance of the flesh of man' (2.xiii.2; fol. 84v). It is only by partaking of human embodiment, and becoming 'subject to hungre, thirst, colde, and other infirmities of our nature' that Christ could become 'all one with us' (2.xiii.2, 2.xii.2; fols. 85v, 81v). At the same time, Calvin is careful to separate Christ's *divinity* from his physical humanity. His body serves only as a receptacle for his divine nature, and does not form part of it: 'Christ woulde not have called his bodie a Temple, unlesse the Godhed did distinctly dwell therein' (2.xiv.4; fol. 89). Indeed, for Calvin, Christ's 'godhed' is effectively hidden behind 'the veile of the flesh' (2.xiii.2; fol. 85v). Calvin attacks the physician and scholar Michael Servetus – executed as a heretic in Geneva in 1553, partly at the behest of Calvin himself – for implying that '[Christ's] flesh is consubstantiall wyth God'. For Calvin, there is nothing in Servetus' theology to prevent him from claiming that 'the same essentiall Godheade is in stones' (2.xiv.8; fol. 91r) and he insists that the divine cannot reside in the material world.

If the body serves only as a container for Christ's divinity, it is also a mere stage in his victory over sin and death. Christ had to take on a fully physical humanity, and his self-sacrifice necessarily had to be in part bodily, because the body is the medium of sin, and sin therefore has to be conquered at least partly via the body: 'the sinnes of the world should be cleansed in our flesh: whiche Paule playnely affirmeth' (2.xiii.1; fol. 85r). In other words, Christ suffered *because of* the flesh, and his bodily suffering serves to offset his eventual spiritual triumph: 'hee suffered by the weaknesse of the fleshe, and rose againe by the power of the spirite, even so in this place he maketh a dyfference of

---

[36] John Calvin, *The [H] institution of Christian religion, wrytten in Latine by maister Jhon Caluin*, trl. Thomas Norton (London, Reinolde Wolfe & Richarde Harison: 1561) fol. 85v.

bothe natures' (2.xiv.6; fol. 90r). Crucially, Calvin never dwells on the particulars of Christ's bodily suffering, and even claims that they were not sufficient in themselves. Christ's death would have been 'to no effect, yf he had suffred only a corporall death: but it behoved also that he shoulde feele the rigour of Gods vengeance' (2.xvi.10; fol. 99r). In other words, Calvin posits a clear distinction between the two different kinds of pain, mental and bodily, that Christ underwent, and underlines the soteriological necessity of Christ's emotional suffering. Indeed, if Christ's soul had not also been a 'partaker of peyne, he had ben only a redemer for bodies' (2.xvi.12; fol. 100r),[37] and Calvin sees Christ's psychological anguish as the more relevant aspect of his Passion – 'an other greater and more excellent price' (2.xvi.10; fol. 99r) – than the sufferings of his body, since the salvation of the *soul* depends on it. This is underlined by the fact that God's vengeance, too, is directed first and foremost at the soul. For Calvin, Christ's bodily suffering is a mere by-product of his more essential psychological suffering. Louis de Granada, by contrast, presents physical pain as essential to Christ's role as saviour, and even argues that Christ's physical constitution was especially designed to make him uniquely vulnerable to bodily suffering:

> The therde cause of his so grievous paynes was the tendernes of his complexion. [...] [O]ur Saviours bodie was the most best complexioned, and most tender of all bodies that ever were, or shal be[.]
>
> And not onely the composition of his bodie, but also the matter thereof was very tender: forsomuch as the matter of it was wholly most pure virgins fleshe, taken of the most pure and virginall bowels of our blessed Lady, without anie other kinde of mixture. And for this cause (as S. Bonaventure saiethe) his bodie was the more tender, and of a more perfecte sense in feelinge.[38]

---

[37] It is worth noting that, in Norton's translation, the phrase 'partaker of peyne' has an ambiguity which it lacks in the Latin and French originals. In Calvin's French version the phrase reads 'participante du chastiment' (John Calvin, *Institution de la réligion chrestienne*, 2 vols. [Paris: 1859] vol. I 292), while the full Latin sentence is as follows: 'Et sane nisi poenae fuisset particeps anima, corporibus tantum fuisset redemptor' (John Calvin, *Institutio Christianae religionis* [London, Thomas Vautrollerius: 1576] 239). Both 'chastiment' and 'poena' mean 'punishment' rather than pain. In sixteenth- and seventeenth-century English, both 'punishment' and 'pain or suffering' were common meanings of 'pain' (see *OED*, s.v. "pain" 1a, 3a).

[38] Louis of Granada, *Of prayer, and meditation Wherein are conteined fowertien devoute meditations for the seven daies of the weeke, bothe for the morninges, and eveninges*, trl. Richard Hopkins (Paris, Thomas Brumeau: 1582) fol. 310r–v.

The extent to which Calvin, in Norton's translation, emphasizes Christ's mental torments at the expense of his physical anguish is captured in the following description of Matt. 27:46 (when the crucified Christ cries out to God: 'My God, my God, why hast thou forsaken me?'):

> [W]hen he felt himselfe as it were forsaken of God, yet he did nothyng at all swarve from the trust of his godnesse. Whiche is proved by that his notable callyng upon God, when for extremitie of peyne he cryed out, My God, my God why hast thou forsaken me? For though he was above measure greved yet he cesseth not to call him his God, of whome he cryeth out that he was forsaken (2.xvi.12; fol. 100v).

The gospel text itself does not provide any motivation for Christ's outcry, but simply states that 'about the ninth hour Jesus cried with a loud voice'. If in Calvin's commentary, the phrase 'extremitie of peyne' may suggest that Christ cried because of his bodily suffering,[39] the passage as a whole swiftly turns attention away from this, and presents Christ's cry of anguish primarily as evidence of His continuing trust in God. By contrast, De Villacastin's description of this central moment in the Crucifixion stresses the physicality of Christ's pain in much more detail, and, far from reading Christ's words as a sign of his unbroken faith, makes abundantly clear that it is bodily pain that causes Christ to cry out:

> He could not leane his head on any side without increase of payne and greeve, the thornes thursing in deeper thereby: of his hands he had no help, because he could not wipe away the drops of bloud which ran downe from his head upon his face, nor the tears which he did shed from his eyes, they being nailed fast to the Crosse. Neither of his feet, for they were not able to sustaine the poyse of his body, but rent themselves with greater payne. Wherfore our Lord seeing himselfe so afflicted, cryed

[39] In the Latin and French versions of the *Institutions* the phrase reads 'doloris vehementia' (Calvin, *Institutio Christianae religionis* vol. I 240) and 'véhémence de la douleur' (John Calvin, *Institution de la rélígion chrestienne* vol. I 293) respectively. Once again, the English phrase may have been ambiguous in sixteenth-century English (see also n. 37): when Robert Burton described the condition of melancholy as 'such extremity of paine and grief', he was clearly talking about suffering rather than punishment Robert Burton, *The anatomy of melancholy what it is. With all the kindes, causes, symptomes, prognostickes, and seuerall cures of it* [Oxford, John Lichfield: 1621] 276), while Elizabeth I's orders that the execution of the Babington conspirators in 1586 be 'protracted to the extremitie of payne' could have been read as an instruction to carry out 'the utmost punishment' rather than inflict the maximum amount of pain (quoted in Hamilton D.B., *Anthony Munday and the Catholics, 1560–1633* [Aldershot: 2005] 62).

> unto his Eternall Father and sayd: My God, why hast thou forsaken me? (432–433).

Calvin is also preoccupied with the question of whether humans can share in Christ's Passion, and his attitude towards this issue is ambivalent. This appears, for example, from his discussion of three moments in the epistles of St Paul that seem to equate the suffering of Christians with that of Christ: the remark in the Second Epistle to the Corinthians that Christians are 'always bearing about in the body the dying of the Lord Jesus (2 Cor. 4:10); St Paul's related wish in the Epistle to the Ephesians to know 'the fellowship of [Christ's] sufferings' and to be made 'conformable unto his death' (Phil. 3:10); and his claim in Colossians 1:23–24 that he 'fill[s] up that which is behind of the afflictions of Christ in my flesh for his body's sake, which is the church'.[40] Calvin is anxious to deny that Paul confers any soteriological efficacy to suffering. While for Teresa of Avila, pain had its place in an economy of punishment, and while Louis of Granada states explicitly that Mary was eventually glorified *because* she had suffered so much during her life, Calvin points out that 'there is no worthinesse of merit' (3.xviii.7; fol. 206v) involved in the sufferings referred to by St Paul in Corinthians. Similarly, the verse from Colossians does not suggest that suffering can in itself contribute to salvation. Rather, St Paul implies that suffering is the inescapable condition of a Christian's earthly life. The 'afflictions' of which he speaks are to be understood as 'those afflictions wherwith all the memb[er]s of Christ [...] must be exercised, so long as they shall be in this fleshe' (3.v.4; fol. 154r), and these can be as much psychological as physical. For Calvin, the idea that physical suffering can have an effect on the fate of a Christian's soul is an intolerable impingement on Christ's unique role as Saviour, and on his unique bodily suffering, and in this respect he undermines the assumptions behind the *imitatio Christi* found in Teresa of Avila: 'what is this els but to leave Christ only his name, otherwise to make him but a common pet[t]y saint [...]? He only, only should have bene preached, he only set fourth, he only named, he only ben loked unto, when the obteining of forgivenesse of sinnes, satisfaction, and sanctification are entreated of' (3.v.3; fol. 153v).

---

[40] The quotations are taken from the King James Bible. The phrase 'that which is *behind* of the afflictions of Christ' seems deliberately vague about the relationship between Paul's suffering and that of Christ. The Douay-Rheims version, by contrast, suggests more openly that Christ's sacrifice was incomplete, and can be reenacted by humans who 'fill up those things that are *wanting* of the sufferings of Christ'.

In spite of this, the idea that humans should strive for conformity with Christ plays an important part in Calvin's theology. It is the 'apointed end for all the children of God', he writes, 'to be fashioned lyke unto him', and this is achieved to a significant extent by 'communicat[ing] with the suffringes of Christ'. Indeed, the idea that adversity and suffering are a form of 'fellowship with Christ' serves to assuage the 'painefulnese of the crosse' that humans have to bear. Moreover, Calvin's claim that bearing affliction will 'help us to the furtherance of our salvation' (3.viii.1; fol. 164r) seems to be in direct conflict with his denial of the soteriological power of suffering elsewhere in the *Institutes*. Yet he points out that it is not so much humans *themselves* who achieve anything through suffering. The initiative lies with God, and this is where he departs most radically from the Catholic writers discussed above, for whom humans have a clearly active role as pain sufferers:

> [W]hen we suffer tribulations for the name of Christe, there are as it were certayne markes printed upon us, wherewith God useth to marke the shepe of hys flock. After this manner therefore we are accompted worthy of the kingdome of God, bicause we beare in oure body the markes of oure lord & master which are the signes of the children of God. To this purpose make these sayengs, That we beare about in our body the mortifications of Jesus Christ and his life maye be shewed in us (3.xviii.7; fols. 206v–207r).

In this passage, human beings play only a passive part, form only a conduit for God's actions. Something is done *to* them by God; they *are* marked by God with the imprint of suffering, they *are* subsequently 'accompted worthy' by God. If suffering has any soteriological efficacy, this is created only by God, and, as Theodore Minnema argues, suffering even serves to engender 'deeper self-knowledge by awakening human *dependence* on God's power'.[41] In addition, even if Calvin shares the idea of participating in the pains of Christ with the Counter Reformation texts we have considered, and in spite of his indebtedness to St Paul's idiom of experiencing Christ's suffering in the body itself, conformity to Christ is, for him, ultimately a non-bodily affair. His references to physical anguish remain generalized and gestural, and never seem to show an interest in the body as a material entity, or in the phenomenology of pain, and it is in the end only by the 'secret effectuall workinge of the Spirite' that we are 'grafted into' Christ (3.i.1.; fol. 106v).

[41] Minnema Th., "Calvin's Interpretation of Human Suffering", in Holwerda D.E. (ed.), *Exploring the Heritage of John Calvin* (Grand Rapids, MI: 1976) 156, my italics.

It is worth noting, in this context, that Calvin explicitly warns against self-inflicted physical suffering as a form of Christian penance, since this will draw attention away from what is really at stake, namely the salvation of the soul: 'when they [...] advaunced that bodyly discipline, this indeede they obteyned, that [...] they in a manner darkned that, which ought to have ben of much greater importance' (3.iii.16; fol. 132v).[42] We might add that self-inflicted pain also places the initiative too squarely with man himself: only God can operate through suffering. Moreover, as Minnema writes, it is only Christ who suffers voluntarily:

> Obedience is what makes the suffering of Christ fundamentally different from the suffering of the sinner. Fallen man must suffer because of disobedience, but Christ suffers because of obedience. Involuntary suffering is what befalls sinners in this world. Voluntary suffering is what Christ chooses in this world.[43]

What remains for Christians themselves, according to Calvin, is to find a purpose for pain outside the experience of pain itself. The meaning of 'hardinesse in povertie', 'peyne in sickenesse', 'grefe in shame', and 'horrour in death' (3.viii.8; fol. 166r) is that they provide an opportunity for the Christian to demonstrate his faith sand Christian valour, and to bear his anguish calmly: 'His cherefulnesse appereth herein, yt beyng wounded with sadnesse and sorrowe, he resteth upon the spirituall comfort of God' (3.viii.8; fol. 166r).

I have outlined two competing religious conceptions of pain that circulated in early modern European religious culture, and specifically in England during approximately the first eighty years after the Elizabethan Settlement: Thomas Norton's translation of Calvin dates from 1561, while Toby Matthew's translation of *The Flaming Hart* was published in 1642, on the eve of the English Civil War. We have seen that Teresa of Avila, Louis of Granada and Ignatius of Loyola, in spite of their different positions within the Catholic Church, share an understanding of pain that revolves first and foremost around the physical human body. They are overwhelmingly preoccupied by the details of Christ's

---

[42] John T. McNeill argues that this passage is an implicit rejection of 'medieval handbooks of penance, the *libri poenitentiales*, in which severe physical penalties were sometimes prescribed' (See McNeill J.T. [ed.] *Calvin: Institutes of the Christian Religion*, trl. Battles F.L. [Philadelphia: 1960], 2 vols., vol. I 610, n. 34).

[43] Minnema, "Calvin's Interpretation of Human Suffering" 150.

physical suffering, which they offer up as an object of sustained meditation, and by the specifics of human physical suffering. They see bodily pain suffered by humans as a way of participating in Christ's Passion, and hence as a way of becoming one with Christ, and present physical anguish as a central element in Christian devotion, and as something to be cultivated and actively sought. Even if pain serves for them as a way of subduing the sinful body, that same body is still their principal devotional instrument – the body is fought through the body. Similarly, those who suffer pain in this world will be rewarded in the next by being given a weightless, immaterial, yet physically intact body, impervious to pain: the afterlife is defined as a bodily state. Moreover, Avila, De Villacastin and Granada do not differentiate clearly between physical and mental pain or between psychological and bodily areas of religious experience, and their rhetoric even actively works to blur any distinctions between the two.

In his views on the theological meaning of suffering, Calvin rejects a number of these assumptions. He posits a clear distinction between Christ's bodily and mental suffering, and sees the mental anguish that Christ suffered as ultimately more important for the atonement of human sin, just as he locates Christ's divinity outside his physical humanity. While he reiterates the idea that humans can imitate Christ's suffering, and that suffering is a crucial aspect of Christian identity, he denies the soteriological effect of this, and maintains that it is only God who works through pain, not humans themselves. Suffering, bodily or mental, should not, therefore, be actively sought, but only accepted when it presents itself; only Christ suffers voluntarily. Moreover, pain is not productive in itself, does not have any *inherent* efficacy, but serves as an opportunity to cultivate *mental* attitudes of temperance and acceptance. In sum, Calvin's interest in the meaning of pain is primarily doctrinal, not experiential or phenomenological. As opposed to his Catholic Reformation counterparts, Calvin never presents the human body and its pain as a crucial channel of religious experience, and the body is in many ways absent from his understanding of suffering. Bodily suffering does not have a special relevance or efficacy for him, and he seeks to disentangle mental from physical anguish. In Calvin, the human body never forms the theological touchstone capable of conferring its quality of 'incontestable reality' on theological concepts that it is in the Catholic texts we have considered.[44]

[44] The formulation is borrowed from Scarry, *The Body in Pain* 27.

If Calvin's understanding of pain is in some ways diametrically opposite to what we have found in Avila, Granada and Ignatius, the parameters of his thinking in themselves also reveal a remarkable continuity with these writers, and with the Catholic discourses in which they operated: the role of suffering in the shaping of a Christian identity, the relation between Christ's pain and human pain, the question of the soteriological power of pain, and the relation between pain and the theological role of the human body. Indeed, Calvin's emphasis on human dependence on God, and on the idea that God confers meaning and efficacy on pain, rather than humans, finds an unexpected parallel in Teresa's repeated insistence that her mystical experiences come from God and not from herself, that she is 'absolutly without anie merit of mine' (458), and that her mysticism is in part *about* becoming fully dependent on God: 'in this discourse, which Almightie God makes to the Soule, there is no remedie at all, but they make me harken to them, whether I will, or no' (336).[45]

Neither of the two models of pain that I have outlined held a clear position of dominance in England between the accession of Elizabeth I and the Civil War. Norton's 1561 translation of the *Institutes* helped to inaugurate the relative official dominance of Calvinist theology in the first decades of Elizabeth's reign, and served as a key statement of doctrine; yet, as the translated works by the Spanish writers discussed in this article show, and as historians of the English Reformation have frequently pointed out, competing forms of spirituality remained present. The position towards the Catholic Church of both the Church of England and the state, moreover, continued to shift between the Elizabethan Settlement and the English Civil War. Exiled on the continent in 1642, Toby Matthew appears to have felt that dedicating his translation of *The Flaming Hart* to the Catholic Queen Henrietta might be a way of reversing his political fortunes.

This religious hybridity is also borne out by the English translation history of Louis of Granada's *Libro*. The first recusant editions of Hopkins' translation, printed on the continent, contain an intensely anti-Protestant prologue by the translator that is steeped in the language

[45] A. de Reuver points to the links between Calvin's spirituality and the late medieval mysticism of Thomas a Kempis in *Calvijn, breuk of brug? Over de spiritualiteit van Thomas a Kempis en Johannes Calvijn* (Utrecht: 1995), and locates these links partly in their shared insistence on human inadequacy and dependence on God.

of apocalypticism and is unambiguous about his overall aims.[46] Hopkins exhorts his readers 'to resiste faithfullye against all Satans wylye deceytefull temptations in this our daungerous age, approchinge so neare towardes the comminge of Antichriste, and the ende of the Worlde' and expresses his 'verie great hope, that with the grace of God theise godlie Meditations will woorke muche good effecte for the conversion of manie of them'.[47] Yet between 1599 and 1634 this once openly seditious work was printed in England in a series of Protestant editions, including the one I have quoted from in this article, that reproduce Hopkins' translation almost verbatim (although they do not refer to Hopkins; the original chapter division has also been rearranged, possibly to make this translation look like an entirely new publication).[48] Maria Hagedorn lists a number of small yet significant alterations – 'the Catholicke Church' has been changed to 'the Church of Christ', for example, while a reference to prayers for the souls of the dead has been removed – and argues that, in order to make the *Libro* palatable for English Protestant readers, Granada's 'besondere Vorliebe für das Emotionale' has been curbed, for example in a reduced emphasis on Christ's suffering.[49] Yet even if Hopkins' translation was adapted to some extent, what is striking is rather how much of his text remains unchanged in the post-1598 editions, and how much of Granada's Counter Reformation sensibility was apparently not seen as directly problematic.

The ambivalence of English theological attitudes towards physical suffering during this period is captured in a Protestant devotional work by the preacher Lawrence Bankes, *The safegard of the soule* (1619), written during his old age as a work of consolation for his parishioners.[50] Unlike Calvin, Bankes goes to considerable lengths in describing the minutiae of Christ's physical agony:

---

46 I borrow the term 'recusant editions' from Hagedorn, *Reformation und Spanische Andachtsliteratur* 30.

47 Granada, *Of prayer, and meditation* (1582) fols. Aiiv; aviiv.

48 See also Hagedorn, *Reformation und Spanische Andachtsliteratur* 41.

49 Hagedorn, *Reformation und Spanische Andachtsliteratur* 43.

50 I have been unable to find any biographical information about Bankes, other than that he was a 'preacher of the word of God: and parson of Staunton, in the county of Glocester', as the title page of *The safegard of the soule* informs us, and that he had preached in 'Drowf[ie]ld, in the Countie of Darby' before this (Lawrence Bankes, *The safegard of the soule. Declaring sundry soueraigne salues tending to the comfort and saluation of the same* [London, G. Purslowe: 1619] fol. A2r–v). He does not seem to have published any other works.

> Behold his tender body how it is scourged, his naked brest is stricken & beaten, his bloudy side is thrust thorow with a speare, his heart panteth, his sinewes bee stretched forth, his christall eyes dazell and lose their sight, his princely face is wan and pale, his pleasant tongue is enflamed with paine, his inward parts waxe dry and starke, his armes both blue and blacke, his bones sore, his comely legges be feeble and weake, and the streames of bloud gush out of his side downe to the ground (134–135).

Read in isolation, this passage could have been lifted from Louis of Granada or Ignatius. Yet here it is not the Christian reader who is urged to behold and ponder Christ's pain, but God himself. The passage is part of a prayer in which Bankes asks God to consider the full weight of Christ's Passion, and to see it as 'sufficient recompence for all our misdemeanour towards thy Majesty' (136). In other words, Christ's pain is evoked in such detail not with the aim of inviting the reader to share in it – Bankes remarks that 'no paine shall bee found like unto his paine' (134) – but to point to God's exclusive soteriological agency, and to underline human dependence on God's judgment, and this is where Bankes departs from Catholic models of pain. Bankes sees the minister as a 'Physicion of the soule' (24), and explicitly states that he should ultimately be unconcerned with the body: 'hee may the better apply his exhortation to the comfort of [the sick person's] Conscience' (24–25). This separation between the domains of the body and the soul can be seen as part of an increasing disentanglement of medicine and religion, analysed by Andrew Wear, that English Protestantism was bringing about in the earlier seventeenth century, and that can clearly be related to the separation between the realms of the body and the soul in Calvin's *Institutes* that I have outlined.[51] As Wear notes, 'Calvin's intellectual preferences and religious doctrines were [...] useful resources in bolstering the claims of the learned physicians, and in attacking not only healers who claimed divinely given powers, but also clergymen who practised medicine. The secular tendency that many have seen in Calvinism seems again apparent, if we interpret such doctrines as limiting the scope or ambit of religion'.[52] Lawrence Bankes' evocation of Christ's pain suggests that this new Protestant understanding of the role of religion, and of the theology of suffering, also drew on, and

---

[51] Wear A., "Religious Beliefs and Medicine in Early Modern England", in Marland H. – Pelling M. (eds.), *The Task of Healing: Medicine, Religion and Gender in England and the Netherlands, 1450–1800* (Rotterdam: 1996) 145–169.

[52] Wear A., "Religious Beliefs and Medicine in Early Modern England" 161.

appropriated, earlier as well as contemporary, post-Tridentine Catholic models of pain, in which the body is at the centre of theological attention.

In all of the religious texts I have considered, the meaning of pain is bound up with the relation between mind and body. Teresa of Avila wonders whether her mystical pains are primarily bodily or mental, and concludes that they are both, and cannot be classified in dualist terms, while in De Villacastin and Louis of Granada the language of bodily and mental suffering flow into each other. Calvin, by contrast, differentiates between physical and mental pain, and presents the suffering of the mind (both in Christ and in humans) as the more relevant and powerful. As a result, in Calvin's *Institutes*, despite its author's preoccupation with issues of suffering, bodily agony disappears into the theological background: it becomes disconnected from salvation, loses its position as an authoritative spiritual experience, and even becomes a potential source of distraction from the more pressing issue of the state of one's soul. When, approximately a century after Calvin, Descartes, in the *Meditations*, defined pain in terms of an epistemological mind-body problem, and saw it as a particularly significant example of the body's infringement on the mind, and therefore as a source of doubt rather than certainty, he was building on and furthering a development that had its origins partly in sixteenth-century Reformed theologies of pain. At the same time, the Descartes' investigation of pain in the *Meditations* suggests that by the mid-seventeenth century, the distinction between mental and bodily suffering that Calvin constructed in the *Institutes*, and that also informs Lawrence Bankes' *The safegard of the soule*, was still not self-evident or unproblematic, and that pain had retained its ability to challenge dualist assumptions.

Selective Bibliography

Bending L., *The Representation of Bodily Pain in Late Nineteenth-Century English Culture* (Oxford: 2000).

Calvin John, *The [H] institution of Christian religion, wrytten in Latine by maister Jhon Caluin*, trl. Thomas Norton (London, Reinolde Wolfe and Richarde Harison: 1561).

Glucklich A., *Sacred Pain: Hurting the Body for the Sake of the Soul* (Oxford: 2001).

Hagedorn M., *Reformation und Spanische Andachtsliteratur. Luis de Granada in England* (Leipzig: 1934).

Howells E., *John of the Cross and Teresa of Avila: Mystical Knowing and Selfhood* (New York: 2002).

Louis of Granada, *Of prayer and meditation contayning foureteene meditations, for the seauen dayes of the weeke, both for mornings and euenings*, trl. Richard Hopkins (London, Edward White: 1611).

Minnema Th., "Calvin's Interpretation of Human Suffering", in Holwerda D.E. (ed.), *Exploring the Heritage of John Calvin* (Grand Rapids, MI: 1976).

Morris D.B., *The Culture of Pain* (Berkeley – Los Angeles: 1993).

Perkins J., *The Suffering Self: Pain and Narrative Representation in the Early Christian Era* (London: 1995).

Porter R. – Porter D., *In Sicknesss and in Health: The British Experience, 1650–1850* (London: 1988).

Scarry E., *The Body in Pain: The Making and Unmaking of the World* (Oxford: 1985).

Silverman L., *Tortured Subjects: Pain, Truth, and the Body in Early Modern France* (Chicago: 2001).

St Teresa of Avila, *The flaming hart, or, The life of the glorious S. Teresa*, trl. Toby Matthew (Antwerp, Johannes Meursius: 1642).

Villacastin Tomas de, *A manuall of devout meditations and exercises instructing how to pray mentally*, trl. Henry More (Saint Omer, English College Press: 1618).

Wall P., *Pain: The Science of Suffering* (London: 1999).

Walsham A., *Church Papists: Catholicism, Conformity and Confessional Polemic in Early Modern England* (London: 1993).

Wear A., "Religious Beliefs and Medicine in Early Modern England", in Marland H. – Pelling M. (eds.), *The Task of Healing: Medicine, Religion and Gender in England and the Netherlands, 1450–1800* (Rotterdam: 1996) 145–169.

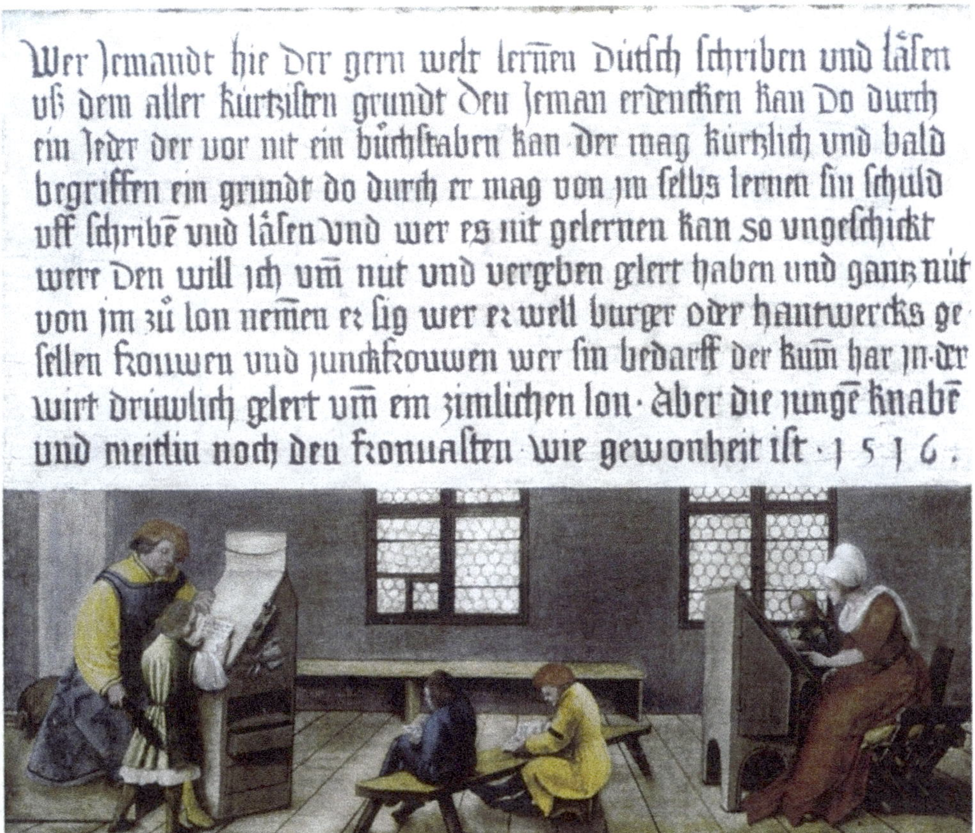
Wer Jemandt hie der gern welt lern̄en dütsch schriben und läsen
uß dem aller kürtzisten grundt den Jeman erdencken kan Do durch
ein Jeder der vor nit ein büchstaben kan der mag kürtzlich und bald
begriffen ein grundt do durch er mag von jm selbs lernen sin schuld
uff schribē und läsen und wer es nit gelernen kan so ungeschickt
were Den will jch um̄ nut und vergeben gelert haben und gantz nüt
von jm zů lon nem̄en er sig wer er well burger oder hantwercks ge
sellen frouwen und junckfrouwen wer sin bedarff der kum̄ har jn der
wirt drüwlich gelert um̄ ein zimlichen lon · aber die jungē knabē
und meitlin noch den fronvasten wie gewonheit ist · 1 5 1 6 .

[Plate II. Enenkel – Fig. 2, p. 99]

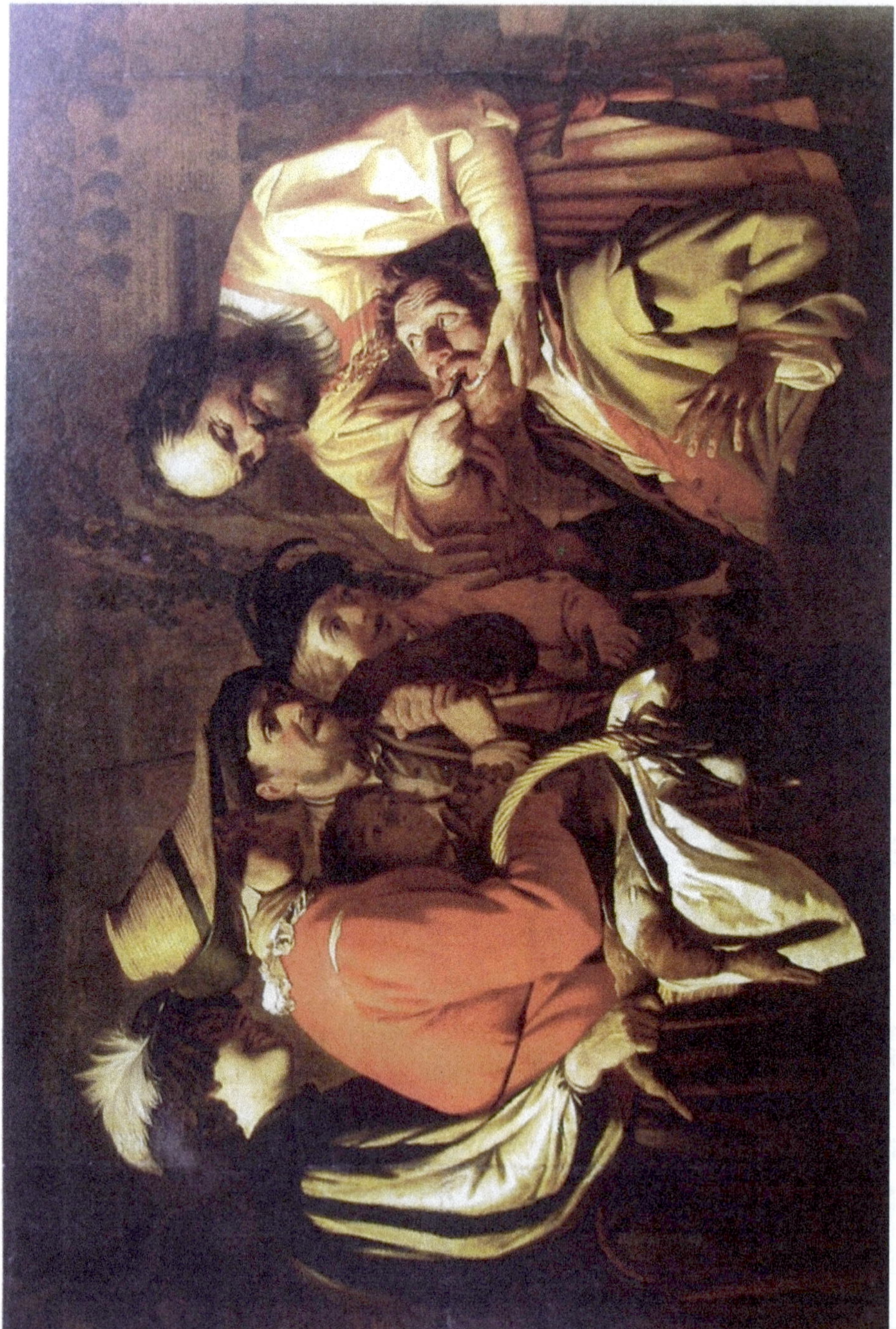

[Plate III. Enenkel – Fig. 3, p. 100]

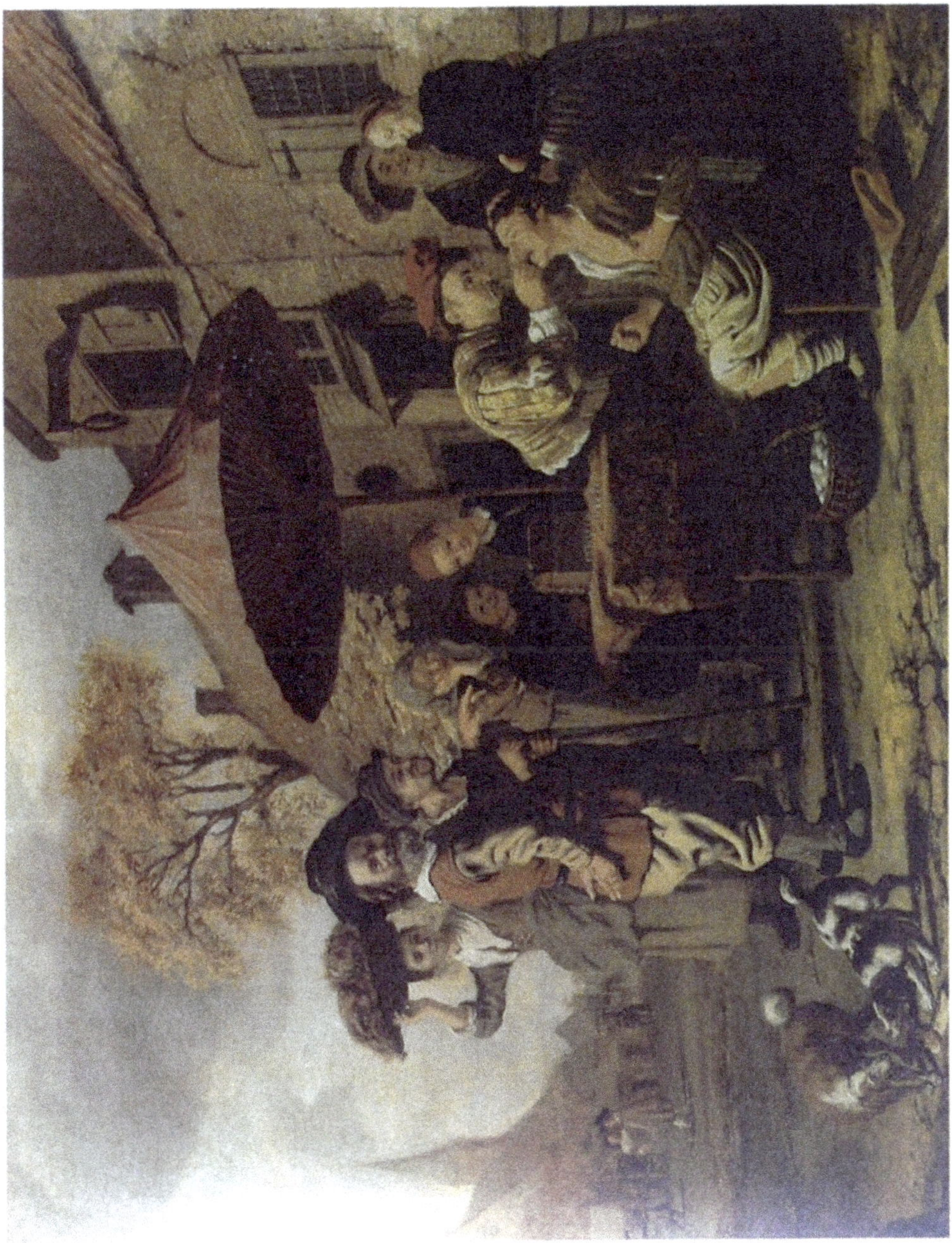

[PLATE IV. ENENKEL – Fig. 4, p. 101]

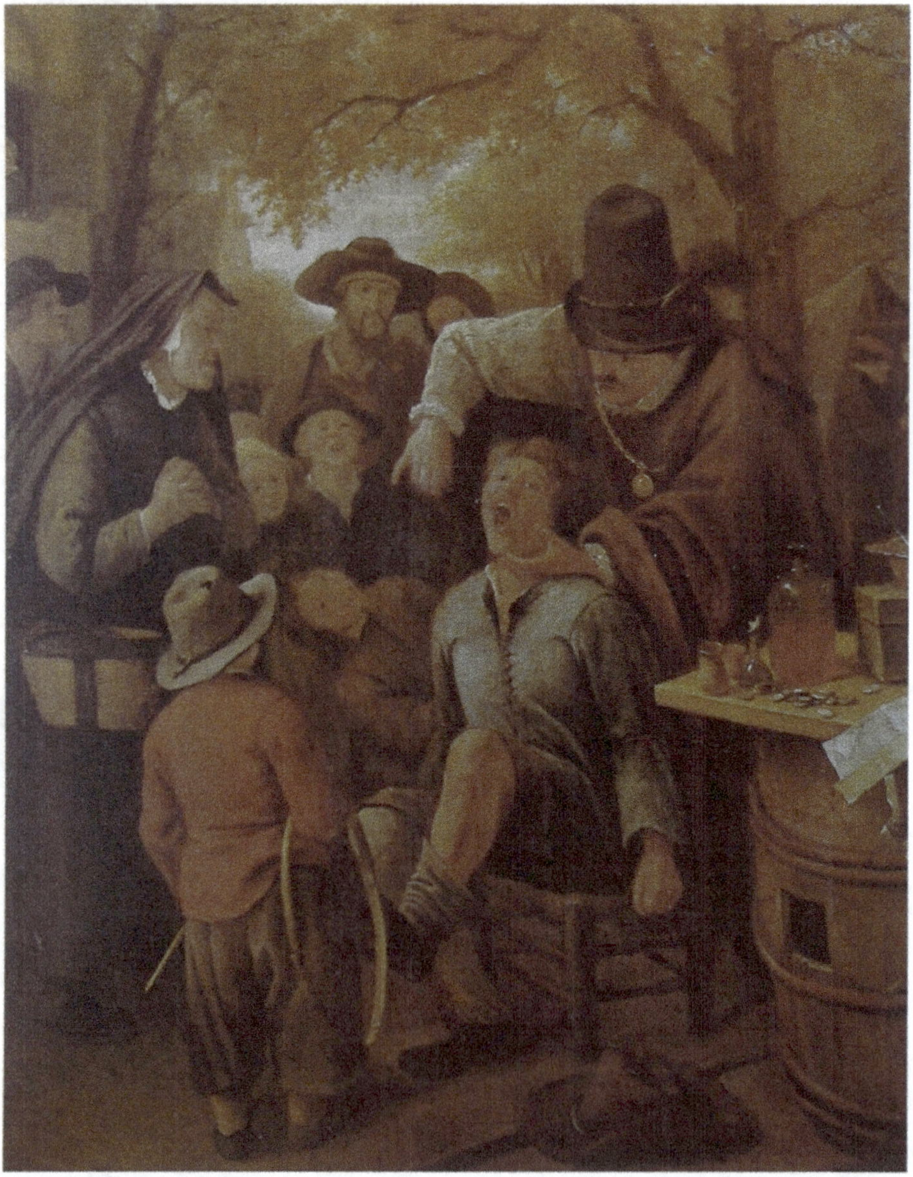

[PLATE V. ENENKEL – Fig. 6, p. 104]

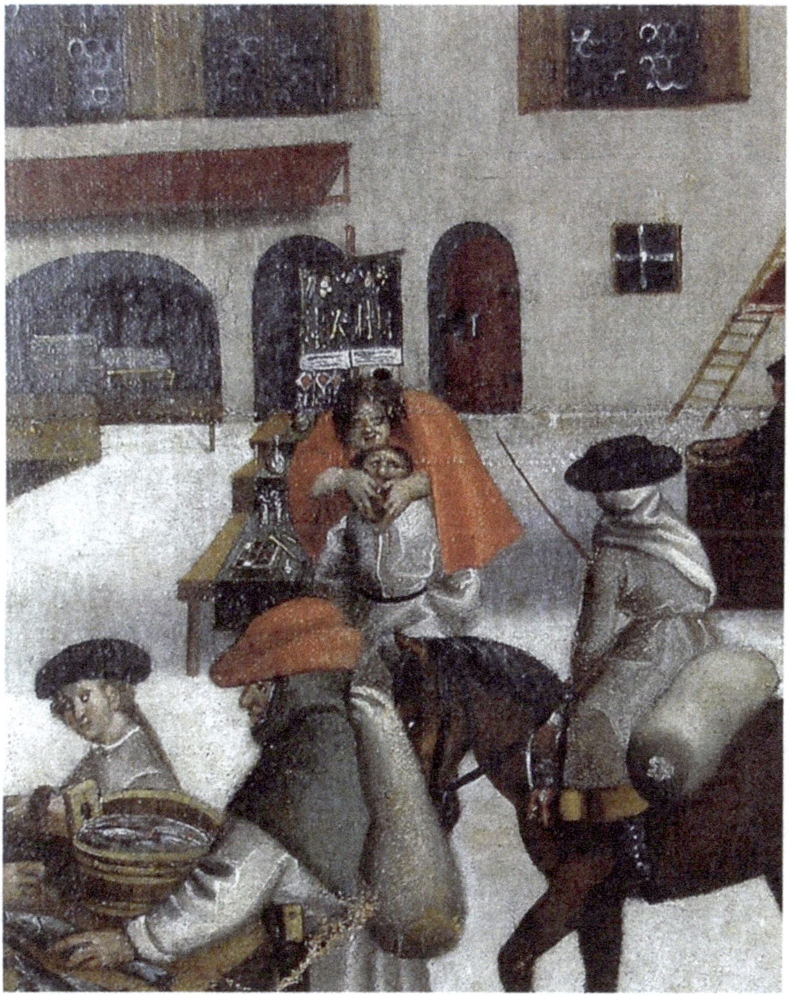

[Plate VI. Enenkel – Fig. 28, p. 141]

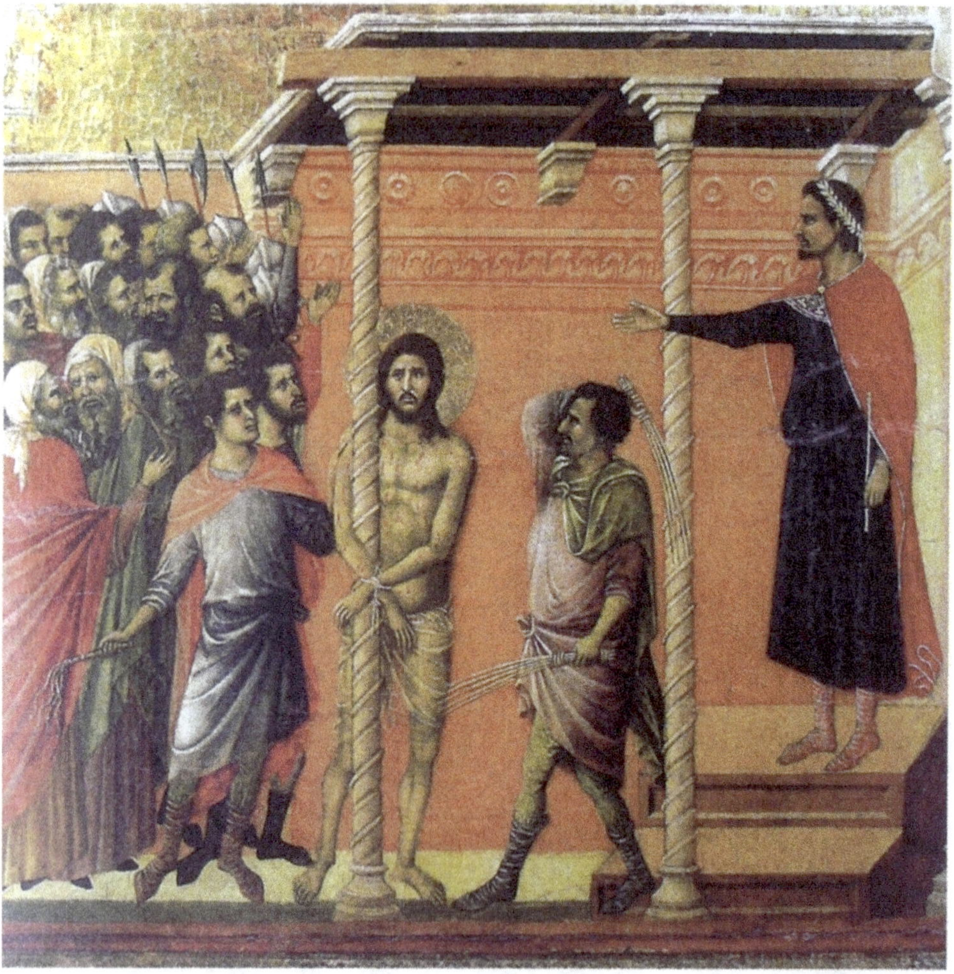

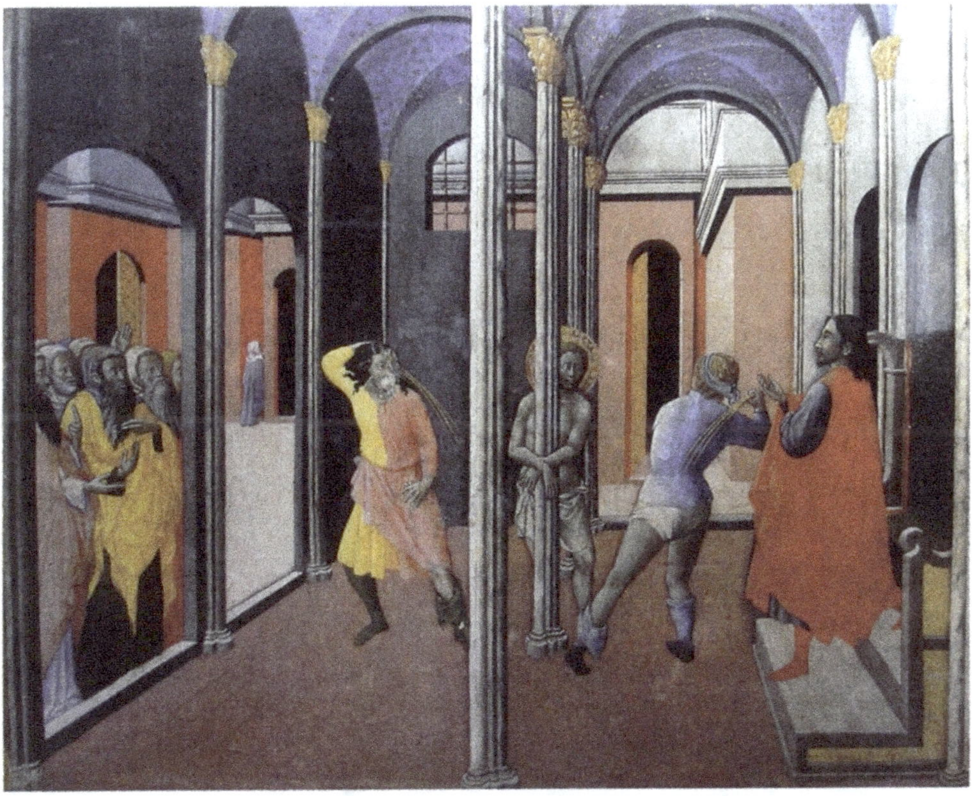

[Plate VIII. Enenkel – Fig. 33, p. 153]

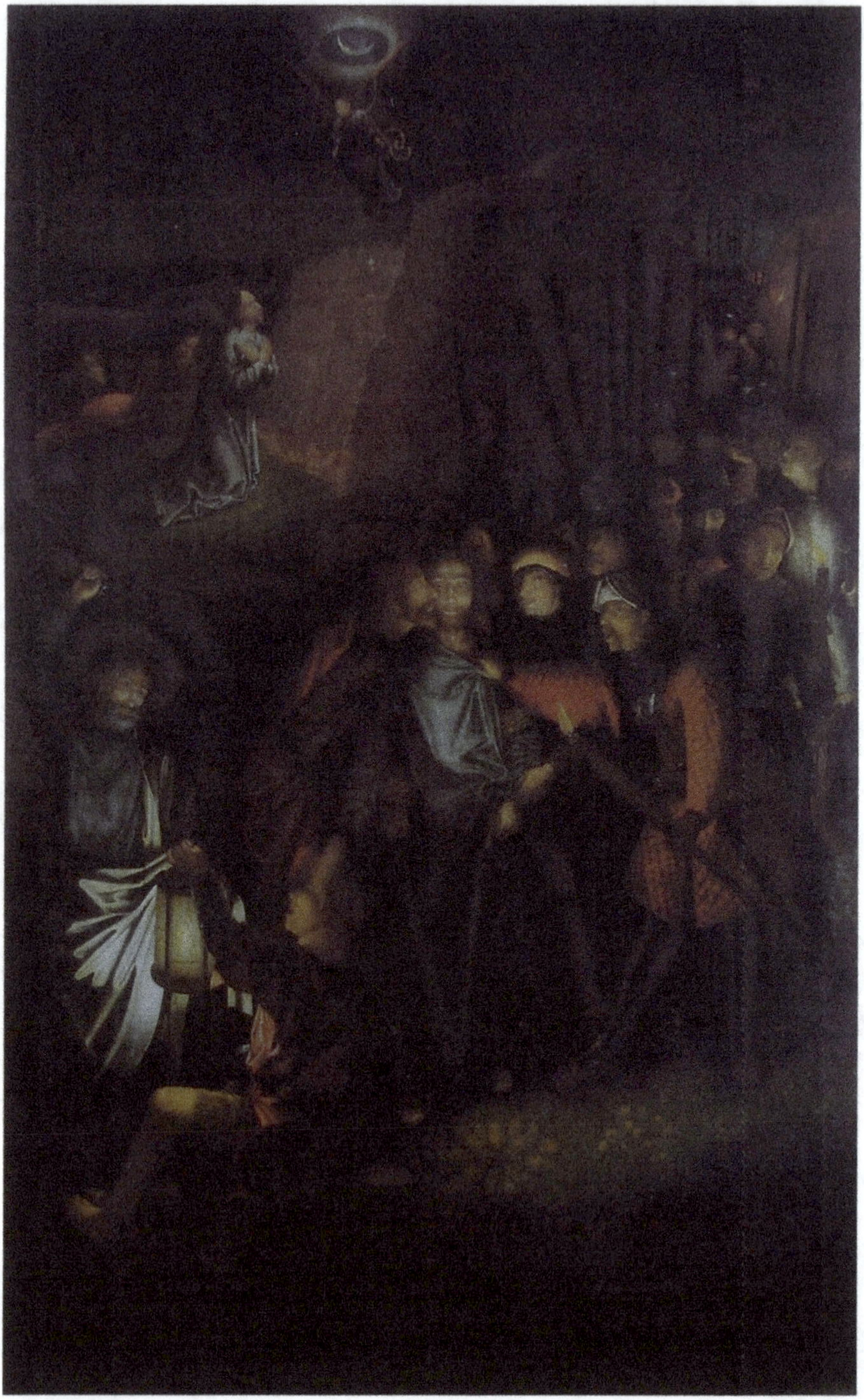

[PLATE IX. ENENKEL – Fig. 34, p. 155]

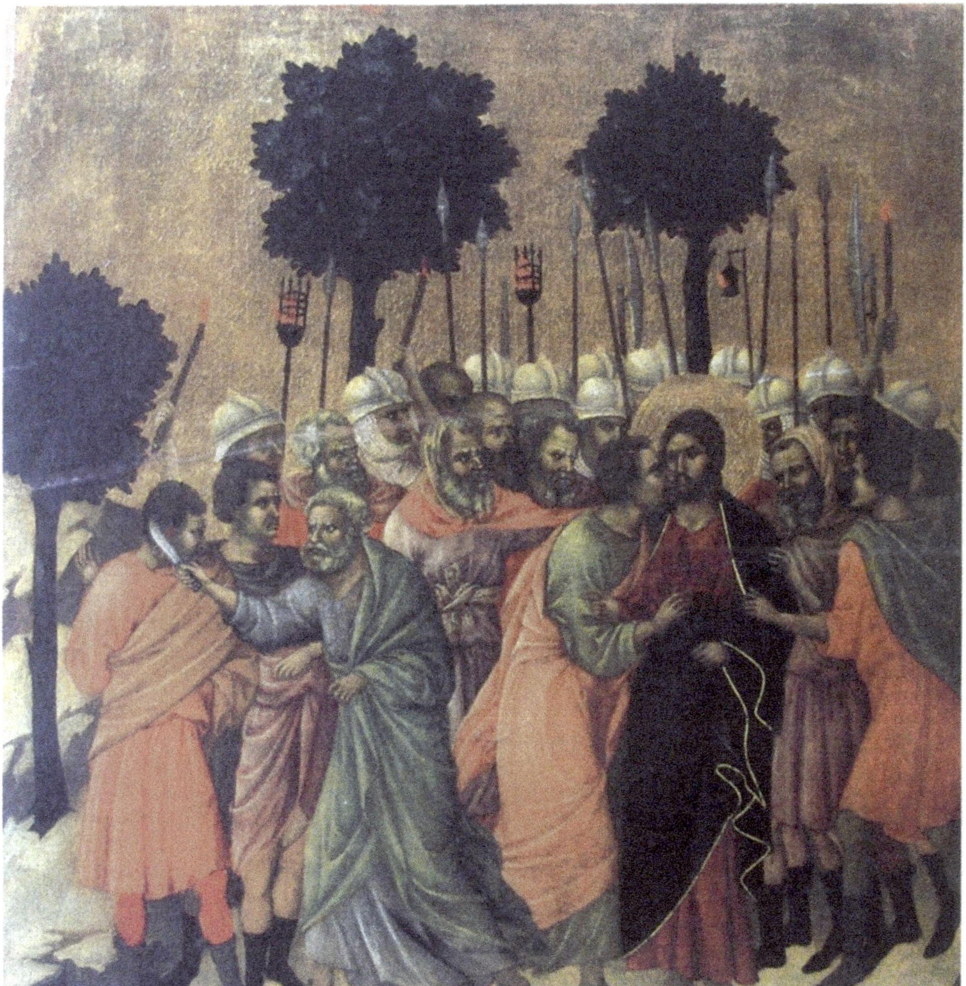

[PLATE X. ENENKEL – Fig. 35, p. 156]

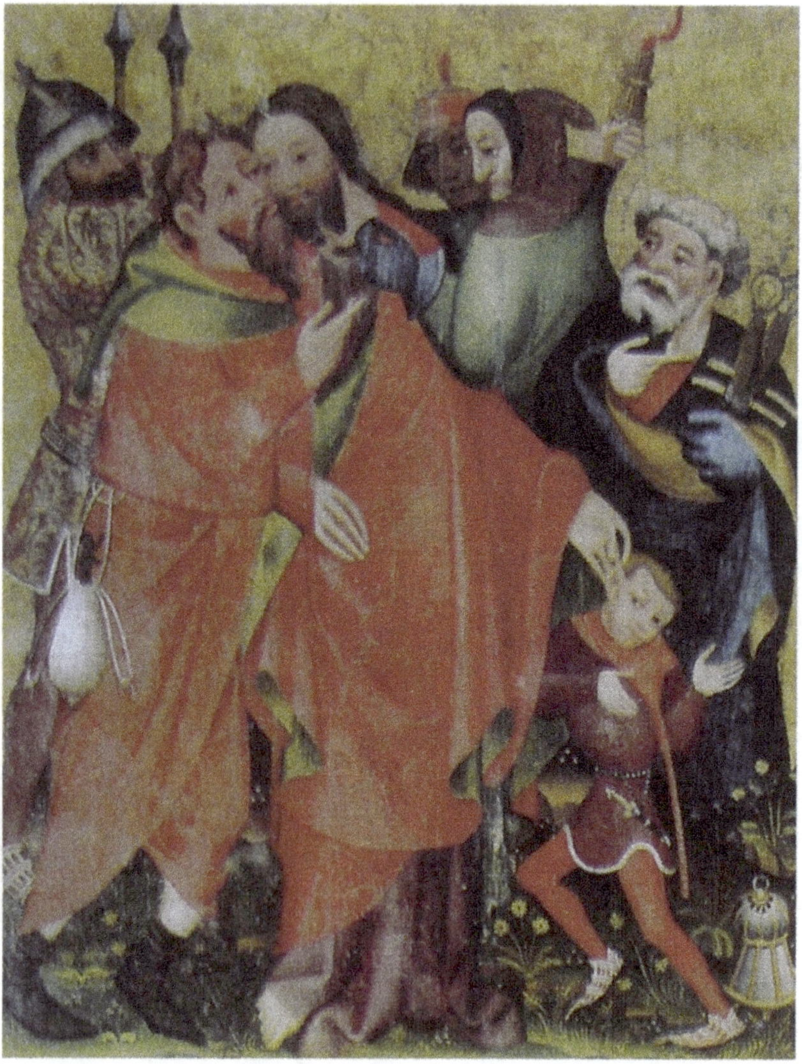

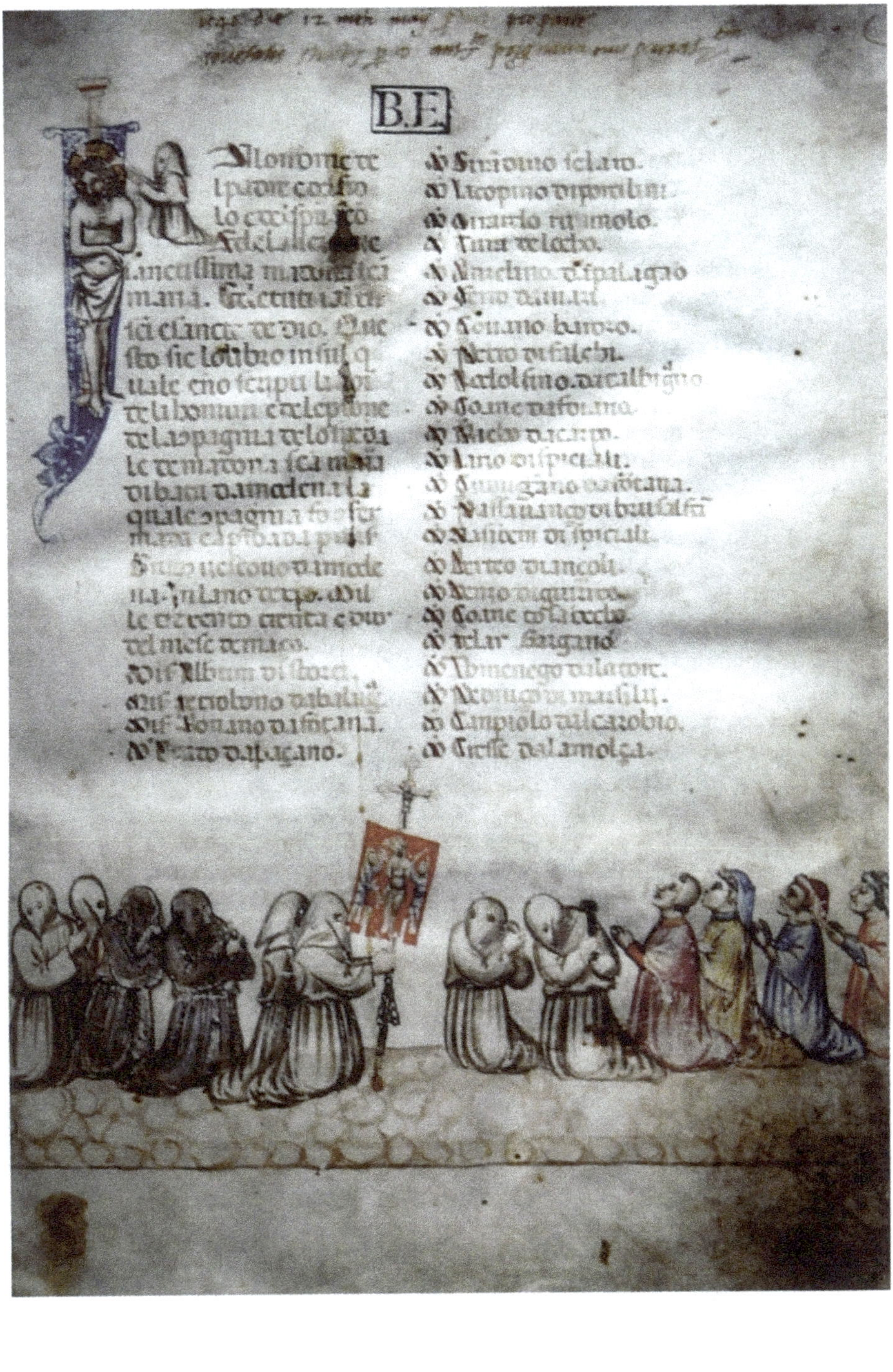

[Plate XII. Dehmer – Fig. 2, p. 236]

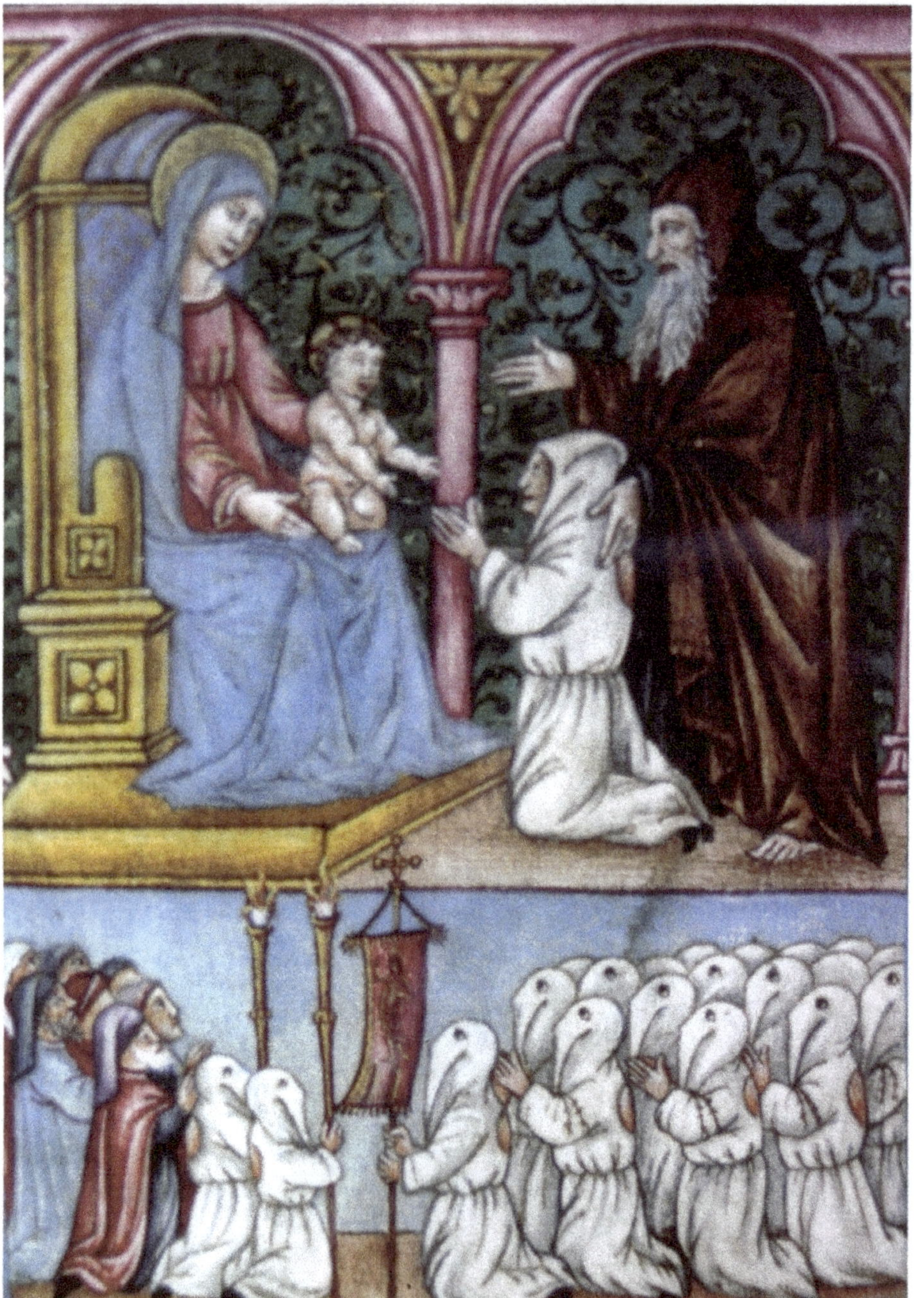

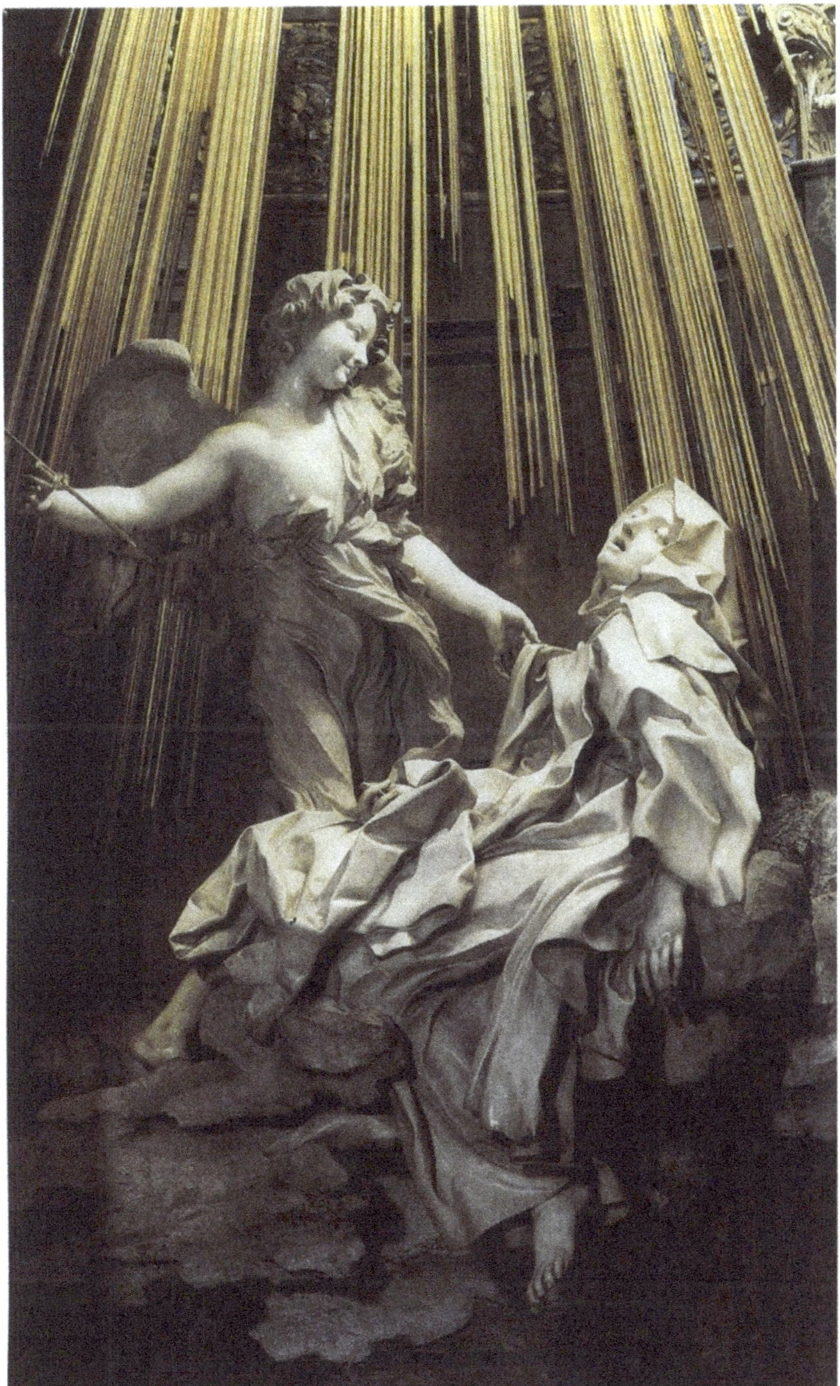

[Plate XIV. Berbara – Fig. 6, p. 284]

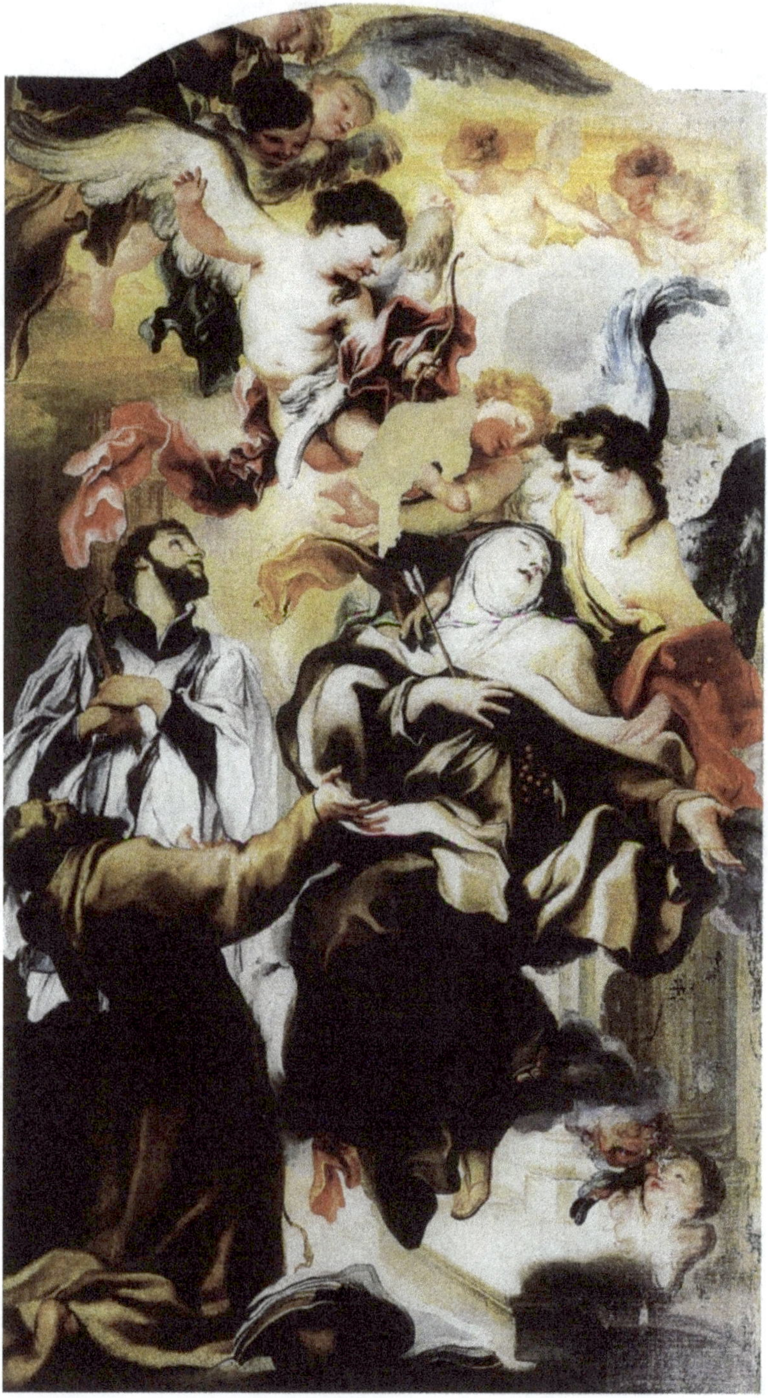

[Plate XV. Berbara – Fig. 7, p. 286]

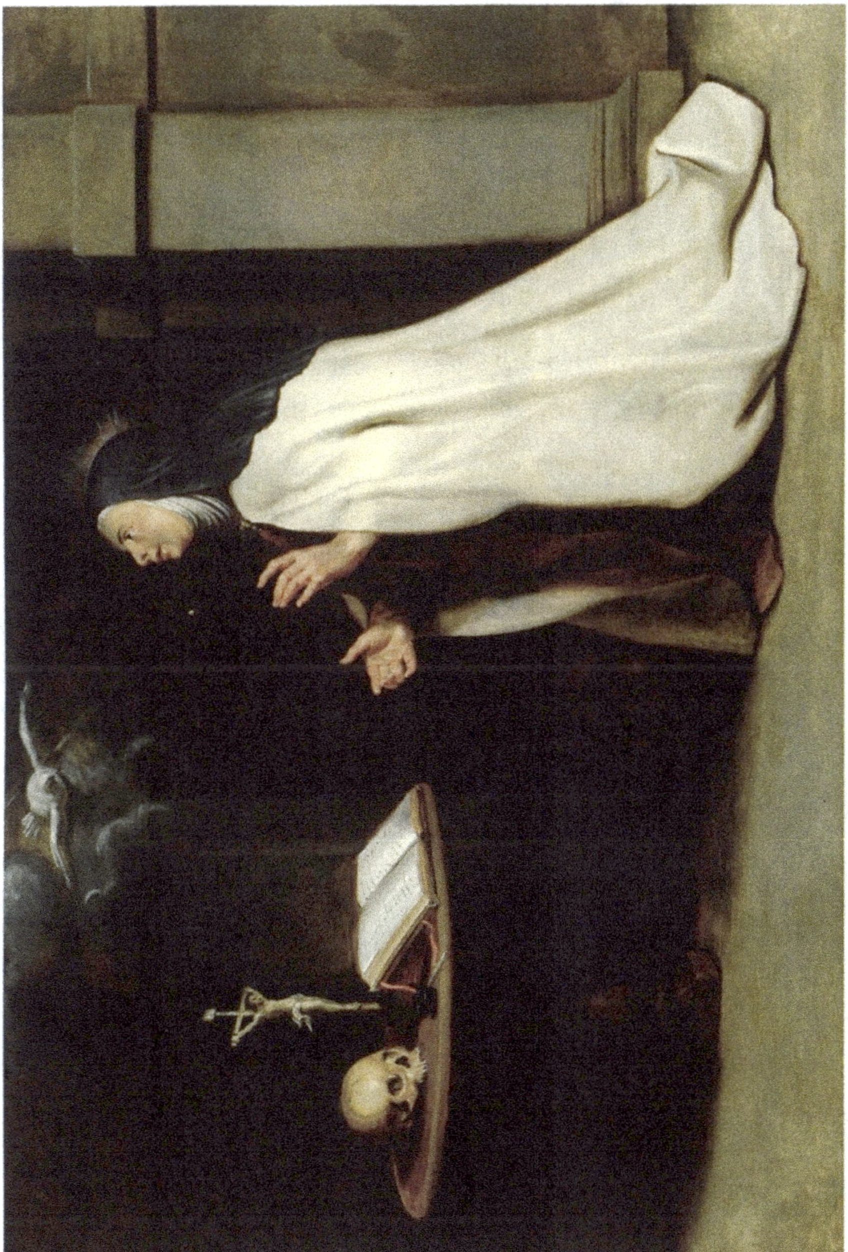

[Plate XVI. Berbara – Fig. 12, p. 296]

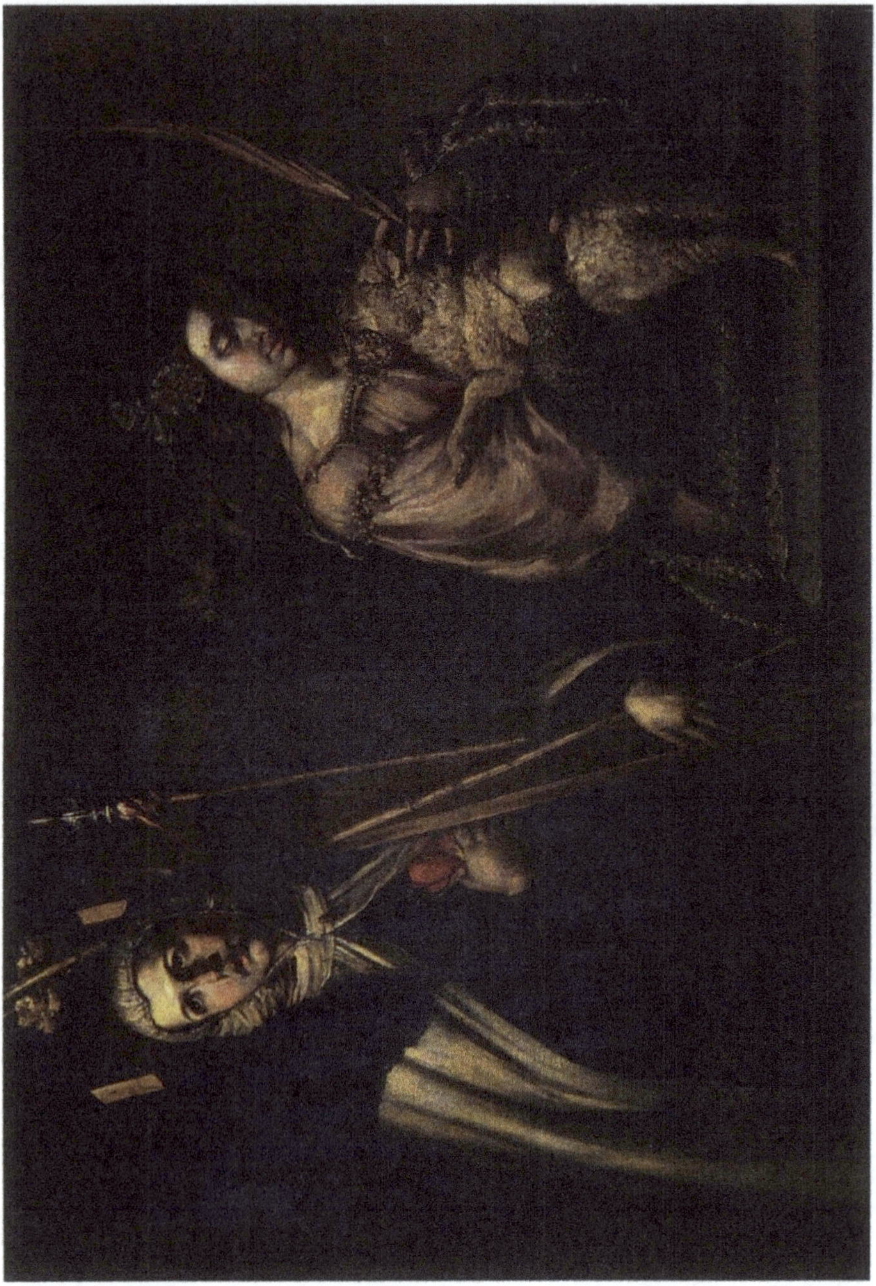

PASSIO UND *COMPASSIO*: GEISSELUNGSRITUALE ITALIENISCHER BUSSBRUDERSCHAFTEN IM SPÄTEN MITTELALTER

Andreas Dehmer

Spätmittelalter und Renaissance gehören in Europa, vor allem aber in Italien, zur Blütezeit religiöser Laiengemeinschaften – allgemein bekannt und subsumiert unter dem Begriff ‚Bruderschaften'. Innerhalb dieses bevölkerungsumgreifenden Phänomens übte die vom Schmerz, von der Passion Christi geprägte Devotion spezieller Buß-Bruderschaften seit jeher eine große Faszination aus, zumal sie auch durch zahlreiche literarische und bildkünstlerische Zeugnisse eindrucksvolle Spuren hinterlassen hat. Allein ein kurzer Gang über den Pisaner Camposanto gewährt einen ersten Einblick in die Geschichte von vierzehn verschiedenen Geißlervereinigungen, die dort im Trecento ihre Grablegen unterhielten.

Die insbesondere von den jungen Bettelorden seit dem 13. Jahrhundert beförderte ‚Passionsfrömmigkeit'[1] wurde von diesen Sozietäten weitläufig propagiert. Anhand dokumentarischer, literarischer und visueller Zeugnisse – vor allem Statuten und Laudentexte, Miniaturen und Gemälde – soll im Folgenden versucht werden, konkrete Abläufe der kollektiven Bußübungen italienischer Bruderschaften zu rekonstruieren. Umfassende Untersuchungen gibt es dazu kaum, obwohl sie für verschiedene Geschichtswissenschaften durchaus von Bedeutung sind: In dem synchronen Zusammenwirken von Aktion, Wort und Bild treffen Religions- und Sozialgeschichte mit Literatur- und Kunstgeschichte in bemerkenswerter Weise aufeinander. Der Beitrag bietet jedoch weniger

[1] Vgl. dazu u.a. Haug W. – Wachinger B. (Hrsg.), *Die Passion Christi in Literatur und Kunst des Spätmittelalters* (Tübingen: 1993); Köpf U., Artikel „Passionsfrömmigkeit", in *Theologische Realenzyklopädie*, Bd. 27 (Berlin – New York: 1997) 722–764; MacDonald A.A. u.a. (Hrsg.), *The Broken Body. Passion Devotion in Late-Medieval Culture* (Groningen: 1998). Vor kurzem war die Passionsfrömmigkeit auch Inhalt verschiedener Beiträge zu der Publikation Blume E. u.a. (Hrsg.), *Schmerz. Kunst + Wissenschaft* (Ausstellungskatalog Berlin 2007) (Köln: 2007) 89 ff.; 153 ff. Die folgenden zentralen Aspekte – Christi Geißelung und die Selbstgeißelung christlicher Laien – sind in diesem umfassenden Katalog jedoch außer Acht gelassen.

einen repräsentativen Überblick, als vielmehr exemplarische Fallstudien, in denen diese Rituale körperlicher Schmerzerfahrung im Nachvollzug der Leiden Christi detailgenau beleuchtet werden sollen.

Die Disciplinati

Ein entscheidendes Datum der Geißlerbewegung im späten Mittelalter war das Jahr 1260, der Beginn einer von Fra Raniero Fasani († vor März 1282) in Perugia ausgelösten, öffentlichen Flagellationswelle, die sich innerhalb kürzester Zeit in zahlreichen Regionen Italiens und darüber hinaus verbreitete.[2] Hintergründe des Massenphänomens waren religiöse ebenso wie soziale Unsicherheiten und eine allgemeine, vor allem mittels Volkspredigten und populärer Schriften propagierte Bußdevotion; aus dem franziskanischen Umfeld seien nur die beiden einflussreichen Passionstraktate *Meditationes Vitae Christi* und *De Meditatione Passionis Christi* genannt.[3] Hauptthema dieser weitläufigen Laien-Frömmigkeit waren die Menschwerdung und die Passion Christi – ihr zentrales Anliegen, seinem Leiden nachzufolgen.[4]

Weitere Geißlerzüge fanden im Trecento einen prominenten Berichterstatter in dem Florentiner Stadtschreiber Giovanni Villani (um 1280–1348), der über eine Bewegung des Jahres 1310 informierte: „zahlreiche Personen aus dem niedrigen Volk ließen ihre Arbeit liegen und kümmerten sich nicht um ihre Bedürfnisse, und mit den Kreuzen voraus marschierten sie sich geißelnd von Ort zu Ort". Die illuminierte Fassung seiner *Nuova Cronica* in einem Kodex der Vatikanischen Bibliothek, aus der zweiten Hälfte des 14. Jahrhunderts, illustriert diesen Bericht. Eine der Miniaturen aus dem Umkreis des Pacino di Buona-

---

[2] Ein kurzer und klarer geschichtlicher Überblick „Sui flagellanti del 1260" stammt von A. Frugoni in ders., *Incontri nel medioevo* (Bologna: 1979) 179–202. Neueren Datums ist der Aufsatz von G. Dickson, „The Flagellants of 1260 and the Crusades", *Journal of Medieval History* 15 (1989) 227–267, der die religionshistorische Betrachtung der Geschehnisse durch soziologische und politische Gesichtspunkte erweitert. Zu Fasani s. den Artikel „Fasani, Raniero", von R. Orioli, in *Dizionaro Biografico degli Italiani*, Bd. 45 (Rom: 1995) 206–209.

[3] Vgl. Derbes A., *Picturing the Passion in Late Medieval Italy. Narrative Painting, Franciscan Ideologies, and the Levant* (Cambridge: 1996).

[4] Dazu u.a. auch Weissman R.F., *Ritual Brotherhood in Renaissance Florence* (New York: 1982) 50 ff.; Henderson J., *Piety and Charity in Late Medieval Florence* (Oxford: 1994) 113–114; Largier N., *Lob der Peitsche. Eine Kulturgeschichte der Erregung* (München: 2001) 83–143.

guida zeigt detailfreudig und im Einklang mit dem Autor eine öffentliche Prozession von halb entblößten, sich mit dem *flagellum* kasteienden Büßern. Doch statt der von Villani erwähnten Tragkreuze sieht man ein blaugrundiges, figürlich bemaltes Banner, auch *gonfalone* oder *vexillum* genannt, auf dem eine Geißelung Christi dargestellt ist.[5] Das mobile Gemälde führt die bußfertigen Gläubigen in ihrer öffentlichen Reue an.

Bereits kurz nach den ersten Geißlerumzügen bildeten sich ab den sechziger Jahren des 13. Jahrhunderts ähnlich gesinnte Flagellantenbruderschaften – vornehmlich zu spirituellen, aber auch zu karitativen Zwecken gegründete und kirchlich approbierte Laienvereinigungen – in Städten wie Perugia, Siena, Bologna, Padua, Vicenza und Bergamo. Die Gründungen der ersten venezianischen ‚Scuole' sind ebenfalls auf den Einfluss jener Massenbewegung von 1260 zurückzuführen.[6]

Allerdings erfuhren die volkssprachlich überwiegend „Disciplinati" oder „Battuti" genannten Vereinigungen erst im Laufe des 14. Jahrhunderts – vor allem infolge verheerender Naturkatastrophen und Epidemien wie der Schwarzen Pest und tiefgreifender Veränderungen der sozialen und politischen Verhältnisse – eine rasche Verbreitung und erfreuten sich bis ins 15. Jahrhundert einer stetig steigenden Popularität. Das frühe öffentliche Auftreten einer solchen Bußbruderschaft in Pavia schilderte um 1330 der Kleriker Opicino de Canistris (1296- um 1352):

> Auch gibt es hier eine Vereinigung von Laien, was sehr lobenswert ist, die an bestimmten Tagen und Nächten, und insbesondere in der hohen

[5] „molta gente minuta [...] sanza numero lasciavano i loro mestieri e bisogne, e co' le croci innanzi s'andavano battende di luogo in luogo"; Villani G., *Nuova Cronica*, hg. v. G. Porta (Parma: 1990/1991) IX, 121. Vgl. Giles Arthur K., „Cult Objects and Artistic Patronage of the Fourteenth-Century Flagellant Confraternity of Gesù Pellegrino", in Verdon T. – Henderson J. (Hrsg.), *Christianity and the Renaissance. Image and Religious Imagination in the Quattrocento* (Syrakus: 1990) 336–360, besd. 337 und 349, Abb. 13.7. Die Handschrift Chigi L.VIII. 296 wurde veröffentlicht von Magnani L., *La cronaca figurata di Giovanni Villani. Ricerche sulla miniatura fiorentina del Trecento* (Vatikanstadt: 1936). Die Miniatur befindet sich auf Fol. 197v. Neueste Forschungen zu dem Kodex stammen von V. Gebhard in ihrer online publizierten Münchner Dissertation von 2007: http://edoc.ub.uni-muenchen.de/archive/00007085.

[6] Wegweisende Studien über italienische Geißlerbruderschaften enthält der Sammelband *Il movimento dei Disciplinati nel settimo centenario dal suo inizio (Perugia-1260)* (Convegno internazionale, Perugina, 1960) (Spoleto: 1962). Zu den „Disciplinati nel Duecento" s. auch Meersseman G.G., *Ordo fraternitatis. Confraternite e pietà dei laici nel medioevo*, 3 Bde. (Italia Sacra 24–26) (Rom: 1977) 451–512.

> Woche, die auch die heilige genannt wird, durch die Stadt zu Kirchen und Predigten ziehen, voran das Kreuz, der nackte Körper von Sackleinen bekleidet, das Gesicht verhüllt und der Rücken entblößt, sich mit eisernen Ketten oder Lederriemen geißelnd und dazu vor den Altären niedergeworfen die Worte einer Andacht singend [...].[7]

Confraternitates Laicorum

Frühe organisierte Assoziationsformen weltlicher Frömmigkeit hatten in Europa zahlreiche Wurzeln. Ausschlaggebender Faktor für den freiwilligen Zusammenschluss Gleichgesinnter war anfangs ein fundamentales menschliches Bedürfnis: die gemeinsame Suche nach Schutz und gegenseitiger Unterstützung innerhalb eines Gemeinschaftswesens. Die zusätzliche religiös-devotionale Komponente, die zu der Ausprägung frommer Laienbruderschaften im heute bekannten Sinne geführt hatte, war vor allem von dem Verlangen nach spiritueller Heilsversicherung bedingt. Nachdem im 12. Jahrhundert die Entwicklung und Ausbreitung der Pfarreien weitgehend abgeschlossen war, konnten, auf diesen Strukturen fußend, aus jeder noch so kleinen oder abgelegenen Gemeinde laikale Glaubensvereinigungen hervorgehen.

Seit dem späten Mittelalter waren religiöse Bruderschaften in der italienischen Gesellschaft weiträumig und fest etabliert. Ihre Grundzüge erfuhren zwischen dem fortgeschrittenen 13. und dem frühen 16. Jahrhundert nur geringe Veränderungen. Stark vereinfacht waren es die zwei Komponenten der caritas, die allen religiösen Konfraternitäten zugrunde lagen, in ihnen institutionalisiert waren und dort mit Demut bzw. *humilitas* verübt werden sollten. Durch das Lesen von Messen, paraliturgische Zeremonien und schließlich durch die Zusicherung von Begräbnis und Kommemoration sollte das Bedürfnis der Mitglieder nach dem eigenen Seelenheil gestillt werden. Dieses Streben nach dem *Amor Dei* ging einher mit dem den Mitmenschen entgegengebrachten *amor proximi*. Die Nächstenliebe artikulierte sich in Hilfeleistungen für

[7] „Est autem ibi quedam societas laycorum, quod laudabilius est, qui certis diebus et noctibus, et maxime in ebdomana maiori, que dicitur sancta, procedunt per civitatem ad ecclesias et predicationes, precedente cruce, amicti sacco super nudo, facieque velata et detectis scapulis, se cathenis ferreis vel corrigiis verberantes, ac ac ante altaria prostrati quedam devotionis verba cantantes [...]"; zit. in Grignani M.A. – Stella A. (Hrsg.), *Antichi testi pavesi* (Pavia: 1977) 12, Anm. 9. Bei der Bruderschaft handelte es sich wahrscheinlich um die Raccomandati della Beata Vergine.

Bedürftige und Kranke und in anderen wohltätigen Werken gegenüber Außenstehenden sowie in gegenseitiger Unterstützung innerhalb der Gemeinschaft. Der letztgenannte Umstand indiziert eine weitere Gemeinsamkeit aller Konfraternitäten, die bereits aus ihrem spezifischen Namen heraus ersichtlich ist: *fraternitas*.

Eben diese drei komplementären Ideale fanden seit dem beginnenden 13. Jahrhundert ihre Verkörperung vor allem in den Bettelorden, die sich ihrerseits außerordentlich stark in der Förderung und Anleitung des Bruderschaftswesens engagierten. Dennoch wäre es falsch, religiöse Laienvereinigungen nur als paramonastische Ableger anzusehen bzw. generell den Einfluss der Orden überzubewerten. Dagegen spricht schon allein die enge Anlehnung zahlreicher früher Bruderschaften an die Pfarreien des jeweiligen Gemeinschaftswesens, innerhalb welcher sie ins Leben gerufen wurden.

Religionshistorisch definiert sich also eine Konfraternität in vorreformatorischer Epoche als verschiedengradig autonome Gemeinschaft gläubiger Laien, die sich vorrangig zu frommen und karitativen Zwecken zusammengeschlossen hatten. Sie wurde durch Regelbücher institutionalisiert und organisiert, bedurfte aber der Anerkennung von kirchlichen Autoritäten, d.h. einer offiziellen Approbation. Durch die entschieden spirituell-religiöse Ausrichtung waren die laikalen Glaubensvereinigungen stark mit den Vertretern der Geistlichkeit verbunden, jedoch standen sie gleichzeitig, durch ihr Verbleiben in der Profanität, in engem Kontakt zu den weltlichen Gemeinschaftsstrukturen. Nicht ohne Grund waren ihre inneren Organisationsformen den Verfassungen der Kommunen oder der Zünfte ähnlicher gestaltet als denjenigen der Orden.[8]

Wie jede religiöse Laienbruderschaft versammelten sich auch die Geisselbrüder regelmäßig zum gemeinsamen Gebet und frommen Wirken in einem Oratorium, einer Kapelle oder einem ihnen zugewiesenen Ort innerhalb einer Kirche. Und wie die meisten spätmittelalterlichen Gebetsvereinigungen weihten sie sich Christus, der Gottesmutter oder anderen heiligen Patronen. An bestimmten, zumeist festgeschriebenen Tagen ließen sie in der Regel ebenfalls Predigten und Messen lesen,

---

[8] Erst das Konzil von Trient versuchte in der zweiten Hälfte des 16. Jahrhunderts die religiösen Laienverbände unter stärkere kirchliche Kontrolle zu bringen und setzte der Eigenständigkeit früher Konfraternitäten bischöfliche Aufsicht entgegen; zusammenfassend zu dieser Entwicklung s. Dehmer A., *Italienische Bruderschaftsbanner des Mittelalters und der Renaissance* (München – Berlin: 2004) Kap. 2. Weitere Abschnitte des vorliegenden Textes entstammen ebenfalls dieser Publikation.

veranstalteten öffentliche Prozessionen oder auch theatralische Mysterienspiele bzw. beteiligten sich daran.

Durch ihr äußeres Erscheinungsbild unterschieden sich die Disciplinati jedoch sehr deutlich von den anderen religiösen Konfraternitäten. Neben Kutte und Kapuze mit Augenschlitzen kennzeichnete sie speziell ein Rückenausschnitt im Gewand, wie es in zahlreichen von ihnen in Auftrag gegebenen Gemälden und Bildwerken überliefert ist. Die Verhüllung diente dem Schutz der Anonymität, welche davor bewahren sollte, dass fromme Taten mehr für die persönliche Eitelkeit als für den spirituellen Gewinn verübt wurden. Zusätzlich blieb die Gleichheit unter den Mitgliedern gewährleistet. Die Öffnung des korporativen Habits hatte hingegen einen handfesteren Grund: Sie enthüllte den Körper zur Geißelung.[9]

Über Jahrhunderte hinweg erfuhr dieses Erscheinungsbild nur geringfügige Veränderungen, die nicht selten jedoch weltlichen Bedürfnissen geschuldet sein konnten; so schrieben die Statuten der prestigereichen venezianischen Scuola di S. Rocco aus dem späten 15. Jahrhundert vor,

> dass alle unsere Brüder der heiligen Disziplin in Sackleinengewändern mit Ärmeln gehen sollen, mit der Kapuze über dem Kopf sowie bedecktem Gesicht, mit blauen Strümpfen und weißen Schuhen, und die Nierengegend hinten unbekleidet, um die Disziplin vollziehen zu können.[10]

Die Disciplina

Die gemeinschaftliche Selbstkasteiung, die ‚Sancta Disciplina',[11] war das hervorragende Charakteristikum der Bußbrüder und ihrer

---

[9] Vgl. u.a. Barr C., *The Monophonic Lauda and the Lay Religious Confraternities of Tuscany and Umbria in the Late Middle Ages* (Kalamazoo – Michigan: 1988) 31–59; Schiferl E., „Corporate Identity and Equality: Confraternity Members in Italian Paintings, c. 1340–1510", *Source* 8,2 (1989) 12–18.

[10] „che tutj j nostri fradeli de la sancta disciplina uadano uestidi de sacho con le maneghe e con el suo Capuçino in cauo etiam con el uolto couerto e con le calçe beretine e con le scarpe bianche e con le rene nude dedriedo per poter far la disciplina"; zit. in Tonon F., *Scuola dei Battuti di San Rocco. Documenti sulle origini e illustrazione dei Capitoli delle Mariegole* (Venedig: 1998) 44.

[11] Der auf eine paraliturgische Auffassung des Bußrituals hinweisende Begriff wurde bereits im 14. Jahrhundert verwendet, vgl. z.B. Grignani – Stella (Hrsg.), *Antichi testi pavesi* 24. Zu der seit dem 8. Jahrhundert belegbaren monastischen Tradition der ‚Disciplina' als freiwillige Bußübung s. auch Largier, *Lob der Peitsche* 43 ff.

christozentrisch ausgerichteten Devotion. Sie bildete den konstitutiven Bestandteil einer Andachtsform, die nicht nur (wie bei den zeitlich früheren Laudenbruderschaften) auf Lob und Erhöhung Gottes, Marias und der Heiligen abzielte, sondern auch auf die eigene Erniedrigung – die im Sinne der Imitatio Christi zugleich als Erhöhung gedeutet werden kann – durch den Akt der Flagellation.[12] Der allgemein übliche Aufruf zur rituellen Selbstzüchtigung, „Apprehendite disciplinam ne quando irascatur Dominus et pereatis de via iusta", basiert auf Ps. 2, 12 – „damit er nicht zürnt und Euer Weg nicht in den Abgrund führt" – und steht programmatisch für das kollektiv verfolgte Ziel nach Erlösung in der Endzeit.

In der Karwoche kulminierte die Geißlerfrömmigkeit. Der Leidensweg Christi wurde durch das Lesen von Predigten und die kollektive Durchführung verschiedener Zeremonien den Mitgliedern solcher devotionalen Vereinigungen eindringlich in Erinnerung gerufen und von ihnen nachempfunden. Jährlicher Höhepunkt war der Gründonnerstag, als Christus beim Letzten Abendmahl sich vor seinen Jüngern herabsetzte, indem er ihnen die Füße wusch. Damit gab er das Vorbild wahrer Demut, dem die Bruderschaften an diesem Tag nacheiferten.[13] Die um 1319 vom dominikanischen Bischof Giacomo Benfatti († 1332) kompilierten Satzungen der Disciplinati di S. Maria della Misericordia in Mantua beinhalten zum Ablauf dieser gemeinschaftlichen Devotions- und Bußübung ausführliche Anweisungen: Als Stellvertreter Christi beschloss der Vorsteher der Vereinigung das von Gesang und Flagellation begleitete rituelle *pedilavium* mit dem Bruderschaftsbanner, das mit Sicherheit auch figürlich bemalt war. Ein während der Fuß-

[12] Henderson, *Piety and Charity* 41–42 und 113 ff.; vgl. ders., „The Flagellant Movement and Flagellant Confraternities in Central Italy, 1260–1400", *Studies in Church History* 15 (1978) 147–160, bes. 158. Largier, *Lob der Peitsche* 9, interpretiert in der „öffentlichen Inszenierung des Körpers" als weitere Absicht die Angleichung von Gott und Mensch. Zur Frühgeschichte von Bußbruderschaften in Mittelitalien s. auch Frank T., *Bruderschaften im spätmittelalterlichen Kirchenstaat. Viterbo, Orvieto, Assisi* (Tübingen: 2002) 60–88; 259–267; 304–316.

[13] Henderson, *Piety and Charity* 128. Ein im englischen Withyham aufbewahrter Zyklus von vier toskanischen Leinwandbildern mit Szenen der Fußwaschung, des Judasverrats, der Verspottung und Geißelung Christi (um 1390, St. Michael and All Angels) wurde möglicherweise innerhalb solcher paraliturgischer Zeremonien während der Karwoche verwendet; s. Villers C., „Paintings on Canvas in Fourteenth Century Italy", *Zeitschrift für Kunstgeschichte* 58 (1995) 338–358; bes. 354.

waschung zu sprechender Gebetstext – das *mandatum* – vervollständigte ein zeitgleiches Zusammenspiel von Wort, Tat und Bild.[14]

Buße und Bilder

Im Mittelpunkt der Gebete und Gesänge der Disciplinati standen Tod, Gericht und Strafe, häufig basierend auf den sieben Bußpsalmen.[15] Ähnliche Thematiken tauchten auch im visuellen Vokabular der Geisselbrüder auf. Natürlich waren zwar ebenso Darstellungen heiliger Patrone und vor allem der Gottesmutter überaus populär, außerdem die Werke der Barmherzigkeit als Programmbilder der kollektiv praktizierten Nächstenliebe,[16] doch den zentralen Kern bildeten wesensgemäß Gemälde mit den Szenen der Passion Jesu Christi.[17]

> Die Bilder spiegelten das vor ihnen stattfindende rituelle, kultische und karitative Leben wider und forderten gleichzeitig zu entsprechendem Verhalten auf, ob zu Andacht, Geißelung, Bildkult oder karitativer Tätigkeit: Bild und Realität konzipierten sich gegenseitig.[18]

Gerade in den einer Bruderschaft und ihren Bußpraktiken vorbehaltenen Bereichen dürften Darstellungen der Leidensgeschichte zum

---

[14] Thompson A., „New Light on bl. Giacomo Benfatti OP, Bishop of Mantua, and the Mantua Disciplinati", *Archivum Fratrum Praedicatorum* 69 (1999) 147–179; Dehmer, *Italienische Bruderschaftsbanner* 115; 266.

[15] Weissman, *Ritual Brotherhood* 57; Barr, *The Monophonic Lauda* 7–8. Zum Einfluss der Passionslauden der Disciplinati auf die italienische Malerei und Skulptur s. Belting H., *Das Bild und sein Publikum im Mittelalter. Form und Funktion früher Bildtafeln der Passion* (Berlin: 1981); Pochat G., *Theater und bildende Kunst im Mittelalter und in der Renaissance in Italien* (Graz: 1990) 52–85.

[16] Vgl. u.a. Dehmer, *Italienische Bruderschaftsbanner* 26–28; Lee E.-K., „Art and Ritual Drama of the Flagellant Confraternities in 13th–15th Century Italy", *Arte medievale* IV,2 (2005) 69–81; Ritzerfeld U., *Pietas – Caritas – Societas. Bildprogramme karitativer Einrichtungen des Spätmittelalters in Italien* (Diss. Bonn: 2007) [http://hss.ulb.uni-bonn.de/diss_online/phil_fak/2007/ritzerfeld_ulrike] 67–75; 180 ff.; 201–203.

[17] Lindemann B.W., „Die Bildlichkeit des Schmerzes in der alten Kunst", in *Schmerz. Kunst + Wissenschaft*, 99–105, über Darstellungen infolge ‚im Spätmittelalter sich intensivierender Passionsfrömmigkeit' (100): „Der Leichnam Christi sollte zu Tränen rühren, der seelische Schmerz der Muttergottes, Johannes' und der anderen Zeugen des Kreuzestodes waren Vorbild für die angemessene Reaktion des Betrachters, der es ihnen gleichtun sollte. Wir wissen in der Tat, dass vor solchen Bildern geweint wurde, dass die Bilder als Aufforderung zur Compassio, zum Mit-Leiden begriffen wurden".

[18] Ritzerfeld, *Pietas – Caritas – Societas* 217.

unverzichtbaren Inhalt malerischer Dekorationen gehört haben.[19] Ferner zählten zu dem Bildinventar der Geißlerbruderschaften verschiedene sowohl kontemplativ als auch didaktisch intendierte Sujets wie der Schmerzensmann, die Pietà bzw. Beweinung Christi und sinnverwandte Themen, die Madonna dell'Umiltà, Totentanz, Triumph des Todes etc.

Diesbezüglich exemplarische Wanddekorationen italienischer Bruderschaftsoratorien sind aus dem 15. Jahrhundert überkommen: Freskenzyklen in Urbino (Oratorio di S. Giovanni, um 1416 ausgeführt von den Brüdern Lorenzo und Jacopo Salimbeni), in Assisi (Oratorio di S. Francescuccio, 1430er Jahre, zugeschrieben Giovanni di Corraduccio und Pietro di Giovanni Mazzaforte), in Serravalle in der Provinz Treviso (S. Lorenzo dei Battuti, nach 1438, verschiedene Maler)[20] und insbesondere in Clusone nahe Bergamo (Oratorio dei Disciplini, 1470–85): Die Giacomo Borlone (dokumentiert 1462–1471) zugeschriebenen Freskomalereien zeigen Darstellungen des Triumphs des Todes und eines Totentanzes an der Außenfassade sowie Szenen aus dem Leben Jesu Christi im Inneren des Oratoriums.[21]

Frühere Bildausstattungen dieser Art sind offenbar nur fragmentarisch erhalten, wie die Wandgemälde der Bruderschaftskirche S. Maria Maddalena in Bergamo oder des Oratorio dei Battuti Bianchi di S. Maria Novella in Ferrara aus dem 14. Jahrhundert.[22] Ebenso wie in

[19] „Whereas a laudesi or devotional image is intended to reflect the image of the saint being venerated, the flagellant artwork has a more active role: that of stimulating the viewer's identification with the suffering and sacrifice of Christ"; Giles Arthur, „Cult Objects and Artistic Patronage" 337. Ähnlich dazu Black C.F., *Italian Confraternities in the 16th Century* (Cambridge: 1989) 102: „A visual reminder and encouragement for brethren to practice flagellation appeared in the miniatures decorating rule-books, or membership books, or on the processional standards (*gonfaloni*) and altarpieces they commissioned". Vgl. Bascapé G., „I sigilli delle confraternite", in *Il movimento* 591–596, bes. 591–592; Prandi A., „Intorno all'iconografia dei Disciplinati", ebd. 496–508.

[20] Weiterführend dazu: Bucci C., „Vicende del ciclo dei Salimbeni in San Giovanni Battista a Urbino", *Proporzioni*, N.S. 2/3 (2001–2002) 42–58; Ritzerfeld, *Pietas – Caritas – Societas* 127–140, 258–264; Fossaluzza G., *Gli affreschi nelle chiese della Marca Trevigiana dal Duecento al Quattrocento*, I. 2, Tardogotico e sue persistenze (Treviso: 2003) 81–240.

[21] Vgl. Cortesi L. – Mandel G., *Affreschi ai disciplini di Clusone. Storie di Gesù (1470–1471). Danza macabra (1485)* (Bergamo: 1972).

[22] Vgl. Dehmer A., „‚Sub Vexillo Sanctae Mariae Magdalenae' – Bilder, Banner und Bruderschaften der hl. Maria Magdalena im Bergamaskischen", *Das Münster* 58 (2005) 206–214; bes. 207–209; Guerzi C., „Frammenti di una decorazione confraternale trecentesca: l'oratorio dei Battuti Bianchi a Ferrara", *Bollettino d'Arte* 87 (2002) 85–118. Eine heute noch in der Vatikanischen Pinakothek aufbewahrte Madonnentafel des Vitale da Bologna (um 1345) diente dort wohl als Altar- und Prozessionsbild. Weitaus anspruchsvoller waren die um 1338 begonnenen Malereien im Oratorium der

den vier Beispielen aus dem Quattrocento zog auch in letzterem eine monumentale Kreuzigung den Blick jedes Eintretenden sogleich auf sich. Zweifellos diente diese prominente Platzierung unter anderem dazu, die Gläubigen auf die Buße einzustimmen und vorzubereiten.

Festgelegte Regeln über den Verlauf des Geißelrituals selbst, inner- und außerhalb der Bruderschaftslokale, variieren in ihrer Ausführlichkeit von Fall zu Fall;[23] nur selten wird eine Miteinbeziehung von Bildern in das Zeremoniell erwähnt. Dennoch ist davon auszugehen, dass visuellen Medien gerade hierbei eine wesentliche Bedeutung zukam, wie es unter anderem die Statuten der Mailänder Raccomandati di S. Maria aus der zweiten Hälfte des 15. Jahrhunderts nahe legen – Kapitel VII enthält präzise Vorschriften zum Ablauf des Rituals, „per fare disciplina in quella caxa a reverentia de la passione de Christo e de la glorioxa vergene Maria“: So sollten die Mitglieder unmittelbar nach Eintreten in ihr Oratorium, vor dem Altar oder dem Vortragekreuz der Bruderschaft niederkniend, ein Vaterunser und ein Avemaria sprechen. Hatten sich alle versammelt, begann die ‚disciplina‘ wiederum mit Fokus auf den Altar. Gingen die Brüder hingegen in Bußprozession, sollte dabei ein Banner vorangeführt werden, das zudem in den zu besuchenden Kirchen vor dem Altar zur Schau gestellt wurde – offenbar als Stellvertreter des eigenen, zurückgelassenen Altarbildes.[24]

Bereits die im mittleren 14. Jahrhundert verfassten Statuten der Fraternita di S. Croce in Urbino schrieben für deren Versammlungsort das Vorhandensein eines Bildes mit dem Kruzifixus zwingend vor. Zudem wurde ausdrücklich festgelegt, ein Tragkreuz oder aber ein tragbares Gemälde mit dem Gekreuzigten in das Zeremoniell der gemeinschaftlichen Selbstzüchtigung miteinzubeziehen:

Compagnia di S. Maria di Mezzaratta, an denen Vitale ebenfalls beteiligt war; s. Volpe A., *Mezzaratta. Vitale e altri pittori per una confraternita bolognese* (Bologna: 2005). Die Reste der umfangreichen Dekoration befinden sich in der Pinacoteca Nazionale in Bologna.

[23] Beispiele für ausführliche Geißelungsvorschriften des 14. Jahrhunderts in Meersseman, *Ordo fraternitatis* 639 (Kapitel IX der Statuten der Compagnia dei Disciplinati in Prato, 1335) 658–659 (Kapitel XXI der Statuten der Compagnia dei Disciplinati di S. Domenico in Campo Regio in Siena, 1344–48). Trotz eines oftmals hohen Grades an Konformität weisen Vorschriften zu bruderschaftlichen Ritualen durchaus auch zahlreiche Unterschiede auf; vgl. Dehmer, *Italienische Bruderschaftsbanner* 94. Grundlegende Richtlinien für die ‚disciplina‘ sind sich jedoch in vielen Fällen sehr ähnlich.

[24] „Statuti de la Fraternitade d'i Recomendati a Madona Sancta Maria in la citade de Millano“ (Mailand, Biblioteca Braidense, *AC. VIII. 2*); zit. in Grignani – Stella (Hrsg.), *Antichi testi pavesi* 95–99; vgl. Dehmer, *Italienische Bruderschaftsbanner* 268–269.

> [...] dass in unserem Ort ein Bild Unseres gekreuzigten Herrn Jesus Christus sein muss, vor welchem Bild sich alle, die diesen Ort betreten, mit aller Ehrfurcht niederknien und ein Vaterunser sprechen und den Altar küssen und dann sagen sollen: Gesegnet sei der Name Unseres gekreuzigten Herrn Jesus Christus; und die anderen sollen antworten: für immer sei gepriesen und gesegnet sein allerheiligster Name [...]. Und wenn es Zeit ist, sich zu geißeln, müssen der Prior, Subprior oder der Vikar jene bestimmt haben, die drinnen und draußen für den Gesang und das Offizium zuständig sind, und jenen, der das Bild oder das Kreuz tragen wird [...].[25]

Die Statuten der toskanischen Disciplinati di S. Michele Arcangelo in San Godenzo von 1415 liefern diesbezüglich zusätzlichen Nachweis – sie schreiben ausdrücklich die Durchführung der internen Flagellation im Beisein einer Christusdarstellung (*imagine*) vor, während bei öffentlichem Auftreten der Gemeinschaft die Funktion des Andachtsbildes von einem Banner (*insegna*) zu übernehmen sei:

> Wo sich die Compagnia zu versammeln hat und warum.
>
> Es wird festgelegt, dass sich diese Compagnia an einem möglichst abgelegenen, geheimen und ehrbaren Ort versammeln soll. Und an diesem Ort bewahre sie ein Christusbild auf, und ihre Kutten halte sie geordnet, und keiner berühre die des anderen, und jede sei von weißer Farbe. Jeden Freitag kommen alle an den bestimmten Ort, und dort halten sie Ruhe, solange sie die Disziplin zu tragen und zu tun gedenken. Nach dem Ankleiden stehe einer von ihnen vor dem Christusbild, mit geschlossenen und erhobenen Händen, bekreuzige sich und sage jene in Gelb geschriebenen Worte: *Adiutorium nostrum in nomine domini. qui fecit celum et terram.* Und alle anderen heben die gefalteten Hände und antworten *Amen.* Sodann heben sie die Geißeln vom Boden auf, und derselbe, der Adiutorium sprach, sage *Adprehendite disciplinam ne quando irascatur dominus. ne pereatis de via iusta.* Darauf gebe er sich einen kräftigen Hieb, und alle anderen tun dies ebenso und antworten *Deo gratias.* Zwei seien dazu angewiesen, dass der eine *Iube domipne benedicere* spreche und der andere antworte *Benedictus cristus qui pro nobis est crucifixus.* Schließlich lese jener,

[25] Kapitel III („del modo de fare la disciplina e de retenere el capitolo"): „Ancho dicemo e ordenamo che en lo luoco nostro debia essere la ymagine del nostro signore ihesu cristo crucefixo, ale quale ymagine tucti l'entranti en esso luoco con onni reuerentia s'enginochie e dicano el pater nostro e bascino l'altare e po dicano: benedecto sia el nome del nostro signore ihesu cristo cruce fixo; e li altri rispondauo: per senpre sia laudato e benedecto el suo nome santissimo [...]. E quando fosse el tenpo de fare la disciplina, el priore, el supriore ouero el uicario debia auere ordenato coloro i quali fanno el canto e l'officio dentro e de fore, e cului el quale portarà la ymagine ouero la cruce [...]"; ausführlich zit. in Grimaldi G., „I capitoli della Fraternita di Santa Croce d'Urbino", *Le Marche illustrate nella storia, nelle lettere, nelle arti* 5 (1905) 256–273, hier 260; vgl. Dehmer, *Italienische Bruderschaftsbanner* 267.

der iube domipne benedice sprach, eine der folgend aufgeschriebenen Lektionen, und jemand anderer, der eine Laudenstanze kennt, sage diese auf, und nachdem dieses auf fromme Weise geschehen ist, entkleiden sich alle in Schweigen und kehren auf geheimem Wege nach Hause zurück [...].

Ebenso wird festgelegt, dass zu allen Hauptfesten der Kirchen innerhalb der Pfarrei, die in den Statuten oder durch den Vorsteher genannt werden, öffentliche Disziplin begangen wird. Und wenn sie eine solche Kirche erreichen, vollziehen sie an sich öffentliche Geißelung mit möglichst frommem Gesang und tragen ihr Zeichen.[26]

Mehrere in diesem kollektiven Ritual zu verlesene Lektionen, im Anhang der Satzungen niedergeschrieben, sind als komplementäre Aussagen zu der Frömmigkeitsübung zu verstehen. Die visuelle Präsenz des leidenden Heilands an Ort und Stelle des Bußrituals entsprach dem am Schluss jeder Lesung ausgesprochenen Verlangen und Vorsatz, eins zu werden mit seiner Passion und durch sie Erlösung zu finden („Die Passion unseres Herrn Jesus Christus sei stets in unseren Herzen"; „Das Feuer seiner Passion entzünde Gott in unseren Herzen"; „Die schmerzensreiche Passion Christi sei unsere Befreiung").[27] Bei derartigen Kombina-

---

[26] „Dove la compagnia si debba ragunare e quando e 'l perché".
„Item e ordinato che questa conpagnia si debba raunare. la ove ella puo piu rimotamente et secretamente et in onesto luogo. et in esso luogo tenghino una imagine di cristo. elle loro veste tenghino ordinatamente e non tocchino l'una l'altra e sieno bianche ciascheduna. Et ciascuno venardi si venghino alluogho ordinato tutti quanti. et ive tenghino silençio tanto quanto intendino al vestire effare la disciplina. E quando sono vestiti e uno di loro stia dinançi alla imagine di cristo tenendo le mani chiuse et alte e segnandosi e poi dicha questo che e scritto di ginabro. *Adiutorium nostrum in nomine domini. qui fecit celum et terram.* E tutti gli altri lievino le mani alte e giunte e rispondino. e dichino. *Amen.* E poi lievino le discipline di terra. E poi quello medesimo che disse. adiutorium dicha chosi *Adprehendite disciplinam ne quando irascatur dominus. ne pereatis de via iusta.* E detto questo si dia una di força. e tutti si dieno allora e rispondino. cosi. *Deo gratias.* E poi due sieno ordinati accio. e dica l'uno *Iube domipne benedicere.* E l'altro dica e risponda chosi. *Benedictus cristus qui pro nobis est crucifixus.* E allora quello ch'a detto iube domipne benedicere dicha una delle lectioni che scripta qui dirieto a questi capitoli. poi alchuno altro che sappia dicha una stança di laude divotamente fatto questo si spoglino et in silençio e tornino a chasa secretamente. [...] Item e ordinato che a tutte le feste principali delle chiese del pivieri le quali seranno nominate per li capitoli overo per lo priore. si vadano a disciplina palese. e quando seranno a quella cotale chiesa si faccino la disciplina palese. col canto detto quanto piu divotamente si puo. e portino la ‚nsegna loro"; Florenz, Archivio di Stato, *Capitoli delle compagnie religiose soppresse da Pietro Leopoldo* 136, Kapitel II, Fol. 4v–5v.

[27] „Passio dominis nostri iesu cristi sit semper in cordibus nostris"/„Ignem sui passionis accendat deus in cordibus nostris"/„Dolorosa cristi passio sit nostra liberatio"; ebd. Fol. 15r und v; vgl. Dehmer, „Mobile Passionsdarstellungen als Leitbilder kollektiver Geißelungsrituale im spätmittelalterlichen Italien", *Das Münster* 55 (2002) 200–207; hier 204.

tionen von stationär abgehaltenen und ambulanten Andachtspraktiken erwiesen sich die beweglichen Banner der Bruderschaften als ideales Zubehör. Als isolierte und somit besonders eindrückliche Bilder, als visuelle Fokuspunkte kamen sie bei dem kollektiven Vollzug der Geißelung offenbar bevorzugt zum Einsatz und ergänzten dadurch den die Büßenden umgebenden, kulissenhaften Bilddekor der Wände.[28]

Das Regelbuch der Compagnia di S. Maria dei Battuti in Modena aus dem 14. Jahrhundert gibt über den Einsatz solcher Einzelbilder näheren Aufschluss. Einer Zusammenfassung der wichtigsten historischen Fakten zu der Marienbruderschaft aus dem 18. Jahrhundert kann entnommen werden, dass sich diese um 1296 unter der Bezeichnung ‚Compagnia del Cristo flagellato' gegründet hatte und auf ihrem Banner eine Geißelung Christi führte.[29]

Eine Miniatur auf der Titelseite ihrer trecentesken Statuten illustriert sehr anschaulich und realitätsgetreu die gewünschte stimulierende Wirkung eines figürlich bemalten Gonfalone im Verlauf der ‚disciplina' (Ende 14. Jh.) [Abb. 1]:[30] Vier Angehörige in weltlicher Kleidung in der rechten Bildhälfte sprechen baren Hauptes Gebete, während vor ihnen sechs verhüllte Gestalten die Passion körperlich nachvollziehen. In ihrer Mitte halten zwei ihrer Mitbrüder ein rotgrundiges Banner mit dem gegeißelten Christus. Der Bildinhalt konzentriert sich auf das Hauptgeschehen der Passionsszene, in klarer und frontalsymmetrischer

---

[28] Ritzerfeld, *Pietas – Caritas – Societas* 214 (über „Vermittlungsmodi korporativer Ziele"): „Die Isolierung spezieller Ausschnitte entsprach der Predigttechnik der Bettelorden, mentaler Devotionspraxis und der Vorgehensweise in Meditationsschriften und Laudengesängen". Zu affektiven und imaginativen Meditationstechniken vgl. auch Largier, *Lob der Peitsche* 53.

[29] „Nello Stendardo di questa Ammirabile Radunanza dipinta contemplavasi l'immagine del nostro Salvator Giesu Cristo flagellato alla Colonna, in memoria della sua acerbissima passione, percio la Compagnia del Cristo flagellato appellavasi; communemente pero dalla maggior parte del volgo era nomata la Compagnia delli battuti, attesoche li fratelli d'essa facendosi vedere in abito penitente, con capsa ben grossa di tella da Sacchi coperti, e cinti con ruida Corda, si battevano con una sforza di ferro".; Wives G.B., „Narrazione d'alcune cose rimarcabili della Confraternita di Sta Maria de Battuti di Modena", in *Libro delle memorie. Ricordi, brevi pontificij, partiti, e narazione delle cose piu rimarcabili della Compagnia de' Battuti di S. Maria della Neve, o del Confalone di Modena*; Modena, Biblioteca Estense, *Campori* 161 (= γ.I.4.21) 29–49, hier 30. Zur Frühgeschichte dieser Gemeinschaft s. Soli G., *Chiese di Modena*, Bd. 2 (Modena: 1974) 441–443. Dort ist auch deren Sitz besprochen, das „Ospedale e Oratorio di S. Maria della Neve". Soli zufolge wurde die Bruderschaft erst 1332 gegründet.

[30] Modena, Biblioteca Estense, *Congregazione della Carità*, Ms. Nr. 2, Fol. 1r; vgl. *Il patrimonio storico-artistico della Congregazione di Carità in Modena* (Modena: 1920), Abb. LXIII; Dehmer, *Italienische Bruderschaftsbanner* 115–116.

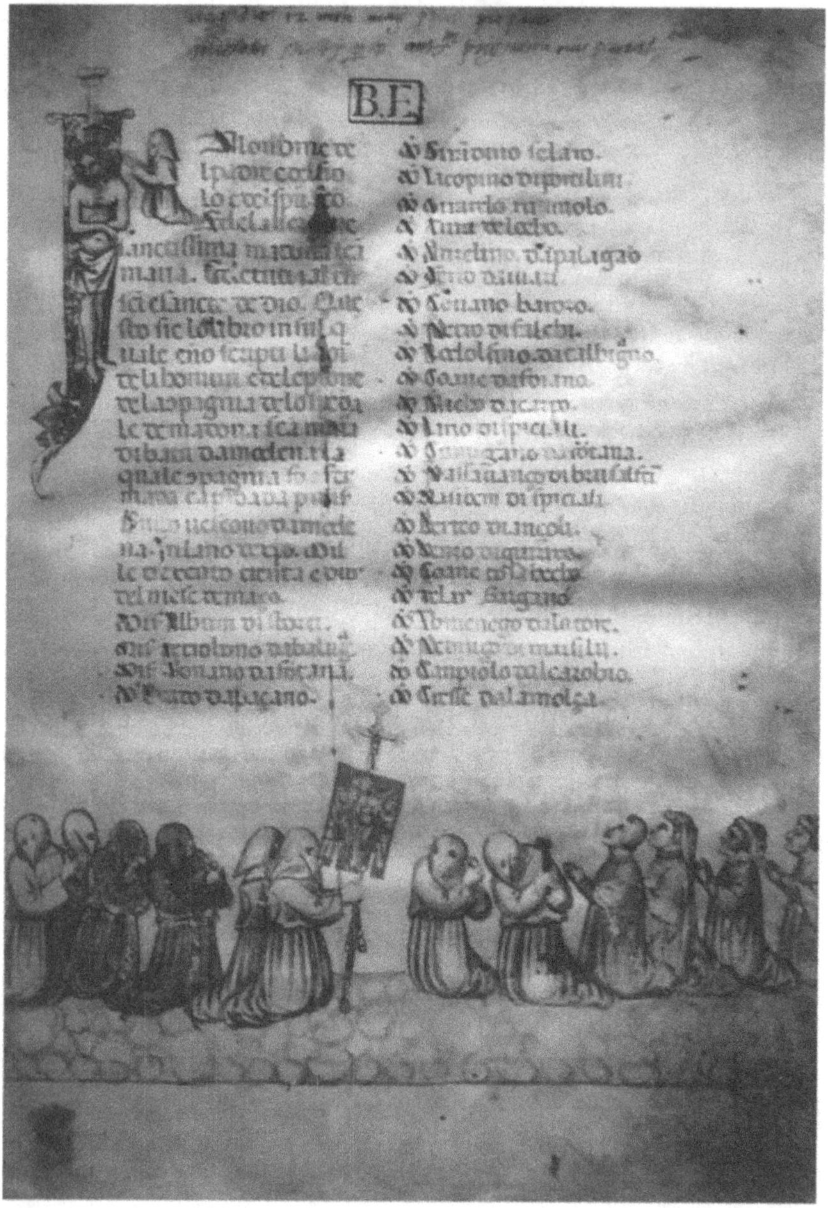

Abb. 1 [Col. pl. XI]. Modenesisch, *Geißelungsritual.* Miniatur (letztes Viertel des 14. Jahrhunderts). Modena, Biblioteca Estense (Congregazione della Carità, Ms. 2) (A. Dehmer, mit freundlicher Genehmigung der Biblioteca Estense).

Form wird es den kniend büßenden und betenden Betrachtern unmittelbar vor Augen geführt. Kapitel XIII der 1334 approbierten Bruderschaftsstatuten erteilt zu der Bußübung einige mit der Miniatur übereinstimmende Anweisungen:

> Diejenigen, welche die Disziplin empfangen und der Passion unseres Herrn Jesu Christi gedenken, haben sich mit einem Bußgewand zu kleiden. Diejenigen, welche sich nicht züchtigen, haben in der Nähe der anderen zu bleiben und zur Vergebung ihrer Sünden mehrere *Vaterunser* und *Avemaria* zu beten.[31]

Eine dazugehörige achtteilige Fürbittenfolge enthält das Laudarium der Gemeinschaft aus dem Jahr 1377. Nach jeder einzelnen Strophe dieser so genannten „Reccomendationes" verabreichten sich die Beteiligten einen Hieb, um ihren Bitten und Gebeten mehr Nachdruck zu verleihen. Den Abschluss des Rituals bildete ein gemeinsamer Umzug, offenbar unter der Führung des Banners: „Und damit Christus unser Beten erhöre, gehen wir dieses achte Mal in Prozession".[32]

Der Modeneser Miniatur kompositionell verblüffend ähnlich erscheint die untere Zone eines zweigeteilten, in gotisierender Formensprache ausgeführten Aquarells, das einem 1567 begonnenen Kompendium zur Geschichte der Veroneser Confraternita di S. Maria del Domo beigefügt ist [Abb. 2]. Bei genauerer Lektüre der Handschrift lässt sich nachweisen, dass es sich um eine Kopie der Statuten von 1392 handelt.[33]

---

[31] „E quili chi voram recevere disiplina e fare memoria de la passione del nostro Segnore misser yhu xpo se debian vestire de vestimenta de penetecia. Et quili che no se vorano disciplinare si dibiano stare apresso de quili e dire *Paltri nostri* et *Ave Marie* in remissione di soi peccati"; zit. in Veratti B., „Monumenti antichi di dialetti volgari. Capitoli de' Battuti di Modena", in *Opuscoli religiosi, letterarj e morali* IV,12 (1858) 366–392, hier 378–379.

[32] „Et a ço che Christo exolda questa nostra oratiom. Nu farem questa octana volta procession"; zit. in Bertoni G., *Il laudario dei Battuti di Modena* (Beihefte zur Zeitschrift für Romanische Philologie 20) (Halle: 1909) 6–11, hier 11. Eine kritische Neu-Edition stammt von Elsheikh M.S., *Il laudario dei Battuti di Modena* (Collezione di opere inedite o rare 156) (Bologna: 2001).

[33] Die Präsentationsszene leitet sich von dem mit demselben Bildmotiv illuminierten Frontispiz der Statuten von 1392 ab, gestiftet von einem Mitglied der Vereinigung, „il devoto Disciplino, et Battuto di essa Compagnia Francesco figliolo di maestro Leone dalle calze"; Verona, Archivio di Stato, *Ospedale di S. Bovo* 1, Fol. 9v: „Costui anchora fu quello, che fece fare, et scrivere il libro delle devote loro constitutioni, et ordini l'anno precedente 1392 cioe mille trecento et nonantadoi nel mese di Luggio, come manifestamente consta nell'istesso libro nella prima charta doppoi la bella figura della santissima Vergine, et di santo Rainero loro Advocato et Protettore". Bereits zu Beginn wird darauf hingewiesen, dass sich die Schrift auf ein altes Regelwerk der im 14. Jahrhundert gegründeten Compagnia di S. Maria del Domo beruft (ebd. Fol. 4r).

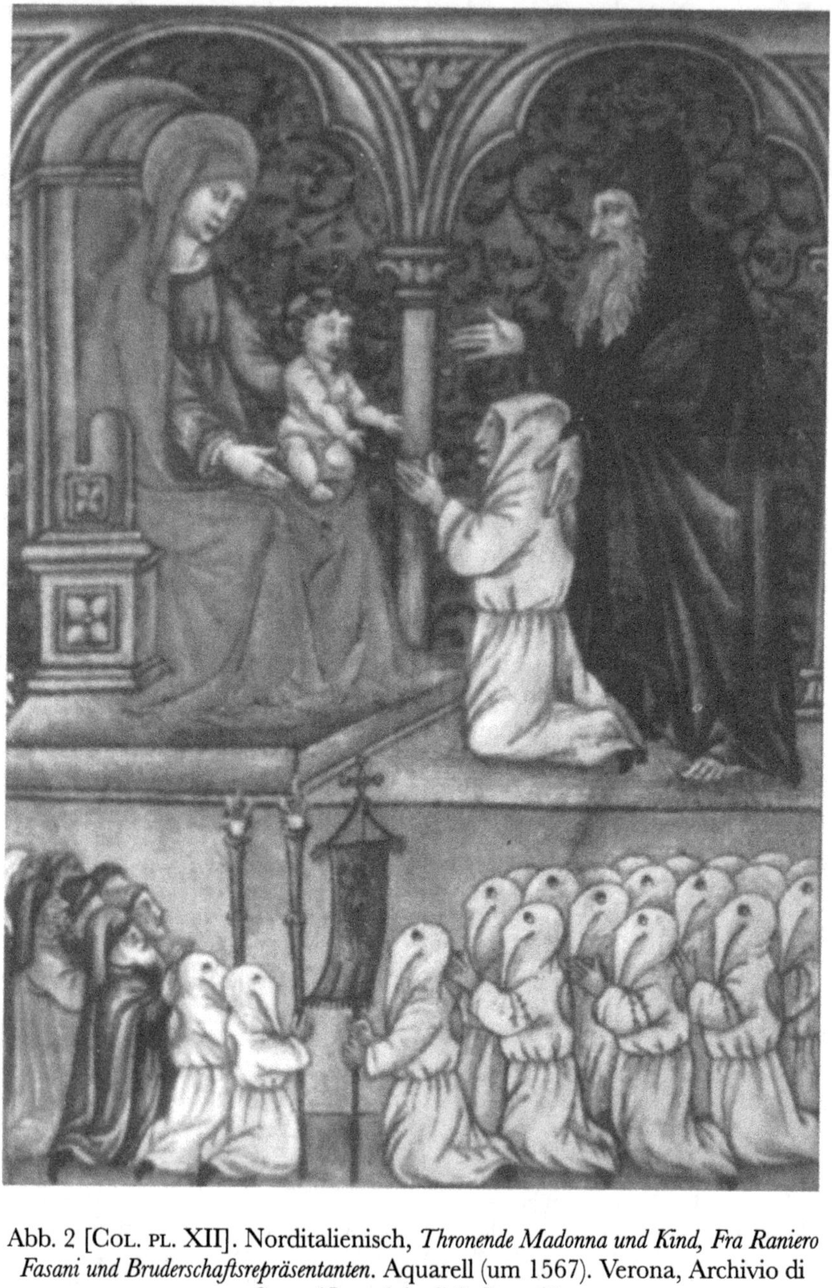

Abb. 2 [Col. pl. XII]. Norditalienisch, *Thronende Madonna und Kind, Fra Raniero Fasani und Bruderschaftsrepräsentanten*. Aquarell (um 1567). Verona, Archivio di Stato (Ospedale di S. Bovo 1).

In derselben Quelle wird auch ein Wandgemälde mit der Gottesmutter, ihrem Sohn und dem Seligen Raniero in der Kirche erwähnt, für welches eine ähnliche bildliche Umsetzung anzunehmen ist.[34]

Zeigt das besagte Aquarell im oberen Register die Empfehlung eines einzelnen Geißelbruders durch Fra Raniero Fasani an die thronende Madonna mit dem Jesuskind, haben sich im unteren Bildfeld weitere Vertreter der Disciplinati versammelt: links weltlich Gewandete – möglicherweise von der Kasteiung befreit[35] –, rechts eine in weiße Kutten gehüllte Gruppe, und dazwischen, zusammen mit zwei Trageleuchtern, ein wiederum auf rotem Stoff figürlich dekorierter Gonfalone. Dass das Bannerbild in diesem Fall keinen gegeißelten, sondern den auferstandenen Christus darstellt, könnte auf einen später erfolgten Motivwandel, auf eine den ursprünglichen Sinn neu interpretierende Wiedergabe von Seiten des Kopisten oder aber auf das grundsätzliche Verlangen der Büßenden nach endzeitlicher Erlösung zurückzuführen sein.

Die alten Satzungen der seit 1341 dokumentierten Flagellantenbruderschaft weisen eine starke Abhängigkeit auf zu jenen der Bologneser

---

Der Beiname der Vereinigung rührt von ihrem ursprünglichen Wirken – bis zum Bau einer eigenen Kirche ab 1342 – in der damaligen Kathedrale von Verona, S. Stefano, her (ebd. Fol. 6v). Laut De Sandre Gasparini G., „Confraternite e ‚cura animarum' nei primi anni del Quattrocento: I disciplinati e la parocchia di S. Vitale a Verona", in Sambin P. (Hrsg.), *Pievi, parrocchie e clero nel Veneto dal X al XV secolo* (Venedig: 1987) 289–360; hier 294–295, stand die Korporation in direktem Kontakt mit der Bologneser Confraternita di S. Maria della Vita.

[34] Verona, Archivio di Stato, *Ospedale di S. Bovo* 1, Fol. 5v. Ein vergleichbar gestaltetes Wandgemälde aus dem 15. Jahrhundert befindet sich in Berzo Inferiore (Val Camonica), S. Lorenzo; s. Mazzini F., *Affreschi lombardi del Quattrocento* (Mailand: 1965) 617, Abb. 378.

[35] In einem Bußbruderschaftsstatut des 14. Jahrhunderts aus Belluno wird diese Möglichkeit für jene, „qui expoliari non possunt", in einem eigenen Kapitel abgehandelt: „lxiiij. Item statuimus et ordinamus quod quilibet homo et persona fraternitatis predicte qui non poterit se expoliare quando vadunt processionaliter, habentes causam legiptimam, volentes stare in loco fraternitatis, quod dare teneantur massario fraternitatis sex parvulos pro quolibet et qualibet vice pro suo offertorio; et si voluerint cum fratribus suis ire inducti vadant et ire debeant de ante verberantes post illos portantes crucem et confallonum, facientes ipsimet suum offertorium si se senciverint faciendum; et si se non senciverint faciendum quod non teneantur ad aliquod bannum, habentes sacramentum per gastaldiones fraternitatis se expoliari non posse".; zit. in De Bortoli G., *Statuto della Scuola dei Battuti bellunesi* (Belluno: 1978) 130 – Natürlich spielten ebenso weltliche Interessen in solche Bilder mit hinein, ist die unterschiedlich gehandhabte Wiedergabe von Bruderschaftsmitgliedern auch darauf zurückzuführen, dass die maßgeblichen Stifter der Kunstwerke nicht auf eine standesgemäße Abbildung verzichten wollten. Mit einer akkuraten Reproduktion der stattlichen Gewänder sollte ihr sozialer Status bewusst hervorgehoben werden.

Confraternita di S. Maria della Vita.[36] Diese kurz nach 1260 gegründete Marienbruderschaft in Bologna führte wohl bereits seit jeher ein Banner[37] und war zudem eine der einflussreichsten Konfraternitäten in der nördlichen Hälfte Italiens: Die ursprünglich „Congregatio devotorum civitatis Bononie et diocesis" bezeichnete Vereinigung übte aufgrund ihres Alters und ihrer kirchlichen Privilegien eine große Anziehungskraft auf jüngere und weniger dotierte Gemeinschaften aus.[38] So vereinigten sich mit ihr am 28. Oktober 1339 auch die Disciplinati von Piacenza und Brescia, und zwar – einer zeitgenössischen Miniatur zufolge – abermals unter einem rotgrundigen Passionschristus-Banner,[39] das wohl ebenso in den Bußritualen der Bruderschaft zum Einsatz kam.

Passio und Compassio

Die wirkungsmächtigen Bologneser Statuten hallen zudem in einem späteren Regelwerk der Scuola di S. Maria Maddalena in Bergamo wider.[40] Diese Bußbruderschaft nahm während des 14. Jahrhunderts in der nordwestitalienischen Region eine ähnlich zentrale Rolle in der organisierten Laienfrömmigkeit ein. Ihren 1336 redigierten Satzungen ist ein mehrteiliger vulgärsprachlicher Laudentext beigefügt, in dem man eine prägnant formulierte Strophe in Form eines Responsoriums

---

[36] Vgl. De Sandre Gasparini, „Confraternite e ‚cura animarum'" 295.

[37] Die Gonfaloni der Bruderschaft durften bei ihrer öffentlichen Zurschaustellung nur von Vorstehern der Korporation getragen werden, „Quod vexilla congregationis semper portentur per guardianos"; zit. in Fanti M., „Gli inizi del movimento dei Disciplinati e la confraternita di Santa Maria della Vita", *Bollettino della Deputazione di Storia Patria per l'Umbria* 66 (1969) 181–232, hier 191, Kap. XXXVII (aus den Statuten in der Redaktion von 1286). Der Autor zitiert auch eine Quelle aus dem 16. Jahrhundert, die eine von roten Bannern angeführten Prozession der Bologneser Disciplinati nach Modena im Jahr 1262 erwähnt, „vexilla purpurea praeferentes"; ebd. 223, Anm. 53.

[38] Eine solche selbstgewählte oder aber auferlegte Anlehnung äußerte sich v.a. in Imitationen von Gründungsverfahren, Regelverfassungen, Ritualen, Gebetstexten und anderen Schriften. Longo P.G., *Letteratura e pietà a Novara tra XV e XVI secolo* (Novara: 1986) 104 ff. gibt einige Beispiele als Beweise dafür, dass die Konstituierung von Bruderschaften in der Lombardei weitgehend von mittelitalienischen Vorbildern (vor allem aus Rom, Siena und Bologna) beeinflusst war. Vgl. Dehmer, *Italienische Bruderschaftsbanner* 20–22.

[39] Medica M., „Il santo patrono in miniatura. Gli esordi di una tradizione iconografica", in Buscaroli B. (Hrsg.), *Petronio e Bologna. Il volto di una storia* (Ausstellungskatalog Bologna 2001/02) (Ferrara: 2001) 141–147, hier 141–142. Das Pergament enthält u.a. eine Auflistung von Privilegien und Indulgenzen, die den Bologneser Bußbrüdern gewährt wurden.

[40] Vgl. Meersseman, *Ordo fraternitatis* 472–473.

liest. Für den Ablauf der korporativen ‚Disciplina' sind diese kurzen Sätze ein eindrucksvoller früher Beleg:

Versammelt Euch Genossen
Schlagt Euch hart und unverdrossen *Und man tu' es froh gestimmt.*
Die Passion Gottes unser Banner

Das hier ebenso wie in zahlreichen anderen Lauden zu konstatierende Verlangen nach Allgemeinverständlichkeit war ein generelles Charakteristikum der Laienbruderschaften, die in ihren Schriften das populäre Volgare dem gelehrten Latein vorzogen. Durch den Verzicht auf die lateinische Sprache wurde ein direktes Verständnis der gesprochenen Zeremonien gewährleistet. Bewusst sind daher auch die folgenden Laudenstrophen im Volgare bzw. sogar in einem dialektalen Italienisch gehalten. Überliefert aus verschiedenen Epochen und verschiedenen Bereichen Norditaliens, sind sie dennoch in sich fast identisch und rezipieren den oben zitierten Text aus Bergamo beinahe wörtlich.

Versammelt Euch, o Genossen
Schlagt Euch hart und unverdrossen
Jesu Christi Passion
Sei für uns der Gonfalone
Auf dass er uns erlöse.

Nun versammelt Euch alle
Schart Euch vor dem Banner
Schlagt Euch hart und unverdrossen
Schonet Euren Körper nicht
Denn vor Euch wird das Kreuz sein.

Gemeinsamer Inhalt dieser Strophenvarianten[41] ist der eindringliche Aufruf zur tatkräftigen, vielmehr schonungslosen Selbstkasteiung im Angesicht und unter der spirituellen Führung des gepeinigten Heilands. Das kollektive Nachvollziehen der Passion an sich sollte den Texten zufolge (obwohl es sich in den späteren Versionen bereits um einen Topos handeln könnte) – wie gehabt – vor einem für jedermann sichtbar exponierten Gonfalone stattfinden. Das Banner barg für die Betrachterschar das Vor-Bild des leidenden Christus, dem es sich anzugleichen galt und das den Weg zum endzeitlichen Heil wies. Dieser Weg führte jedoch nur über das Mit-Leiden im eigenen körperlichen

[41] Wortlaute und Quellennachweise in Dehmer, *Italienische Bruderschaftsbanner* 182–183.

Schmerz. Noch deutlicher bringt dies eine Strophe aus der Umgebung von Padua zum Ausdruck. Der Passus stammt aus den Orationen und Lauden der Compagnia di S. Maria dei Battuti in Castelbaldo, im Anhang ihrer Satzungen von 1425 (Redaktion von 1560).

Mutter Gottes

Wohlan Brüder, schlagt Euch kräftig.
Diese Schläge mögen Euch nicht schmerzen,
da Ihr offen finden werdet die Tore
zum Eintritt in das Paradies.

Mutter Gottes

Wohlan Brüder, von Schar zu Schar,
schlagt Euch hart und unverdrossen.
Das heilige Kreuz ist unser Banner
und unser aufgerichteter Gonfalone.[42]

Das erwähnte Prozessionszeichen ist auch in den Statuten der Vereinigung nachweisbar; dort sind sein Besitz sowie seine motivische Gestaltung explizit vorgeschrieben: „Und sie sollen ein Kreuz haben, und einen bemalten Gonfalone mit dem geschlagenen Christus an der Säule".[43] Dass das Bild in dem das Geißelungsritual selbst betreffenden Kapitel nicht erwähnt ist,[44] verdeutlicht, wie oft solche Zeremonien nur vage skizziert sind, ihre Rekonstruktion aus verschiedenen Quellen gespeist werden muss.

---

[42] „*Madre de Dio* – Horsu fratelli battevi forte/Ne non ve do[gl]ia queste botte/Che voi troverete aperte le porte/Dello entrare al paradiso./*Madre de Dio* – Horsu fratelli di schiera in schiera/Battevi forte e volentiera/La santa Croce e nostra bandiera/E nostro dritto gonfalone"; Venedig, Biblioteca del Museo Civico Correr, *Cl. IV.* 168, nicht paginiert [Fol. 37 r].

[43] „Et che li habbino una Crose: et uno Confalone depento con xpo battudo alla colonna"; ebd. (Fol. 10v/Kapitel XII).

[44] „Item Statuimo, et Ordinemo che tutti quelli che faranno la disciplina: si la debbia fare humilemente, et soavemente: cum le sue cappe honeste et lo buso de le spalle convenientemente grande: et che loro si possino percuodere et battere suso la carne sença camisa cum una cadena o laççi gropposi deputadi a questo servigio. Et andando non vagando, murmurando, ne favellando l'uno cum l'altro. Et vagano a dui a dui devota et honestamente, aço che li non façςi far beffe de loro. Et se alcuno fara alcuna cosa disonesta: cada alla pena de soldi. ij"; ebd. (Fol. 8r/Kapitel III: „Della Disciplina che si die fare").

Abbild und Vorbild

Viele dieser Bruderschaftsbanner wurden mit zwei unterschiedlichen Schauseiten ausgeführt: Das vordere Bild war hauptsächlich für das den rituellen Umzügen beiwohnende Publikum bestimmt, mit der identitätsstiftenden Figur der bzw. des Titelheiligen oder -mysteriums; das rückwärtige Bild dagegen enthielt häufig eine Passionsdarstellung, welche die dahinter marschierenden Büßer in ihrer Reue anspornen und anleiten sollte. Durch das in präsenter, lebensnaher Bildgestalt vor Augen geführte, somit vergegenwärtigte Leiden Christi sollten die Bußbrüder zur umfassenden *compassio* – zu mental kontemplativer *commemoratio* und körperlich tätiger *imitatio* – angeregt bzw. aufgefordert werden. Für Miniaturen, die in den Satzungen von Geißelbruderschaften eine ähnliche Funktion ausübten, prägte Hans Belting einen treffenden Begriff: Er bezeichnete sie als „Leitbilder".[45] Ohne Probleme lässt sich die Charakterisierung ebenso auf Malwerke großen Formats übertragen, die in der Öffentlichkeit präsentiert wurden.

Um sowohl die Bruderschaften selbst als auch das Publikum ihrer Prozessionen auf Anhieb anzusprechen, bedienten sich die zur Dekoration der Gonfaloni beauftragten Maler häufig einer komprimierenden Darstellungsweise. Sie bestand vor allem in der bewussten Anwendung einer veranschaulichenden, klaren Raum- und Figurenkonzeption. Überflüssige Ablenkung der Betrachter durch Detailschilderung oder narrative Elemente wurde weitgehend vermieden – ergreifende Emotionalität war ein vorherrschendes Gestaltungsprinzip und eine Grundvoraussetzung für aktive Mimesis und Empathie. Diese eindringliche Methode der nachdrücklichen Vermittlung von „Glaubensinhalten" lässt sich ferner daran erkennen, dass die Motive oft als griffige Formeln frontalsymmetrisch und nahsichtig angelegt sowie plakativ an die Bildoberfläche gesetzt, im planen Vordergrund verhaftet sind.[46]

Zu den populärsten christologischen Motiven auf bemalten Bruderschaftsbannern des späten Mittelalters zählt die Passionsszene der

[45] Belting, *Das Bild und sein Publikum* 210 ff.; darüber hinaus erkennt er in diesem Kontext in der Geißelung Christi zu Recht ‚nicht nur ein Meditationsbild, sondern auch ein Programmbild' (ebd. 211).

[46] Obwohl bewährte Bildlösungen vielfach kopiert bzw. mit wenigen spezifischen Veränderungen übernommen wurden, konnten dabei durchaus künstlerisch eigenständige, qualitätsvolle und innovative Resultate erzielt werden; Dehmer, *Italienische Bruderschaftsbanner* 230–235; Ritzerfeld, *Pietas – Caritas – Societas* 213–218.

Geißelung.[47] Ihr Erscheinen steht stets in einem unmittelbaren Zusammenhang mit der spezifischen Devotion der Auftraggeber: Bereits die überlieferten Statuten der Confraternita di S. Maria della Scala in Siena von 1295 legten den Gebrauch ihres Gonfalone ausschließlich für jene Versammlungen fest, in denen die kollektive Flagellation durchgeführt wurde.[48] Dasselbe Zeichen taucht in einem Inventar von 1325 ohne weitere Ausführungen auf, könnte aber mit einem 1492 registrierten Objekt noch identisch sein, nämlich ein „alter Gonfalone, darin gemalt als unser Herr an die Säule gebunden und geschlagen ward, mit einem Holzkreuz auf der Spitze".[49]

Ein Leinwandgemälde, das auf grünem Grund eine Christusfigur an der Geißelsäule zeigte, verzeichneten auch in einem Inventar von 1350 die Disciplinati di Gesù Pellegrino in Florenz. Ob man es für Prozessionen verwendete, ist ungewiss; mitunter diente es zur Verhüllung der Altartafel (einem Madonnenbild), wurde also als Velum verwendet – vermutlich ebenso anlässlich der Durchführung der gemeinsamen Bußübungen.[50] Ein großformatiges Bild, das sowohl mobil als auch stationär genutzt wurde, führt hingegen das 1388 datierte Inventar der Peruginer Confraternita dell'Annunziata auf: Christus an der Geißelsäule auf der Rückseite, recto die Verkündigung.[51] Es ist das

[47] Dass das Motiv auch von den Franziskanern frühzeitig propagiert wurde, dokumentiert ein etwa 1300 datiertes, beidseitig bemaltes Prozessionskreuz in Perugia (56,7 × 38,3 cm; Galleria Nazionale dell'Umbria). Zeigt die Vorderseite den Gekreuzigten mit zwei Stifterfiguren in Minoritentracht zu seinen Füßen, ist das Hauptfeld der Rückseite – in ungewöhnlicher Weise – vollständig der Darstellung der Geißelung Christi gewidmet; vgl. Frenzel A., *Die Darstellung der Geißelung Christi in der italienischen Kunst von den Anfängen im 11. Jahrhundert bis ins 17. Jahrhundert* (Diss. Frankfurt am Main: 1998) 109–110. Dort wird auch die Verbindung des Sujets mit der Frömmigkeit der Bußbruderschaften angesprochen (22–25; 44–51; 188). Ergänzend dazu: Schiferl E., „Caritas and the Iconography of Italian Confraternity Art", *Studies in Iconography* 14 (1995) 207–246, bes. 220–223 und 234 (Beispiele aus dem 14. und 15. Jh.); Dehmer, „Mobile Passionsdarstellungen" 200–207.

[48] „Anco, che in niuna andata, la quale non si facesse generalmente per tutti e' frategli a disciplina, si possa portare lo gonfalone; e che 'l Priore di ciò non possa dare licenzia"; zit. in Bianchi L., *Capitoli della Compagnia dei Disciplinati di Siena nei secoli XIII, XIV e XV* (Siena: 1866) 30, Kap. XXXVII.

[49] Dehmer, *Italienische Bruderschaftsbanner* 179–180: „gonfalone antico, dipèntovi quando il nostro signore fu legato e battuto a la colonna, con una croce da capo in legno".

[50] Giles Arthur, „Cult Objects and Artistic Patronage", 337 ff. Grundlegende Daten zu der 1334 in S. Maria Novella gegründeten Bruderschaft, bei Henderson, *Piety and Charity* 455, Nr. 60.

[51] Rihouet P., „‚Societas Anuntiate fecit fieri hoc opus': The Gonfalone dell' Annunziata (1466) in Perugia and its Patrons", *Bollettino della Deputazione di Storia Patria per l'Umbria* 103,1 (2006) 303–375, hier 343: „I tavola grande portareccia, da una

einzige registrierte Gemälde mit diesem Sujet, dürfte also ebenfalls bei den Bußritualen der Disciplinati zum Einsatz gekommen sein. Als ein frühes erhaltenes Beispiel dieser Art lässt sich das Prozessionsbanner von Spinello Aretino (um 1346–1410) im New Yorker Metropolitan Museum anführen (Ende 14. Jh.).[52] Gemalt für die 1334 in Borgo Sansepolcro gegründete Confraternita di S. Maria Maddalena, kam auf der Vorderseite die thronende Patronin der Vereinigung zur Abbildung; den vier ihr zugewandten Geißelbrüdern in Adorationsgestus hält die Bußheilige einen kleinen Kruzifixus entgegen. Die Rückseite zeigt den von zwei Schergen gegeißelten, duldend den Betrachter anblickenden Gottessohn an der Säule.

Neben Christi Geißelung war insbesondere die Kreuzigung ein populäres Motiv für Banner von Bußbruderschaften (von den bereits erwähnten, in Prozessionen stets vorangeführten Tragkreuzen ganz abgesehen). Wie die Geißelung sollte es den Betrachtern das Leiden des Erlösers verdeutlichen und sie zur heilbringenden, kollektiven *compassio* veranlassen. So führt ein 1421 datiertes Banner aus dem märkischen Sestino, S. Maria della Misericordia [Abb. 9 und 10], die Darstellung einer Schutzmantelmadonna, die als Patronin zahlreiche schwarz gekleidete Repräsentanten einer Bußbruderschaft unter ihrem Umhang geborgen hat – Angehörige der Confraternita di S. Maria della Misericordia –, mit dem Bild einer Kreuzigungsgruppe zusammen. Die kompositionelle Gleichsetzung der Bußbrüder recto und der am Kreuzesstamm den Kruzifixus verehrenden Maria Magdalena verso ist frappierend und liegt zweifellos in der Vorbildfunktion der Bußheiligen und ihres Mitleidens begründet.[53] Ähnliche Intentionen ließen bereits in einem Barnaba da Modena († nach 1383) bzw. seinem Umkreis zugeschriebenen zweiseitigen Bruderschaftsbanner im Londoner Victoria & Albert Museum (letztes Viertel 14./Anfang 15. Jh.) den hl. Antonius Abbas nicht nur recto in thronender Gestalt neben dem hl. Eligius darstellen, sondern auch verso am Fuße des Kreuzes kniend und Christi Füße küssend.[54]

parte ci è penta la Nonçiata coll'agniolo e da l'atro el nostro singnore Eddio leghato a la cholonda (grande)".

[52] Tempera/Leinwand, 175 × 119 cm; s. Dehmer, *Italienische Bruderschaftsbanner* 168; 180 und 324; Nr. 62.

[53] Tempera/Leinwand, 68,5 × 59,5 cm; s. Dehmer, *Italienische Bruderschaftsbanner* 141 und 345; Nr. 99.

[54] Tempera/Leinwand, 197 × 128 cm; ebd. 173–174; 202 und 318; Nr. 50. Der Auftraggeber, mit Sicherheit eine Antoniusbruderschaft, ist bislang nicht endgültig identifiziert worden.

Von eminenter Bedeutung war das Sujet des Gekreuzigten schließlich auch bei der letzten großen Geißelbewegung in Italien, die der so genannten ‚Bianchi' um 1399/1400: „zu jener Zeit zogen sich Personen beiderlei Geschlechts, Männer und Frauen, weiße Gewänder aus Sackleinen an und trugen durch die Landschaften Gonfaloni mit dem Gekreuzigten oder mit anderen Heiligen vor sich her".[55] In ihren Prozessionsgesängen findet sich ein weiterer Beleg für die allgegenwärtige Bildpräsenz Jesu Christi bei kollektiven Bußveranstaltungen des späten Mittelalters. Die folgende Lauden-Terzine wurde von dem Chronisten Giovanni Sercambi aus Lucca (1348–1424) notiert und betont – wörtlich genommen – abermals die Funktion mobiler Christusdarstellungen als Leitbilder gemeinschaftlicher Geißelungsrituale:

> Die gesamte Menschheit,
> alle gehen mit seiner Schar,
> tragen Christus als Banner.[56]

Christi Geißelung und Kreuzigung waren allerdings nicht die einzigen Darstellungen Jesu, vor denen Bußrituale vollzogen werden konnten. So stammt aus dem umbrischen Bettona (Pinacoteca Comunale) einer der frühesten erhaltenen Gonfaloni, in denen die Kreuzigung mit einer Imago Pietatis kombiniert wurde.[57] Das Werk ist in das letzte Viertel des 15. Jahrhunderts zu datieren und greift unter anderem auf Masolinos

[55] „Chronicon Fratris Hieronymi de Forlivio ab anno MCCCXCII usque ad MCCCCXXXIII", in *Rerum Italicarum Scriptores*, hg. v. L.A. Muratori, Bd. XIX (1731) 873–908, hier 873–874: „tempore illo, utriusque sexus, scilicet homines & mulieres induerunt se saccis, seu linteaminibus albis, portantes ante se per regiones Vexilla Crucifixi, vel alterius Sancti". – Weiterführend dazu Frugoni, *Incontri nel medioevo* 203–214 („La devozione dei Bianchi del 1399"). Bornstein D.E., *The Bianchi of 1399. Popular Devotion in Late Medieval Italy* (Ithaca-London: 1993) bes. 62ff., informiert ausführlich über Verlauf und Verbreitung dieser Massenzüge. Die ausführlichste und dazu reich illustrierte Chronik der Bewegung stammt aus ihrem Ursprungsort; vgl. Sercambi G., *Le illustrazioni delle chroniche nel codice Lucchese*, hg. v. O. Banti – M.L. Testi Cristiani, 2 Bde. (Genua: 1978).

[56] „L'universo populo,/Tucti vanno con sua schiera,/Portan Christo per bandiera"; zit. in *Le croniche di Giovanni Sercambi Lucchese*, Bd. 2, hg. v. Bongi S. (Rom: 1892/Neudruck 1969) 300 f. (Kap. DCXVIII). – Ungefähr zur selben Zeit hielt der Dominikanerprediger Vinzenz Ferrer (1350–1419) in Südfrankreich zahlreiche Bußsermone, in deren Folge ebenfalls Umzüge veranstaltet wurden. Dabei traf das Publikum auf bildliche Illustrationen seiner Worte, wiederum in Form von Bannern, deren Bemalungen die einzelnen Stationen der Passion Christi sowie die *Arma Christi* didaktisch vorführten; Amtmann R., *Die Bussbruderschaften in Frankreich* (Wiesbaden: 1977) 425–426.

[57] Tempera/Leinwand, 140 × 151 cm; s. Dehmer, *Italienische Bruderschaftsbanner* 187 und 292; Nr. 8. Ausführlich zu Begriff und Bildform der Imago Pietatis s. Belting, *Das Bild und sein Publikum* 53 ff.

Beweinung in der Collegiata zu Empoli (1424/25) zurück. Eindeutig ist auch hier die *compassio* der zentrale Bildvorwand. Die dramatische Kreuzigungsgruppe auf der einen, auf der anderen Seite die hinter Christi Leichnam am Kreuzbalken befestigten Geißeln dürften von dem Auftrag einer Flagellantenbruderschaft herrühren.[58] Der dunkle Bildgrund lässt zudem annehmen, dass das Banner bei Begräbnisgängen der Bruderschaft mitgeführt worden sein könnte.[59]

Bereits in einem Tafelbild aus dem frühen 15. Jahrhundert – es wurde wohl von Niccolò di Pietro Gerini (1345–um 1415) im Auftrag der Disciplinati di Gesù Pellegrino in Florenz gemalt – ist der aufrecht im Grab stehende, seine Wunden weisende tote Christus zusammen mit den Passionswerkzeugen abgebildet, dazu zwei am Querbalken des Kreuzes befestigte Geißeln. In der Predella darunter wird ein unmittelbarer Zusammenhang zwischen dem Motiv und dem kollektiven Gedenken der verstorbenen Angehörigen hergestellt: Sie zeigt das offizielle Begräbnis eines Mitbruders durch die versammelte Büßergemeinschaft (Florenz, Accademia).[60] Dieselbe gedankliche Verbindung von Schmerzensmann und Totengedächtnis birgt ein Wandgemälde mit einer von den *Arma Christi* umgebenen *Imago Pietatis* am Triumphbogen

---

[58] Eine solche Vereinigung ist dokumentiert bei Santucci F., „I disciplinati a Bettona nel sec. XIV“, *Quaderni del Centro di Documentazione sul Movimento dei Disciplinati* 19 (1977) 11–16, bes. 12–13: Die seit 1338 nachweisbare Korporation der ‚disciplinatorum alborum sancte Marie de Bictonio‘ besaß ein eigenes Hospital „prope ecclesiam sancte Marie de Bictonio“.

[59] Ein solcher Verwendungszweck war für Bruderschaftsbanner nicht unüblich; s. Dehmer, *Italienische Bruderschaftsbanner* 116–118.

[60] Gesamtmaße 353 × 152 cm (der Aufsatz stellt Christus als Pilger, vier Heilige und zwei Repräsentanten der Bruderschaft dar); vgl. auch Giles Arthur, „Cult Objects and Artistic Patronage“ 337 ff. und 350 f., Abb. 13.1 und 13.7. Auf die Besitzer verweist eine Inschrift: „QUESTA TAVOLA E DELLA CONPAGNIA DELLA DISCIPLINA DEL PELLEGRINO [...]“, von Lee, „Art and Ritual Drama“ 77, falsch um das Jahr 1341 datiert. Beide Autorinnen besprechen auch das Predellenbild von Bartolomeo da Camoglis Madonna dell'Umiltà aus dem Jahr 1346 (Palermo, Galleria Nazionale). Dort werden die *Arma Christi* auf einer weißen Bildfläche zwischen den zwei Gruppen von Angehörigen einer Flagellantengemeinschaft zur Schau gestellt. Das Bild im Bild zeigt die Geißelsäule, die Lanze, in der Mitte das Kreuz mit Nägeln, Dornenkrone, Geißeln und Essigbehälter, den Schwamm und eine Leiter. Vgl. De Floriani A., *Bartolomeo da Camogli* (Genua: 1979) 5–22. Es stellt sich die Frage, ob diese Darstellung nicht auch als das Banner der Konfraternität gedient haben könnte. Aus Südfrankreich weiß man von Bußprozessionen des frühen 15. Jahrhunderts, deren Gonfaloni ebenfalls die Arma Christi wiedergaben; Amtmann, *Die Bussbruderschaften in Frankreich* 425–426.

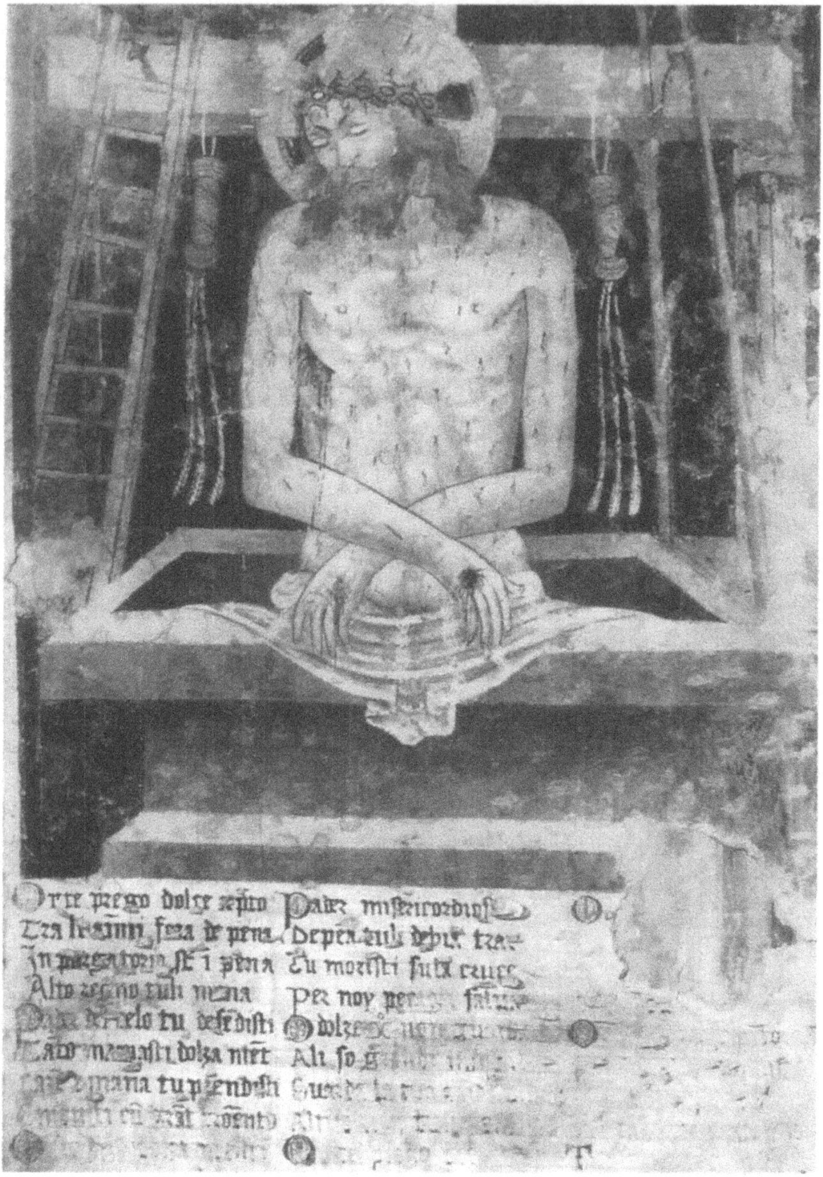

Abb. 3. Norditalienisch, *Imago Pietatis*. Fresko, 140 × 85 cm (Ende des 14./Anfang des 15. Jahrhunderts). Bergamo, S. Maria Maddalena (Archiv des Autors).

der ehemaligen Kirche der bereits erwähnten Scuola di S. Maria Maddalena in Bergamo (Ende 14./Anfang 15. Jh.) [Abb. 3].[61] Die Arme des Schmerzensmanns sind – in enger Anlehnung an die Geißelung – vor seinem Körper überkreuzt. Die Abbildung der Geißeln am Kreuzbalken ist als Hinweis auf die Bußdevotion der Magdalenenbrüder zu verstehen; durch einen unter die Figur gesetzten Text in Volgare wird das Gemälde konkret auf den Inhalt eines Bittgesangs für die Armen Seelen bezogen, der Lauda „Or te prego, dolzo Cristo".[62] Ob das Fresko in die Rituale der Bruderschaft auch miteinbezogen wurde, ist aufgrund seines Standorts hoch über dem heutigen Bodenniveau ungewiss – aber es reflektiert die Einbettung der gemeinschaftlichen *commemoratio* der Verstorbenen in die kollektive *compassio* der Lebenden (in Form von Fürbitten innerhalb der Bußgesänge oder durch Seelenmessen).[63]

Die motivische Parallele zwischen Geißelchristus und Schmerzensmann begegnet im Übrigen ebenso in einer vorangestellten Miniatur der schon angesprochenen Statuten der Disciplinati in Modena. Sie enthält eine interessante Mischform aus Christus an der Geißelsäule und *Imago Pietatis*: den gestorbenen Christus vor einer Säule stehend. Beiden Sujets ist gemein, das Leiden Christi in einer einfachen und prägnanten, Mitleid erregenden sowie zur Empathie auffordernden Bildformel vorzuführen.[64]

---

[61] Dehmer, „Sub Vexillo Sanctae Mariae Magdalenae" 207–208.

[62] Ciociola C., „Una lauda dipinta: il titolo dell'Imago pietatis nell'ex chiesa di S. Maria Maddalena in Bergamo", in *2° Convegno Internazionale di Studi sulla Danza Macabra* (Clusone: 1987) 65–66; ders., „*Visibile parlare*": *Agenda* (Cassino: 1992), Paragraph 22. Zu dem Bild s. Dell'Acqua G.A. (Hrsg.), *I Pittori bergamaschi dal XIII al XIX secolo. Le origini* (Bergamo: 1992) 467; Nr. 45 [L. Tognoli Bardin], Abb. auf 516.

[63] Geißelung und Gebete für die Toten einer Bruderschaft waren mitunter statuarisch festgelegt; s. Henderson, „The Flagellant Movement and Flagellant Confraternities" 158; Giles Arthur, „Cult Objects and Artistic Patronage" 350; Schiferl, „Caritas and the Iconography of Italian Confraternity Art" 220–223.

[64] Frenzel, *Die Darstellung der Geißelung Christi in der italienischen Kunst* 62–66; vgl. auch Belting, *Das Bild und sein Publikum* 283–284. Die Austauschbarkeit beider Motive zeigt sich zudem in zwei Totentafeln aus Sizilien. Ist auf dem 1388 von Antonio Veneziano gemalten Beispiel die Geißelung Christi im aktiv mitleidenden Beisein der auftraggebenden Bruderschaft – der Confraternita di San Niccolò Reale in Palermo – abgebildet (Palermo, Museo Diocesano), stellt ein acht Jahre jüngeres Bild mit gleicher Funktion, entstanden im Auftrag der Confraternita dei SS. Simone e Giuda in Martorana, eine von vier Disciplinati verehrte Imago Pietatis über die Liste der verstorbenen Mitglieder (Palermo, Galleria Nazionale); vgl. Bresc-Bautier G., *Artistes, patriciens et confréries. Production et consommation de l'œuvre d'art à Palerme et en Sicile occidentale (1348–1460)* (Rom: 1979) 209–210, Abb. 2 und 4.

Bild und Spiegelbild

Eines der ältesten erhaltenen italienischen Bruderschaftszeichen schließlich – eine in kleinem Format zweiseitig auf Holz ausgeführte ‚Bandinella' in Pisa (Museo Nazionale di San Matteo)[65] – stammt aus der Mitte des 14. Jahrhunderts und kombiniert eine vielfigurige Kreuzigungsszene auf der einen Seite mit der Geißelung Christi, zusammen mit zwei Heiligen und vier Flagellanten, auf der anderen. Die Identität der auftraggebenden Bußbruderschaft war mangels eindeutiger Attribute der seitlich zur Geißelungsszene postierten Heiligen, ein Papst und ein Bischof, bislang nicht geklärt. Doch handelt es sich hierbei um die Pisaner Disciplinati di S. Gregorio Papa in S. Zeno, die seit dem 14. Jahrhundert – und damit verbinden sich die abschließenden Ausführungen mit den einleitenden Zeilen der Untersuchung – durch eine Gemeinschaftsgrabplatte auf dem Camposanto inschriftlich nachweisbar sind. Für diese Identifizierung spricht nicht nur die Darstellung eines Papstes und eines Bischofs zu Seiten der Geißelungsszene, sondern ebenso der eindeutige Bezug der Raumarchitektur im Bild auf die reale, spätgotische Fassade der Abteikirche S. Zeno – des Versammlungsortes der Bruderschaft.

Durch die Reproduktion des eigenen Betlokals ist die historische Szene explizit in einem zeitgenössischen Kontext verortet, der den vor dem Gemälde vereinten Disciplinati ein unmittelbares Hineinversetzen in das Leiden Christi erleichterte. Auch die abgebildeten Bruderschaftsrepräsentanten, in Adorationsgestus und kleinem Maßstab eingefügt, dienten als hilfreiche Identifikationsfiguren für die vor dem Bild betende und büßende Gemeinschaft.[66] So ließen sich bereits 1318 die Battuti von Teramo (Abruzzen) in dem auf beiden Seiten mit einem „gegeißelten Jesus Christus an der Säule" bemalten Banner abbilden. In der Gestalt als kniende Bußbrüder, in ihrer distinktiven Tracht und

[65] Tempera/Holz, 69 × 59 cm; s. Savettieri C., „Zeugnisse der Volksfrömmigkeit", in Burresi M. (Hrsg.), *Schätze sakraler Kunst aus dem Pisa des 14. Jahrhunderts* (Ausst.-Kat. Unna 1999) (Pisa: 1999) 21–44, hier 27–29, Nr. 2. Dort ist sie Giovanni di Nicola zugeschrieben.

[66] Vgl. dazu Schiferl, "Corporate Identity and Equality" 12–13; Ritzerfeld, *Pietas – Caritas – Societas* 217. Bis weit ins 16. Jahrhundert hinein blieben solche Darstellungsformen eine weithin geläufige Tradition: Allein im nordostitalienischen Raum wurde noch im Cinquecento zahlreichen Aufträgen für Bruderschaftsbanner der Festlegung des zu malenden Bildmotivs oftmals ein kurzer Zusatz beigefügt, unter die heilige Hauptfigur Angehörige der bestellenden Gemeinschaft zu setzen, „e sotto i confratelli battuti"; vgl. Dehmer, *Italienische Bruderschaftsbanner* 130–131; 216.

mit Peitschen in der Hand, wohnten sie als verehrende Zeugen dem leidvollen Geschehen bei.[67]

Das Bemerkenswerte dabei ist – und dieser Gedanke führt wieder unmittelbar zurück zu dem Thema des Sammelbandes –, dass die Disciplinati weder in der Pisaner Standarte noch in den meisten anderen erhaltenen Bruderschaftsbildern mit schmerzverzerrten Gesichtern oder gar vor Pein sich windenden Körpern dargestellt sind. Dies überrascht umso mehr, als die zuweilen blutüberströmt gemalten Rückenansichten entsprechende Reaktionen durchaus nahe legen würden.

Vor diesem Hintergrund erscheint die bereits zitierte trecenteske Laudenstrophe aus Bergamo als eine durchaus ambivalente Handlungsanleitung zur ‚Sancta Disciplina' – nicht nur als Aufruf zum kollektiven Mit-Leiden („Versammelt Euch Genossen"), sondern ebenso als eindringlicher Appell, den Schmerz beim schonungslosen Vollzug der Imitatio Christi („Schlagt Euch hart und unverdrossen") ohne Klagen vertrauens- und hoffnungsvoll zu ertragen („Und man tu' es froh gestimmt"), und zwar in ähnlich demütiger Duldsamkeit, wie es das nachzuahmende Vorbild erforderte („Die Passion Gottes unser Banner"). Doch der Körpereinsatz lohnte sich, wie auch die Laudenstrophe aus Castelbaldo erläuterte: Der in Gottergebenheit ertragene Schmerz öffnete „die Tore zum Eintritt in das Paradies".

Ausblick

Seit dem 15. Jahrhundert vollzogen sich vielerorts Veränderungen auch in den öffentlichen Auftritten der Bußbruderschaften, welche symptomatisch waren für den allgemeinen Wandel der Form von Prozessionen

[67] Die Überlieferung des verlorenen Bannerbildes stammt aus dem späten 16. Jahrhundert; zit. in Savini F., „Sui flagellanti, sui fraticelli e sui bizochi nel teramano durante i secoli XIII e XIV e una bolla di Bonifacio VIII del 1297 contro i bizochi ivi rifugiati", *Archivio Storico Italiano* 5,35 (1905) 82–90, hier 83–84: „1318 era in Teramo istituita la Fraternita de' Battuti, la quale fece compire in quest'anno il Gonfalone, e dipingere nel diritto e nel rovescio Cristo Gesù flagellato alla Colonna [...], e vi fece effigiare i Confratelli ginocchiati, e vestiti di sacco colle discipline in mano. [...]". Ein späteres, noch erhaltenes Bild des Christus an der Geißelsäule mit adorierenden Bruderschaftsrepräsentanten (Leinwand auf Holz, 202 × 76 cm) stammt aus den Jahren um 1500 von Angelo Bizamano (1467–1532), gemalt für den Altar der Confraternita del Salvatore in der Franziskanerkirche von San Mauro Forte; s. Gelao C. (Hrsg.), *Confraternite, arte e devozione in Puglia dal Quattrocento al Settecento* (Ausstellungs-Katalog Bari 1994) (Neapel: 1994) 215, Nr. III. 3.

während der italienischen Renaissance. Nicht zuletzt in Gestalt von lebendigen Bildern wurden sie zunehmend dramatisiert und dynamisiert.[68] Von einer durchgreifenden Ablösung der Rituale zu sprechen – „wenn im Laufe des 13. Jahrhunderts die blutgetränkte Episode der Passion Jesu Christi unmittelbar von den Geißelbrüdern verkörpert wurde, beschränken sich diese gegen Ende des 15. Jahrhunderts darauf, sie darzustellen"[69] –, wäre aber zu rigoros. Soweit dies anhand schriftlicher Quellen überhaupt nachvollziehbar ist, wurde die körperliche Anteilnahme am Leiden Christi durch theatralische, spektakuläre Inszenierungen nicht unbedingt durchweg ersetzt, sondern oft nur weiter ergänzt. Der (ohnehin seit jeher mit performativen Spiel-Arten eng verwobene) Akt der ‚Disciplina' blieb – wie unter anderem 1575 von Karl Borromäus aus der Diözese von Bergamo berichtet wird – in vielen Bußbruderschaften auch weiterhin ein zentraler Bestandteil ihrer paraliturgischen Praktiken.[70]

[68] Helas P., *Lebende Bilder in der italienischen Festkultur des 15. Jahrhunderts* (Berlin: 1999) 50–58. Vgl. dazu u.a. auch Wisch B., „The Passion of Christ in the Art, Theater, and Penitential Rituals of the Roman Confraternity of the Gonfalone", in Eisenbichler K. (Hrsg.), *Crossing the Boundaries. Christian Piety and the Arts in Italian Medieval and Renaissance Confraternities* (Kalamazoo: 1991) 237–262.

[69] „se nel corso del ‚200 il sanguinoso episodio della passione del Cristo veniva ‚impersonato' direttamente dai confratelli, alla fine del ‚400 essi si limitano a ‚rappresentarlo' "; Rusconi R., „La religione dei cittadini: Riti, credenze, devozioni", in Chiabò M. – Doglio F. (Hrsg.), *Ceti sociali ed ambienti urbani nel teatro religioso europeo del '300 e del '400* (Convegno di studi, Viterbo 1985) (Viterbo: 1986) 17–40, hier 32.

[70] Largier, *Lob der Peitsche* 138; 142–143. Vgl. Black, *Italian Confraternities in the 16th Century* 100–103.

Auswahlbibliographie

Modena, Biblioteca Estense, *Congregazione della Carità*, Ms. Nr. 2
Venedig, Biblioteca del Museo Civico Correr, *Cl. IV.* 168
Verona, Archivio di Stato, *Ospedale di S. Bovo* 1

AA. VV., *Il movimento dei Disciplinati nel settimo centenario dal suo inizio (Perugia–1260)* (Convegno internazionale, Perugia 1960) (Spoleto: 1962).
AMTMANN R., *Die Bussbruderschaften in Frankreich* (Wiesbaden: 1977).
BARR C., *The Monophonic Lauda and the Lay Religious Confraternities of Tuscany and Umbria in the Late Middle Ages* (Kalamazoo – Michigan: 1988).
BELTING H., *Das Bild und sein Publikum im Mittelalter. Form und Funktion früher Bildtafeln der Passion* (Berlin: 1981).
DEHMER A., „Mobile Passionsdarstellungen als Leitbilder kollektiver Geißelungsrituale im spätmittelalterlichen Italien", *Das Münster* 55 (2002) 200–207.
——, *Italienische Bruderschaftsbanner des Mittelalters und der Renaissance* (München – Berlin: 2004).
——, „‚Sub Vexillo Sanctae Mariae Magdalenae' – Bilder, Banner und Bruderschaften der hl. Maria Magdalena im Bergamaskischen", *Das Münster* 58 (2005) 206–214.
FANTI M., „Gli inizi del movimento dei Disciplinati e la confraternita di Santa Maria della Vita", *Bollettino della Deputazione di Storia Patria per l'Umbria* 66 (1969) 181–232.
FRENZEL A., *Die Darstellung der Geißelung Christi in der italienischen Kunst von den Anfängen im 11. Jahrhundert bis ins 17. Jahrhundert* (Diss. Frankfurt am Main: 1998).
FRUGONI A., *Incontri nel medioevo* (Bologna: 1979).
GILES ARTHUR K., „Cult Objects and Artistic Patronage of the Fourteenth-Century Flagellant Confraternity of Gesù Pellegrino", in Verdon T. – Henderson J. (Hrsg.), *Christianity and the Renaissance. Image and Religious Imagination in the Quattrocento* (Syrakus: 1990).
GRIGNANI M.A. – STELLA A. (Hrsg.), *Antichi testi pavesi* (Pavia: 1977).
HENDERSON J., *Piety and charity in late medieval Florence* (Oxford: 1994).
——, „The Flagellant Movement and Flagellant Confraternities in Central Italy, 1260–1400", *Studies in Church History* 15 (1978) 147–160.
LARGIER N., *Lob der Peitsche. Eine Kulturgeschichte der Erregung* (München: 2001).
LEE E.-K., „Art and Ritual Drama of the Flagellant Confraternities in 13th–15th Century Italy", *Arte medievale* 4,2 (2005) 69–81.
MEDICA M., „Il santo patrono in miniatura. Gli esordi di una tradizione iconografica", in Buscaroli B. (Hrsg.), *Petronio e Bologna. Il volto di una storia* (Ausstellungs-Katalog Bologna 2001/2002) (Ferrara: 2001) 141–147.
MEERSSEMAN G.G., *Ordo fraternitatis. Confraternite e pietà dei laici nel medioevo*, 3 Bde. (Italia Sacra 24–26) (Rom: 1977).
RITZERFELD U., *Pietas – Caritas – Societas. Bildprogramme karitativer Einrichtungen des Spätmittelalters in Italien* (Diss. Bonn: 2007) [http://hss.ulb.uni-bonn.de/diss_online/phil_fak/2007/ritzerfeld_ulrike].
DE SANDRE GASPARINI G., „Confraternite e ‚cura animarum' nei primi anni del Quattrocento: I disciplinati e la parocchia di S. Vitale a Verona", in Sambin P. (Hrsg.), *Pievi, parrocchie e clero nel Veneto dal X al XV secolo* (Venedig: 1987) 289–360.
SCHIFERL E., „Corporate Identity and Equality: Confraternity Members in Italian Paintings, c. 1340–1510", *Source* 8,2 (1989) 12–18.
——, „Caritas and the Iconography of Italian Confraternity Art", *Studies in Iconography* 14 (1995) 207–246.
WEISSMAN R.F., *Ritual Brotherhood in Renaissance Florence* (New York: 1982).

SELF-FLAGELLATION IN THE EARLY MODERN ERA

Patrick Vandermeersch

Self-flagellation is often understood as self-punishment. History teaches us, however, that the same physical act has taken various psychological meanings. As a mass movement in the fourteenth century, it was primarily seen as an act of protest whereby the flagellants rejected the spiritual authority and sacramental power of the clergy. In the sixteenth century, flagellation came to be associated with self-control, and a new term was coined in order to designate it: 'discipline'. Curiously, in some religious orders this shift was accompanied by a change in focus: rather than the shoulders or back, the buttocks were to be whipped instead. A great controversy immediately arose but was silenced when the possible sexual meaning of flagellation was realized – or should we say, constructed? My hypothesis is that the change in both the name and the way flagellation was performed indicates the emergence of a new type of modern subjectivity. I will suggest, furthermore, that this requires a further elaboration of Norbert Elias's theory of the 'civilizing process'.

A Brief Overview of the History of Flagellation[1]

Let us start with the origins of religious self-flagellation. Although there were many ascetic practices in the monasteries at the time of the desert fathers, self-flagellation does not seem to have been among them. Without doubt many extraordinary rituals were performed. Extreme degrees

[1] The following historical account summarizes the more detailed historical research presented in my *La chair de la passion. Une histoire de foi: la flagellation* (Paris: 2002). For this reason, footnote references have been restricted to the most essential ones. The original research project had a broader scope: starting with an observation of contemporary forms of self-flagellation in a Spanish village, I argue that a psychological hermeneutic of this practice involves doing historical research. This insight stems from psychoanalytical experience, which demonstrates that individuals cannot understand themselves without performing an anamnesis. The same applies to social phenomena; this opens up the reverse question of the psychological efficacy of historical research in general.

of fasting would give rise to intense debates concerning, for example, whether eating three or four olives a day was still compliant with the ascetic ideal, as such a small number could encourage the sin of pride. Painful situations were purposely sought, with ascetics praying in spaces filled with stinging insects, bathing in icy water or rolling in thorns. However, as far as we know, whipping oneself was not among the practices, although scourging was a common punishment, even for monks. Historians might argue that self-flagellation is so obviously classifiable as an ascetic practice that this could be the reason it is not mentioned explicitly, but from a psychological point of view this is questionable. In any case, it was certainly experienced as a different form of ascetic behaviour as soon as its practice became a public issue.

The eleventh-century monastic leader and Church reformer Peter Damian seems to have been the initiator of the practice and wrote much about it. In the monastery of Fonte Avellana, where he was prior, monks were expected to whip their naked bodies and to do this together, without being ashamed of each other's nakedness. He wrote so prolifically on the topic that many historians have assumed that, from this moment on, the practice spread throughout the monasteries and until recently was a well-established custom. However, careful reading of other sources leads us to consider that this was not the case. The Franciscans may have been an exception during the first decades of their establishment, as they are said to have influenced a first wave of public, group flagellation in Perugia in 1260. However, they then seem to have abandoned the practice for a few centuries. Lay people who flagellated themselves in public were swiftly referred to lay confraternities of 'penitents', where they could continue the practice under clerical supervision and hidden from the public.

Thus, it appears that the practice was neither widespread nor well known until the rise of an extensive flagellant movement in 1349. In the summer of this year, many large groups of flagellants wandered throughout Europe before gathering in Tournai, the seat of an important diocese in the south of present-day Belgium. The local abbot, Li Muisis, wrote in his chronicle that he had never seen such a practice.[2] This is even more remarkable when we consider the fact that a few

---

[2] *Chronica Aegidii Li Muisis*, in De Smet J.J., *Recueil des chroniques de Flandre*, Collection des chroniques belges inédites, publiées par la Commission Royale d'Histoire (Brussels, M. Hayez: 1841) II, 344–359.

years earlier he had written on the customs in his abbey and described the *disciplina*, another form of whipping.[3] In the latter case, however, a monk was whipped by another monk, even when the whipping was not imposed as a punishment but freely chosen as devotion.[4] Asking to be whipped by someone else and whipping oneself were clearly considered to be very different.

Indeed, closer research does not give the impression that the practice of self-flagellation was understood as self-punishment. More precisely, it was not, in any case, an expression of humility or self-abnegation. The flagellants formed a seditious movement. They reacted against the rising power of the parish clergy, against the newly established sacrament of confession and against the withdrawal of the Eucharistic wine, Christ's blood, from the lay community. Undoubtedly, they experienced pain and inflicted it on their own bodies. In doing so, they felt superior to others, since during flagellation they experienced in themselves the suffering of Christ, as though Christ's blood was present in their bodies. Moreover, they rejected the practice of priestly mediation that the Church was trying to establish. They spoke of sin and of God's anger in order to warn others of the need to renounce their sinful lives or face the consequences in times of spreading plague, but they did not provoke confession to a priest. Thus, there was much pride in their behaviour, even a form of 'narcissism' which I will specify below, in the sense that the self-infliction of pain seemed to strengthen narcissistic feelings rather than weaken them.

The flagellant movement was brought to an end while its followers were on their way to Avignon, where they hoped to speak with the Pope, who had just issued a condemnation of the practice. The French king sent his troops to disperse them and what was left of the movement headed north, surviving for a while in the region of Erfurt, where Protestantism would later emerge. There were revivals in Spain and France, with the famous Dominican missionary Vincent Ferrer (1350–1419), accompanied by a group of flagellants, preaching from town to town. Such acts irritated the bishops meeting at the Council of Constance (1414–1418), who were trying to end the Western schism which saw two popes, one in Avignon and one in Rome, disputing the

---

[3] Li Muisis A., *Tractatus de consuetudinibus*, in "Le Tractatus de consuetudinibus de Gilles Li Muisis (1347)", *Bulletin de la Commission Royale d'Histoire – Handelingen van de Koninklijke Commissie voor Geschiedenis* 124 (1959) 193–194.

[4] Li Muisis A., *Tractatus de consuetudinibus* 193–194.

Papal See. Jean Gerson, the famous Parisian theologian and initiator of a deliberate pastoral approach to lay people, was particularly upset. One of the direct causes may have been that during the Holy Week of 1416, Ferrer had convinced many of the Toulouse hierarchy, including members of the theological faculty, to participate in a procession in which they whipped themselves. However, attacking Ferrer too directly was hazardous. He was a mighty figure both in the Church and in secular politics, having convinced the Castilians to withdraw their support from the third pope, Peter of Luna, who had been chosen in the hope that the other two would then resign. Nevertheless, Gerson wrote a famous treatise, the 1417 *Contra sectam flagellantium*, against Ferrer[5] that seems to have been effective, since Ferrer continued his preaching without his company of flagellants. We do not know if he intended to dismiss them permanently, as he died soon after in Vannes in 1419, where he is buried in the cathedral.

Moving from the public manifestation of flagellation by wandering groups that accompanied preachers, we find that the discreet practice persisted in confraternities of pious lay people. Genoan sailors introduced flagellation into Spain and France – more precisely into Valencia and Marseille – at the end of the fifteenth century, and suddenly it began to flourish. Franciscans were especially active in its propagation. Several fraternities of penitents sprang up both in the Papal States surrounding Avignon and in Spain. In France, however, the lay confraternities did not practise flagellation. Some groups tried to introduce the practice with a limited amount of success, with self-flagellation being somewhat secretly inaugurated into the practices of the Blue Penitents of Bourges in 1584, and into the private *Confrérie de la mort* of King Henry III, established in 1585. The king was murdered in 1589 and Henry IV of Navarre was not in favour of such Catholic devotions, so this seems to have marked the end of lay flagellation in France.

Later, we still find some rare examples of public flagellation. At the beginning of the seventeenth century, a huge controversy arose in Germany, when the Catholics announced their presence in Augsburg – a town stiff with the symbolism of the Protestant *Confessio Augustana* – with processions that included public flagellation. This gave birth to an enormous literary production on the topic, especially by the Jesuit

---

[5] In Jean Gerson, *Œuvres complètes*, vol. X *L'œuvre polémique* (Paris: 1973) 46–51.

James Gretser (1562–1625),[6] indicating that there was clearly no fear of public discussion of the topic. These kinds of procession would, however, soon disappear, even in Spain, where Charles III forbade public flagellation in 1777.

The practice of flagellation was nevertheless kept alive in most religious orders and congregations, especially in newly created orders such as the Jesuits. They practised flagellation in a less harsh manner, using whips that did not hurt excessively. Significantly, the name was also changed; instead of flagellation the term 'discipline' was reintroduced, but with a notable shift in meaning, as the term 'discipline' previously referred specifically to being scourged by someone else, whereas flagellation specifically meant whipping oneself. There was also a second significant change. In the monasteries and convents where the practice was adopted or readopted, it was often not the back but the buttocks that became the object of flagellation. It is debatable whether this reorientation was commonplace, especially as recent interviews conducted by Emke Bosgraaf, who is completing a PhD thesis on the subject at the University of Groningen, have indicated that various parts of the body, including the back, the arms, the shoulders and the legs, could have been used for flagellation until the middle of the twentieth century.

We are well informed on the topic by a book by the Parisian canon, Jacques Boileau (1635–1716), the brother of Nicolas, the great poet, who sneered at the 'newly introduced practice' in the convents. His *Histoire des flagellants*, published in 1700 in Latin and a year later in French, for a long time remained the standard book on the topic.[7] It was immediately followed by a reply written by another Parisian canon, Jean-Baptiste Thiers (1636–1703), who published his *Critique de l'histoire des flagellants, et justification de l'usage des disciplines volontaires* in 1703. While the latter book is poor with respect to its argument, the list of all the religious orders and congregations that adopted flagellation and the dates of its introduction is instructive. Against Boileau, Thiers attempted to prove

[6] James Gretser S.J., *De spontanea disciplinarum seu flagellorum cruce* (1606), in *Opera omnia*, vol. IV (Regensburg, J.C. Peez and F. Baader: 1743).

[7] Jacques Boileau, *Historia Flagellantium, de recto et perverso flagrorum usu apud Christianos. Ex antiquis Scripturae, Patrum, Pontificum, Conciliorum et Scriptorum Profanorum monumentis cum cura et fide expressa* (Paris, Jean Anisson: 1700); French translation: *Histoire des flagellants. Le bon et le mauvais usage des flagellations parmi les chrétiens* (Amsterdam, François vander Plaats: 1701). A new edition, with an introduction by C. Louis-Combet but without the original notes: Montbonnot-St-Martin: 1986. The text is available on the internet at <www.eros-thanatos.com>.

that self-flagellation was not a recent practice, but he was unable to find any earlier example of the practice than that of the Capuchins in 1529, who, he had to admit, were somewhat reluctant, with the practice having to be reintroduced in 1536.[8]

The changed site of discipline gave the sarcastic Boileau the perfect argument to deride the practice. The reason used to justify this type of 'discipline', he said, was that it helped to restrain lust. However, he continued by claiming that medical knowledge revealed that being beaten on the buttocks produced the opposite. It is with his book that the possible sexual interpretation of flagellation became apparent. Religious flagellation was then treated by sexology and taken as proof that sexual masochism had always existed, something that is actually disputable. As a result of this insinuated interweaving of sexual feelings and pain in the experience of being flogged, religious flagellation was no longer discussed openly, as it had been in Gretser's time. Nevertheless, the practice continued in secret. Young nuns and brothers entering a religious congregation were mostly not aware before the end of their novitiate that they would have to submit themselves to it once they had taken their vows.

How did the practice finally come to an end? While my own book on the history of self-flagellation, *Chair de la passion*, concludes that this still required investigation, the research undertaken since then by Emke Bosgraaf has shown that it disappeared quite suddenly in the 1950s and 1960s. This was a time in which there was an expectation of a radical change in spirituality as the Church prepared itself for the Second Vatican Council. In this context the meaning of self-flagellation was no longer obvious. Did it have to do with pain, with the act of flogging, or with the self? Let us add psychology to historical research.

The Disciplined Self and Its Body

Since the publication of *The Civilizing Process* by the sociologist Norbert Elias (1897–1990),[9] we expect a given culture to evolve from a phase of

[8] 'Mais leur première ferveur s'étant un peu ralentie depuis cette première congrégation, on ne les a obligés qu'à se discipliner trois fois la semaine', et ceci par une adaptation de la règle en 1536.' Jean-Baptiste Thiers, *Critique de l'histoire des flagellants, et justification de l'usage des disciplines volontaires Critique* (Paris, Jean de Nully: 1703) 354–355.

[9] Elias N., *The Civilizing Process* (Oxford: 2000).

restraint imposed by others to one of self-restraint. In this process there is also a transition from shame to guilt. In the first phase individuals feel shame only when other people witness their wrongdoing. This phase is followed by one in which they feel guilty even if nobody is aware of their faults. A typical experience of this distinction in culpability can easily be had in relation to encountering a red traffic light on an empty road at night. Do you respect this sign, which an all-seeing authority would do better to switch off?

In the history of European culture the rise of modernity in the sixteenth and seventeenth centuries has often been conceived of as the turning point in the shift from external to internal control. During this period, an increasing awareness of the value of personal life developed and, as a consequence, the individual was expected to attain a higher level of self-control. The process began in towns in the higher Middle Ages but became more manifest, and a more frequent object of reflection, in modernity. The process shows that the degree of evaluation of the individual and the propensity for feelings of personal guilt increased proportionally.

One of the first philosophers to be concerned with these issues is Michel de Montaigne (1533–1592), who in his *Essays* reflects on the knowledge to be gained from personal observation, including observations of bodily experiences. Montaigne examines everything from his kidney stones to political events. In accordance with the ideas developed in *De la servitude volontaire* by his dear friend Etienne de la Boétie (1530–1563), he is struck by the fact that human beings enjoy being guided and dominated, and further notes that the achievement of freedom is not easy. Of course, the most important herald of this new awareness of the value of personal life is Descartes, who starts his *Discours sur la méthode* with the proclamation that he will never accept as truth anything that he cannot prove starting from his own experience. Modern man is convinced that the value of life begins with the individual.

The same phenomenon can be observed in the religious realm, with the Jesuits being the clearest representatives of the new cultural atmosphere. Earlier, the ultimate Christian ideal clearly consisted in a monastic life for all, although it was accepted that most were bound to adopt a more limited ideal. The Jesuits, however, were convinced that there was no universal ideal and that every human being should discover the particular divine plan made for their own life. The famous *Exercises* of Ignatius of Loyola were precisely aimed at discovering God's very special purpose for the individual. Somewhat ambiguously, individual freedom was also stressed; however, in this context this did not mean being free from feelings of guilt, as we would think today, but in fact quite the opposite. Catholicism established the practice of confession extensively, with people being taught to confess more frequently and more broadly, including the lesser sins along with the 'mortal'. They were required to provide all the details of their sins, including the inner motives and the degree of free will involved. Thus, for Catholic countries, confession was an important instrument in achieving self-control, in that to become a responsible individual, one had to rely on an authority figure.

Considered from a psychoanalytical point of view, we here confront the emergence of the superego structure that would continue to grow in Western culture until it fostered paralysing guilt, hampering both the enjoyment of life and the strength to act. The fear of possibly doing something wrong could even hamper an attempt to achieve the good. Sigmund Freud's work can be understood as the elaboration of a technique for reducing the repressing power of the hypertrophied superego. If the superego can be understood as a mechanism of self-punishment whereby the individual's aggression is turned back against their own person, the interpretation of self-flagellation seems obvious: it is a perfect symbol of the internalization of punishment. Things are not so simple, however, and both Freud's view on the superego and our naive presupposition that pain lies at the real core of self-flagellation need more elaboration.[10] Elias was to an extent aware of this, as he frequently puts 'superego' between quotation marks in *The Civilizing Process*, and seems to suggest that a more precise elaboration of the Freudian concept is needed before we can use it in a sociohistorical analysis. Let us proceed in that direction.

According to Freud, the superego's self-punishing function presupposes a deeper psychological structure, that of narcissism. It is for this reason that Freud originally coined a different term for the superego, the ego ideal, which he continued to use as a synonym later. Individuals want to act in a certain way because they consider themselves appealing when they do so. Thus, for Freud, self-love as a form of being in love

[10] For the psychological theory and especially the way American Ego Psychology has dismissed essential parts of the original Freudian insights, see Vandermeersch P., "Het narcisme. De psychoanalytische theorie en haar lotgevallen", in Huijts J.H. (ed.), *Ik zei de gek. Tussen zelf-ontkenning en zelf-verheerlijking* (Baarn: 1982) 32–58 and Vandermeersch P. – Westerink H., *Godsdienstpsychologie in cultuurhistorisch perspectief* (Amsterdam: 2007).

with an image of oneself – an essential experience which is required to establish one's own individuality and to escape psychosis – is the basis of the ego ideal or superego.

We must emphasize two elements in this narcissism. The first is sexuality: we essentially love the image of ourselves as an image of someone with a particular sexual identity. We love ourselves as male or female – something which seems to be a basic experience required at a bodily level. Secondly, narcissism is closely related to identification with others, in that the image of our sexual ego that we adopt as 'our beautiful ego' in narcissism is borrowed from other human beings. We love ourselves as if we were the other. This event of 'transitivism' is part of narcissism, and implies that self-love involves love of an alter ego.

We see how a more complete outline of Freud's superego theory puts many elements of the history of self-flagellation into perspective: the psychological structure which promotes the value of morality to an individualized subject is not just the result of an internalized fear of painful punishment. It consists primarily of internalized self-love, consequently making it possible to overcome the continuous need to be admired by others. Thus, a circular 'empathetic' drive in the identification process is established that enables individuals to experience themselves as if they were the other, without losing the feeling of being themselves.

Is Guilt the Feeling of Internalized Pain?

Using Elias's scheme, we can investigate the extent to which the introduction of self-flagellation as discipline was a sign of a broader turn to self-restraint. Let us start with the common assumption that flagellation is the self-infliction of pain and consequently a form of self-chastisement. We know, however, that the painful element was restricted precisely at the time that this internalization is presumed to have occurred. I have already mentioned that flagellation was performed in a less harsh manner when the practice was adopted by the Jesuits, exactly those who insisted on using the term 'discipline'. Ignatius even invented a new type of whip that was not so harmful and could be used more frequently. The two aspects are, of course, linked from a practical point of view: if you perform the ritual more regularly, you cannot be so aggressive. However, changing the frequency of the exercise and flattening the whip changed its psychological meaning. As the pain is no longer so great and no bleeding is provoked, it is no longer the intrusion of something alien into the body. Rather, flagellation becomes a self-provoked awareness of being a mind within a skin. The body is yours and that you can appropriate it. By doing this regularly, it becomes an exercise for the self, and not a demonstration addressed to others. Rather than a form of self-rejection on the basis of one's faults, flagellation developed into a means of enhancing a narcissism of a more reflective nature. This pertained first and foremost to the psychological event of experiencing one's own body, as opposed to medieval flagellation, which fundamentally involved others in its need for a public.

Let us pay more attention to the topic of the public exhibition of flagellation, which was discredited with the rise of modernity. The members of the religious congregations that favoured the practice seem to have been faintly aware of the importance of withdrawing the element of public performance so predominant in the Middle Ages. What struck the public most in the procession on Maundy Thursday 1583 in Paris, where some flagellation was performed, was not the peculiar gesture, but the fact that the participants were wearing masks. The explanation given to the amazed spectators was that the penitents were to show humility through their anonymity.[11] However, people knew that there were those of high rank involved and that the king was quite surely among them, as his chapel choir was taking part. This gave rise to a very interesting debate about whether it was good for officials, especially the king, to adopt such a humble position.

Indeed, this was the very reason why priests had already been forbidden to take part in public manifestations of penance. If a priest positioned himself among the sinners, how could he be expected to preserve his authority over his parishioners? The same remark could be applied to civil authorities. However, the Jesuits and Franciscans, who were among the zealous initiators of public flagellation, replied that a distinction should be made between a penance imposed for the expiation of a personal sin, and a penance freely chosen to sharpen one's consciousness of universal human sinfulness. The latter testified precisely to the moral *sensitivity* of the penitent. Therefore a nobleman

[11] De Cheffontaines C., *Apologie de la confrairie des pénitents érigée et instituée en la ville de Paris par le tres chrestien roy de France et de Pollogne, Henry troisième de son nom* (Paris, M. Julian: 1583).

participating in such a penitential ritual should be recognized as being extremely trustworthy.

We might wonder about the actual reactions of ordinary people witnessing such processions. We know from popular songs that people mocked this kind of devotion. Nevertheless, the Jesuits continued to stress the ideal of humility in the private flagellation rituals they introduced into the confraternity of the Blue Penitents of Bourges and into the private confraternity of the king. The rule stipulated that the members had to whip themselves in the dark and then leave on their own, without talking to each other. In the rules of the Spanish confraternities of disciplinants of the sixteenth century we find the same insistence on leaving individually and in silence. Thus, flagellation was to be performed in a humble manner, privately and in silence, without reducing the intensity of the bodily experience by putting it into words and sharing it with others.

To summarize, the repeatedly performed ritual of flagellation is indeed an exercise, but is more psychologically complex than the repetitive infliction of punishment through pain; rather it incorporates both an experience of pain and a sensation of being alive. While being scourged by someone else is a reminder of the requirement to do what is socially expected, self-flagellation stresses the experience of remaining an 'I' on a fundamental level, even if this identity is no longer supported by the social structure. Those who whipped themselves in the dark and left without speaking were experiencing in common a primary awareness of being a meaningful body. Regression into that primitive layer of narcissism gave them the support which allowed them to question their social identity without confronting the anxiety of becoming 'nobody', partly in the sense of literally becoming 'no body'. The silent togetherness of the event accentuated this process of regression into the primitive experience of being an 'I' linked to a body. It was a form of male bonding which ignored social distinctions.

Let us return, to our main question of whether flagellation was accepted because it was an impressive symbol of the turn to self-control. The answer seems to be that this was indeed the case to some extent, but not in any simple sense, since flagellation involved the internalization of a painful punishment. Self-flagellation came to display the fact that the body can resist the deconstruction of the subject and that the 'I' can emerge even when its identity is no longer assured by self-evident customs and rules. In this sense, self-flagellation expresses the basic autonomy of the individual that is necessary for internalization.

It does not, however, automatically enact the internalization of the will of the other. Self-flagellation is completely different from being scourged or caned.

We should not forget, finally, that the history of self-flagellation is confined to religious contexts. The fact seems so obvious that we hardly wonder why similar practices did not appear in the secular world which, much more than monasteries and convents, needed to establish self-control. Have there been similar rituals? Elias points to the influence of the French royal court, where new manners had to be learned and where it became a skill to foresee how someone in power would act in particular circumstances. However, perhaps we should direct our attention to rituals of a more basic bodily nature, providing support to modern minds that are increasingly expected to become 'themselves'. The French sociologist David Lebreton has shown how such rituals still function today, ranging from fitness centres to tattoo shops and extreme sports.[12] It might be worthwhile to investigate the prehistory of these modern lifestyles. It would surely be enlightening to grasp more precisely why the history of religiosity has taken a different direction to that of the secular *mentalité*.

---

[12] Le Breton D., *Passions du risque* (Paris: 1991); *Signes d'identité. Tatouages, piercings et autres marques corporelles* (Paris: 2002); *La peau et la trace. Sur les blessures de soi* (Paris: 2003).

Selective Bibliography

Boileau Jean, *Historia Flagellantium, de recto et perverso flagrorum usu apud Christianos. Ex antiquis Scripturae, Patrum, Pontificum, Conciliorum, et Scriptorum Profanorum monumentis cum cura et fide expressa* (Paris, Jean Anisson: 1700). French translation: *Histoire des flagellants. Le bon et le mauvais usage des flagellations parmi les chrétiens* (Amsterdam, François vander Plaats: 1701).

de Cheffontaines Chr., *Apologie de la confrairie des pénitents érigée et instituée en la ville de Paris par le tres chrestien roy de France et de Pollogne, Henry troisième de son nom* (Paris, M. Julian: 1583)

Foucault M., *The History of Sexuality: An Introduction* (Harmondsworth: 1984).

Freud S., *The Ego and the Id*, in *The Standard Edition of the Complete Psychological Works of Sigmund Freud* (London: 1953–1974) XIX, 1–66.

Gerson Jean, *Contra sectam flagellantium* (1417), in *Œuvres complètes* X: *L'œuvre polémique* (Paris: 1973) 46–51.

Gretser James, *De spontanea disciplinarum seu flagellorum cruce* (1606), in *Opera omnia*, vol. IV (Regensburg, J.C. Peez and F. Baader: 1743).

Le Breton D., *Passion du risque* (Paris: 1991).

——, *Signes d'identité. Tatouages, piercings et autres marques corporelles* (Paris: 2002).

——, *La peau et la trace. Sur les blessures de soi* (Paris: 2003).

Li Muisis A., *Chronica*, in De Smet J.-J., *Recueil des chroniques de Flandre* (Brussels: 1841; Collection des chroniques belges inédites, publiées par la Commission Royale d'Histoire) II, 344–359.

——, *Tractatus de consuetudinibus*, in "Le Tractatus de consuetudinibus de Gilles Li Muisis (1347)", *Bulletin de la Commission Royale d'Histoire – Handelingen van de Koninklijke Commissie voor Geschiedenis* 124 (1959) 193–194.

Thiers Jean-Baptiste, *Critique de l'histoire des flagellants, et justification de l'usage des disciplines volontaires* (Paris, Jean de Nully: 1703).

Vandermeersch P., *La chair de la Passion. Une histoire de foi: la flagellation* (Paris: 2002). Spanish translation: *Carne de la Pasión. Flagelantes y disciplinantes: contexto historico-psychologico* (Madrid: 2004).

'ESTA PENA TAN SABROSA': TERESA OF AVILA AND THE FIGURATIVE ARTS IN EARLY MODERN EUROPE

Maria Berbara

Spiritu intelligentiae replevit illam*

This paper will focus on Teresa of Avila[1] and her representation in visual arts during the early-modern period, especially the first half of the seventeenth century, with an emphasis on her experience of pain. How did Teresa describe her own pain during ecstasies and higher levels of prayer, and what did this suffering mean to her? Was Teresa's construction of pain in tune with that of most sixteenth-century Catholic saints and with the medieval tradition? Did her texts somehow influence, and/or were influenced by, contemporary visual arts? To what extent was there a correspondence between Teresa's iconography and her writings, as far as pain was concerned? How were Teresa's writings on pain interpreted by early modern artists?

From the very beginnings of Christianity, ecstatic experiences described by mystics had a physical dimension in which pain frequently played a part. As a member of this long lineage, Teresa of Avila is no

---

* See Fig. 9, p. 289 below.

[1] Teresa de Cepeda y Ahumada (Avila, 1515 – Alba de Tormes, 1582) entered the Carmelite Convent of the Incarnation (Avila) in November 1535, and made her vows two years later. From 1560/62 onwards, she worked actively in the foundation of several convents for the reformed order of the Discalced Carmelites. Teresa wrote five complete books (*Libro de la Vida*, 1562–1565; *Camino de perfección*, 1565–1566; *Meditaciones sobre los Cantares*, 1566–1567; *Libro de las fundaciones*, 1573–1582; and *Castillo interior o las moradas*, 1577) as well as various collections of poems, letters and writings related to her reform (*Constituciones*, 1563; *Visita de Descalzas*, 1576). Her complete works, edited by the Augustinian Fray Luis de León, were first published – with important omissions – in 1588 (in Salamanca), although copies of some of her writings started to circulate in Spain soon after her death, and independent editions of the *Maxims* and *Way of Perfection* appeared between 1583 and 1585. Further editions and translations followed rapidly (Zaragoza: 1592; Madrid: 1597; Naples: 1604; Brussels: 1604; Valencia: 1613, among others). She was beatified by Paul V in 1614 and canonized by Gregory XV in 1622, together with Ignatius of Loyola, Francis Xavier, Filippo Neri and Isidro. At the time of her canonization she received the appelative *de Avila*, which in more recent times has served to distinguish her from Teresa of Lisieux, her French namesake. The saint herself used to sign her writings as Teresa de Jesús, a name by which she is also occasionally referred to (especially by Spanish-language writers).

exception. Her discourses on pain, different as they are from late antique and medieval ones, keep this strong traditional intermingling of body and soul. The suffering she experiences during ecstasy is overwhelmingly physical, and she usually describes it by pointing out specific parts of her body, as well as objects – such as arrows and spears – which cause her pain. This mystical suffering affects her body directly, leaving her often with bruises and wounds;[2] on the other hand, it also fosters a transient improvement of her natural aches.[3] Physical as its manifestations may be, Teresa's pain during mystical experiences is a function of the soul, and it differs from mundane bodily aches.[4]

The pain which Teresa felt during ecstasies and higher levels of prayer was not of a moral quality. She did not suffer from remorse, guilt for her own or for other people's sins, as could happen in other historical contexts; her suffering was totally individual and formed an intrinsic part of the joy of revelations. Particular to Teresa's conceptions of this kind of pain is not its bodily dimension, nor the fact that she endured suffering – a common characteristic of Christian saints and martyrs of all times – but that it was, in Teresa's own words, *in itself* blissful, delightful, delectable. In what she calls the third and, especially, fourth level of prayer, pleasure and pain unite and heighten each other generating a feeling of rapture whose intensity Teresa finds difficult to describe. Ecstasy itself is a foretaste of Heaven; in no other earthly moment can the soul be as close to God. This apparent paradox of simultaneous pleasure and pain comes out many times in Teresa's writings. As Robert Petersson notes, they "yield a product which exceeds the sum of both. A third kind of experience is created which is different from both; not pleasure-pain but a nameless something".[5] Other saints before her, such as Catherine of Siena (1347–1380), spoke about the sweetness of the pain they experienced during ecstasies or higher levels of prayer. For some medieval saints, the experience of pain during ecstasies, eucharistic frenzy, fasting and mortifications was deeply connected with the idea of embracing Christ through the sharing of His suffering.[6] This

---

[2] *Interior Castle*, chapter 6, 11,4.

[3] Cf. for instance *Vida* 20; 21.

[4] Cf. *Interior Castle*, chapter 6, 11, especially 2–3.

[5] Petersson R., *The Art of Ecstasy. Saint Teresa, Bernini and Crashaw* (London: 1970) 33.

[6] For Catherine of Siena, for example, her own pain could have an expiatory quality; she spent the last years of her life experiencing intense physical sufferings caused by a vision she had of the weight of the ship of the Church descending on her shoulders.

embrace is delicious, since it elevates and purifies the soul, bringing it closer to Christ and his sufferings.[7] For Teresa, however, the pain she senses during ecstatic experiences – which always comes from God, never from herself – is an intrinsic aspect of the soul's elevation itself, and it may be understood positively as a sign of her spiritual development. It does not have an expiatory or redemptive function, nor is it conceived as a punishment; on the contrary, it is a privilege, a blessing, a gift from God. It can be dangerous, as she describes in the *Interior Castle*, because during ecstasy the soul is so strongly attracted to God that it can become detached from the body and the person in question may die.[8] At this level, it becomes one with delight – and therefore can be as dangerous as any other kind of sensual seduction. There are several passages in her writings in which she describes the ambiguity of the experience:

> No words will suffice to describe the way in which God wounds the soul and the sore distress which He causes it, so that it hardly knows what it is doing. Yet so delectable is this distress (*es esta pena tan sabrosa*) that life holds no delight which can give greater satisfaction. As I have said, the soul would gladly be dying of this will.[9]
>
> The other [peril of the spiritual road] is of excessive rejoicing and delight, which can be carried to such an extreme that it really seems as if the soul is swooning, and as if the slightest thing would be enough to drive it out of the body.[10]

Thus, Teresa inherited from medieval traditions the physicality of pain during intense religious experiences and its intrinsic connection with pleasure, but not its ultimate meaning.

Teresa insists on what seemed to be common knowledge about ecstasies in her days: they were the product less of a spiritual elevation achieved through individual effort than of a grace granted by God: 'It is not we who put on the fuel; it seems rather as if the fire is already kindled and it is we who are suddenly thrown into it to be burned up'.[11] If, for the Platonist humanist Marsilio Ficino in the previous century, beatific vision was the ultimate degree of intellectual contemplation,

---

[7] For examples cf. Bynum C. Walker, *Holy Feast and Holy Fast: The Religious Significance of Food to Medieval Women* (University of California Press: 1987), chapter 8.

[8] 6, 11. Cf. also *Meditaciones sobre los Cantares* 7,2.

[9] *Vida*, chapter 29 (For the English translation cf. Peers E.A. [ed.], *The Complete Works of Saint Teresa of Jesus*, 3 vols. (London – New York: 1950), vol. I, 191).

[10] *Interior Castle*, chapter 6, 11; trl. Peers, vol. II, 328.

[11] *Ibidem*.

achieved through the dominion of reason over the body, and through an effort to liberate oneself from its prison,[12] for Teresa it was a divine gift solely bestowed by the will of God. Visions and ecstasies where not achieved through intelligence and meditation, but through faith, and they were attributable to Divine Love only. In many passages of her biography, she claims to be an unlearned woman (she cannot read Latin or Greek; in fact, she cannot read any foreign language at all), and sometimes she clearly states her disbelief in those who intend to achieve the grace of God through erudition and intellectual meditation.[13] When Don Fernando de Valdés, grand inquisitor of Spain, published an index of forbidden books that included some of Teresa's favorites, she had a vision of Christ saying to her: 'Be not distressed, for I will give thee a living book'.[14]

In her writings, she uses the image of an arrow to explain how God strikes her with Divine Love:

> [...] an arrow is driven into the very depths of the entrails, and sometimes into the heart, so that the soul does not know either what is the matter with it or what it desires. It knows quite well that it desires God and that the arrow seems to have dipped in some drug which leads it to hate itself for the love of this Lord so that it would gladly lose its life for Him.[15]

The word 'rapture', '*arrobamiento*' (or '*arrebatamiento*'), is often equated to a 'flight of the spirit' during which the soul is transported with overwhelming intensity and extreme velocity: Teresa uses the image of a ship lifted by a powerful wave, and of a bullet leaving a gun when the trigger is pulled.[16] Contemporary saints, such as Catherine of Genoa, also employ visual metaphors to describe how it is God's love that lifts their spirit: the Italian mystic speaks of a golden chain with which the

---

[12] Cf. *Theologia Platonica* XIII, 2: 'Magnum certe est mentis imperium, quae virtute sua a compedibus corporis solvitur'.

[13] For example *Life*, chapter 40,4. This had been a *locus communis* among mystics at least since Saint Bonaventura, who insists on the suspension of intellectual activities of any kind for the soul to be reached and transformed by Divine Love. Cf. Treffers B., "Gettarsi nel niente. Immagini ed esperienza mistica", in Morello G. (ed.), *Visioni ed Estasi. Capolavori dell'arte europea tra Seicento e Settecento* (Milan, Skira: 2004) 51. In a similar vein, Ugo di San Vittore affirms the superiority of spirituality over erudition.

[14] *Vida*, chapter 26; trl. Peers, vol. I, 168.

[15] *Ibid.* See also *Interior Castle*, chapter 6, 11,2.

[16] *Interior Castle*, chapters 6, 5 and 5, 3.

Christ Child, helped by Mary, pulls her towards Himself, uniting her soul to Divine Love.[17]

According to her own account and that of her biographers, Teresa was a very sick woman in her youth, and she describes in several passages of the *Vida* the horrors of her intense pains. In one occasion she suffered from a seizure that lasted four days, during which she was totally paralysed and unconscious. The nuns thought her to be dead, and a grave was prepared. Teresa tells that, when she woke up, she had wax on her eyelids. After that, she was paralysed for three years, at the beginning of which she could only move some of her fingers.[18] Her descriptions of the physical pain she experienced are vivid and graphic, yet they are of another kind to those connected to mystical ecstasies. In the last chapter of the *Vida*, she even describes how the ordinary bodily pain and the 'usual vomiting' distracts her from prayer and prevents her from experiencing visions and other higher levels of beatific contemplation (40,20).

Concepts such as sacrifice and martyrdom acquired a new meaning in Teresa's experiences and writings. Every Spaniard knows the story of how a seven-year-old Teresa and her favorite brother, Rodrigo, planned to escape home in order to search for martyrdom in Africa:

> We used to read the lives of saints together; and, when I read of the martyrdoms suffered by saintly women for God's sake, I used to think they had purchased the fruition of God very cheaply; and I had a keen desire to die as they had done, not out of any love for God of which I was conscious, but in order to attain as quickly as possible to the fruition of the great blessings which, as I read, were laid up in Heaven. I used to discuss with this brother of mine how we could become martyrs. We

---

[17] The *catena d'oro* is represented in iconography, for instance, by Domenico Piola in a painting of ca. 1675, presently in the Church of St Francis, Genoa; cf. Magnani L., "Nele ceneri del volto esprimeva l'incendio, che covava nel core', vista immaginaria tra descrizione verbale e raffigurazioni: l'esperienza genovese", in *Visioni ed Estasi* 45 ff. Like Teresa, Catherine feels she is close to death during these kind of ecstasies: 'Io mi sento tagliare a poco a poco le radici della vita', i.e. 'I feel the roots of life being slowly cut'. The dissemination of Teresa's iconography in Europe was very much connected to the establishment of the reformed Carmelite order. In places such as Genoa – the first region outside Spain where the order was established – images of Teresa where particularly abundant even before her canonization in 1622.

[18] Some scholars believe that Teresa might have suffered from meningitis; cf. Steggink O., *Libro de la vida* (Madrid: 1986) 132, notes 2 and 4.

> agreed to go off to the country of the Moors, begging our bread for the love of God, so that they might behead us there.[19]

According to Francisco de Ribera, her first biographer, Teresa and Rodrigo were found by an uncle and brought home before they could reach the outskirts of Avila.[20] In Teresa's juvenile dreams, the heroic trip to the pagan country was meant not as a contribution to the war against the infidels, nor as a proof of faithfulness to God, an expiation of sins, an imitation of Christ's Passion, and not even as a display of civil courage; she simply wanted to suffer and to die gazing upon the heavenly reward which safely awaits the martyrs. Both her own writings and those of her biographers often refer to martyrdom and sacrifice not in a literal sense, but as alternative ways of pursuing a saintly life.[21] That Christian virtues such as patience, abnegation and devotion were considered as forms of martyrdom was not something new among spiritual writers, but Teresa goes as far as to affirm indirectly the superiority of a long and virtuous monastic life to a brief martyrdom: 'And do you know, sisters, that the life of a good religious, who wishes to be among the closest friends of God, is one long martyrdom? I say 'long', for, by comparison with decapitation, which is over very quickly, it may well be termed so'.[22] The idea of the prevalence of a certain attitude or virtue over actual martyrdom is present in Spanish authors contemporary to Teresa, such as Antonio de Guevara, for whom 'Martyrs were not martyrs because of the labors they suffered, but because of the patience they showed in them'.[23] For Teresa, this alternative type of martyrdom was not characterised by pain, but by a loving self-offering.

---

[19] Trl. Peers, vol. I, 11. Rodrigo de Ahumada would emigrate to America in 1535; when Teresa heard he had died in a battle against the payagua Indians, close to the desert of Chaco, in 1557, she reportedly said that she considered him to be a martyr (María de San José Salazar, *Libro de recreaciones*, VIII, 67).

[20] *La vida de la Madre Teresa de Jesús* (Salamanca, Pedro Lasso: 1590; new edition by Pons J., Barcelona, Gustavo Gili: 1908, I, 4).

[21] For references in Ana de San Bartolomé, Francisco de Ribera and Diego de Yepes, cf. Eire C., *From Madrid to Purgatory: The Art and Craft of Dying in Sixteenth-Century Spain* (Cambridge University Press: 1995) 402 ff.

[22] *Way of Perfection*, chapter 12,2. The idea that actual martyrdom, because of its quickness, is a very 'cheap' way of buying paradise is a *topos* among early Christian writings; cf. for example the Martyrdom of Polycarp, 2: 'Fixing their eyes on the favour of Christ, they (the martyrs) despised the tortures of this world, in one hour buying themselves an exemption from the eternal fire'; see Musurillo H. (ed.), *Acts of the Christian Martyrs* (Oxford: 1972) 3–5.

[23] *Epistolas Familiares* 13; 211, in Eire, *From Madrid to Purgatory* 403.

Gregory XV, who established the *Sacra Congregatio de Propaganda Fide*, also in 1622, made sure that the episode would be quoted in Teresa's bull of canonization, emphasising her innate vocation to martyrdom. Her biographers, on the other hand, stressed Teresa's heroic deeds and sacrifices during the trips she made while establishing convents for the newly reformed order.[24] Teresa herself, in the opening chapter of the *Foundations*, parallels her work with that of Christian missionaries in the New World; both are imbued by a spirit of self-sacrifice and devoted to save souls through the propagation of the Christian faith.[25]

In the visual arts, Teresa has been almost invariably depicted during one of her several ecstasies; the visions she herself so graphically describes in her books are the main elements of the saint's iconography.[26] Her persuasive texts, written in a light and fluid oral style,[27] displayed a notable ability to create visual metaphors for her ecstasies and mystical experiences that often allude to traditional iconography; sometimes, there is an intense similarity between her visions and specific works of art she had seen.[28] One of Teresa's main books, the *Interior Castle*,

---

[24] For references cf. Gutiérrez Rueda L., "Ensayo de iconografia teresiana", *Revista de Espiritualidad* 23, 90 (1964), chapter 8.

[25] In a sense, Teresa's own profession as a nun can be considered a kind of self-imposed sacrifice, since, as she herself explains in the *Vida*, as a young woman she was not at all inclined to religious life.

[26] The only exception of a non-ecstatic moment consistently represented in visual arts is her abortive journey to Africa, engraved by Collaert and Galle, who also depicted other earthly moments of Teresa's life, such as her entry in the convent, and copied by others (for example in a wooden frieze in the Augustinian convent of Ghent). A representation of her coordinating the construction of a reformed convent sometimes appears in the background, for instance in plate XIV of the *Vita B. Virginis Teresiae a Iesu ordinis carmelitarum excalceatorum piae restauratricis* (illustrated with 25 engravings by Adrien Collaert and Corneille Galle, published in Antwerp in 1613). Although more than 500 miracles were listed during the ecclesiastical procedures that led to Teresa's canonization, only some of them are represented, very ocasionally, in iconography (cf. Gutiérrez Rueda, *iconografia teresiana*, chapter 9).

[27] Teresa's writings do not seem to have any preconceived narrative or rhetorical structure; especially her *Vida*, the main source for artists who represented her, is written as a kind of stream of consciousness.

[28] The link between pictorial representations and visionary mystical experiences is quite frequent in Teresa's writings, as for instance in the description of a vision she had of the Virgin and angels descending from heaven towards the Prioress's stall, exactly where a picture of Mary was situated (*Cuentas de conciencia*, 22a, January 1579). As Viktor Stoichita points out in *Visionary Experience in the Golden Age of Spanish Art* (London: 1995) 48 ff., there is an obvious similarity between Teresa's vision and Pedro Berruguete's *Apparition of the Virgin to a Dominican Community*, now in the Prado but in Teresa's times in the monastery of St Thomas in Avila, which she visited many times. In a passage of the *Relations* (58), she writes that 'Cristo se puso en mis brazos como

is built upon a visual metaphor in which the saint compares the soul to a diamond castle divided into seven courts, through which the soul must journey in order to reach, in the last chamber, total communion with God.

Teresa's descriptions of her visions also create a pattern of devotional images that were in conformity with the main artistic tendencies of post-Tridentine Spain: plain, pious, emotional, essential, almost palpable, they generate a feeling of compassion which, in contemporary mysticism, was the first step towards spiritual elevation.[29] Those descriptions were frequently seized on by artists who sought to reproduce them after the saint's own words. An interesting example is Alonso Cano's *Vision of St Teresa* (ca. 1629) presently at a Spanish private collection. Basing himself on Teresa's description of a vision of Christ she had during mass on the feast of St Paul – 'indescribably beautiful and majestic as he is depicted in paintings of him resurrected' – Cano appealed to the traditional iconography of the Resurrected in order to create a victorious Christ: not suffering and wounded, but strong, beautiful and firm.[30]

Teresa recalls moments in which the sight of sculptures or paintings reaffirmed her own faith, for example in the ninth chapter of her *Vida*, in which the vision of an *Ecce Homo* moved her to the greatest devotion. Some lines further, she states:

> As I could not reason with my mind, I would try to make pictures of Christ inwardly; and I used to think I felt better when I dwelt on those parts of His life when He was most often alone. It seemed to me that His being alone and afflicted, like a person in need, made it possible for me to approach Him.[31] [...] I had so little ability for picturing things in my mind that if I did not actually see a thing I could not use my imagination [...]. It was for this reason that I was so fond of pictures. Unhappy are those who through their own fault lose this blessing! It really looks as if they do not love the Lord, for if they loved Him they would delight in looking at pictures of Him, just as they take pleasure in seeing pictures of anyone else whom they love.[32]

---

se pinta habitualmente la angustia de la virgen'. Unlike Teresa, St John of the Cross believed that mystical experiences could never be related to anything visual – paintings included (cf. Stoichita, *Visionary Experience* 60 ff.).

[29] One can easily find parallels between Teresa's prose and the naturalistic elements of Italian and Spanish paintings, especially in the first half of the seventeenth century.

[30] The painting is reproduced by Stoichita, *Visionary Experience*.

[31] Here and elsewhere, Teresa's compassion is much more connected to love than to the traditional *imitatio Christi*.

[32] Trans. Peers, vol. I, 54–56.

In a period during which the legitimacy of religious images was continuously questioned and debated, Teresa fervently reaffirmed their power to purify, reveal, teach and, last but not least, delight. According to a widespread idea divulged mainly by Paleotti in his 1582 treatise *Discorso intorno alle imagini sacre e profane*, artists' main concern when producing religious images should be their capacity to 'move the affections' of the viewer. Also in Spain, writers like Jusepe Martínez (1602–1682) emphasised that Christian piety could be inspired by a well-painted picture.[33] In total opposition to Calvinist conceptions, Catholic art sought to fuel the sensual exchange between paintings or sculptures and the viewer by 'putting in front of his eyes' episodes of the life of Christ and Christian martyrs. Their sacrifice and mercy, their love and the grace bestowed upon mankind, were not to be understood intellectually, but felt sensually in a process of deep emotional and mental identification between themselves and the faithful.[34]

In prints[35] and paintings, as well as in literary sources such as Francisco de Ribera or Diego de Yepes' biography, conventional martyrological typology[36] was employed not only in reference to Teresa's death, but also to the mystic union she achieved during ecstasy, often described by her as a kind of death. In Teresa's case, however, martyrdom had different reasons and meanings than those connected either with ancient or contemporary Christian martyrs. As I. Lavin aptly summarizes it in his classic work on Bernini, Teresa did not feel that she was dying physically *for* her faith, but dying spiritually *of* her faith.[37] It was not martyrdom in the literal sense of the word, but mystical martyrdom, in which she was symbolically wounded by Divine Love. Her martyrdom for love was made visually explicit by Anton Wierix in a curious engraving of the early seventeenth century showing the Christ Child,

---

33 Stoichita, *Visionary Experience* 67 ff.

34 Identification, however, does not necessarily mean sharing, in the sense that it does not imply any soteriological efficacy of pain or other affections. Identification may simply be connected to compassion, understood as an experience of love; see above, note 31.

35 Prints played a very important role in the diffusion of Teresa's images, especially in the Low Countries and the Americas. A very important work in this sense is the aforementioned *Vita B. Virginis Teresiae a Iesu*.

36 Martyrological typology appear also in contemporary representations of ecstasies and stigmatisations of other saints; cf. for instance Francesco Baratta's *Ecstasy of St. Francis* in the Raimondi chapel (San Pietro in Montorio, Rome), in which an angel is represented holding the palm of martyrdom.

37 *Bernini and the Unity of the Visual Arts*, 2 vols. (Oxford: 1980) vol. I, 114.

helped by Mary and Joseph and obviously paralleled to Cupid, preparing to launch an arrow at Teresa, while angels fly down to bring her the palm frond and the flower wreath [Fig. 1].[38] A hymn in the divine office for Teresa's feast day, composed by Urban VIII, speaks directly of a mortal wound produced in her by the dart of Divine Love – she was meant to die a sweeter death, says the hymn, than the one she longed for as a child, in barbarous lands.[39]

Typologically, seventeenth-century gestures and postures signaling ecstasies and visions are very similar to the ones connected to representations of martyrdoms: head turned to heaven, slightly opened mouth, opened arms, and a general attitude of patience. If previously, saints had their eyes mostly opened towards heaven in a heroic affirmation of their own will, seventeenth-century ecstatic saints had them partly shut in their trance.[40] This strengthens both passiveness and internalisation. On the other hand, seventeenth-century martyrs were not so frequently represented when they are being tortured and killed, but as they are being cured or consoled by other saints or angels. Artists were not so often interested in their heroism or the pain they endured, but in the acts of love to which they were bound. Culturally, these two moments – ecstasies and martyrdoms – were intrinsically united, as both of them represent the earthly encounter between men and God.[41]

The transverberation, the piercing of Teresa's heart, may be not the most frequently represented of her ecstasies, but because of Bernini's extraordinary marble group in Rome, it is certainly the better-known

[38] The metaphor of the 'wound of love' caused by an arrow, both in literature and in arts, precedes Christianity – it goes back to Greek and Roman images, and became extremely popular during the seventeenth century, together with a renewed cult of the heart conceived as a center of both physical and spiritual life. The identification of the Child Christ with Cupid, on the other hand, has of course Neoplatonic echoes. Wierix' model was followed by others; cf. Gutiérrez Rueda, *Iconografia teresiana* 114–115.

[39] The hymn is quoted and translated in full in Lavin, *Bernini and the Unity of the Visual Arts*, vol. I, 116–117.

[40] Cf. for instance Francesco Cairo's *Santa Caterina of Siena*, ca. 1645, Brera (Milan).

[41] In Spanish iconography, particularly during the first half of the seventeenth century, representations of saints in ecstasies of pure love abound, for example in Ribalta's St Bernard in the Prado (1625–1627). By means of an extreme naturalism comparable to Teresa's literary style, Ribalta creates a deeply devotional image whose central theme is the highest expression of love.

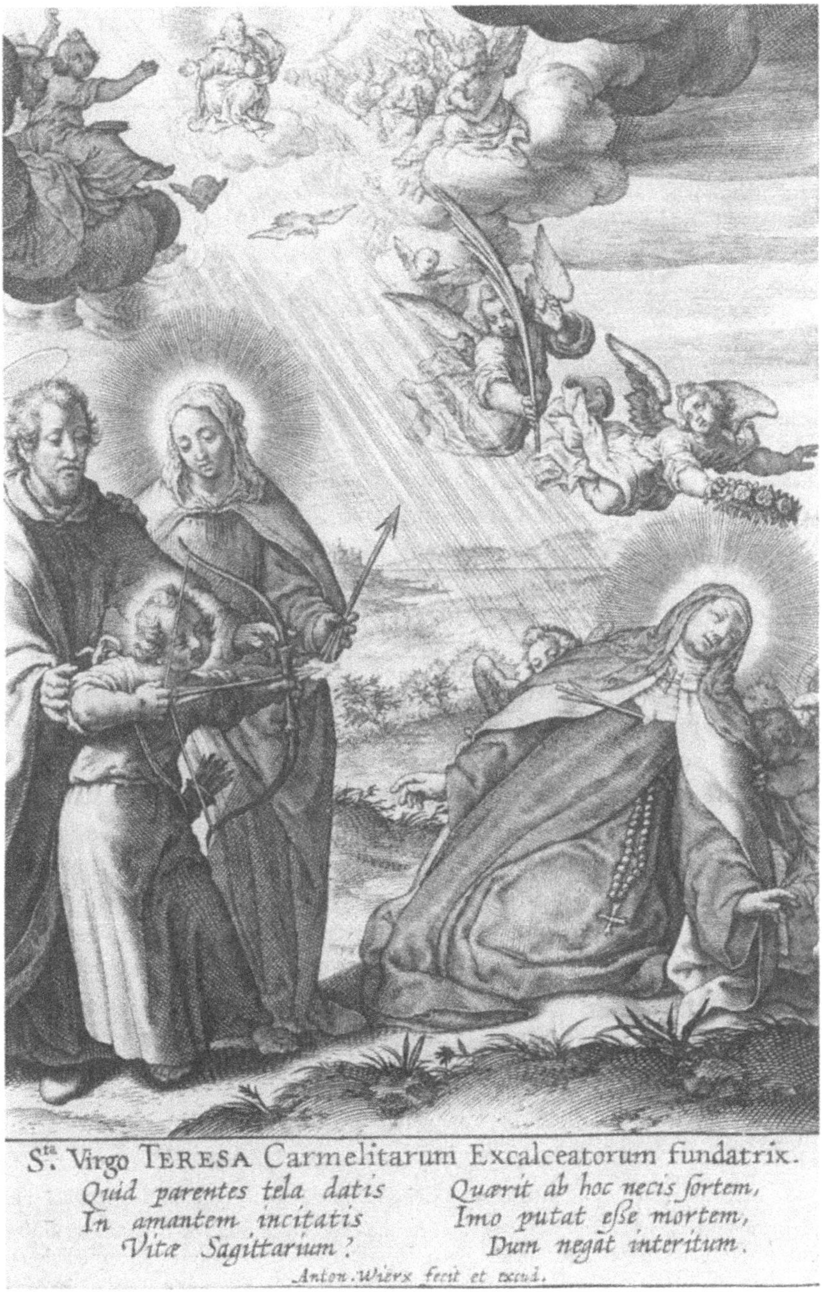
Sta. Virgo TERESA Carmelitarum Excalceatorum fundatrix.
Quid parentes tela datis
In amantem incitatis
Vitæ Sagittarium?
Quærit ab hoc necis sortem,
Imo putat esse mortem,
Dum negat interitum.
Anton. Wierx fecit et excud.

Fig. 1. Anton Wierix, *Mystic Transverberation of St Teresa* (ca. 1622–1624). Engraving, New York, The Metropolitan Museum of Art, The Elisha Whittelsey Collection, The Elisha Whittelsey Fund, 1951 (51.501.6213). Image © The Metropolitan Museum of Art.

moment of her life [Fig. 2 and 3].[42] The source is a passage of the *Vida*, which took place in Avila around 1559:

> It pleased the Lord that I should see this angel in the following way. He was not tall, but short, and very beautiful, his face so aflame that he appeared to be one of the highest types of angel who seem to be all afire [...]. In his hands I saw a long golden spear and at the end of the iron tip I seemed to see a point of fire. With this he seemed to pierce my heart several times so that it penetrated to my entrails. When he drew it out, I thought he was drawing them out with it and he left me completely afire with a great love for God. The pain was so sharp that it made me utter several moans; and so excessive was the sweetness caused me by this intense pain that one can never wish to lose it [...]. It is not bodily pain, but spiritual, though the body has a share in it – indeed, a great share.

That this episode exerted a strong impact on her contemporaries is clear; the bull of her canonization mentions it explicitly, and the arrow became Teresa's principal iconographical attribute shared with Saint Sebastian, Saint Augustine, Saint Giles (Egidius), Saint Canute, Saint Christina of Bolsena and Saint Ursula. In a painting by Antonio Bisquert now in the Cathedral of Teruel (1628), Teresa is placed, next to St Ursula holding an arrow, among the eleven thousand virgins of the latter's retinue who were massacred by the Huns and, therefore, equated to those women who suffered the martyrdom of the arrows.[43]

Teresa is usually represented during the transverberation itself, which is performed by the seraph. Mainly in Italian works, a second angel often helps her not to fall, holding her gently in his arms. Although the transverberation was a physical act, in iconography no apparent wound is ever to be found in her. Although the angel is very seldom depicted as actually piercing Teresa's heart – he is more often holding the dart as if about to do it – the saint is invariably represented as already in a state of ecstasy. Alternatively, she may be depicted holding the arrow, or

[42] The transverberation had been quoted in the bull of canonization, and emblems depicting it were placed all over St Peter's basilica the day Teresa was canonized. Visions are traditionally divided into three categories: corporeal, imaginary and intellectual. In spite of Teresa's total involvement – sensual and spiritual – her transverberation belongs to the latter class. Cf. Petersson, *The Art of Ecstasy* 38 ff.

[43] Teresa's iconography also borrows the attribute of the protecting cloak, common to the Madonna of Mercy and St Ursula; cf. for example an engraving by Adrien Collaert and Corneille Galle in the *Vita B. Virginis Teresiae a Iesu* (XIX).

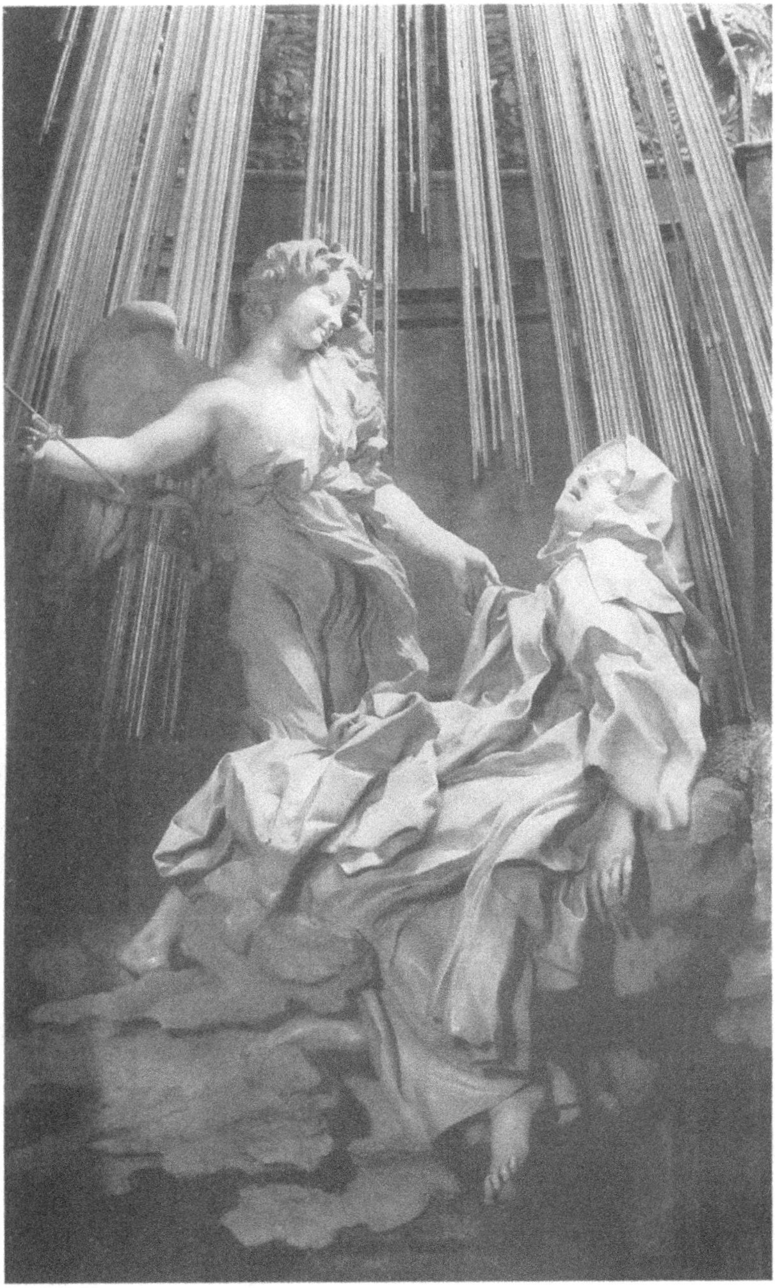

Fig. 2 [Col. pl. XIII]. Lorenzo Bernini, *Transverberation of St Teresa*. 1647–1652. Sculpture from marble. Rome, Santa Maria della Vittoria, Cornaro Chapel.

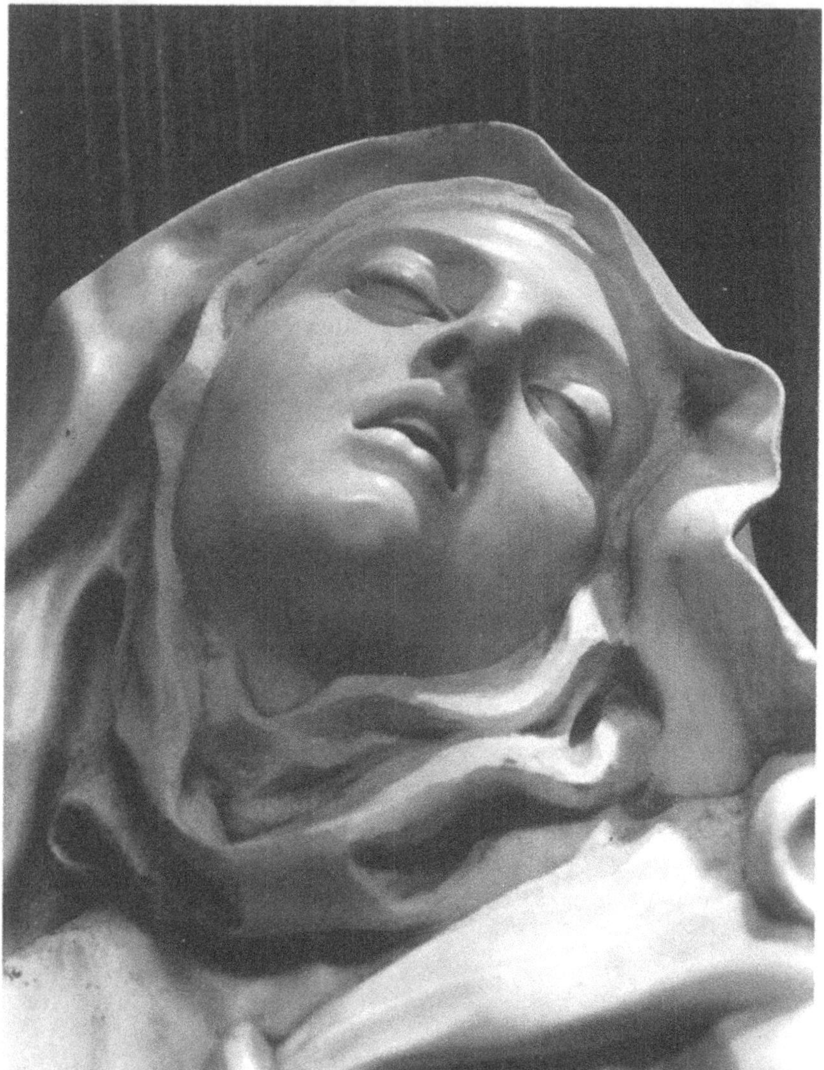

Fig. 3. Lorenzo Bernini, *Transverberation of St Teresa*. Detail. National Italian Photographic Archive.

holding her inflamed heart and offering it to an altar in front of her.[44] She is always alone with the divine; the transverberation is a private moment. Teresa does not specify the place where it occurred, but artists often place her in front of an altar, which stresses the sacrificial aspect of the scene (Palma Giovane [Fig. 4], for example, emphasises the correspondence of Teresa's and Christ's wound, in this case the metaphorical "wound of love"). In this painting, the transverberation implicitly alludes to Teresa's mystical marriage to Christ. The transverberation also serves as a marital metaphor in other representations of the theme, for example in a second Anton Wierix engraving, in which angels shower Teresa with blossoms, while an inscription below quotes a passage form the Song of Songs: 'Surround me with flowers, strengthen me with apples, for I am faint with love' [Fig. 5]. The transverberation is understood as a consummation of Teresa's spiritual marriage to God, celebrated by the angels. It should be noted that the seraph is also often paralleled to Cupid, example in Gregorio de Ferrari's canvas in Genoa, Church of Maria Misericordia [Fig. 6].

The most frequently represented of Teresa's ecstasies is not the transverberation, but the dove she sees during one of her visions:

> One day – it was the vigil of Pentecost (*víspera del Espiritu Santo*) – I went, after Mass, to a very solitary spot, where I used often to say my prayers, and began to read about this festival in the Carthusian's *Life of Christ*. As I read about the signs by which beginners, proficients and perfect may know if the Holy Spirit is with them, it seemed to me, when I had read about these three states, that by the goodness of God, and so far as I could understand, He was certainly with me then [...]. While I was meditating in this way a strong impulse seized me without my realizing why. It seemed as if my soul was about to leave my body, because it could no longer contain itself and was incapable of waiting for so great a blessing [...]. While in this condition, I saw a dove over my head, very different from those we see on earth, for it had not feathers like theirs but its wings were made of little shells which emitted a great brilliance. It was larger than a dove; I seemed to hear the rustling of its wings. It must have been fluttering like this for the space of an *Ave Maria*.[45]

This moment was represented many times by artists, for instance by Rubens, in a painting of ca. 1614, presently conserved at the Boijmans

[44] For example a statue in the Church of Rongy or an engraving from the *Konste der Konste* (in the latter Teresa's heart is light by an intense light emanating from the wafer).

[45] *Vida*, chapter 38; trans. Peers, vol. I, 270–271.

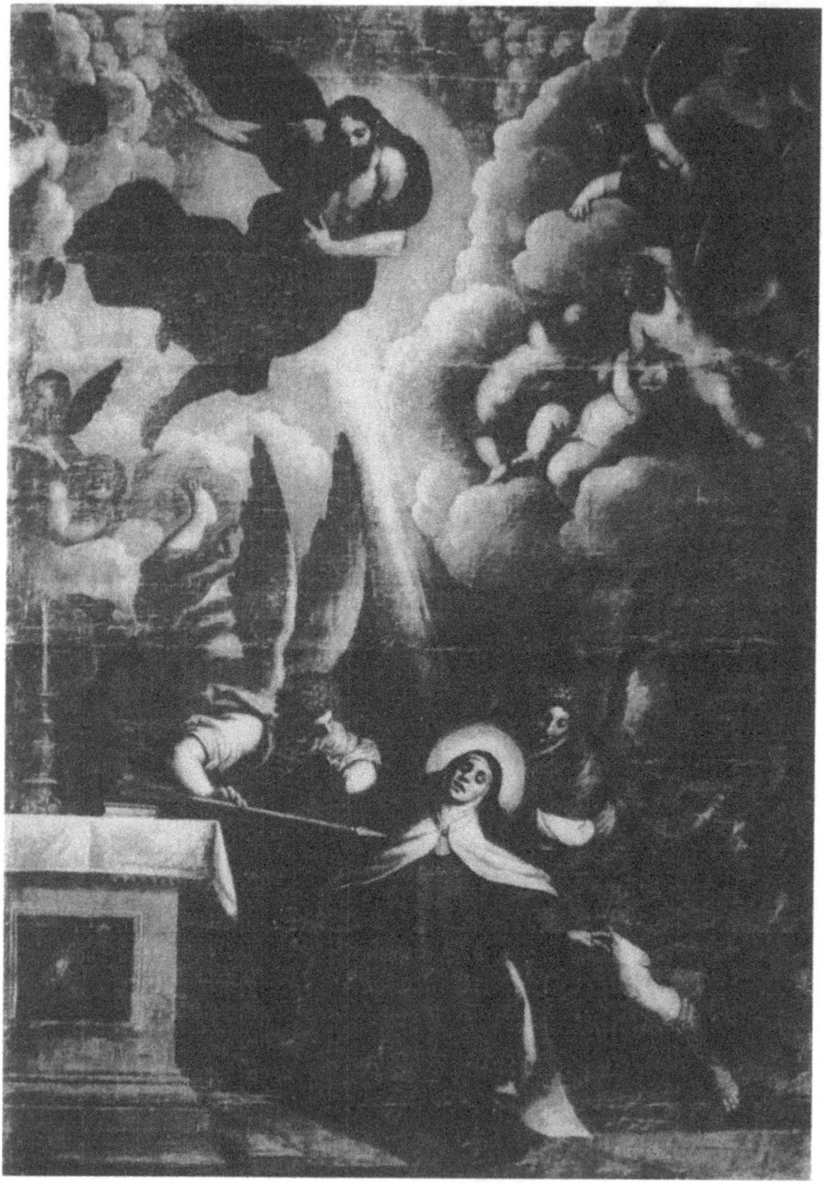

Fig. 4. Palma il Giovane, *Transverberation of St Teresa*, 1615. Oil on canvas. Rome, Basilica di San Pancrazio.

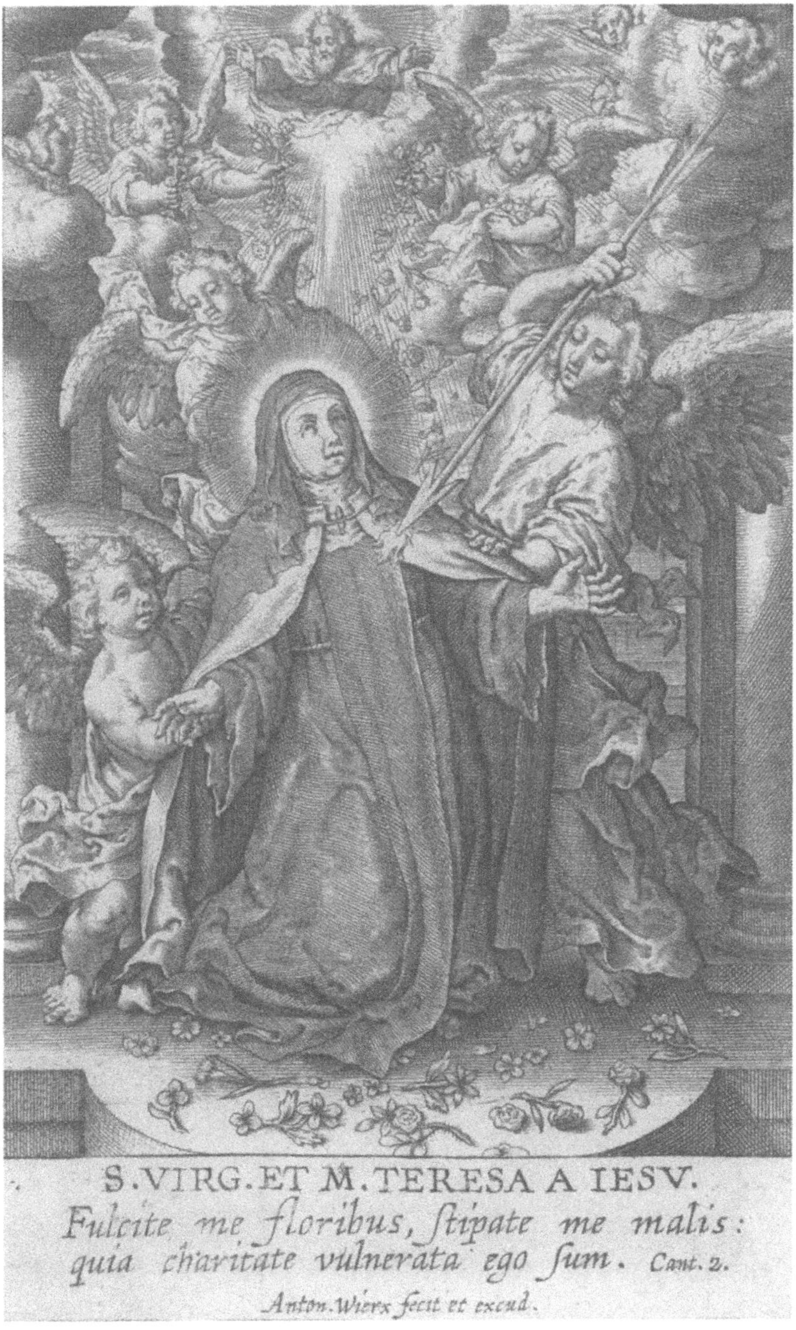
S.VIRG.ET M.TERESA A IESV.
Fulcite me floribus, ſtipate me malis:
quia charitate vulnerata ego ſum. Cant. 2.
Anton.Wierx fecit et excud.

Fig. 5. Anton Wierix, *Transverberation of St Teresa* (ca. 1614–1622). Engraving, New York, The Metropolitan Museum of Art, Harris Brisbane Dick Fund, 1953 [53.601.19(143)]. Image © The Metropolitan Museum of Art.

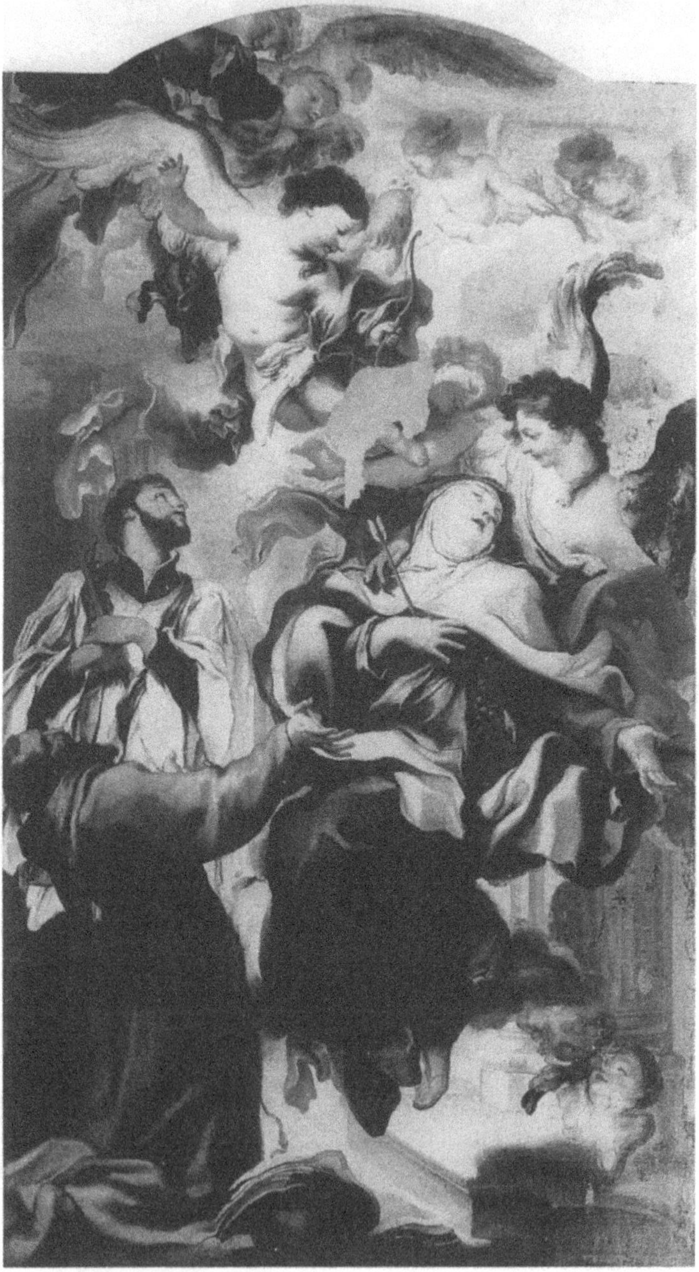

Fig. 6 [Col. pl. XIV]. Gregorio de Ferrari, *Transverberation with St Francis and St Francis Xavier*, ca. 1680–90. Oil on canvas. Genoa, Church of Maria Santissima della Misericordia e di Santa Fede.

van Beuningen Museum in Rotterdam [Fig. 7]. Teresa relates the dove to the Holy Spirit, and in iconography, its presence suggested that she was a doctor of the Church – which was not the case at the time these works of art were produced. Very soon, the dove of Teresa's vision was substituted by the dove-shaped Holy Spirit that inspires doctors of the Church, a transformation made possible by the subtlety of showing Teresa writing, instead of reading, as she says she was doing (for example the Ribera in the Museum of Valencia).[46] Centuries later, in 1970, she would be the first woman to be officially declared a doctor of the Church.[47] The introduction to the commemorative volume of the *Ephemerides Carmeliticae* claims that, in spite of the novelty of Teresa's doctorate, 'da la impresión de ser cosa familiar y vieja'; 'one has the impression that it is something familiar and old'. The reason for this is that from the very beginning, Teresa was represented as a Doctor of the Church by artists.[48]

The dove is Teresa's primary attribute: it appears in the portrait made from life by Fr. Juan de la Miseria[49] [Fig. 8]. In an engraving by Collaert and Galle for the *Vita B. Virginis Teresiae a Iesu*, a dove flies towards Teresa as she is writing at a table on which some of her books

[46] A painting by a disciple of Zurbarán in the Cathedral of Seville employs the same iconographical scheme.

[47] Fray Luis de León already argued that Teresa wrote under the inspiration of the Holy Spirit – and for this reason she was able to teach, despite St Paul's prohibition ('mulieres in ecclesia taceant', I Cor. 14:34). The presence of the dove, in this sense, might serve the purpose of legitimising Teresa's writings by suggesting that she had been invested with the authority of the Church. Teresa was declared a doctor of the church by Paul VI on September 27th, 1970; Catherine of Siena followed shortly after. Teresa had previously been declared a doctor of theology by the University of Salamanca, which surely aggravated the confusion.

[48] In fact, one of the oldest descriptions of Teresa's iconography, Diego de San José's account of the festivities held throughout Spain to commemorate her beatification, speaks of 'una imagen de nuestra Santa Madre Teresa vestida ricamente: en la mano izquierda, libro y palma; en la derecha, una pluma, insignias de Virgen y Doctora' (quoted by Gutiérrez Rueda, "Ensayo de iconografia teresiana" 64). Teresa herself suggests, if not directly, that the Holy Spirit had guided her writings; for references cf. Jean de la Croix, "L'iconographie de Therese de Jesus", *Ephemerides Carmeliticae* 21 (1970) 222. In the city decorations and poems composed in Spain to celebrate Teresa's beatification, the dove she saw was already identified with the Holy Spirit; cf. Diego de S. José (Jean de la Croix, *L'iconographie de Therese de Jesus* 224, note 13).

[49] Jean de la Croix (*L'iconographie de Therese de Jesus* 229) suggests – probably to safeguard Teresa's humility – that the dove of Juan de la Miseria's portrait was inserted *a posteriori*, after Teresa's death, but does not present any grounds for this suggestion. There are several copies made after this portrait, some by Juan de la Miseria himself. For the artist's biography cf. Benezit, 8, 209, and Thieme-Becker, vol. XXIV, 590.

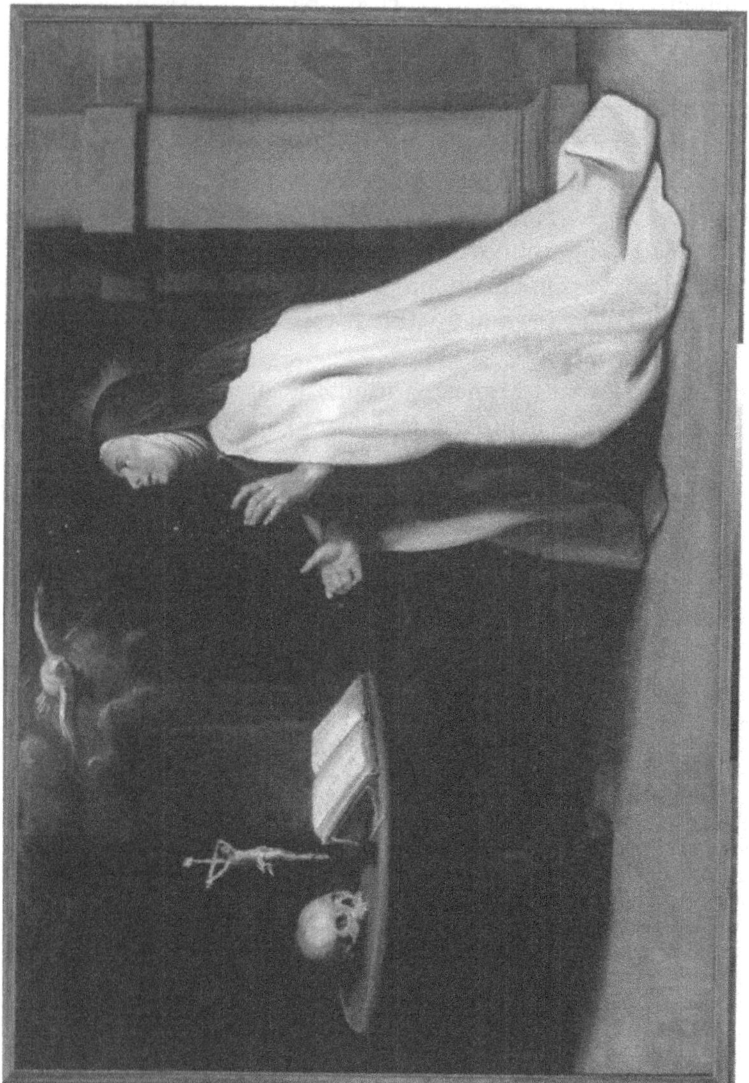

Fig. 7 [Col. pl. XV]. Peter Paul Rubens, *Vision of the Dove* (ca. 1614). Oil on canvas. Rotterdam, Museum Boijmans van Beuningen.

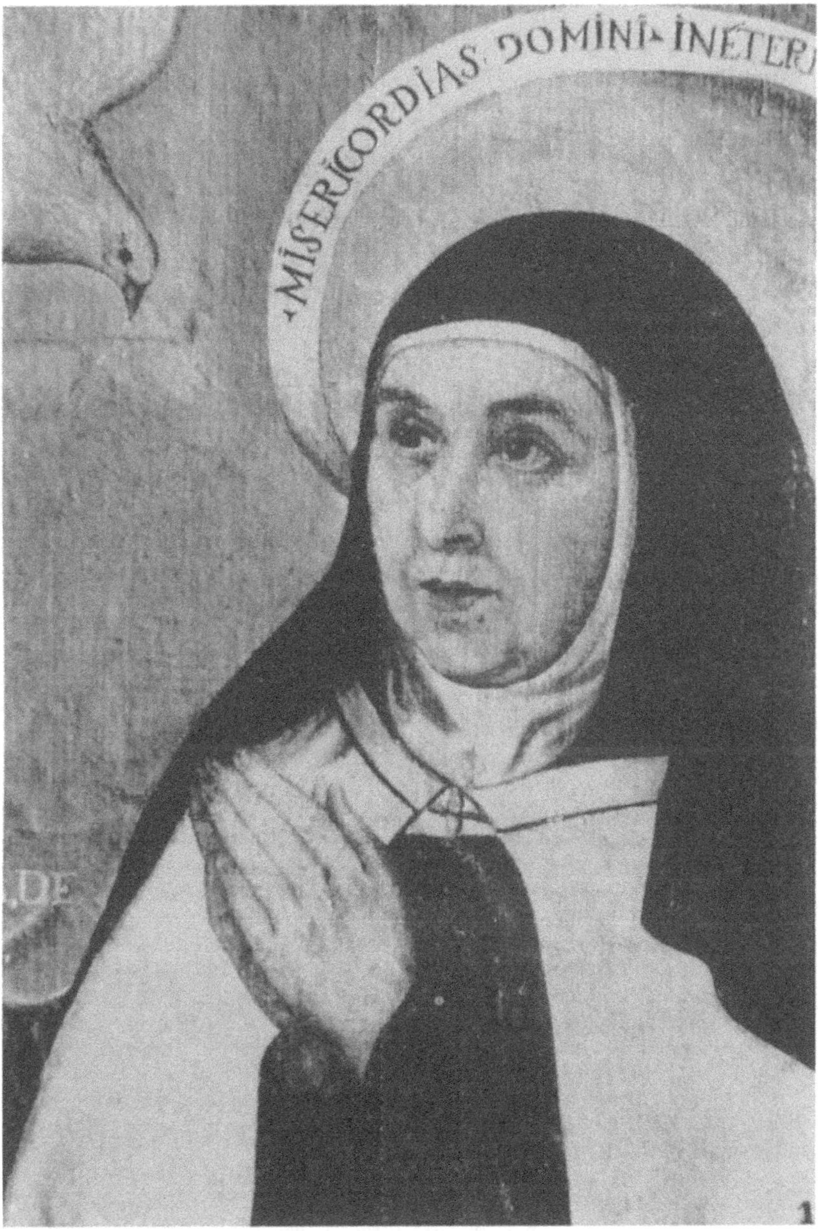

Fig. 8. Juan de la Miseria, *Portrait of St Teresa*. 1576. Seville, Convent of the Discalced Carmelites. Detail.

are displayed. One of the rays emanating towards her contains the words *spiritu intelligentiae replevit illam*, an adaptation of a passage from the bull of canonization: *adimplevit enim eam spiritu intelligentiae* (Fig. 9; *Acta Sanctorum*, p. 418, 1394).[50] The dove traditionally symbolises the Holy Spirit and the idea of unity, either between Father, Son and Holy Ghost, or between God and (holy) men and women.[51] Indeed, as early as in Paul's I Cor. 2,10 mystical knowledge is linked to a revelation operated by the Holy Spirit.[52] It also emphasises implicitly the true value of the Eucharistic sacrament; this is corroborated by Teresa herself, as she recalls that the vision of the dove occurred just after Communion. Finally, the dove also stresses the union between the observer and Teresa, who becomes, like Mary, a link between the earthly and heavenly levels of existence. The dove also sometimes appears in images of the transverberation, for instance in the aforementioned engraving by Wierix and others, where it probably carries the same sense.

Between 1576, when Juan de la Miseria painted his portrait, and the second decade of the seventeenth century, when Teresa was beatified, all of her representations derived from that first original portrait. She was represented in prayer, with the dove and the phylactery with the first words of Psalm 89: '*Misericordias Domini in aeternum cantabo*'. This is how she appears in the prints accompanying the editions of her

---

[50] The dove also appeared as an attribute of Saint Catherine of Siena during the fifteenth century, and during the first half of the seventeenth century. In these cases, it was connected to a vision which Catherine's father had of a white dove flying above her head while she was praying; he had opposed his daughter's religious life until this vision. In southern Spanish art of the *Setecento*, however, there appeared some representations of Catherine, with the four-pointed biretta, holding a feather and an open book; in one of them, she is also inspired by the Holy Spirit in the shape of dove. That this was a borrowing from Teresa's iconography is corroborated by the fact that Catherine is painted as a *pendant* to Saint Tomas Aquinas, a frequent partner of Teresa; cf. Bianchi L. – Giunta D., *Iconografia di Santa Caterina da Siena* (Rome: 1988) 114.

[51] In the *Vida* (though not in Teresa's later writings), *unión mistica* is the same as ecstasy. Teresa is not a scholar; she did not have any formal training in theology, and her use of specific terms is not particularly coherent. In the *Vida*, words such as ecstasy may appear almost interchangeably with 'vision', 'trance' or 'rapture' ('*arrobamiento*'). Cf. Tomás de la Cruz, "L'extase chez Sainte Thérèse D'Avila", *Dictionnaire de Spiritualité, Ascetique, et Mystique* (Paris: 1960), vol. IV, 2100–2160, who demonstrates how the words used by Teresa to describe mystical ecstasy are unsystematic. The same is true for words such as 'mind', 'soul' or 'spirit', to quote a few examples. On the other hand, some words in the teresian lexicon have an idiosyncratic meaning, for example 'sensuality', '*sensualidad*', by which she meant the senses and sensibility (for Teresa's lexicon cf. O. Steggink's edition of the *Vida*, 563–690).

[52] Cf. *Visioni ed Estasi* 51.

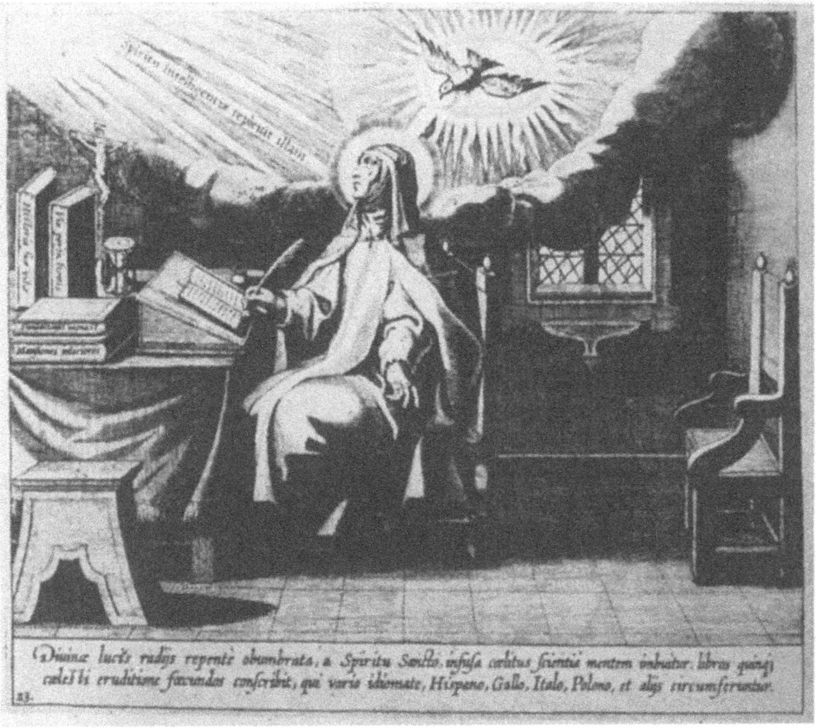

Fig. 9. Adrien Collaert and Corneille Galle, engraving, from *Vita B. Virginis Teresiae a Iesu* (Antwerp: 1613), fig. 23.

writings published in Spain and abroad during the following decades. Both the philactere and the dove, therefore, had become a standard element in Teresa's iconography many years before her beatification. It is in the first Italian edition of the *Vida* (1599) that Teresa is first represented with a book and pen in front of her, as well as a Latin inscription; this strengthens her image as a Doctor of the Church [Fig. 10]. The opened book bears the words '*Vivo sin vivir en mi, y muero por que no muero*', an abbreviation of the first verses of her most famous poem: '*Vivo sin vivir en mí, y tan alta vida espero, que muero porque no muero*'.[53] In

[53] According to Peers's translation (vol. III, 277): 'I live, yet no true life I know/ And, living thus expectanly/ I die because I do not die'. The poem also appears in her open book in an engraving from a Flemish 1620 edition of the *Vida*, and in a Venetian 1619 edition of the *Way of Perfection*. Juan de la Cruz openly alludes to this poem in his 'Vivo sin vivir en mi/y de tal manera espero/ que muero porque no muero' (cf. De la Iglesia R. (ed.), *Obras completas de San Juan de la Cruz* (Madrid: 2005) 77–78).

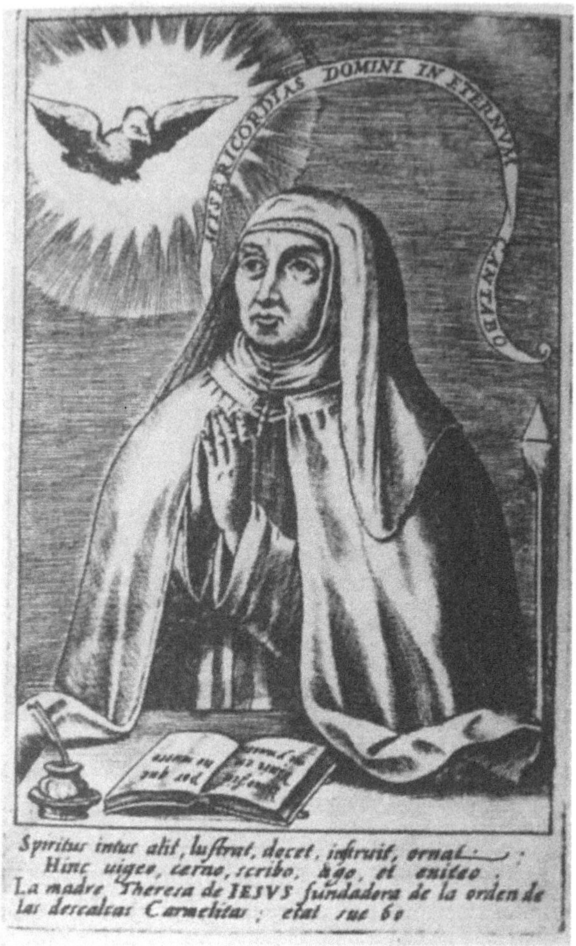
DOMINI IN ETERNVM
CANTABO
Spiritus intus alit, lustrat, docet, instruit, ornat:
Hinc uigeo, cerno, scribo, ago, et eniteo.
La madre Theresa de IESVS fundadora de la orden de
las descalcas Carmelitas; etat sue 60

Fig. 10. Page from the front matter of *Vita della M. Teresa di Giesù*, translated by Francesco Bordini (Rome, Guglielmo Facciotto: 1599).

the *Vida* published in 1606 in Zaragoza by Diego de Yepes, the book laid open in front of Teresa bears the words '*Aut mori, aut pati*' ['to die, or to suffer'], which would become her famous motto [Fig. 11]. These derive from a passage of the last book of her *Vida*: 'I sometimes say to Him with my whole will: 'To die, Lord, or to suffer! I ask nothing else of Thee for myself but this'. It comforts me to hear a clock strike, for when I find that another hour of life has passed away, I seem to

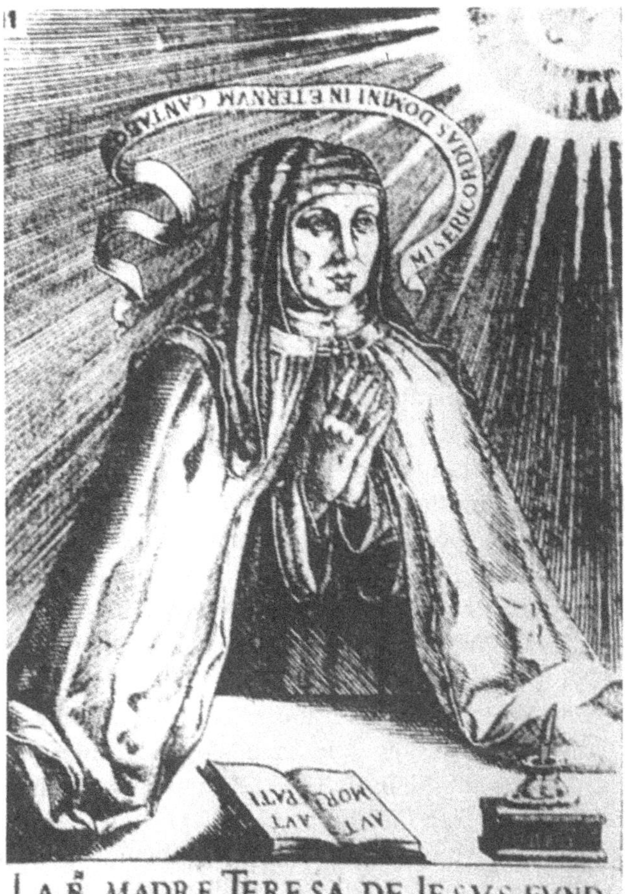
LA B. MADRE TERESA DE IESVS FVNDA
DORA DE LOS DESCALÇOS CARMELITAS

Fig. 11. Page from the front matter of *Vida, virtudes y milagros de la B.V. Teresa de Jesús* (Zaragoza, Diego de Yepes: 1606).

be getting a little nearer to the vision of God'.[54] The words also relate directly to her afore-mentioned poem and to many other passages of her writings in which she expresses her intense longing for death.[55] Teresa manifests repeatedly her melancholy in the face of a life which she likens to a long exile and which she sees as a bitter separation from her beloved. Earthly life is contraposed to true life, a taste of which she

[54] Trans. Peers, vol. I, 297.

[55] For example *Vida*, chapter 29, 8; *Exclamations* 6, and *Interior Castle* chapter 6, 11, 9.

experiences during ecstasies. Those sentiments are in conformity with a general insistence on the transitoriness of life, and with contempt of worldly things; in contemporary Spanish visual arts, few subjects are as frequently depicted as *vanitas* and its derivations.

In spite of the clarity of Teresa's conceptions, the bull of her canonization reverses the order of the words – 'aut pati, aut mori' – and this is how they would appear in iconography from this moment onwards.[56] A seventeenth-century engraving,[57] for example, shows Teresa inspired by the dove and playing a lute in front of an altar. A Christian virtue is written on each pair of strings (humilitas, patientia, mansuetudo, etcetera), and the words '*aut pati aut mori*' emanate from the instrument. This motto, associated with Teresa until the present days, was also connected to Teresa's Italian counterpart, Maria Maddalena Pazzi, who would reportedly repeat the words 'Non mori, sed pati', i.e. not to die, but to suffer. Both sayings are often quoted together in literary sources. In one of Antonio Vieira's beautiful sermons, for example, Maddalena's words are interpreted as going one step further than Teresa's motto: 'Santa Teresa herself used to say: *Aut pati, aut mori*: to suffer, or to die, because she would not dare to live without suffering. And Santa Maddalena Pazzi, perhaps with more energy: *Pati, non mori*: to suffer, yes, and not to die, because in death the exercise of suffering ends, while in life it lasts and perseveres'.[58] In Maddalena's writings, in fact, pain has a different meaning than in Teresa's. Maddalena identifies deeply with Catherine of Siena (her born name is Catherine), and from the very beginning her visions and ecstasies were mainly connected with Christ's sufferings.[59] In iconography, Maddalena is almost invariably

---

[56] *Acta Sanctorum*, p. 418, 1394: 'Invictam autem hujus Sanctae Virginis patientiam illa vox attestatur qua saepius ad Dominum exclamabat: 'Domine, aut pati aut mori'".

[57] Reproduced by de la Croix, *L'iconographie de Therese de Jesus*, nr. 66.

[58] 'A mesma Santa Teresa dizia: *Aut pati, aut mori*: ou padecer, ou morrer, porque se não atrevia a viver sem padecer. E Santa Madalena de Pazzi, não sei se com maior energia: *Pati, non mori*: padecer sim, morrer não, porque na morte acaba-se o exercício de padecer, e na vida dura e persevera' (*Sermão de Todos os Santos*, VIII).

[59] Shortly after her profession as a Carmelite nun (1584), Christ offered her the crown of thorns – one of her most frequent attributes – and the pain it causes her would be felt throughout her life. She received the (invisible) stigmata, and had two long ecstatic experiences during which she participated in the sufferings of Christ's Passion. She led an ascetic life, fasting for extremely long periods. In 1595, she reportedly begged the Lord for 'pure suffering' – a wish which would be granted in 1604, when she started to suffer from the long and painful disease that would kill her three years later. The motto *non mori, sed pati*, seem to derive from the biography written by her confessor, Vincentio Puccini, and published in Florence in 1609: 'She was further so greedy

connected to mortification instruments or to the imitation of Christ through pain.[60] The reversing of the motto 'aut mori aut pati' does makes sense if it is applied to her, rather than to Teresa, since she saw "pure suffering" as the main goal of her life, and she wished to delay death in order to suffer more.[61]

Contrary to Maddalena's, Teresa's iconography does not include elements connected to mortification or to self-inflicted suffering. In fact, she seems always to have been reluctant to adopt practices of mortification, or to attribute to these any effective role in saving her soul or that of others. She does not mention mortifications often,[62] and when she does, it is usually in connection with the Jesuits, for example in *Vida*, 23,16, when she explains how her Jesuit confessor told her: 'I was not working upon a good foundation, nor had I begun to understand the nature of mortification (which was true: I did not even know the meaning of the word)'. According to her confessor, the origin of her visions could very well be diabolical:

---

of suffering that she would often say that she wished not do die so soon, because in heaven there is no suffering' (quoted from the 1619 English translation republished by Scolar Press in 1970, chapter 47, 178–179. The first page bears the inscription *Si compatimur, et conregnabimus*, with the English translation *If we suffer with Christ, we shall raigne with him* – a passage from Paul's epistle to the Romans (8,17). The link between suffering and glory appears many times in the New Testament, for instance in Paul's own epistle to Timothy, (II, 2,11–13: 'If we have died with him, we shall live with him. If we endure, then we shall reign with him'; cf. also Lk. 24, 26, or I Pet. I:II; 4,13; 5,1; 10), and is repeated many times by saints and mystics (for example Bernardo di Chiaravalle in the 11th century, and St Ignatius in the *Spiritual Exercises*; for references cf. *Visioni ed Estasi* 52).

[60] Important for the definition of Maddalena's iconography is a graphic cycle from the first decades of the seventeenth century by an anonymous Florentine artist, which was published in its entirety by Pacini P., "Contributi per l'iconografia di S. Maria Maddalena Pazzi", *Mitteilungen des Kunsthistorischen Institutes in Florenz* 28,3 (1984) 279–350. From the 87 sanguines representing her life, at least 10 are directly connected to self-mortification or painful ecstasies in which she relived the sufferings of Christ (nos. 2; 13; 16; 21; 29–31; 43; 47 and 76). In these images and the texts which accompany them, Maddalena's pain can be seen as an *imitatio Christi*, as a means of fighting temptations, or as self-inflicted punishment.

[61] The process of Maddalena's beatification begun in 1611, under the same pope (Paul V) that beatified Teresa; her beatification was proclaimed by Urban VIII in 1626. In iconography, there seems to have been a fusion between Teresa's arrow and the spear as symbol of Maddalena's sharing in Christ's passion – for example in Valdés Leal's painting at the Carmelite Church of Córdoba. The two saints are sometimes represented together, as in a Cagnacci canvas of *ca.* 1640 presently in Rimini.

[62] Padre Yepes, however, speaks of disciplines and mortifications, and some seventeenth-century prints represent her with mortification instruments; cf. Gutiérrez Rueda, *iconografia teresiana* 108–109.

> when, in order to obtain light from him, I told him of the graces which God was bestowing upon me, he warned me that these two things were not consistent, that such favors were given to persons who were very far advanced and mortified, and that he could not help having misgivings lest in some of these matters an evil spirit might be at work in me [...]. This caused me such distress and fear that I did not know what to do. But while I was in an oratory, in great affliction, and not knowing what was to become of me, I read in a book, which it seemed as if the Lord had put into my hands, those words of Saint Paul, that God is very faithful and never allows people who love Him to be deluded by devil (23,11; 23,15).

Finally, she recalls how her confessor substituted her own method of prayer by a program of 'certain mortifications which I did not find very agreeable' ('mortificaciones no muy sabrosas para mi'). The more she tried to resist God's consolations and favors, though, 'the more completely the Lord enveloped me in that sweetness and glory until I felt so completely surrounded by it that I could not flee from it in any direction. [...] Resistance was no longer in my power' (24,2–3).

Teresa was one of those rare personalities that combine intellectual fertility with an unrestrained practical working energy. In spite of her vast spiritual experience, she could be rightly considered as a woman of action. Whereas a saint like Maddalena Pazzi spent her entire adult life inside a convent, Teresa traveled the whole of Spain while supervising the foundation of Discalced Carmelite convents. As a true reformer, she had a profoundly political nature. Always availing herself of an impeccable rhetoric of humility, she managed to achieve her goals without ever clashing directly with established religious authorities. In her spiritual path, in spite of many attacks equating her visions and ecstasies to those of *alumbrados* and similar heretics, she does not seem to have had great difficulties in avoiding problems with the Inquisition.[63]

[63] When she was called by the Inquisition in Seville to testify about her visionary experiences (*Spiritual Testimonies* 57, dated 1576), she stressed the fact that she had been in touch with 'spiritual people from the Society of Jesus'. It is worth noting that there had recently been a clash between Augustinians and Dominicans, on the one hand, and Jesuits on the other, at the university of Salamanca, where the Jesuits had been trying to impose themselves. Luis de Leon, an Augustinian, had suppressed all references to the Jesuits in his 1588 edition of the *Vida*. Recent scholarship has been increasingly critical of the view that Teresa represents the quintessence of the Counter Reformation sensibility as diametrically opposed to Protestantism. Scholars have pointed to the controversial aspects of her writings, and have questioned the notion of a strict division between Protestants and Catholics insofar as religious ideas were concerned (Cf. Pérez-Romero A., *Subversion and Liberation in the Writings of St. Teresa of*

Her writings are in tune with some of the major artistic trends of the first half of the seventeenth century, with their emphasis on simplicity and essentiality, and on the inspiration, through empathy, of both reader and viewer. In iconography, Teresa was never represented in pain, but in a state of bliss that corresponds quite well to her own accounts of her ecstatic experiences. As well as her writings, her visual representations emphasise her own understanding of perfection as total communion with Christ. Stress is put not on the painful aspect of her visions and ecstasies – the self-mortification, abnegation, patience and self-sacrifice connected to her monastic life – but on the delightful and sensual nature of her mystical experiences and on her conceptions of prayer and meditation as dialogues of friendship and love. In this sense, her iconography differs from that of traditional counterparts such as Catherine of Siena and Maddalena Pazzi, most often represented with stigmas and mortification instruments (as for instance in a Valdes Leal canvas representing Maddalena in the Carmelite convent of Cordoba [Fig. 12], which could not be further away from Teresa's glorious ecstasies). Teresa's main iconographic attribute, the arrow, is connected to an experience of love rather than to the infliction of pain.

Teresa's pain is sensual, blissful, and seductive, and one could even question whether it should be classified as pain. In Teresa's days, however, pain was not always considered as something negative – especially in religious contexts. Moreover, pain could be connected to feelings that would nowadays be considered its opposite. Teresa generally differentiates mundane from heavenly pain. The former – which she experiences mainly in her youthful diseases – is negative and debilitating. The latter – sensed during ecstasies and higher levels of prayer – is positive, not because of any effectiveness in theological terms, but because it is intimately connected to Divine Love. She sees no contradiction between bodily pain and spiritual joy; what amazes her, as she herself states at the very beginning of chapter 30 of the *Vida*, is that such an intense physical and spiritual pain can be intrinsically bound to a 'grandisimo gusto', an intense delight. At this point of her life, says Teresa, 'no one understood me'. The pain she felt was not caused by mortification, nor by remorse. It did not serve as a means of purging her own sins, or

---

Avila (Cleveland: 1996), for an updated bibliography on this matter). The Spanish religious landscape of her time seemed to be distinguished more by clashes among conflicting Catholic orders and forms of spirituality than by a clear-cut struggle between Protestants and Catholics.

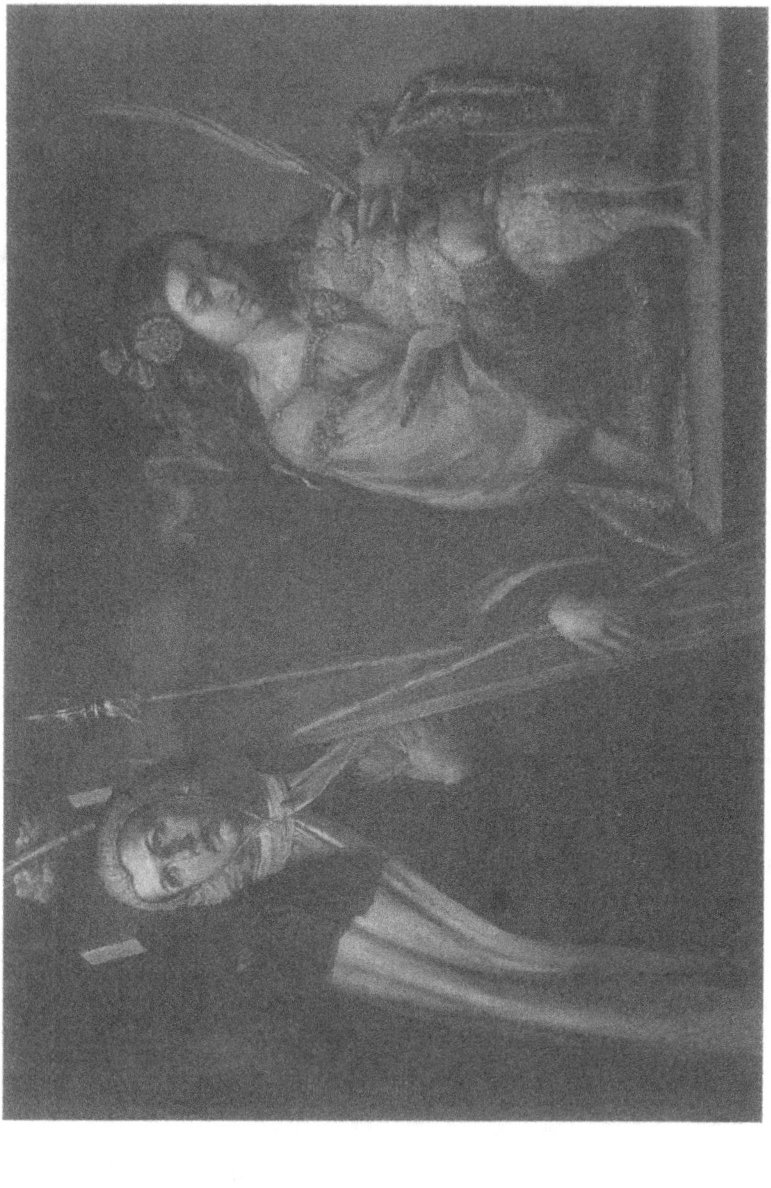

Fig. 12 [Col. pl. XVI]. Valdes Leal, *Maria Maddalena Pazzi*. Oil on canvas. Cordoba, Carmelite Church. Detail.

those of others, nor was it, in itself, the cause of her spiritual progress. Rather, it formed an organic unity with the bliss caused by her visions of Heaven. This subtle yet decisive rethinking of the cause/effect relation between pain and pleasure – pleasure is not caused *by* pain, but is at one with it – was particular to Teresa's discourse of mystical experience. Not surprisingly, artists always perceived the ambiguous qualities of these feelings, producing works which, far from inspiring fear, remorse or horror, represent glorious raptures in which Teresa seems very close to Heaven.

Selective Bibliography

Bianchi L. – Giunta D., *Iconografia di Santa Caterina da Siena* (Rome: 1988).
De la Iglesia R. (ed.), *Obras completas de San Juan de la Cruz* (Madrid: 2005).
Efren de la Madre de Dios – Steggink O. (eds.), *Obras completas de Santa Teresa de Jesus* (Madrid: 2006).
Eire C., *From Madrid to Purgatory: The Art and Craft of Dying in Sixteenth-Century Spain* (Cambridge: 1995).
Gutiérrez Rueda L., "Ensayo de iconografia teresiana", *Revista de Espiritualidad* 23, 90 (1964) 5–168.
Jean de la Croix, "L'iconographie de Therese de Jesus", *Ephemerides Carmeliticae* 21 (1970) 219–260.
Lavin I., *Bernini and the Unity of the Visual Arts*, 2 vols. (Oxford: 1980).
Morello G. (ed.), *Visioni ed Estasi. Capolavori dell'arte europea tra Seicento e Settecento* (Milan: 2004).
Musurillo H. (ed.), *Acts of the Christian Martyrs* (Oxford: 1972).
Pacini P., "Contributi per l'iconografia di S. Maria Maddalena Pazzi", *Mitteilungen des Kunsthistorischen Institutes in Florenz* 28,3 (1984) 279–350.
Peers E.A. (trsl.), *The Complete Works of Saint Teresa of Jesus*, 3 vols. (London – New York: 1950).
Pérez-romero A., *Subversion and Liberation in the Writings of St. Teresa of Avila.* (Cleveland: 1996).
Petersson R., *The Art of Ecstasy. Saint Teresa, Bernini and Crashaw* (London: 1970).
Steggink O. (ed.), *Libro de la vida* (Madrid: 1986).
Stoichita V., *Visionary Experience in the Golden Age of Spanish Art* (London: 1995).
Walker Bynum C., *Holy Feast and Holy Fast. The Religious Significance of Food to Medieval Women* (Berkeley: 1987).

GODLY BEDS OF PAIN: PAIN IN ENGLISH PROTESTANT MANUALS (*CA.* 1550–1650)

Jenny Mayhew

According to the Protestant divine Samuel Ward of Ipswich (1577–1640), writing in 1622, religious belief can transform agony into ecstasy.[1] 'Faith', Ward states, 'turneth feares into hopes, sighings and groanings, into wishings and longings, shaking and trembling into leaping and clapping of hands'.[2] With this claim as my starting point, I wish to examine in some detail how the groaning or trembling of an afflicted body could be turned into sensations of elation. I approach the 'turning' or transformation as a rhetorical process; a persuasive and self-persuasive activity. Suffering believers used godly books and godly brethren to manipulate their own understanding of pain. In doing so, the faithful appear to have succeeded in changing their actual experience of pain. This second proposition, impossible to prove, rests on the supposition that cognition and sensation are so tightly interrelated that the manipulation of thoughts can affect what a person physically feels. Arguments have been made by social scientists that pain 'occurs' not only in the nerve endings, but in the cognitive, linguistic and cultural activities that give pain meaning.[3] According to Mark Turner, only 'a very few and very simples responses are controlled way down in the spinal cord'; whereas 'anything that has bodily meaning for us happens not in the torso or the appendages or on our skin, but in the mappings of the body that exist in the brain'.[4] From this perspective, pain may be changed and re-directed by rhetorical devices that make bodily sensations significant.

---

[1] My thanks to Jonathan Charteris-Black and Mary Ann Lund for their helpful comments on this paper.

[2] Samuel Ward, *The Life of Faith in Death* (London, John Marriot and John Grismand: 1622) 4.

[3] Good M. – Brodwin P. – Good B. – Kleinman A. (eds.), *Pain as Human Experience: An Anthropological Perspective* (Berkeley: 1992), chapter 1. Rey R., *The History of Pain*, trans. L. Wallace, J. and S. Cadden (Cambridge, Mass.: 1995) 5.

[4] Turner M., *Reading Minds: The Study of English in an Age of Cognitive Science* (Princeton: 1993) 34.

Many Protestant handbooks of the late sixteenth and early seventeenth centuries, which I am calling godly manuals, were designed to alleviate suffering – or more accurately, to guide readers to a faithful and productive experience of suffering. Their authors, usually clergymen with Calvinist leanings, sometimes referred to these small books as 'salves'. The function of a 'salve' seems clear from its title; but godly manuals define suffering – and its cure – in ways that differ significantly from our modern categorisation of conditions as either physical or mental. In the example given above, Samuel Ward's depiction of suffering as 'sighings and groanings', or 'shaking and trembling', emphasises the visible and audible properties of distress. In a popular guide to dying by William Perkins (1558–1602), to be discussed at greater length below, there is a similarly striking evocation of the noise of suffering, the 'sobs, sighs and groans' of a repentant sick man.[5] Typically for godly authors, among whom he was in the Elizabethan era an acknowledged leader, Perkins conflates physical and spiritual kinds of suffering in describing their manifest expression. Whereas we would habitually identify and rank symptoms according to their cause and degree of severity, distinguishing physical pain from psychological anxiety, godly authors show more interest in what symptoms communicate.

Certain that all forms of affliction derive from original sin, divines see pain in general as a sign of the spiritual sickness that is mankind's condition. Particular pains may derive from personal faults, or may be morally 'benign' to the extent that they result from other physical conditions. In either case, what pain communicates to – and through – the body of a sick creature is an urgent need for the individual to mend the rift with his or her divine Maker. As it is not in the Calvinist believer's power to make amends for his sins, godly prescriptions for remedial action reveal a tension between the impulse to improve one's own or one's neighbour's condition, and the need to submit to God's will; a point to which I shall return.

A contemporary of Ward and Perkins, Nicholas Byfield (1578/9–1622), explains in *The Promises* of 1619 that 'all afflictions are eyther outward, or inward'. Outward afflictions include 'wants, losses, wrongs, troubles, exile, imprisonment, sickness, feares, poverty, or any other

[5] A longer discussion of this point is made in Mayhew J., *English Godly Art of Dying Manuals, c. 1590–1625* (Ph.D. thesis, Oxford Brookes University: 2007; available from British Library Dissertations) 89.

thing, wherewith the life of man is molested in any condition'; and inward afflictions are temptations of Satan or troubles of conscience.[6] What we call bodily pain could apparently manifest itself in either of Byfield's categories as a result of external tribulation or inner troubles of conscience. In either case, bodily pain functions as a messenger to the sufferer and his community, signalling the severity of his spiritual endangerment. A sick or poor man is not to blame for his 'outward' affliction, though he must strengthen his faith to endure it; but a conscience-stricken individual is in critical danger until he repents.

Again, it is possible to detect a conflict in Byfield's outlook between his assumption of human corruption and dependency on divine will, and his apparent offer of help to the afflicted. Does *The Promises* promise to guide people to their own health and salvation? On the contrary, Byfield would surely argue; it is God who has promised to cure his elected. The manual's author is merely helping readers to recognise and take comfort from that divine promise. An anthology of consoling biblical phrases, Byfield's *Promises* shares with many conduct manuals, pious regimens and godly books of household management published in the Tudor-Stuart period the idea that individuals have a duty to preserve the bodies that have been lent to them; much as a gardener is obliged to tend plants that are temporarily in his care.[7] God's children are responsible for maintaining what belongs to their heavenly father, and for applying the Scriptural resources granted to them to the trials and duties of earthly life. Using the language of husbandry, William Perkins explains that spiritual and medicinal remedies must both be followed, in the 'right manner', with repentance as the necessary first step, since until 'the *root* of sicknesse be cured, phyisick for the body is nothing' (my emphasis).[8]

Godly manuals teach readers to fulfil God's prescribed actions, rather than to be self-willed actors, in the management of their bodily lives. However tenuous that distinction might seem under scrutiny, it justified an active, self-disciplined approach to sickness and dying. The manuals urge readers to steer themselves, somewhat paradoxically, to a state of utter submissiveness to divine will. Believers are taught to enact their predetermined roles in the divine drama – and especially

---

[6] Nicholas Byfield, *The Promises* (London, Ralph Rounthwaite: 1619) 26; 48.

[7] Several medical regimens of the period are discussed in Healy M., *Fictions of Disease in Early Modern England: Bodies, Plagues and Politics* (Basingstoke, Palgrave: 2001).

[8] William Perkins, *A Salve for a Sicke Man* (Cambridge, John Legate: 1595) 61.

in the culminating trials of sickness and pain – with zealous obedience. They are led to expect, and so to effect, a transition from fear to exhilaration in the final moments of life. The small size of these manuals (typically a few inches) presumably added to the attractiveness of their reassuringly tangible, authoritative, didactic guidance. Eminently portable, godly handbooks could be kept under a pillow, taken on a journey, or drawn from a pocket and cited at an appropriate moment in conversation with pained or anxious friends. Perkins' *A Salve for a Sicke Man* of 1595, published in small octavo format, is directed on the title page to three specific types of reader: mariners going to sea, soldiers going to battle, and women approaching childbirth.[9] For such people, faced with the prospect of certain pain and possibly imminent death, a small pocketbook of pastoral advice would provide more than vague comfort: it offers a kind of script, albeit sketchy and terse. The unequivocal nature of Perkins' righteous convictions makes his formula for 'the right manner of dying well' a useful clutch for those in desperate or disordered states of mind.[10]

The ease with which these portable texts could be given, borrowed and discussed must also have contributed to the godly community's involvement in the pain of individual brethren. This social aspect of pain is hinted at in my title, *Godly Beds of Pain*. The metonym of a 'sick bed' evokes a particular set of societal relations between the patient and his or her visitors, most obviously imagined as nursing attendants and family members. Emphasising the patient's condition, this image tends to obscure the many other kinds of social relationship which would typically be conducted in, on and by the same bed in normal conditions – and perhaps continued there in parallel with the sickness. With the phrase 'godly beds of pain', I hope to suggest that sites of sickness in Protestant households were equally and at the same time sites of pious ministration, instruction and performance. Godliness is not a separate and secondary focus of attention to suffering believers, to judge by contemporary descriptions of illness in religious families.[11]

[9] The book 'may serve for spirituall instruction to 1. Mariners when they goe to sea. 2. Souldiers when they goe to battell. 3. Women when they travell of child' (Perkins, *Salve*, title page).

[10] The subtitle of Perkins' *Salve*, which runs across the top of every page, is 'The right way of dying well'.

[11] A wide range of primary material is discussed in Houlbrooke R., *Death, Religion, and the Family in England, 1480–1750* (Oxford: 1998).

Godly beliefs and habits inform the patient's expression of pain, just as his or her pain provokes and informs the didactic encouragement given by godly visitors. The term godly, used not infrequently within or on the title pages of Protestant books, denotes those Protestants, and specifically Calvinists, who shared a distinct sense of religious identity; an expectation of predestined election; habits of pious self-discipline and didacticism; and a moralised understanding of physical life. The godly regarded their bodily symptoms as signs of moral import. Pain could not be morally neutral to the godly; nor could it be solitary and private. As an aspect, symptom and signifier of the broader religious category of 'affliction', pain in this community demanded recognition. Responses could take the form of bedside fellowship and pious supervision, facilitated by godly manuals. Pain was rhetorical; it required and involved an audience. Godly guides to affliction helped the sick and their companions to read, transpose and respond to the signs manifested in their bodies.

In *A Salve for a Sicke Man*, William Perkins gives directions to those who suffer, and to those who witness suffering, thereby involving the sick man's friends in his condition as interpreters, lay ministers and fellow 'patients' in the fullest sense of that term. Determined to ensure that these participants interpret pain correctly, Perkins warns that the 'writhing of the lippes, the turning of the neck, the buckling of the joints and the whole body' must not be assumed to be signs of spiritual torment prior to damnation. Such symptoms 'proceed of cramps and convulsions, which follow after much evacuation'.[12] Visitors at the bedside participate in the experience of suffering, helping to determine its meaning and perhaps to modify its intensity: this they must do conscientiously, using approved godly semiotics. In his anxiety to prevent casual or presumptuous misdiagnoses, Perkins reveals how far a system of religious interpretation can shape the significance and management of pain.

Pain relief is an important objective of Protestant manuals, and various persuasive 'medicines' are supplied for use by sufferers, though never simply for the sake of their bodily comfort alone. Seen as a significant, expressive force communicating spiritual needs, pain has several uses to the godly. It has the potential to clarify, discipline, refine and elevate

[12] Perkins, *Salve* 16.

the sinful self, bringing a suffering individual closer to the community and to the divine. Indeed, some degree of pain is positively welcome to the godly, as a spur to the activities of penitent prayer and faithful testifying by which a suffering body will incidentally find relief. Manuals that offer 'comfort' to the afflicted do not seek to eradicate pain altogether, but aim rather to manage suffering, by controlling its significance and exploiting its utility. The management of pain, through linguistic performance, by godly believers, is what interests me here.

How exactly could Perkins' *Salve*, or any similar godly manual, help those going into labour or lying injured or fevered, by providing nothing more than a set of godly words? Could these words induce change in a reader's physical sensations, alleviating her pain to some degree and turning her 'shaking and trembling' into 'leaping and clapping of hands'?

Four strategies of pain management, as I see it, recur frequently (by other names) in godly manuals. Firstly, demonstrative rhetoric is used by tortured martyrs and their ordinary imitators to defy the meaning of inflicted harm and so to alter its felt significance. Secondly, the device of internal dialogue is used to divide a pained body from its superior, soulful occupant. A third strategy is the contemplative use of metaphors to 'turn' the experience of pain, figuratively, into another kind of experience. Finally, inuring the mind to the prospect of pain (or death, or other affliction) in advance of its onset is expected to strengthen the believer's physical and spiritual capacity to endure – or even enjoy – its actual occurrence.

Considering these tactics in a small sample of godly manuals, I am guided by the question of how language might affect what a suffering body feels.

Demonstrative Rhetoric, or, Fighting Talk

The language of insult or affirmation, of invective or encomium, provides afflicted individuals with an opportunity to 'turn' their suffered pain into speaking performance. Persecuted martyrs in Foxe's *Acts and Monuments* defy their persecutors in the midst of torment, responding with courage and celebratory assertions of faith, and thereby gaining vocal control of a situation in which they are otherwise unwilling victims. John Knott has called this tendency 'bold speaking', giving us a more suggestive term than the classical *apatheia*.[13] The martyrs' apparent enthusiasm for demonstrative speaking during moments of intense physical pain suggests that this action is effectively therapeutic for those individuals in agony; it is not only effective in encouraging their fellow witnesses. This at least is the impression created by Samuel Ward's abbreviated tales of heroic Christian dying in *The Life of Faith in Death* (1622). Ward's manual, quoted at the start of this paper, condenses into single lines the last dying words and actions of more than seventy Christian martyrs. In emblematic moments, voices call out from the flames in pious delight at the prospect of meeting their Maker, providing a kaleidoscope of believers overcoming pain with demonstrative rhetoric. By testifying aloud in excruciating circumstances, Ward's martyrs – selected from the *Acts and Monuments* and from other Protestant martyrologies – appear to transmute their physical sensations of suffering into amusement, aggression or euphoria.

Ward's *Faith in Death* helps to solidify the belief of his godly contemporaries in the special ability of the Protestant faithful to withstand torment. Selecting from Foxe's narrative those moments of agony which seem to be transformed in and by declarations of faith, Ward intensifies an implied connection between vocal testifying and physical fortitude. Rhetoric at the stake appears in this manual to be a mode of pious behaviour, a way of bearing witness that has direct relevance and utility for readers suffering in ordinary circumstances. Ward explicitly recommends the analgesic properties of martyrs' speeches, advising readers to repeat the quoted phrases aloud to suffering friends. 'Read them over to a sicke or to a dying Christian', he instructs; 'if they quicken not, if they comfort not, it is because there is no life of Faith in them'.[14] With this prescription, Ward claims that the martyrs' exemplary responses to persecution can effectively revive or 'quicken' ordinary, bedridden believers. The combination of theatricality and practicality in this godly manual is striking; and it may help us to understand how Protestants of this period directed themselves and each other to acts of responsive, demonstrative and affective testimony.

An early entry in Ward's 'living speeches of dying Christians' cites Lawrence as saying, whilst being burnt on coals, 'Turne the other side

[13] Knott J., *Discourses of Martyrdom* (Cambridge: 1993) 8.
[14] Ward, *Faith in Death* 10.

also, least raw flesh offend'.[15] Here an imperative verb, 'turn', is used by a burning man to reject the meaning of pain that is being imposed or branded on him by his persecutors. What is meant to be insufferable is in fact so easily endured, the speaker insists, that he is prepared to repeat the experience on the other side of his body. Ward's godly readers would recognise the rhetorical game being played here, since irony and logical reproofs are standard tools of dialectical argument. Lawrence's command to 'turn the other side', like Christ's instruction to turn the other cheek, rejects the opponent's insult by reversing its significance. An inventive tactic, it requires the speaker to find a contrary meaning in his suffering. The suggestion that the sight of 'raw flesh' might offend onlookers achieves its ironic effect by giving precedence to an aspect of human 'flesh' that is not implied by the context of torture: its shameful nakedness, or its resemblance to inedible, uncooked meat. Ward's martyr, in this example, manipulates the semantics of a painful situation. Reversing his inflicted injuries through irony, and so wresting verbal control from a tormenter, the afflicted man has the satisfaction of seeing or imagining his opponent baffled. Whether or not such a retort was actually made, and whether or not Lawrence's pain was dulled as a result of it, are matters of doubt: but what seems certain is that the retelling of the jest in a spiritual guidebook offers godly imitators a way to make new sense of their pain.

The bold talk exemplified in Ward's manual needs an audience to be effective, I suggest. By playing silently with words in his mind, a martyr could perhaps reorder the syntax of his suffering; but without a human response to this linguistic trickery, his changed consciousness of pain seems unlikely to amount to the 'leaping and clapping of hands' described by Ward (at the start of this paper) as the action of faith. Rhetoric is an interpersonal system, in which speaker and listener affect one another. The sense of an audience is implicit in almost all of Ward's 'lively testimonies', and explicit in the prescription (quoted above) by which he introduces them to readers. For instance: '*Marcus* of *Arethuse*, hung up in a basket, annoynted with hony, and so exposed to the stinging of Waspes, and Bees [said] to his persecutors that stood and beheld him; *How am I advanced, despising you that are below on earth*'.[16] Caged in a humiliating fashion and half stung to death, this martyr

[15] Ward, *Faith in Death* 15.
[16] Ward, *Faith in Death* 16.

uses his proximity to death to joke at his persecutors' expense, by contrasting his elevated position with their worldly lowliness. The speaker stimulates his resistance to pain by revelling in the witty provocation of his enemies. Arousal of the audience here facilitates another sort of arousal in the suffering speaker.

Raimie Targoff describes a similar rebounding effect in the public performance of prayer. Despite their opposition to set prayer and ritual, the godly prayed aloud in more or less extemporaneous fashion because they believed that the presence of their brethren would increase the truthfulness, efficacy and emotional arousal of the individual at prayer.[17] Declarations spoken aloud in prayer, and rebuttals cried out in persecution operate alike to cause beneficial change in the speaker's whole person. On this effective basis, a martyr's speech made in extraordinary historical circumstances can provide a template for godly conduct in ordinary pain or illness. Whatever the affliction, believers could comfort themselves by demonstrating to others their acceptance of it. This helps to make sense of Ward's decision to present the last cries of dying Christians as a 'posy' of 'flowres' to his 'loving Mother'.[18] He clearly intended his anthology to be a comforting, remedial gift. The aim of godly aids to affliction such as *Faith in Death* is not to rid sufferers of their symptoms; but rather to help them incorporate pain into their experience of faith, and vice versa.

To present this remedial use of demonstrative rhetoric as an exclusively godly art would be false. Protestant authors who deny or ignore their debt to Catholic writers and to the shared religious tradition, sometimes grudgingly admit that pre-Christian Stoics were expert at using oratory to turn feelings of pain into feelings of indifference. Thomas Lupset's *A Compendious and a very Fruteful Treatise teachynge the waye of Dyenge well* (1541) opens with the example of Cato, who committed suicide 'bothe with swerde, and his nayles, tearynge out his owne bowelles'.[19] This drastic action is, if silent, unmistakably rhetorical, persuasively demonstrating to observers Cato's contempt for his body. At greater length, Lupset admires Canius, who 'from a noble stomacke' gave witty retorts to the Emperor Caligula on being sentenced to death.

[17] Targoff R., "The Performance of Prayer: Sincerity and Theatricality in Early Modern England", *Representations* 60 (1997) 49–65.

[18] Ward, *Faith in Death* fol. A1r–v.

[19] Thomas Lupset, *A Compendious and a very Fruteful Treatise teachynge the waye of Dyenge well* (London, Thomas Berthelet: 1541) 3.

With vocal displays of indifference, Canius appears to have bolstered his own unflinching resilience. Moments before death, according to Lupset, Canius continued to speak eloquently to observers, maintaining 'a wonderfull caulme stomake in the myddest of so stormy a tempest'.[20] 'Stomach' is used by Lupset to denote courage; and this application of the term, conventional in the sixteenth century, gives a visceral quality to the ideal disposition of endurance that Lupset portrays. The gutsy talk of a Cato, a Canius, a St Paul, or St Lawrence emerges from the speaker's body and creates resilience in that body.

What Lupset calls a 'valiant stomach' is an evident, if unacknowledged, feature of what Ward calls faith. Faith in God turns a shaking body to a leaping one, Ward says. His dying Christians, joking and testifying under torture, demonstrate faith not only in divine deliverance but in the power of human speech and companionship. The verbal responses to pain admired in these manuals are equally remarkable for their godliness and their manliness.

Internal Dialogue

If bold speech-making is put to use in godly manuals as an effective response to suffering, silent internal dialogue is similarly promoted as an aid to endurance. In this technique, a pained, complaining or fearful inner voice is contradicted – that is, made to contradict itself – by one of spiritual calm. Dialogues between two objectified aspects of a single person, typically rendered as the Soul and the Body, or the Spirit and the Flesh, had a long literary history in Pauline Christianity before being applied in this explicitly therapeutic way. An older devotional use of internal dialogue, to dramatise and personify the Christian afterlife, is illustrated by William Crashaw's 1622 translation of a Latin ballad, supposedly written by St Bernard from a vision of his, as *The Complaint or Dialogue, betwixt the Soule and the Bodie of a damned man*. Written in verse, this terrifying night vision gives voice to a 'dead carcasse' in 'bitter paine':

> No tongue of living man
> Hath power to tell
> One of the smallest torments I sustaine,

[20] Lupset, *Waye of Dyenge Well* 7.

Where (which is worst)
I must forever dwell.[21]

Hell, according to the testimony of this pained body or 'carcasse', is not a place so much as a state of endless pain. The pain is delineated in a description of the dreamer's Soul being tortured by two fire-breathing, pitchfork-wielding devils. Both damned to suffer the same torment (because they are, after all, the same person), Soul and Body blame each other for their fate. Their brief but impassioned debate effectively splits the character of the dreamer, a typical sinner, into two sub-characters. Making two distinct selves or voices out of one is a rhetorical device which helps the author or dreamer to make sense – or more accurately, senses – out of his torment. While it could be argued that St Bernard's vision and Crashaw's translation of it more of less consciously deploy a conventional mode of philosophical debate in order to dramatise religious dogma, I want to argue that this same dialectical form or genre is activated in godly manuals as a direct, active method of easing a person's discomfort.

Frequent use of the dialogue form in works of practical divinity, such as Thomas Becon's *The Sicke Mans Salve* (1561), Arthur Dent's *The Plaine-Mans Pathway to Heaven* (1601) or Robert Hill's The *Pathway to Prayer and Pietie* (1609), may have conditioned godly readers to structure their devotional thinking in an interrogative pattern. Once learned, this dialogic mode of thought could be internalised still further by a believer seeking to make sense of his or her pain, as suggested by John Donne's use of questions and self-rebuke in the *Devotions Upon Emergent Occasions*, and by George Herbert's stylised self-interrogation in *Affliction (I)*: 'My flesh began unto my soul in pain/ "Sickness cleaves my bones [...]"'. The artistry of individual poets is not my focus here, however: I am proposing that godly manuals teach a wide range of readers, prosaically and effectively, to use the rhetorical device of a soul-body debate as a method of pain management. Authors offer internal dialogue, that is, as a curative tool. They do so directly, by instructing readers to talk to themselves; and indirectly, by citing hypothetical or supposedly reported internal dialogues for comfort and inspiration. Readers of these dialogues are thereby encouraged to split themselves

[21] William Crashaw, *The Complaint or Dialogue, Betwixt the Soule and the Bodie of a damned man* (London: 1622) verse 10.

imaginatively into two selves, and with the spiritual self to thwart the complaints of the flesh.

Throughout Bartholomew Robertson's death preparation manual, *The Crowne of Life* (1618), the interlocutor 'Flesh' challenges his opposing 'Spirit' on points such as 'how I may resist Sathan in my sicknesse'.[22] Reflecting the godly preoccupations of his author, 'Flesh' rarely inquires about matters of the flesh, as we would understand them, being anxious only to ward off the greater infliction of spiritual despair that may be triggered by prolonged bodily suffering. 'Shew mee some comforts if sicknesse continue long with mee', the Flesh pleads, 'that so I may not despaire in Gods mercie'.[23] Robertson's Flesh teaches readers by example to perceive their physical discomfort as an early symptom of the condition of despair; and to dread it for this reason alone. The 'Spirit' character reinforces this message by insisting that 'as death is the wages of sinne, so likewise are all sicknesses, Gods punishments, whereby hee brings us to him, when wee have gone astray by sinne'.[24] To the reader, the combined effect of these two voices is of a godly duet rather than a polarised debate. Told again and again that pain is a form of divine summons, and that his soul and body are calling him to repent, a godly reader is led to feel – in every sense – that he will comfort his body and soul by answering the call. The 'pill' of godly pain relief may indeed work, if faithfully swallowed.

Another godly manual written, like Robertson's *Crowne*, by a Scottish divine indicates in its title a more dynamic use of the internal dialogue device for self-persuasion. Zacharie Boyd's *The Last Battell of the Soule in Deathe* (1628) opens with a sick man's cry of a pain. It is distinctly godly pain, combining spiritual fear with bodily discomfort.

> My Bodie is sicke, my Soule is wounded: Gods wrath is fearfull; it burneth to the bottome of Hell. The heate thereof already maketh my Soule to sweate: I can find no Skrine or Sconce to set betweene mee and this fire: Oh, in all appearance I shall shortlie bee dissolved, for to be brought before that great Tribunall.[25]

The man's sensations of burning and sweating are experienced as divine scorching, anticipations of hellfire. This fearful discomfort prompts

---

[22] Bartholomew Robertson, *The Crowne of Life* (London, John Marriot: 1618) 204.
[23] Robertson, *Crowne* 178.
[24] Robertson, *Crowne* 173.
[25] Zacharie Boyd, *The Last Battell of the Soule in Deathe* (Edinburgh, Heirs of Andro Hart: 1628) 3.

eight long 'conferences' at the sick man's bed involving a pastor and spiritual friend who seek to educate the sufferer out of his agony, in conventional godly fashion. Towards the end of Boyd's (relatively long) manual, this bedside colloquium gives way to an internal dialogue, which Boyd more accurately terms 'A Soliloquee, Or a privie conference betweene the Soule and the bodie of the sicke Man lying in a sowne'.[26] Here the man's bodily self regrets his soul's departure, while the soul promises a reunion at the Resurrection. Valedictory rather than antagonistic, this reported inner debate ends peacefully, leaving visible signs of godly relief on the sick man's body. The watching Pastor comments: 'His eyes stirre a little, they are full of *teares the tribute of Repentance*: He beginneth to shake, he now seemeth to bee wakened out of his *traunce*'.[27] Physical recovery communicates to Boyd's readers that the sick man's truly dangerous, Life-threatening spiritual agony has been successfully resolved by this faithful inner dialogue. The length of the passage, and indeed of the whole manual, indicates that readers must make sustained efforts to prepare and repent in order that a final 'soliloquy' be effective.

On the evidence of these two manuals, the therapeutic method of inner debate or soliloquising varies to some extent with each prescription in a godly text, much as medical treatment varies with the outlook of individual doctors and patients. In Samuel Ward's collection of 'the Living speeches of dying Christians', discussed above, several martyrs in circumstances of actual torment appear to address their divided selves in order to moderate their pain. Characteristically, Ward's selections favour aggressive soliloquies. Hilarion complains: 'Soule, get thee out, thou hast seventie yeares served Christ, and art thou now loath to dye, or afrayd of Death?'.[28] By treating his soul in this way as a distinct entity with its own motivations, Hilarion is apparently able to find refuge from, and in, physical discomfort. Barlaam, holding his hand in a flame over the altar and quoting Psalm 144, 'Thou teachest my hands to warre, and my fingers to fight', appears to dull his consciousness of pain by generating a hierarchical sense of his body parts as Christian troops.[29] Tankerfield, putting one leg into the fire, alienates his body from a spiritual self in this reported commentary:

[26] Boyd, *Last Battell* 1132.
[27] Boyd, *Last Battell* 1149.
[28] Ward, *Faith in Death* 14.
[29] Ward, *Faith in Death* 15.

> The Flesh shrinkes and sayes, Thou foote, wilt thou burne and needest no? The spirit sayes, Hell fire is sharper, and wilt thou adventure that? The flesh saies, 'Wilt thou leave thy Friends?' The Spirit answers, 'Christ and his Saints society is better'.[30]

Leaving aside the awkward question of how Ward knows what Tankerfield's 'flesh' and 'spirit' say, this passage suggests that the soliloquiser gains physical relief by reinventing his pain as an argument and resolving it in the mind by dialectical means. Verbs in the present tense, 'shrinks', 'says', 'answers', increase the immediacy of the dialogue and may thereby intensify its secondary therapeutic effect, on readers or imitators.

One of Ward's martyrs, Julian Palmer, comments on the technique I have called internal dialogue, observing that 'if one be able to separate soule and body, then by the helpe of Gods spirit it [death] is no more mastery for such a one, then for mee to drinke this Cup'.[31] The clinical detachment of Palmer's phrase 'if one be able' suggests that suffering soliloquisers, or their authors, master this therapy with difficulty, practice, and divine grace.

Metaphor

The most common way in which physical suffering appears to be 'turned' – to repeat Ward's suggestive verb – into resignation or celebration in godly manuals is through metaphor. To say that metaphors change the significance of what they represent is merely to state the most obvious feature of figurative language. Here I want to penetrate more deeply (as it were) into the affective psychological action of metaphors on those who invent or (again, as it were) absorb them. The difficulty of discussing metaphors without using metaphors is, here as everywhere, confirmation of the extent to which they permeate our language and thinking. Can literary tropes induce psychotropic transformation? Do godly metaphors for pain turn physical sensations, as well as concepts, from one domain of experience to another?

Authors of godly manuals certainly expected the faithful contemplation of Scriptural metaphors to bring about spiritual and bodily change.

---

[30] Ward, *Faith in Death* 24.
[31] Ward, *Faith in Death* 24.

As university-trained practitioners of rhetoric in an era of intense fascination with the persuasive arts, godly divines paid thorough, if not thoroughly consistent, attention to their self-appointed task of using words to direct the thoughts, feelings and actions of their audiences. Nicholas Byfield's *The Promises* of 1619 aims to show 'how a godly Christian may support his heart with comfort' against 'all distresses' with a collection of topical 'places' selected from the Scriptures and 'orderly digested'.[32] This reader's digest is effectively a little book of comforting metaphors. Applying the single curative strategy of metaphorical comfort to both 'inward' and outward' forms of affliction, Byfield selects Scriptural verses for each sort of distress much as a physician or apothecary might select medicines from a cabinet. The dominant metaphors by which Byfield describes his pastoral activity and his afflicted reader's response are of reaching, clutching and swallowing the holy Word. In adversity, we must 'cast the anchor of our hope' upon God's promises (p. 22). Fed with the 'bread of affliction, and the water of adversity' (p. 58), suffering believers will be refreshed by drawing 'the water of life' from 'wells of salvation' (fol. A4r). God's promises, more precious than jewels, should be kept hidden in our hearts (p. 4). These metaphors for Bible-reading create an expectation – which might in itself bring some physical relief to the believing reader – that divine love can be ingested in the body, inscribed on the body, or used in other ways by the faithful to ease personal discomfort.

In Byfield's *Promises*, as in other godly manuals, the border between bodily pain and spiritual regeneration, between one kind of experience and another, is blurred by insistent use of curative metaphors. Repetition diminishes the figurative quality of Scriptural tropes, making them appear to be literal representations of the natural order. Told again and again that they are being nourished by contemplation of the Word, afflicted readers would have little encouragement to resist this figuration, and an obvious incentive to believe it and feel changed by it. A common and particularly irresistible metaphor in manuals such as Byfield's *Promises* represents affliction as a divine gift, a sign of God's especial concern, and a mark of distinction and election. The problem of pain or other affliction is in this way metaphorically transposed, at least on the page, into a desirable good. Refiguring suffering as privilege, godly authors attempt an ambitious rhetorical manoeuvre, as they persuade

[32] Nicholas Byfield, *The Promises* (London, Ralph Rownthwaite: 1619), title page.

readers not to seek relief from pain but on the contrary, to experience pain itself as a cordial. To this end, an anonymous funeral sermon, *The Profit of Affictions*, insists that affliction is:

> Profitable, as physicke to the body, to purge out the malignant humours. Profitable, as sope to the cloth, to fetch out the staines [...] Profitable, as the pruning knife to the tree, to make it more fruitfull.[33]

Reading this incremental list of pain's benefits, the godly reader is led imaginatively and emotively, by a rhythmic procession of similes, to the sense that suffering is good. One of the most alluring tropes of this sermon represents affliction as a perfecting process: 'Afflictions and chastisements, they become profitable, as the furnace to the gold, to purge out the drosse, to make a separation between the pure mettall, and the ore' (p. 581).[34] By figuring affliction in this way as a process of purification or improvement, godly texts make repeated attempts to change the reader's dominant metaphor for his or her suffering. Manipulating the reader's metaphoric structuring of pain, manuals provide an intimately controlled remedy.

The unknown author of *The Profit of Afflictions* recognises explicitly that he is offering, as a cure, the instrumental use of metaphors. He follows a long catalogue of similes and analogies for affliction with the comment: 'These, and the like metaphors we have, by them wee are to conceive of the good, and benefit that comes to us by Gods' castigation [...]'.[35] In this godly viewpoint, Biblical metaphors have practical utility and are to be used accordingly by believers to bring relief. The process seems remarkably clear to the authors of Protestant manuals. There is one source of medicinal metaphors, which is the Bible; and one condition necessary for their successful action, which is faith.

If Christians need only to meditate faithfully on Scriptural metaphors to be healed, can we then assume that these little books of metaphors were effectively remedial? Samuel Ward's anthology of martyrs' last words in *The Life of Faith in Death*, presented as a posy of 'flowres' to his mother Susan, is to some extent an anthology of Christian metaphors used *in extremis*. Cyprian thanks God for his 'Gaole delivery' (p. 13).

---

[33] *The Profit of Afflictions* is included in a collection of funeral sermons by Featley D. – Day M. – Sibbs R. – Taylor T., *Threnoikos: the House of Morning* (London, Ralph Mabbe and Nicholas Bourne: 1640) 581.

[34] Anon., *Profit of Afflictions* 581.

[35] Anon., *Profit of Afflictions* 581.

Iubentius and Maximus declare themselves ready to 'lay off the last Garment of the Flesh' (p. 14). Baynaam taunts miracle-loving Papists with the assertion that 'I feele no more paine in the fire, then if I were in a bed of downe, it is as sweet to me as a bed of Roses' (p. 20). How useful were these metaphors to the ageing Susan Ward and other ordinary readers?

It may seem naïve to speculate on the actual effects of godly rhetoric; but I cannot confidently claim to understand how Protestants of this period conceptualised pain, and, at the same time, treat their felt experience as an entirely separate entity. If the godly did not distinguish sharply between knowledge and sensation, why should we impose this distinction on them? Indeed, our tendency to assign metaphorical activities solely to the realm of 'the mind' and to assume that physiological responses belong exclusively to 'the body' is currently under attack from various disciplines. Mark Johnson, co-author of *Metaphors We Live By*, invites us in his new book to take seriously 'the 'embodiment of mind' by recognising the interconnectedness of everything Descartes separated.[36] One advantage of doing so might be to activate a more empathetic response to texts of the past. A Jacobean individual's pain is not necessarily more alien to us than the pain of a contemporary neighbour; and something might be gained by considering how both use metaphors – if not necessarily the same metaphors – to give structure to, or even alter, their suffering. Godly manuals do not give us a brain scan or clinical record of 'early modern' suffering; but they do provide something like an anthropologist's sound-recording of the language patterns used by this religious community to express, evaluate and reform experiences of affliction. These expressions suggest that human thoughts and bodies may be inseparably involved (albeit to differing degrees) in metaphorical processes: it is not necessarily clear where the conceptualisation of a trope ends and a psychotropic or physical shift begins.

Inuring

Finally I would like to consider the Christian practice of inuring the self to pain or death, that is, of repeatedly forcing one's attention to

[36] Johnson M., *The Meaning of the Body: Aesthetics of Human Understanding* (Chicago: 2007).

the brevity and depravity of physical life, as a way of modifying painful sensations by anticipation. Readers of godly manuals are encouraged to endure 'little deaths' in advance of death; to 'die before dying'; to feign a mental combat with 'the Enemy'; to contemplate death-heads; to make use of the deaths of friends, and by various other means to anticipate suffering or annihilation in the midst of life.[37] The logic of these recommendations is that a feared prospect will be easier to endure if expectant victims accommodate themselves in advance to the inevitability and hidden blessings of death and its painful harbingers. 'Thus enuring thy selfe to carry the Calfe', reasons the Protestant divine Samuel Crooke (1575–1649), 'thou shalt not faint under it, when it is growen to an Oxe'.[38]

How exactly are readers to take up the instruction, made in various ways in godly prescriptive literature, to 'exercise and inure our selves in dying by litle and litle';[39] and how effective might such exercise be as a form of pain management? In a collection of funeral sermons by several Protestant divines, published in 1640 as *Threnoikos: The House of Mourning*, the unnamed author of a sermon on Christ's victory over death calls on all believers to subdue the 'sting' of their own deaths by learning to die daily:

> Consider we have many little deaths to undergoe in the world, as we have many delights; Learne to inure and acquaint thy selfe before hand with the patient and quiet bearing and enduring of these many troubles and crosses that befall thee, As Agamemnon first overcame the Lacedemonians by wrestling, and then by fighting, and Bilney first burnt his finger in the Candle, that after he might the better endure the burning of his body at the Stake. So thinke with your selves, If I cannot endure a little, how shall I endure more?[40]

The direction to 'thinke with your selves' is an invitation to practise the kind of internal dialogue previously discussed; an inner dialectic between fearful and determined selves.

Of two cited masters of the art, the exemplary inuring of Thomas Bilney is worth examining, because it used frequently and persuasively

---

[37] Perkins, *Salve* 46–7. These *memento mori* exercises are discussed at greater length in my PhD thesis, *English Godly Art of Dying Manuals*, 126–137.

[38] Samuel Crooke, *Death Subdued, or, The Death of Death* (London, Edmund Weaver: 1619) fol. C5v.

[39] Perkins, *Salve* 46.

[40] Featley et al., *Threnoikos* 278.

in godly manuals. An evangelist with somewhat ambiguous beliefs, Bilney was executed under Mary Tudor for illegal preaching. The Protestant martyrologist John Foxe, apparently struggling to present Bilney as a thoroughly godly martyr, seized on reports that, while in prison awaiting his death, Bilney held his finger in a candle flame. The episode is subtitled in the 1563 edition of *Acts and Monuments*: 'the godly constancy of Thomas Bilney, who being in prison, oftentimes proved the fire with his finger'.[41] With the word 'oftentimes', Bilney's testing of the flame appears to be a repeated, if not habitual, act. Authority for the story comes, in the 1563 edition, indirectly from a fellow prisoner who reportedly asked Bilney what he was doing, and received the reply: 'nothing but trying my flesh by Gods grace, and burning one joynt'.[42] In the 1570 edition, perhaps responding to readers' curiosity, Foxe significantly expands the episode and narrates directly how Bilney sat with his friends in godly talk on the eve of his execution, discussing the heat of the fire he was to suffer the next day, whereupon:

> [...] puttyng hys hand towarde the flame of the candell burning before them [...] and feeling the heate therof, O (sayd hee) I feele by experience, and have knowen it long by Philosophie, that fire by Gods ordinance is naturally hote, but yet I am persuaded by gods holy word, & by the experience of some spoken of in the same, that in the flame they felte no heate [...].[43]

In this expanded version, Bilney comments on his practice of finger-burning, giving it authority and persuasive force. The story, accompanied by a woodcut illustration, is further accentuated with an additional margin note in the 1583 *Acts and Monuments*.

What began, in Foxe's first account, as a singular detail of one man's use of pain became, in Protestant manuals, a method of godly endurance promoted for widespread imitation. William Perkins' *The Salve for a Sicke Man* of 1595, reporting that Bilney 'oftentimes before he was burned, put his finger into the flame of the candle', replaces Foxe's adverbs 'toward' or 'nye to' the flame with the more direct 'into'.[44] This minor substitution intensifies and clarifies Bilney's daring. Perkins also increases the relevance of the episode to readers by providing two

[41] John Foxe, *Acts and Monuments: Varorium Edition* (1563 ed.; Sheffield, hriOnline: 2004) 482.
[42] Foxe, *Acts and Monuments* (1563) 482–483.
[43] Foxe, *Acts and Monuments* (1570) 1151.
[44] Perkins, *Salve* 47–48.

distinct objectives for the martyr's action, claiming that Bilney put his finger into the flame 'to make triall of his abilitie in suffering, but also to arme and strengthen himselfe against greater torments in death'.[45] Self-inflicted pain serves the Christian as a method of self-assessment and as a kind of protective armour against future pain, Perkins implies. Addressing himself, as the *Salve's* title page specifies, to such ordinary readers as pregnant women, soldiers and sailors, Perkins insists that all should 'acquaint our selves with [these] little deaths'.[46] Bilney's flame-testing is a model for common piety.

One way to account for the recurrent instances and recommendations of 'inuring' in godly manuals would be to view this concept as a metonym for Christian courage. Just as Canius' 'stomach' denotes this figure's stoical endurance in Lupset's *Waye of Dyenge Well*, so we might say Bilney's finger represents in one part the entire valour of the man. But it is also possible that brave Bilney, or the authors who embellished his brave character, believed that his repeated practice of fire-testing caused an actual change in his sensory apprehension of the flame; a kind of spiritually induced thermostatic control whereby eventually he, like the anonymous forerunners 'spoken of' in Foxe's 1570 version (cited above), 'felte no heate'. Without explicitly describing Bilney's practice as physically transformative, Foxe and Perkins allow readers to find the story remarkable, and not merely characteristic. This element of wonder or marvel would help to explain how 'inuring' took hold as a popular godly concept.

At risk of overstepping once again the bounds of literary study, I will briefly note that 'extreme swimmer' Lewis Pugh, making a record-breaking swim at the North Pole in July 2007, was reportedly able to change the temperature of his body before entering the icy water by a psychological process of "anticipatory thermogenesis".[47] This term refers to a process of mental preparation whereby Pugh apparently conditions his body, by repeated practice, to respond in specific ways to certain triggers such as visual symbols and vocal incantation.

---

[45] Perkins, *Salve* 48.

[46] Perkins, *Salve* 47.

[47] Butcher J., "Profile: Lewis Gordon Pugh – polar swimmer", *The Lancet* 366 (2005) 23–24. See also www.nationalgeographic.com. I am grateful to Pugh's 'mind coach', David Becker, for explaining to me how he helps individuals to prepare for trials of endurance.

Parallels between modern conditioning techniques and godly faith-based inuring should not, of course, be overstated. But if – and the matter is surely not beyond all doubt – pain, or more broadly sensation, is historically contingent, then this contingency is not its only significant aspect. Godly writing on pain provides evidence not only of 'early modern' thinking, but also of rhetorical activity being used in the expectation of felt effects. The practice of using language to manipulate thoughts and bodily feelings is known to many societies, time periods and literary genres, and offers many avenues of investigation.

Godly manuals, I have suggested, encourage readers to turn passive suffering into active oratory; to turn a spiritual self against a bodily self; to turn one metaphoric conceptualisation of pain into another; and to ameliorate the feared prospect of pain or death by daily practice. To return to a question posed earlier: what gave godly Protestants, believing as they did in man's utter dependency on divine will, the right to manage and manipulate God-given pain?

There can be no doubt that godly authors knowingly advocated the manipulation of felt experience, and used rhetorical techniques to this end with some sophistication. When Jean Guillemard recommends the faithful to 'make a fayned Combat against death', he, like his fellow clergymen in England, knows that he is advising readers to *feign* an activity.[48] Believers are to trick themselves, persuade themselves, and habituate themselves into states of consciousness that are not instinctive. Protestant authors do not see these activities as attempts to take the initiative, or to avoid suffering; but on contrary, as divinely prompted responses to a foreordained trial. William Perkins, discussing 'the right manner of dying well', states: 'Wee are *commanded* to *present our selves* unto God as *free-will* offerings'.[49] This paradoxical notion that believers are self-sacrificing lambs offering themselves willingly for slaughter is Perkins' attempt to resolve the persistent question of whether men are free or compelled. In his rationalisation, they are both. Moreover, there is a causal connection between self-willed and divinely ordained action, in Perkins' logic: because the faithful have been chosen to suffer, they willingly choose to suffer. Godly manuals direct readers to suffer and die 'well', not to escape or negate suffering altogether. Suffering

[48] Jean Guillemard, *A Combat Betwixt Man and Death*, translated by Edward Grimeston (London, Nicholas Okes: 1621) fol. A7v.

[49] Perkins, *Salve* 97 (original italics).

'well', in godly terms, means making a transformation from the basic, animalistic appetite for bodily comfort that constricts 'natural' men to the rapturous desire for eternal life that defines the faithful.

For all their rhetorical ingenuity, godly manuals do not entirely resolve the tension between their theology of dependence and their provision of self-help advice. Nor do these 'salves' provide straightforward therapy to the certain benefit of a person's health, as we would now measure it. At times, godly books celebrate pain, by voyeuristically relaying the tortures of martyrs, or despise and denigrate the human body. 'Preparationists' like Perkins or Sibbes who urge the 'bruising' of the soul as an essential stage of repentance thereby inevitably, if unintentionally, advocate something akin to self-harm. The pervasive godly instruction to search one's mind and deeds for 'marks' of election, which has a literal and punitive counterpoint in the 'pricking' of suspected witches to discover the Devil's 'mark', seems to exert a potentially destructive influence on what might now be called the self-image of believers. Godly 'cures' could cause suffering, as well as relieve it.

On the other hand, the godly understanding of pain as a system of signs which could be read, translated, and 'turned' by the application of tropes to reveal new significance in, and to change the felt experience of, painful symptoms, strikes a modern observer as insightful and productive. Godly authors were alert to categorisation error, and to the possibility of manipulating cognitive categories. Milton knew that the mind could make a heaven of hell, or a hell of heaven. Likewise manuals that urge readers to seize the 'Enemy' before it (death) seizes them demonstrate a keen awareness of the capacity of individuals to train their responses by analogue, visualisation, habit and self-suggestion: the physic of words. Martyrs dying with witty retorts make their pain a persuasive process, co-opting their audience into an exchange of meaning and feeling. Ward's claim that faith 'turneth feares into hopes, sighings and groanings, into wishings and longings, shaking and trembling into leaping and clapping of hands', displays in its linguistic exuberance the potential of human emotions, physical energy and verbal ingenuity to influence one another.

I end with a brief observation on the development of godly 'salves' or manuals promising comfort to the afflicted. As might be expected, the long titles of these publications show increasing concern with social strife as a cause of affliction in the Civil War period, and subsequently offer more in the way of recognisably medical treatments later in the century. William Waldwyn's *Physick for Families* of 1696 is entirely different in tone to William Perkins' *The Salve for a Sicke Man* of 1595, for example. Godly preoccupation with sin and faith seems to give way over the century to an interest in pharmaceutical remedies.

One reason for focusing this paper on examples from late sixteenth and early seventeenth century manuals is that religious anxiety and physical symptoms inform each another most conspicuously in the godly texts of this period. Here also, the transformation of mental states promised or reported in these manuals is extreme. Before being treated by the rhetorical strategies discussed above, pain signals to godly authors the onset of despair; most damnable of all conditions. Once the suffering believer has taken a supervised, sustained leap of faith, however, his pain will seem useful, refining, elevating, reassuring and even delightful. Adam Harsnett's *A Cordiall for the Afflicted* of 1638 declares boldly to prospective purchasers:

> The Necessitie and Utilitie of Afflictions.
> Proving unto us
> The happiness of those that thankfully receive them:
> AND
> The misery of all that want them, or profit not by them.[50]

This advertisement exemplifies the rhetorical skill with which godly authors transform pain into privilege. It tells suffering readers that they are blessed by their affliction, and – with a stress on the second statement – that, by contrast, unaffected neighbours are miserable in their unscathed, worldly skins. Sure knowledge of an enemy's pain is a sweet cordial indeed.

---

[50] Harsnett A., *A Cordiall for the Afflicted* (London: Stephens and Meredith, 1638), title page.

Selective Bibliography

Boyd Zacharie, *The Last Battell of the Soule in Death* (Edinburgh, Heirs of Andro Hart: 1628).

Byfield Nicholas, *The Promises* (London, Ralph Rownthwaite: 1619).

Crashaw William, *The Complaint or Dialogue, Betwixt the Soule and the Bodie of a damned man* (London: 1622).

Crooke Samuel, *Death Subdued, or, The Death of Death* (London, Edmund Weaver: 1619).

Featly Daniel – Day Martin – Sibbs Richard – Taylor, *Threnoikos: The House of Mourning* (London, Ralph Mabbe and Nicholas Bourne: 1640).

Foxe John, *Acts and Monuments: Varorium Edition* (Sheffield, hriOnline: 2004).

Good M. – Brodwin P. – Good B. – Kleinman A. (eds.), *Pain as Human Experience: An Anthropological Perspective* (Berkeley: 1992).

Guillemard Jean, *A Combat Betwixt Man and Death*, trans. Edward Grimeston (London, Nicholas Okes: 1621).

Harsnett A., *A Cordiall for the Afflicted* (London, Stephens and Meredith: 1638).

Houlbrooke R., *Death, Religion, and the Family in England, 1480–1750* (Oxford, Clarendon Press: 1998).

Johnson M., *The Body in the Mind: The Bodily Basis of Meaning, Imagination, and Reason* (Chicago: 1987).

Knott J., *Discourses of Martyrdom* (Cambridge: 1993).

Lakoff G. – Johnson M., *Metaphors We Live By* (Chicago: 1980).

Lupset Thomas, *A Compendious and a very Fruteful Treatise teachynge the waye of Dyenge well* (London, Thomas Berthelet: 1541).

Healy M., *Fictions of Disease in Early Modern England: Bodies, Plagues and Politics* (Basingstoke, Palgrave: 2001).

Perkins William, *A Salve for a Sicke Man* (Cambridge, John Legate: 1595).

Rey R., *The History of Pain*, trans. L. Wallace – S. and J. Cadden (Cambridge, Mass., 1995).

Robertson Bartholomew, *The Crowne of Life* (London, John Marriot: 1618).

Targoff R., "The Performance of Prayer: Sincerity and Theatricality in Early Modern England", *Representations* 60 (1997) 49–65.

Turner M., *Reading Minds: The Study of English in an Age of Cognitive Science* (Princeton: 1993).

Ward Samuel, *The Life of Faith in Death* (London, Marriot and Grismand: 1622).

EXPERIENCING PAIN IN JOHN DONNE'S *DEVOTIONS UPON EMERGENT OCCASIONS* (1624)

Mary Ann Lund

In late 1623 the inveterate gossip and letter-writer John Chamberlain informed a correspondent that London was being swept by 'a contagious spotted or purple fever that reigns much which together with the small pox hath taken away many of good sort as well as meaner people'. John Donne, the renowned preacher and Dean of St Paul's Cathedral, was one of the fever's victims. He was taken ill in late November (at the age of 51) and was for a time 'in great danger', as Chamberlain remarked.[1] Unlike many, though, he was not 'taken away'. During his slow recovery he composed the *Devotions upon Emergent Occasions, and Severall Steps in my Sicknes*, a series of twenty three meditations, expostulations (or debates with God), and prayers in which the writer sifts through the physical experiences of his fever for their spiritual signification. The work was published almost immediately, in late January 1624, at a time when Donne was still not in full health (he would not re-enter the pulpit until late March).[2] The text is thus unique in early modern writing as an artistically shaped, personal account of sickness composed in its immediate aftermath and tracking its onset, progress, crisis, and final subsidence.

Physical experience is at the centre of Donne's text.[3] Although the devotions are acts of worship, this is not to imply that the steps in Donne's sickness are mere starting-points and that physical concerns are replaced by purely spiritual ones. From the first, Donne questions '*My God, my* God, why is not my *soule*, as sensible as my *body*?'; the soul's lack of sensation means that physical feeling instead provides the

[1] John Chamberlain, *The Letters of John Chamberlain* (ed. N.E. McClure), 2 vols. (Philadelphia: 1938) II, 531.

[2] The first known sermon from 1624 was preached at St Paul's on Easter day; John Donne, *The Sermons of John Donne* (ed. G.R. Potter and E.M.S. Simpson), 10 vols. (Berkeley: 1953–1962) VI, no. 2.

[3] This point is made and brilliantly elucidated by Pender S., "Essaying the Body: Donne, Affliction, and Medicine", in Colclough D. (ed.), *John Donne's Professional Lives* (Cambridge: 2003) 215–248.

key to spiritual awareness.[4] Donne regards sickness as the result of sin, as a form of correction from God, and also as a spiritually beneficial process, a view which is typical of mainstream Protestant (and indeed Catholic) thinking.[5] The experience of physical suffering forms part of an essential spiritual process, and in Donne's handling the two are inseparable. The prayer which ends each devotion is not an opportunity to move beyond the sick body but to view it side by side with the soul, as for example in the twenty-first prayer:

> as I acknowledge, that my *bodily strength* is subject to every *puffe of wind*, so is my *spirituall strength* to every *blast of vanitie*. Keepe me therefore still, O my gracious *God*, in such a *proportion* of both *strengths* [...] (115).

Physical experience is therefore important, but pain itself is by no means the most prominent element of the text. Donne does not present himself as being subject to extreme or constant torments, and when he does discuss the nature of physical pain (as he does at the beginning and end of the work) he does so in general terms. Yet personal aspects of the pain of fever do leave their mark, I would argue, in major patterns of imagery he uses in the text. His representation of pain is sophisticated and subtle: metaphors evoke particular qualities of pain, and his recurrent use of that imagery forms an impression on the reader's imagination that a more straightforward account of symptoms might not. Medical historians have remarked that the writers of antiquity – whose works formed the basis of early modern medical thinking – had little to say about the intrinsic qualities of pain. In general they were not interested in pain's theoretical significance except inasmuch as it indicated certain disorders.[6] This lack of theorizing about pain in medical writing means that we have to look elsewhere to uncover its meanings in early modern England. Donne's treatment of pain reveals important aspects of his attitude to medicine and sickness, as well as his theological outlook, while his metaphorical representation of personal

[4] John Donne, *Devotions Upon Emergent Occasions* (ed. A. Raspa) (Oxford: 1987) 8. All quotations from the *Devotions* are from this edition, incorporated in the text.

[5] Jonathan Goldberg stresses the conventional aspects of Donne's treatment of illness, "The Understanding of Sickness in Donne's *Devotions*", *Renaissance Quarterly* 24 (1971) 507–517. See also Melling D.J., "Suffering and Sanctification in Christianity", in Hinnells J.R. – Porter R. (eds.), *Religion, Health and Suffering* (London: 1999) 46–64.

[6] Rey R., *The History of Pain* (trans. by L.E. Wallace – J.A. Cadden – S.W. Cadden) (Cambridge, MA: 1995) 26; Horden P., "Pain in Hippocratic Medicine", in Hinnells – Porter, *Religion, Health and Suffering* 295–315 (esp. 296–297).

suffering shows a deliberately unconventional method of expressing and shaping physical experience.

The *Devotions* is one of very few autobiographical accounts of illness in the seventeenth century; others are found in diaries, letters, and autobiographies.[7] Such writings should not be regarded simply as records, since each writer (consciously or otherwise) employs techniques to structure narrative and selects language to express his or her illness: as David Morris has put it, 'the experience of pain is decisively shaped or modified by individual minds and by specific human cultures'.[8] Early modern medicine has inherently literary and rhetorical qualities which are reflected in accounts by patients. Diseases, Andrew Wear has argued, 'lent themselves to being put into narrative formats', having a beginning, middle and ending (happy or otherwise), and this sense of narrative was strengthened by the physician's interventions for treatment (adding episodes to the story), and also by the medical understanding of the body as an interconnected whole. Both patients and medical practitioners told stories: the patient recounted his or her experience, which then played a part in diagnosis, and the physician gave bedside accounts of what he perceived was happening and would happen to the patient.[9]

Donne makes the literary qualities of early modern medicine an integral feature of his text. Unlike most other seventeenth-century illness narratives, the *Devotions* is an elaborately ordered work, tightly controlled by a literary artist. Donne recognises and takes advantage of the sense of narrative in early modern sickness and its treatment, building an exoskeletal structure out of it in the titles of devotions: "The Patient takes his bed" (14), "Upon their Consultation, they [the physicians] prescribe" (44), "The Sicknes declares the infection and malignity thereof by spots" (67), for example. Lucinda McCray Beier has recognized that 'Taking to bed was and is the signal for alterations in the behaviour of the sufferer and those around him or her', and Donne incorporates this change into the structure of his book, as the first example shows.[10] The unique features of the text should be

[7] McCray Beier L., *Sufferers and Healers: The Experience of Illness in Seventeenth-Century England* (London: 1987) 219.

[8] Morris D.B., *The Culture of Pain* (Berkeley: 1991) 1.

[9] Wear A., *Knowledge and Practice in English Medicine, 1550–1680* (Cambridge: 2000) 133–134; see also 149–153.

[10] Beier, *Sufferers and Healers* 243.

emphasised. While its form has similarities to other devotional writing, Protestant and Catholic, it has no real precedents. Its ideas and images run in patterns throughout the text and hence the reader must view its individual parts in the context of the whole. My analysis of Donne's experience of pain will take such an approach, attending to his language of physical suffering and to the way broader religious and medical meanings collect around his expressions of pain.

The Nature of Pain

Donne's text, intended for the 'holy delight' of others (as he claimed in a letter to Sir Robert Ker),[11] is concerned not simply with his individual experience but with universal meditations. In my discussion of pain I will firstly consider the remarks Donne makes about the nature of pain in general, which feature at the beginning and end of the work, then move on to examine the ways in which his language of pain and affliction develops throughout the text.

From the very beginning, pain forms an important part of the *Devotions*. The first meditation throws the reader into the dramatic present of illness's onset: 'this minute I was well, and am ill, this minute' (7). The writer has been surprised by a 'sodaine change' which has taken him from a state of health or at least neutrality (in Galenic terms) to sickness. The rest of the meditation is not about his own state, however, but that of man in general, and the ruinous consequences of the Fall. Physical suffering takes a significant role:

> now, we doe not onely die, but die upon the Rack, die by the torment of sicknesse, nor that onely, but are pre-afflicted, super-afflicted with these jelousies and suspitions, and apprehensions of *Sicknes*, before we can cal it a sicknes; we are not sure we are ill; one hand askes the other by the pulse, and our eye askes our own urine, how we do. O multiplied misery! we die, and cannot enjoy death, because wee die in this torment of sicknes (7).

The pain of disease, which is depicted here in extreme terms as torment and the torture of the rack, is not only an affliction but an obstacle: it prevents us from a good end. It is noteworthy that Donne associates

[11] Cited in Raspa, *Devotions* xvii.

physical with psychological suffering here. The anxieties – the jealousies and suspicions – which are provoked by the preliminary signs of ill-health precede and accompany the body's torments, layering onto it (as the word 'super-afflicted' suggests). Pain belongs not only to the senses but to the mind as well.

The suffering wrought by illness is hence confronted at the beginning of the *Devotions*, but mainly in general terms: he is describing the experience of illness as all are affected by it. His other comments about the nature of pain occur near the end of the text when, in narrative terms, the patient is still physically weak but showing signs of recovery. It is as if, once the crisis of the fever is past, Donne is free to step back from his own subjective experience to contemplate the broader meanings of pain. So, in the twenty-second meditation, Donne considers the fact that every part of the body is prone to infirmities. It is not merely the major afflictions which are to be dreaded, since 'every *tooth* in our *head*, [hath] such a paine, as a *constant man* is afraid of, and yet *ashamed* of that *feare*, of that sense of the paine' (116). Again, physical affliction and anxiety go hand in hand here. Fear precedes pain – even if our teeth are healthy we may fear toothache – and accompanies it, while also producing another emotional reaction: shame at being scared of pain. It is worth pausing over the phrase 'that sense of the paine'. Donne does not mean simply the sensation of pain but an awareness of pain, even a heightened consciousness of it, whether it is being experienced or merely imagined. He has already used the phrase in the twentieth prayer in relation to Christ, who 'being offered in the way to his *Execution*, a Cup of *Stupefaction*, to take away the sense of his paine, [...] refused that *ease*, and embraced the whole *torment*' (108). The 'sense' is part of the full experience of pain and is partly intellectual. The echoed phrase serves to contrast sinful man's fearful attitude to pain with Christ's 'embracing' of it.

In the last meditation of the work Donne extends his remarks about the nature of pain. One can only truly understand one's own experience of pain, he concludes, never someone else's:

> Even in *pleasures*, and in *paines*, there is a *propriety*, a *Meum & Tuum*; and a man is most affected with that pleasure which is *his*, *his* by former enjoying and experience, and most intimidated with those *paines* which are *his*, *his* by a wofull sense of them, in former afflictions. [...] in *bodily paines*, in a fit of the *stone*, the patient wonders why any man should call the *Gout* a *paine*: And hee that hath felt neither, but the *tooth-ach*, is as much afraid

> of a fit of that, as either of the other, of either of the other. *Diseases*, which we never *felt* in our selves, come but to a *compassion* of others that have endured them; Nay, *compassion* it selfe, comes to no great *degree*, if wee have not *felt*, in some *proportion*, in *our selves*, that which wee lament and condole in another (121).

It might be surprising to find a minister of the church admitting that compassion can be limited, but we must remember the etymological root of the word (*com-* together with; *pati* to suffer). Donne is exploiting the double meaning of compassion, first as 'Suffering together with another, participation in suffering', and second as 'The feeling or emotion, when a person is moved by the suffering or distress of another, and by the desire to relieve it'.[12] The first meaning of the word comes to eclipse the second: without the personal memory of a particular pain, Donne argues, one cannot fully appreciate it when it afflicts another.

Imagining Pain

We have seen how at the beginning and the end of the work Donne meditates on the qualities of pain in general. Physical pain is closely associated with the psychological anxieties of the sufferer; it is an impediment to a good Christian death (partly, it is implied, because pain distorts the mind); it can be caused by almost anything in the body and even seemingly minor complaints can fill one with fear, pain's inevitable companion; and it can only be understood by the one who has experienced it. It is more or less impossible to imagine other people's pain. In the main body of the work, though, Donne's writing encourages the reader to do exactly that: to participate in the experience of a disease which the reader has probably never felt. Donne evokes his pain principally through a series of metaphors. These subtly and gradually convey a sense of the physical affliction the writer suffers and at the same time tie it in with the spiritual process undergone in the text.

The importance of bodily experience in the work is shown by Donne's specific allusions to his physical symptoms. These are, we learn early on, principally fever and sweats, dulling of the senses, loss of strength, and insomnia. Donne subjects each symptom to religious analysis; while

---

[12] *Oxford English Dictionary*, 2nd edition, s.v. "compassion", 1, 2.

his doctors try to identify the illness from the evidence the symptoms present, Donne uses them to reach spiritual interpretations. Hence in the sixth prayer he hopes that God will have 'inflamd, & thawd my former coldnesses, and indevotions, which these heats, and quenched my former heates, with these sweats, and inundations' (34). Donne's high temperature and sweating serve to rebalance his spiritual state, which is prone to insufficient love of God and to bodily lusts. His painful symptoms are not merely symbols for an experience of spiritual correction which he undergoes in parallel, but an integral part of that experience. Donne imagines his soul in terms of bodily temperature and hopes that the sufferings produced by fever will contribute towards restoring spiritual equilibrium. Later on, he declares to God that 'I know that in the state of my *body*, which is more *discernible*, than that of my soule, thou dost *effigiate* my *Soule* to me' (119). Physical sickness is the revealed part of a hidden spiritual process; hence Donne's discourse always remains within the perspective of his sick body, which is a vital indicator of the state of his soul.

Throughout the text, Donne's metaphors for his physical suffering convey a sense of constriction, oppression and suffocation. He introduces this idea subtly. In the third meditation, which is prompted by the patient taking his bed, Donne meditates that humans are the only species to take erect form but that this unique attribute is fragile and threatened by sickness. Part way through, he considers that rulers are subject to illness too:

> And that hand that signed Pardons, is too weake to begge his owne, if hee might have it for lifting up that hand: Strange fetters to the feete, strange Manacles to the hands, when the feete, and handes are bound so much the faster, by how much the coards are slacker; So much the lesse able to doe their Offices, by how much more the Sinnewes and Ligaments are the looser (15).

The most obvious owner of 'that hand that signed Pardons' is James I, the king whom Donne served as royal chaplain and who, Donne claimed, first encouraged him to enter the ministry (as he puts it in the eighth expostulation, James 'descended to an intimation, to a perswasion, almost to a solicitation, that I would embrace that calling', 44). In October 1623 James suffered from a bout of ill-health, with symptoms including 'violent diarrhoea, weakness, piercing pains in the hip, muscular spasms in the right leg'; the king's physician, Theodore de Mayerne, would later attend Donne himself, as the eighth Devotion marks.[13] While Donne's words may refer to James, one must remember that he is also describing his own experience of taking to bed. The specific description of weak sinews and ligaments which paradoxically and oppressively bind their own hands and feet suggests Donne's own symptoms, even though it is applied to another. This impression is strengthened by the fact that, in the next two, final sentences, he shifts to the first person singular for the only time in this meditation: 'Here I am mine own *Ghost*' (15).

The link between this passage and Donne's own symptoms is made explicit in the expostulation section. He echoes his earlier words about the sick ruler as he mourns the fact that he is unable to go to church to worship or preach: 'when I am cast into this bedd, my slacke sinewes are yron fetters, and those thin sheets, yron dores upon me' (17). The experience earlier applied to a ruler figure is reapplied, more forcefully, to Donne himself. As Donne revisits the imagery of the meditation, its overtones of personal pain become more powerful: this time it suggests physical restraint ('fetters') and additionally torture. The sheets which prevent Donne from rising are figured as iron doors, which are not simply weighty objects but instruments of death. The execution method known as pressing to death or *peine forte et dure* involved putting a condemned person under a door and adding weights gradually, often over a period of days, until finally external pressure on the body caused suffocation. It was reserved for those who stood mute and refused to plead in a trial: either the agony would force them to put in a plea or they would die. Well-known examples from Donne's lifetime include Richard Weston, who was tried for the poisoning of Sir Thomas Overbury in 1615 (he eventually pleaded to escape death by the press) and Walter Calverly, who murdered two of his children but refused to plead in his 1605 trial and was hence pressed to death (a decision that ensured his surviving son would inherit his estate).[14] Calverly's crime was the inspiration for *A Yorkshire Tragedy* (1608). Donne uses the image of pressing twice, in one of many instances of the work's formal symmetry: it first appears in the third devotion and reappears in the twenty-first, the third from

---

[13] Trevor-Roper H., *Europe's Physician: The Various Life of Sir Theodore de Mayerne* (New Haven: 2006) 272. James' illness is noted by Raspa in connection with the Ninth Devotion, *Devotions* 147.

[14] For this and other cases see McKenzie A., "'This Death Some Strong and Stout Hearted Man Doth Choose': The Practice of Peine Forte et Dure in Seventeenth- and Eighteenth-Century England", *Law and History Review* 32 (2005) 279–313.

the end. In this latter devotion he meditates on his physical weakness as he attempts to rise from his bed, which leads him to consider the impotence of humankind. Man is so weak that

> when it falls out, (as it falls out in some cases) that more *misery*, and more *oppression*, would bee an *ease* to a *man*, he cannot give himselfe that *miserable addition*, of *more misery*; A *man* that is *pressed to death*, and might be eased by more *weights*, cannot lay those more *weights* upon himselfe (110).

Psychological oppression becomes literal oppression, a slow and agonising fate which cannot be accelerated by one's own efforts.

Why does Donne use this image of pressing to death? A number of reasons are suggested both by the text and by the illness.[15] To start with, Donne's phrase suggests that the sensation of heaviness and weight pressing down is a physical symptom. Edward Edwards' *The Cure of All Sorts of Fever* (1638) lists 'heaviness' and a 'head-ach, very heavy and sleepy' as a symptom of the fever pestilence, while spotted fever – categorised as a type of pestilent fever – causes pains in the head and heart.[16] The pressing image evokes a quality of Donne's pain. Medical practitioners may not have been interested in the intrinsic status of pain but they did make use of it in diagnosis, following the system

---

[15] One reason I would dismiss altogether is that it is linked to Donne's anxiety about converting from Catholicism. John Carey has claimed that an allusion in Donne's poetry to *peine forte et dure* should be seen in the light of his apostasy. According to Carey, it was 'common practice' for Catholics to refuse to plead at trial and the case of Margaret Clitherow, who was pressed to death at York in 1586 for standing mute when on trial for harbouring Catholic priests, found fame throughout England; *John Donne: Life, Mind and Art*, 2nd edn (Oxford: 1990) 26–27. I can find no evidence that there was an association between pressing to death and Catholic martyrdom in the period. The case of Clitherow was not well known in Donne's lifetime: John Mush's brief biography of 1619 appears not to have circulated widely (the English Short Title Catalogue lists only a single copy), and no other printed source in the period reports the form of Clitherow's death. Pressing to death is not mentioned by Peter Lake and Michael Questier in their work on the execution of Catholics, "Agency, Appropriation and Rhetoric in the Gallows: Puritans, Romanists and the State in Early Modern England", *Past and Present* 153 (1996) 64–107. Andrea McKenzie, who has written a detailed study of *peine forte et dure* in the period, makes no case that the punishment was seen as especially "Catholic", and suggests that the government may have deliberately avoided creating 'a second peine forte et dure martyr' when a similar case to Clitherow's arose; "This Death" 301.

[16] Edward Edwards, *The Cure of all Sorts of Fevers* (London, Thomas Harper: 1638) 38–39; 52–53. Interestingly, Clara Lander, who makes the case that Donne had typhus, quotes a nineteenth-century account of the disease which lists among the symptoms 'a sense of weight or load or increased bulk': Lander C., "A Dangerous Sickness Which Turned to a Spotted Fever", *Studies in English Literature, 1500–1900* 11 (1971) 89–108 (99, n. 33).

handed down by Galen: the type of pain experienced was linked to the part of the body afflicted and hence could point to the cause of the disorder.[17] One of the recognised forms of pain was this sense of heaviness. The pressing image also suggests a feeling of suffocation. We find this sense evoked by later images, too, and I will return to it. Donne draws attention to the specific character of his pain because he is distressed by it and perhaps also as it forms part of the illness narrative developed by patient and physicians.

As well as physical suffering, the image of *peine forte et dure* suggests the patient's sense of powerlessness. The action of taking to his bed marks a change as Donne assumes the role of patient, and the sheets pressing down like iron doors further the sense of confinement and imprisonment; indeed, he expresses a fear that he may never get up again. Much of the ensuing action consists of what the physicians do: we see them observing, consulting and prescribing while the patient remains necessarily inactive. At the moment of prescription (in the ninth devotion) Donne meditates that 'They have seene me, and heard mee, arraign'd mee in these fetters, and receiv'd the *evidence*: I have cut up mine own *Anatomy*, dissected myselfe, and they are gon to *read* upon me' (45–46). Again, Donne imagines himself as a fettered criminal, then as a cadaver. There is a grim wit in the idea of the body dissecting itself, suggesting an odd mix of agency and a complete lack of it (similar to the idea of a condemned man adding more weights to press himself to death). This notion that the patient is involved in the process of medical observation and yet detached from it reflects a fact highlighted by Andrew Wear concerning the patient's role. Early modern medicine did not distinguish between subjective symptoms and objective signs. Hence 'The patient's subjective symptoms or feelings about his or her body that led to diagnosis were also part of the expert, objective discourse of medicine, so that what the patient may have experienced appeared to be observed by the physician, whilst the *persona* of the patient could be reduced to a collection of bodily parts'.[18] Wear's comment is strongly reminiscent of Donne's image of himself in the text as the corpse dissecting itself, simultaneously active and passive, alive and dead. While meditation, expostulation and prayer allow Donne to participate in and shape his illness, his physical state

[17] Rey, *History of Pain* 34–35.
[18] Wear, *Knowledge and Practice* 127.

renders him beyond his own control. The image of pressing to death suggests the emotional distress of powerlessness as well as the physical suffering of the illness.

This experience of powerlessness has a related spiritual meaning which is central to the text. The state of illness vividly illustrates for Donne humankind's inability and weakness. It is a physical manifestation of the Lutheran (and Calvinist) doctrine that humans are not capable of achieving good through their own merits: as Donne comments in the twelfth prayer, although God has 'suffred us to destroy our selves' he has 'not given us the power of reparation in our selves' (66). Even animals know how to heal themselves while wounded, while humans cannot recover without the aid of a physician (20). This link between Calvinist theology and medicine is even more forcefully made in a Whitsunday sermon (conjecturally dated to 1624). There Donne argues that we 'have lost our possession, and our possibility of recovering, by *Adams* sin'. He continues by invoking the Paracelsian theory of balsam:

> Every thing hath in it, as Physitians use to call it, *Naturale Balsamum*, A naturall Balsamum, which, if any wound or hurt which that creature hath received, be kept clean from extrinsique putrefaction, will heale of it self. We are so far from that naturall Balsamum, as that we have a naturall poyson in us, Originall sin.[19]

Paracelsus' theory that all bodies (humans' included) contain a balsam with properties to preserve and heal them interests Donne because the medical idea contrasts with Protestant theology, specifically Luther's doctrine of the bondage of the will and Calvin's doctrine of the total depravity of man. In the *Devotions* Donne denies that humans can heal themselves without the help of others, and shows that spiritual recovery is equally impossible of oneself. The experience of illness causes the sufferer to confront the level of his sinfulness and his inability to rise above it through his own means (as he puts it in the second meditation, 'My *body* falls downe without pushing, my *Soule* does not go up without pulling', 11). This does not force him into a position of complete passivity: the reading of his soul through his body and particularly his expostulations with God allow Donne some level of activity, although expostulation can turn into dangerous '*murmuring*' (27) or questioning of God's ways (an act which led some of the Israelites to be swallowed up in the desert, Numbers 16.31–33). Nonetheless, illness and the physical

---

[19] Donne, *Sermons* VI, 116.

suffering which accompanies it reinforce for Donne that humans are unable to act of themselves. The symptoms of fever become demonstrations of theological doctrine.

The sense of powerlessness has a further significance in the context of Donne's vocation. He expostulates that the 'yron dores' of the sheets prevent him from entering the congregation of the church: 'It is not a *Recusancie*, for I would come, but it is an *Excommunication*, I must not' (17). Yet it is not merely that sickness restricts him from the means of public worship; it also bars him from exercising his ministry:

> Why callest thou me from my calling? *In the grave no man shall praise thee*; In the doore of the grave, this sicke bed, no Man shal heare mee praise thee: Thou hast not opened my lips, that my mouth might shew *thee* thy praise, but that my mouth might shew *foorth* thy praise (17).

Where before the sick bed represented oppression and constriction, now it also stands for exclusion from ministry. We see Donne's deanery chamber, the cramped centre of the *Devotions*, suddenly in relation to St Paul's cathedral next door, the principal site of his ministry and a place now inaccessible to him. A similar shift of perspective occurs when Donne meditates on the tolling bells, which bring a message from the outside world and from God (*Devotions* 16 to 18). It is specifically the activity of preaching which Donne is denied. His illness not only confines him to his sickbed but also forces him to remain mute; hence the heavy sheets mimic the punishment inflicted for silence (at trial). While the text publishes the author's private devotions for the 'holy delight' of others, it also records his enforced inactivity. For a minister who repeatedly asserts that sermons are the central act of public worship and the key to salvation (a major tenet of mainstream English Calvinism), the inability to preach is a serious restriction, and the alternative – sickbed meditations – a poor substitute.[20]

The pressing image provides a tangible, external agent – the iron door – for the writer's affliction, whereas in illness there is nothing so palpable. In the twelfth devotion Donne's doctors try to draw damag-

[20] On hearing sermons and salvation, see e.g. Donne, *Sermons* VI, 86. In arguing for Donne's mainstream Calvinism I differ from Richard Strier's claim that the *Devotions* is a work of Arminian polemic, "Donne and the Politics of Devotion", in Hamilton D.B. – Strier R. (eds.), *Religion, Literature, and Politics in Post-Reformation England, 1540–1688* (Cambridge: 1996) 93–114.

ing vapours away from his head, and he meditates on the notion that something as insubstantial as a vapour can kill a human being:

> If this were a violent shaking of the Ayre by *Thunder*, or by *Canon*, in that case the *Ayre* is condensed above the thicknesse of *water*, of water baked into *Ice*, almost *petrified*, almost made stone, and no wonder that that kills; but that that which is but a *vapor*, and a *vapor* not forced, but breathed, should kill [...] (62).

The writer struggles with the idea that air is a deadly weapon, and plays with the Paracelsian idea that stones are made from elements of the air, transformed by violent forces such as thunder.[21] If the air is 'almost made stone', it becomes a plausible agent of death. Elaine Scarry, author of *The Body in Pain*, has commented that 'two and only two metaphors' are ever used to express pain: one which specifies the bodily damage that is pictured as accompanying pain, and the other which specifies an external agent of the pain, a weapon that is imagined to produce it.[22] We have seen how Donne figures the torment of illness early on as a rack, and later as *peine forte et dure*. Both are classic examples of Scarry's latter category of images: an external agent that inflicts pain. However, the vapours which are causing Donne's fever, and the pain that accompanies it, cannot be compared to solid objects: they are not air 'almost made stone', and moreover they are not forced upon the body.

His invocation of a Paracelsian idea at this point is telling, since in Paracelsian medical theory diseases are external forces and are local processes, attacking the body like weapons.[23] According to the much more widely accepted Galenic theory, however, disease is internal, resulting from humoral dyscrasia. Vapours are the result of putrefaction of the humours, in Donne's case melancholy, as his physicians tell him (63). The explanation of his illness is classically Galenic (although the king's doctor Mayerne was a leading Paracelsian physician, there is no mention of any Paracelsian treatments being applied to Donne). Paracelsus' theory views disease in terms of external agency, but it is not a theory Donne adopts. Instead, he wrestles with the Galenic notion

[21] Raspa, *Devotions* 160.
[22] Scarry E., *The Body in Pain: The Making and Unmaking of the World* (New York: 1985) 15.
[23] Debus A.G., *The English Paracelsians* (London: 1965) 30.

of internal cause, a notion that fits in with his spiritual meditation since sin – the cause of all disease – stems from the individual.

The twelfth meditation sees Donne exploring the causes of his physical suffering. It is, as has been suggested, no easy task. The classification and diagnosis of fevers in the early modern period are highly complex; Donne comments that that 'it would overlode, & oppress any naturall, disorder and discompose any artificiall *Memory*, to deliver the names of severall *Fevers*' (46).[24] From early on his sickness is regarded as infectious (he bemoans his necessary solitude in the fifth meditation) and by the twelfth devotion his physicians say that his vapours arise from melancholy, but it is only in the thirteenth that 'The Sicknes declares the infection and malignity thereof by spots' (67). Yet this "declaration" is not, as we might assume, the same as diagnosis. Donne is thankful that the spots enable the physicians to 'see more clearly what to doe' because the rash reveals that the sickness is malign and pestilential, but according to classical medical tradition (followed by many writers on fever, such as the French physician Jean Fernel (1497–1558)) exanthemata are not distinguishing characteristics of different fevers; rather they indicate, as Donne's words suggest, the severity and virulence ('malignity') of the fever.[25] It is not until the twenty-second devotion that the physicians '*consider the root and occasion, the embers, and coales, and fuell of the disease*' (116). Chamberlain's comment about the 'contagious spotted or purple fever' can be misleading for modern readers of the *Devotions*, who might infer that Chamberlain and his contemporaries believe that a single disease with a single cause is sweeping London, as we might think of a cholera or a typhus epidemic. In fact, in early modern medicine individual circumstances are believed to play the principal part in how a disease manifests itself. According to Galenic theory each case of illness is different (depending upon a person's humoral balance) and hence physicians must pay attention to the individual patient in order to observe symptoms and design the necessary personally tailored course of treatment. Early modern books on fever register the wide variation in its forms: Edward Edwards, for example, lists the causes of spotted

---

[24] On theories of fevers in the period see Lonie I.M., "Fever Pathology in the Sixteenth Century: Tradition and Innovation" 19–44, and Bates D.G., "Thomas Willis and the Fevers Literature of the Seventeenth Century" 45–70, both in Bynum W.F. – Nutton V. (eds.), *Theories of Fever from Antiquity to the Enlightenment*, *Medical History* Supplement no. 1 (London: 1981).

[25] Bates, "Thomas Willis" 66.

fever as 'sometimes' blood, choler, melancholy, or all the humours, which are putrified within the veins either in simple or mixed form.[26] This point is important for a reading of the *Devotions* since, as the twelfth devotion shows, the nature of Donne's sickness is not established. His text does not show the benefit of hindsight in its attitude towards his illness but instead registers the mysterious nature of the fever and the effects on the patient as it begins to reveal itself.[27]

Donne confronts the idea that his vapours come from within his own body, that 'our selves are the *Well*, that breathes out this exhalation, the *Myne* that spues out this suffocating, and strangling dampe' (62). Citing the commonplace that a well or mine can exude poisonous airs, Donne once again plays with the paradoxical notion of the patient acting as external agent upon himself. The body produces deadly vapours which suffocate from inside but which function like an external force that chokes it. He is intrigued by the Galenic idea of the body working upon itself from within (again, there is a theological dimension to this in the self-destructive nature of sinful humankind). Soon after, he recounts the tale of a prisoner who committed suicide by strangling himself with his own knees: an example, and a peculiar one at that, of self-suffocation performed entirely by one's own body. Yet this story is not a satisfactory equivalent. Donne cannot escape the fact that the vapour remains an invisible, intangible, and internal cause of this suffocating sensation: 'it is so insensible a thing; so neere *nothing* is that that reduces us to *nothing*' (63). Michael Schoenfeldt has remarked that humoral theories 'describe not so much the actual workings of the body as the experience of the body'.[28] The feeling of suffocation Donne experiences corresponds with its perceived cause: harmful vapours which 'strangle' from within. His understanding in Galenic terms of what is happening inside him affects the way he imagines his pain, and the earlier image of the iron door pressing down and suffocating transforms into the less tangible but more physiological idea of the choking vapour.

---

[26] Edwards, *Cure* 52.

[27] This also problematises the task of diagnosing Donne's illness retrospectively. Critics have scoured the *Devotions* for records of symptoms as if it were a case-history, yet Donne's descriptions reflect the experience of an unfolding illness which is (during its course) unpredictable and undefined. See Shapiro I.A., "Walton and the Occasion of Donne's *Devotions*", *Review of English Studies* 9 (1958) 18–22; Lander, "A Dangerous Sickness" 89–108; Raspa, *Devotions* xiii–xix.

[28] Schoenfeldt M.C., *Bodies and Selves in Early Modern England: Physiology and Inwardness in Spenser, Shakespeare, Herbert, and Milton* (Cambridge: 1999) 3.

The Waters of Affliction

I would like now to turn to a major current of imagery in the *Devotions*: that of water, and particularly flooding water. Water signifies all kinds of affliction for Donne, but the particular power of this imagery stems from its link with the type of physical experience charted in the work. Pressing to death, choking vapours, and deep waters are all linked through the notion of constriction and suffocation. Donne's water imagery conveys a sense of pain which is, I would argue, distinctively early modern, being linked to the amorphous qualities of the vapour and to the Galenic understanding of the sick body. It is also unlike the two metaphors which Scarry claims are the limits of our pain expressions; although water acts as an external agent, it is not a weapon, any more than a vapour is.

From the eighth devotion onwards, Donne's text is full of thoughts about water. The theme arises out of a traditional idea, already examined and re-examined by the author:

> Stil when we return to that Meditation, that *Man is a World*, we find new *discoveries*. Let him be a *world*, and him self will be the *land*, and *misery* the *sea*. His misery [...] as the *sea*, swells above all the hilles, and reaches to the remotest parts of this earth, *Man* (40–41).

The sea stands for misery, and this negative connotation of water is suggested throughout the work; only the waters of baptism have positive force, as he will later argue. The association between water and affliction is an Old Testament one. The most obvious narrative examples are the great flood that destroys all except Noah and the contents of the ark, and Jonah, whose prayer in the belly of the big fish speaks of his affliction when cast into the seas, 'and the floods compassed me about: all thy billows and thy waves passed over me' (Jonah 2.3). Water imagery also recurs in the Psalms, of which number 69 is a prominent example:

> Save me, O God; for the waters are come in unto my soul. I sink in deep mire, where there is no standing: I am come into deep waters, where the floods overflow me.[29]

[29] Psalm 69.1–2. Other references to waters and affliction include Psalm 46.1–3, Psalm 124.3–5, Song of Solomon 8.7, Lamentations 3.54. All Bible quotations are from the Authorised Version.

The association between the miseries of this life and waters hence has a strong Biblical precedent, and is invoked by a number of religious writers contemporary to Donne.[30]

In Donne's handling, however, the image of overflowing waters begins to take on a more specific meaning as he applies it to the experience of illness, with particular connotations of physical pain. It is important to recognise how delicately he unravels the image during the work. In the eighth meditation, from which I have already quoted, misery is the sea, and he goes on to add that 'Scarce any misery equals to *sicknesse*' (41). Having made this suggestion – that sickness is the worst of miseries, the sea that threatens to overwhelm everything – he puts it to one side. The idea of water as a damaging force appears again briefly and sporadically. For example, in the seventeenth meditation, as Donne elucidates the notion that 'No Man is an *Iland*', he adds that 'if a *Clod* bee washed away by the *Sea, Europe* is the lesse, as well as if a *Promontorie* were' (87). The inundating sea of the eighth meditation is brought to the reader's mind again but only briefly, Donne's main subject here being the relationship between the individual and mankind. It is in the nineteenth devotion that the waters of affliction become the centre of Donne's attention, and his ideas about them fully develop. Even then, the full implications of his words only become clear during the rest of the work. In the nineteenth expostulation he remarks that the Bible calls Gennezareth a sea although it is a freshwater lake, and the Mediterranean a great sea although it is only small, because those who lived there had nothing to compare these bodies of water to and thought them bigger than they were. Likewise 'wee that know not the *afflictions* of others, call our owne the *heaviest*' (101). He revisits this idea about the relativity of individual perception in the twenty-third devotion when he comments that those in pain think their own experience the worst because they have not experienced other types of pain. Thus the '*afflictions* of others' become understood in retrospect more specifically as the pain of others, and the association between water imagery and pain is strengthened. Donne draws out images and themes in the *Devotions* slowly and intricately, and their full significance can only be understood in the context of the work as a whole.

---

[30] An interesting case is Timothy Rogers, who like Donne applies the 'waters of affliction' to his own experience of sickness, *Practical Discourses on Sickness and Recovery* (London, Thomas Parkhurst, Jonathan Robinson, John Dunton: 1691) 3; 22; 160.

According to the title of the nineteenth devotion, "At last, the Physitians, after a long and stormie voyage, see land" (97), and may safely purge him. Like Noah, Donne says, the physicians are looking for 'any *land* in this *Sea*, any *earth*, any *cloud*, any *indication* of *concoction* in these *waters*' (97). Donne brings a touch of lightness with this parallelism: the doctors are literally seeking the signs of concoction – the clear, uncorrupt humours that indicate recovery – in the '*waters*' of his urine. By the time of the expostulation, however, his tone has changed:

> wherefore, O my *God*, hast thou presented to us, the *afflictions* and *calamities* of this life, in the name of *waters*? so often in the name of *waters*, and *deepe waters*, and *Seas* of *waters*? must we looke to bee *drowned*? are they *bottomlesse*, are they *boundles*? (100).

They are not, he goes on to conclude, since God has given 'a *Remedie* against the deepest *water*, by *water*' in baptism. Yet this conclusion does not settle his thoughts, and the long expostulation continues to explore the notion that 'affliction is a Sea, too deepe for us' (101). Of the anxious series of questions quoted above, the starkest and most abrupt is 'must we looke to bee *drowned*?'. Donne not only conjures up the dangerous waters but specifies their physical effect on the body. Death by drowning marks another form of suffocation, along with pressing and the vapours. All three convey a sense of the patient's body as afflicted and oppressed. The growing claustrophobia of Donne's sickbed, where he is exiled from church but cannot escape the tolling bell that marks dying and death, mirrors the physical sense of tightness and inward pressure. The idea of drowning furthers this sense even as it casts Donne's experience of illness in the light of biblical affliction.

This notion of drowning can be better understood through comparison. In Act 1 of Shakespeare's *Richard III*, Clarence tells his gaoler about a dream that will prove to be prophetic. He has dreamed that his brother, Richard Gloucester, falls from the deck of a ship and pulls him overboard too into the sea:

> O Lord, me thought what pain it was to drown,
> What dreadful noise of water in mine ears,
> What sights of ugly death within mine eyes.[31]

For Clarence, one aspect of the horror of his dream is the physical effect of drowning on the body. Although he does not feel pain directly

[31] William Shakespeare, *King Richard III* (ed. J. Lull) (Cambridge: 1999) 1.4.21–23.

since he is dreaming (he only thinks of it), the sensations of drowning form an immediate impression on him. Clarence says that he wished to 'yield the ghost',

> ...but still the envious flood
> Stopped in my soul and would not let it forth
> To find the empty, vast, and wandering air,
> But smothered it within my panting bulk,
> Who almost burst to belch it in the sea.[32]

For Clarence, the agony of drowning is not simply the horrors he witnesses but, most of all, the pressing-in of waters on his body. The sea prevents the release of his soul which is trapped within his body, keeping him alive. The soul is smothered even as the body is by the water, the soul being imagined materially as a last breath to be 'belched' out. Clarence wishes to find relief in death but cannot, any more than the man who is being pressed to death can add more weights to hasten his end.

External pressure pushes in on and restricts the body, for Shakespeare's Clarence literally (at least in his dream) and for Donne metaphorically. How can we understand this idea of pain in Donne's illness? Breathlessness and a feeling of stifling may be symptoms of his fever, but early modern perceptions of the body also provide a key. As Michael Schoenfeldt has argued, according to Galenic physiology the body is not a 'seamless corporal enclosure' (a description which Bakhtin identifies with the ideal classical body) but rather a 'dynamic and porous edifice continually producing "superfluous excrements" which must be removed'.[33] The healthy body maintains a constant movement of fluids and a process of outward flow, but Donne's imagery suggests the opposite. His sickness has restricted his body from this healthy function. Instead of allowing release of substances, illness has stopped them in. Vapours have gathered in the head and need to be removed through medicine, while malignity and venom threaten to attack the heart and must be kept away with cordials. Medical treatment in the period commonly aimed at the removal of obstructions which prevent free flow and the expulsion of noxious substances, through procedures such as bleeding and purging. In the case of the spotted fever, Edwards' instructions for cure include 'use diaphoreticks [substances which provoke sweat] to

[32] Shakespeare, *King Richard III*, 1.4.37–41.
[33] Schoenfeldt, *Bodies and Selves* 13–14.

expel the venom', 'open the pore of the skin to breathe vapours', and 'use fit antidotes and cordials to expel the malignitie'.[34]

Donne's use of water imagery in the context of physiology and ill-health forms an important contrast to the figurative language of the French essayist Michel de Montaigne. Jonathan Sawday has observed that 'metaphors of flowing water are scattered continuously throughout [Montaigne's] writings' and he links this with the essayist's condition of the stone, which often made urination difficult or impossible. In the travel journal Montaigne wrote while visiting spas in search of relief, Sawday finds that flowing water is used as a positive image of change, healthfulness and activity, while all blockages and impediments are to be avoided.[35] Montaigne and Donne draw on the same source of imagery to describe contrary internal processes. Whereas in Montaigne water represents the healthy flow of the Galenic body, in Donne water stands for its opposite, the sickness that assaults and hems in the body, preventing it from its usual functions. It is significant that he imagines the waters pressing inwards upon him just before the physicians proceed to purge him in the twentieth devotion, thus restoring healthful outward flow. His employment of a siege metaphor in the nineteenth meditation is telling. All this while, he comments,

> we are but upon a *defensive warre*, and that is but a *doubtfull state*: Especially where they who are *besieged* doe know the *best* of their *defences*, and doe not know the worst of their *enemies power*; when they cannot mend their *works within*, and the *enemie* can increase his *numbers without* (98).

Donne explores and extends the traditional image of the sick body as under siege. At the height of illness, only defence from outward assault is possible, but Donne concludes with thanks that he, unlike others, has physicians who can watch for signs of the enemies' 'weaknesse' and prepare to '*sally*' and fight in the '*field*' (99). The metaphor of going out to attack the enemy mirrors the purging of corrupt humours which the doctors decide to undertake in order to restore health. Soon after, the image of inundating waters which has haunted so much of the text resolves itself:

---

[34] Edwards, *Cure* 53.

[35] Sawday J., "In Search of the Philosopher's Stone: Montaigne, Interiority and Madness", *Dalhousie Review* 85 (2005) 195–220 (esp. 202–203).

> O my *God*, and *affliction* is a *Sea*, too deepe for us, what is our *refuge*? thine *Arke*, thy *ship*. In all other *Seas*, in all other *afflictions*, those *meanes* which thou hast ordained; In this *Sea*, in *Sicknesse*, thy *Ship* is thy *Physitian* (101).

In the case of physical affliction, medical treatment provides safety at last from the threatening waters. Purgation marks a step towards recovery and also reverses the inward pressing and suffocation of his illness.

The images I have explored evoke a particular sense of constricting, suffocating pain. All along the work has focussed on the sickbed, and as the bells toll repeatedly outside, the atmosphere becomes all the more oppressive and confined. This mirrors the sense of pressure closing in on the body: although the suffocating vapours may be within Donne, they affect him as an outside force might, whether an iron door pressing down or waters smothering. The latter image of waters resonates particularly with the physiological understanding of vapours since it suggests their shapeless and unsubstantial nature. His meditation on vapours forces him to consider the causes of disease, and this leads him to a more nuanced – and unusual – metaphor for pain according to the Galenic system. There is, as Donne remarks, a propriety in pain, a *Meum* and *Tuum*. Yet at the same time his text resists the idea that another's pain is unimaginable, by drawing the reader into the experience it depicts, into the sickbed, almost. The images of pain hint at a specific and authentic experience of physical suffering, suggesting the stifling and pressing-in of illness on the body. The subtle, indirect approach Donne uses to convey this sensation means that the reader has to work to uncover this. His imagery of pain is physically specific and spiritually loaded at the same time, and also mirrors wider artistic structures. I have suggested how physical pain can be represented in texts not solely through direct statement but through a range of literary techniques. Donne follows the divine example of speaking 'in a *figurative*, in a *Metaphoricall language*' (100) by richly conveying his own pain through patterns of imagery. Illness permeates every layer of the *Devotions*, and while pain may not always lie at the surface, it underpins a work which has the personal experience of illness at its centre.

Selective Bibliography

Bates D.G., "Thomas Willis and the Fevers Literature of the Seventeenth Century", in Bynum W.F. – Nutton V. (eds.), *Theories of Fever from Antiquity to the Enlightenment, Medical History* Supplement no. 1 (London: 1981) 45–70.

McCray Beier L., *Sufferers and Healers: The Experience of Illness in Seventeenth-Century England* (London: 1987).

Carey J., *John Donne: Life, Mind, and Art* (London: 1981; 2nd edition 1990).

Chamberlain John, *The Letters of John Chamberlain* (ed. N.E. McClure), 2 vols. (Philadelphia: 1938).

Debus A.G., *The English Paracelsians* (London: 1965).

Donne John, *Devotions Upon Emergent Occasions* (ed. Raspa A.) (Oxford: 1987).

——, *The Sermons of John Donne* (eds. G.R. Potter. – E.M.S. Simpson), 10 vols. (Berkeley: 1953–1962).

Edwards Edward, *The Cure of all Sorts of Fevers* (London, Thomas Harper: 1638).

Frost K. Gartner, *Holy Delight: Typology, Numerology, and Autobiography in Donne's 'Devotions Upon Emergent Occasions'* (Princeton: 1990).

Goldberg J., "The Understanding of Sickness in Donne's *Devotions*", *Renaissance Quarterly* 24 (1971) 507–17.

Horden P., "Pain in Hippocratic Medicine", in Hinnells J.R. – Porter R. (eds.), *Religion, Health and Suffering* (London: 1999) 295–315.

Lake P. – Questier M., "Agency, Appropriation and Rhetoric in the Gallows: Puritans, Romanists and the State in Early Modern England", *Past and Present* 153 (1996) 64–107.

Lander C., "A Dangerous Sickness Which Turned to a Spotted Fever", *Studies in English Literature, 1500–1900* 11 (1971), 89–108.

Lonie I.M., "Fever Pathology in the Sixteenth Century: Tradition and Innovation", in Bynum W.F. – Nutton V. (eds.), *Theories of Fever from Antiquity to the Enlightenment, Medical History*, Supplement no. 1 (London: 1981) 19–44.

McKenzie A., "'This Death Some Strong and Stout Hearted Man Doth Choose': The Practice of Peine Forte et Dure in Seventeenth- and Eighteenth-Century England", *Law and History Review* 32 (2005) 279–313.

Melling D.J., "Suffering and Sanctification in Christianity", in Hinnells J.R. – Porter R. (eds.), *Religion, Health and Suffering* (London: 1999) 46–64.

Morris D.B., *The Culture of Pain* (Berkeley: 1991).

Pender S., "Essaying the Body: Donne, Affliction, and Medicine", in Colclough D. (ed.) *John Donne's Professional Lives* (Cambridge: 2003) 215–248.

Rey R., *The History of Pain* (trans. L.E. Wallace – J.A. Cadden – S.W. Cadden) (Cambridge, MA: 1995).

Rogers Timothy, *Practical Discourses on Sickness and Recovery* (London, Thomas Parkhurst, Jonathan Robinson, John Dunton: 1691).

Sawday J., "In Search of the Philosopher's Stone: Montaigne, Interiority and Madness", *Dalhousie Review* 85 (2005) 195–220.

Scarry E., *The Body in Pain: The Making and Unmaking of the World* (New York: 1985).

Schoenfeldt M.C., *Bodies and Selves in Early Modern England: Physiology and Inwardness in Spenser, Shakespeare, Herbert, and Milton* (Cambridge: 1999).

Shakespeare W., *King Richard III* (ed. J. Lull) (Cambridge: 1999).

Shapiro I.A., "Walton and the Occasion of Donne's *Devotions*", *Review of English Studies* 9 (1958) 18–22.

STRIER R., "Donne and the Politics of Devotion", in Hamilton D.B. – Strier R. (eds.), *Religion, Literature, and Politics in Post-Reformation England, 1540–1688* (Cambridge: 1996) 93–114.

TREVOR-ROPER H., *Europe's Physician: The Various Life of Sir Theodore de Mayerne* (New Haven: 2006).

WEAR A., *Knowledge and Practice in English Medicine, 1550–1680* (Cambridge: 2000).

READING BLEEDING TREES: THE POETICS OF OTHER PEOPLE'S PAIN IN "THE LEGEND OF HOLINESS"

Joseph Campana

Near the opening of "The Legend of Holiness", that legend's exemplary figure, the Redcrosse Knight, plucks a branch from a tree in a dark wood to fashion a garland for his ill-chosen beloved, Fidessa, who is, in fact, Duessa the seductive Catholic whore of Babylon and the physical manifestation of sinful carnality in *The Faerie Queene*. As so often is the case in Spenser's poetry, complexity wells up to contaminate obvious surface significance, as errant romance complicates the stricter tendencies of allegory. In Redcrosse's encounter with Fradubio, that complexity wells up as blood: 'He pluckt a bough; out of whose rifte there came/ Smal drops of gory bloud, that trickled downe the same' (1.2.30).[1] Then the tree bleeds and speaks:

> Therewith a piteous yelling voice was heard,
> Crying, O spare with guilty hands to teare
> My tender sides in this rough rynd embard,
> But fly, ah fly far hence away, for feare
> Least to you hap, that happened to me heare,
> And to this wretched Lady, my deare loue,
> O too deare loue, loue bought with death too deare.
> Astond he stood, and vp his heare did houe,
> And with that suddein horror could no member moue (1.2.31).

Ready-made interpretations for even the most marvelous events spring up easily in "The Legend of Holiness", the most commonly read book of *The Faerie Queene*, one all too often read as an emblematic version of allegory written in support of rather obvious Protestant moral impulses. The tree, we learn, was once Fradubio ('brother doubt' or 'amidst doubt'), and his capitulation to Duessa's seduction results in his transformation to a rationally lower, vegetative form of life.[2] Fradubio

[1] All text citations (to book, canto, and stanza) are to Edward Spenser, *The Faerie Queene* (ed. A.C. Hamilton), 2nd ed. (London: 2007).

[2] As Donald Cheney argues, 'Fradubio's human reason is the first to fail him when he chooses Duessa'. Moreover, he provides 'an emblem of man trapped by the flesh'

seems, then, to stand not only as one of the many moral signposts in *The Faerie Queene* but as one pointing directly to Redcrosse, who has been seduced by Duessa and led astray from the path of righteous Protestant truth and violence.[3]

Signposts such as these (Ovidian mythic and Virgilian epic tropes, etymologically instructive names, and monstrous female bodies) seem to instruct us as to what we should do at this moment in the allegory: note Redcrosse's error and ongoing fall into sin; beware the treachery of appearances; vilify Duessa, Catholics, and so forth. However, Redcrosse's encounter with Fradubio, by invoking the trope of the bleeding tree, activates that trope's capacity to consider both the nature of pain and the ramifications of violence. But the essential mystery of the bleeding tree is not just the infliction of violence but the experience of suffering matter, for we must remember that the Greek for 'wood', *hyle*, is also the word for 'matter'. If a tree cries out in pain in a dark forest, is there anyone to hear it? And how can we think of that pain as real? Furthermore, how do we hear and receive other people's pain? How is pain communicated? And does its communicability make us spectators, participants, or even members of a community? This last question is of particular import since so often the tree knows its assailant as brother or brother-in-arms, parent, or friend. Suffering is intimate, elemental, and enigmatic; we might say that trying to understand other people's

---

(Cheney D., *Spenser's Images of Nature: Wild Man and Shepherd in 'The Faerie Queene'* [New Haven: 1966] 37).

[3] Readings of "The Legend of Holiness" tend to contextualize the most obvious moral evaluation of Redcrosse's progress. See, for example, Neill K., "The Degradation of the Red Cross Knight", *English Literary History* 19 (1952) 173–190, and Shroeder J.W., "Spenser's Erotic Drama: The Orgoglio Episode", *ELH: English Literary History* 29 (1962) 140–159. In most readings of the Fradubio episode, Fradubio is merely a moral signpost of the failing knight of holiness. As Maureen Quilligan puts it, 'The Redcrosse Knight meets a character who is a projection of his own psyche' (Quilligan M., *The Language of Allegory* [Ithaca: 1978] 111). William Kennedy confirms this reading as he examines the dialectic of doubt and fear that explains the intersection of rhetorical, dramatic, and allegorical significance in the episode in Kennedy W., "Rhetoric, Allegory, and Dramatic Modality in Spenser's Fradubio Episode", *ELR: English Literary Renaissance* 3 (1973) 351–368, and his entry 'Fradubio' in *The Spenser Encyclopedia* (ed. A.C. Hamilton) (Toronto: 1990) 317. Shirley Clay Scott (Scott S.C., "From Polydorus to Fradubio: The History of a Topos", *Spenser Studies* 7 [1986] 27–57) and Elizabeth Bellamy read the episode in light of a struggle with literary forebears in the epic tradition, while Bellamy also describes an 'ongoing Renaissance battle between the romance and epic genres' that is 'a key to understanding the incompletion of *The Faerie Queene* itself' (Bellamy E., "The Broken Branch and the 'Liuing Well': Spenser's Fradubio and Romance Error in *The Faerie Queene*", *Renaissance Papers* [1985] 2).

pain, even one's own, is like standing in an obscure wood in which an uncanny voice echoes, demanding some response. Does imagination encourage or obstruct a capacity to experience and respond to our own pain or the pain of others?

As Redcrosse makes this seemingly idle gesture, he already signals his unwitting participation in intertwining histories of pain embedded in *The Faerie Queene*. Spenser invokes a literary history of bleeding trees in order to think through the relationships governing pain and the imagination, on the one hand, and beauty and violence on the other. These literary marvels enable Spenser to consider the ethics of witnessing, experiencing, appropriating, or responding to pain and to consider the extent to which it is that *suffering* (not violence) in which both a sense of lived embodiment and the possibility of subjectivity might be rooted. Moreover, this episode is also embedded in Spenser's attempt to account for religious experience in a post-Reformation world in which the lingering desire for sacramentality is as intense as the virulence of Protestant iconoclasm in England, which forbids or neutralizes most traditional late medieval and pre-Reformation religious sensibilities. Spenser translates the bleeding tree from an epic inheritance to a poetic compensation for the loss of the figure of the suffering Christ in the early modern imaginary, a figure that embodies the importance of the lived experience of pain and provides the ground of an ethics rooted in compassion. "The Legend of Holiness" dramatizes as romance adventure the consequences of Reformation religious ideology: (a) the disappearance of the suffering Christ, which produces an emphasis on Christian morality as expressed through heroic masculinity; (b) the conversion of suffering to obedient reception, rendering the body an allegorical signifier of virtue and thus alienating the body from its lived experience, which renders actual suffering inconsequential; (c) a consequent inability to apprehend the suffering of others and to respond compassionately, which derives from the derogation of both pain and the imagination; and (d) the relegation of suffering and compassion to forms of idolatry, which produces a cult of sentimental beauty that incites violence and relegates suffering and sympathy to 'evil characters' vulnerable to iconoclastic attack. The separate adventures of Redcrosse and Una suggest competing economies of idolatrous suffering (and sympathy), on the one hand, and iconoclastic violence (and beauty), on the other. As Redcrosse sinks into idolatrous attachment, we witness not merely a moral lapse but the critique of a heroic masculinity constituted as a form of iconoclastic violence. Redcrosse and a series of 'evil' characters thus return to representation textures of suffering and sympathy that provide an ethical ground for subjects. As we follow Una, we witness her conversion into a figure of sentimental beauty whose appeal and triumph are underwritten by a displaced violence directed at demonized figures of feminine materiality, such as Duessa.[4] While this legend witnesses the correction of Redcrosse by Protestant ideology and the defeat of the problems of pain and sympathy (in the form of Duessa, Orgoglio, and the dragon), it also witnesses in such correction the loss of the lived experience of the body from which emerges an ethics rooted in common experiences of pain and in compassionate responses to the pain of others, pain we can only understand as we peel back the layers of ideological obfuscation that render suffering at best inconsequential and at worst idolatrous.

Pain poses a unique problem in the wake of the Reformation. To a great extent, that wake extends to influential contemporary thinkers on the subject. Like other Christian apologists, C.S. Lewis, in *The Problem of Pain*, relies on 'sin' and 'evil' to justify the often-violent ways of God to men. Pain provides a corrective force that neutralizes sin by inciting benign violence. As Lewis argues, in a phrase worthy of Milton, pain 'plants the flag of truth within a rebel fortress'.[5] Although Lewis argues that pain is central to being created, it is, at best, 'sterile' or 'disinfected' evil.[6] Lewis's *The Problem of Pain* inscribes itself in a long tradition of ambivalence about suffering, which results in a language of pure negativity. Pain is privative, sterile, aversive, evil: its only validity comes when it signifies something other than itself, such as obedience, humility, mortification, or love. The conversion of pain to a signifier without a signified, a *verbum* independent of any *res*, occludes the experience of human suffering as it naturalizes both violence and the patient acceptance of violence. Suffering points away from the lived experience of the body and sympathy (the social) can have no role when pain is righteous violence applied to the fallen. If, for Lewis, pain's fundamentally negative character emerges from the fallen nature of humanity, Elaine Scarry's influential *The Body in Pain* presents a

[4] A tradition of distinguishing sensual beauty, of Duessa's variety, from Platonic beauty, of Una's variety, allows us to ignore the question of how beauty functions by asking us to focus on the source of beauty (the material or the spiritual). See Orange L.E., "Sensual Beauty in Book I of *The Faerie Queene*", *Journal of English and Germanic Philology* 61 (1962) 555–61.

[5] Lewis C.S., *The Problem of Pain* (New York: 2000) 122.

[6] Lewis, *The Problem of Pain* 177.

decidedly secular account of pain that traces its negative character to the fundamental structures of the brain. Pain destroys the capacity for language and consciousness by rendering an individual purely physical with no room for the communicative gestures of civilization, without which one reverts to a 'pre-language of cries and groans' and loses the capacity to project 'the facts of sentience into speech'.[7] The suffering body, unable to exert will on external objects, becomes an object as a consequence of the 'corporeal engulfment', that is, being reduced to 'sheer material factualness' in pain.[8] Pain traps the subject in self-involvement, alienating those who suffer from others. 'Pain's triumph' is the 'temptation to invoke analogies to remote cosmologies' in order to apprehend the pain of others; pain 'achieves its aversiveness. [...] by bringing about, even within the radius of several feet, this absolute split between one's sense of one's own reality and the reality of other persons'.[9] Here, too, suffering prevents signification and renders sympathy a false analogy.

While a reliance on theology in Lewis's *The Problem of Pain* must, at first glance, seem alien to a recourse to cognitive science in Scarry's *The Body in Pain*, these influential views of the nature of pain must also be considered as a consequence not only of the tension between suffering and violence in the history of Christianity but also of the massive sea changes of the Reformation, in which declining representations of the suffering Christ participate in a larger prohibition of representational acts endemic to an iconoclastic spirit reaching back to the Byzantine iconoclastic controversies and, further still, to the early church fathers. Nowhere was the tension between violence and suffering more heightened than in the early modernity of Spenser's England, marked as it was by escalating religious violence, proliferating doctrinal and sectarian differences, and a fundamental ambivalence about theological opinions and ritual practices focusing on the incarnate Christ. Noting the lack of Calvinist passion narratives, Deborah Shuger claims, 'The figure of the crucified Jesus slips to the margins of English Protestantism, which favored dogmatic theology and devotional introspection over retelling the story of Christ's suffering and death – the pervasive focus of late medieval and Tridentine Catholicism'.[10] The move away from 'affective

[7] Scarry E., *The Body in Pain* (Oxford: 1985) 6.
[8] Scarry, *The Body in Pain* 167; 14.
[9] Scarry, *The Body in Pain* 3; 4.
[10] Shuger D.K., *The Renaissance Bible* (Berkeley: 1994) 89.

piety' produces, then, 'curious and problematic texts, particularly in their ambivalent fascination with revenge, torture, and the dialectics of male violence and victimization'.[11] This Calvinist dialectic of violence and victimization conceives of pain only from the perspective of infliction, requiring suffering to be no more than the passive, obedient reception of violence. Thomas Luxon observes, '*Imitatio Christi* gives way to a new form of piety in which the faithful Hebrew prophet (Isaiah, Daniel, and especially David) is the model for Christian faithfulness – wayfaring and warfaring'.[12] A typical iconoclastic gesture of the English Reformation was to remove or replace figures of Christ's Passion in churches, as 'the royal arms' came to be 'substituted for the holy rood'.[13] As such, the virtues associated with the suffering body recede before the power associated with righteous, royal militancy.

The problem of pain in "The Legend of Holiness" is not solely a problem of theology but also one of genre. The varieties of Christian epic romance to which Spenser was indebted tended not only to include *meraviglie* (such as bleeding trees) that had to be justified but also to emphasize spectacular violence, featuring either invading infidels who had to be beaten back by virtuous Christian knights, as in Ariosto's *Orlando Furioso*, or infidels who occupy the holy city of Jerusalem, as in Tasso's *Gerusalemme liberata*. The sanctity of homeland and holy land alike depended upon the successful exercise of righteous violence, which prevented the victimization of Christianity, leaving, it would seem, little room for suffering, charity, or compassion. Moreover, when the poem is read as a Protestant epic defending itself from Catholic as well as Saracen or pagan incursions, another obstacle to our understanding of the role of pain in this poem emerges from the very reading of Spenser's *Faerie Queene* in its purportedly 'Protestant' nature. Such readings emerge early in the history of the poem's reception, as in John Dixon's annotations of a 1590 edition. As Graham Hough relates in his introduction to these annotations, Dixon remains 'interested in Book I almost entirely as an allegory of the English Reformation'. He is, furthermore, 'indifferent to the courtly and romantic aspects of *The Faerie Queene*; like

[11] Shuger, *The Renaissance Bible* 12.

[12] Luxon T., "Allegory and the Puritan Self", *ELH: English Literary History* 60 (1993) 918.

[13] Phillips J., *The Reformation of Images* (Berkeley: 1973) 102. As Mary Aston indicates, 'The contentious rood images are assumed to be gone [by the 1560s] [...] And now, in the central place of the proscribed crucifixion, stood the royal arms' (Aston M., *England's Iconoclasts* [Oxford: 1988] 313).

Milton in the next generation he is inclined to see Spenser as 'a better teacher than Scotus or Aquinas'; and it is the Protestant divinity, the ascetic morality and the national history that concern him. He looks very like a Puritan parson of moderately scholarly tastes'.[14] For the most part, Spenser's identity as not merely Protestant but as a proponent of a fiercely Protestant poetics has remained unshakable. John N. King argues that Spenser began his career articulating 'Reformation themes' in his early poetry and later 'self-consciously adopted the mantle of the Protestant visionary poet'.[15] For all that 'literary historians have', according to Jeffrey Knapp, 'given new life to the subject of religion in Spenser's works' by 'resisting the old urge to enlist Spenser in one sectarian camp or another', many of these 'eclectic' approaches, even Richard Mallette's refusal to locate *any* doctrinal or religious identity, through action or inaction reify Spenser's identity as a Protestant poet.[16] As King puts it, 'Despite the indeterminate open-endedness of Spenserian allegory, consensus exists concerning the reformist Protestantism of Spenser's romantic epic'.[17]

Kenneth Gross, however, has noted the ways in which the violence of religious iconoclasm in Spenser's treatment of religious virtue comes to pose at least as great a danger as idolatry, leading one to 'fear the unstable power mobilized in acts of iconoclasm as much as it does idolatry'.[18] Sean Kane has argued that the true problem for Spenserian Holiness is not the behavior or practices of other religions but the virulence of Protestant, reformist religiosity, which fantasizes the threat of pagans, Saracens, and Catholics to feed its own violent fervor. Kane suggests that Spenser was wary of the 'dependence for definition on the negation of a rival [which] made Protestantism its

[14] Hough G., *The First Commentary on 'The Faerie Queene'* (privately published, 1964) 1.

[15] King J.N., *English Reformation Literature: The Tudor Origins of the Protestant Tradition* (Princeton: 1982) 445; 446. See also Hume A., *Edmund Spenser: Protestant Poet* (Cambridge: 1984). King, quite influentially, defines Spenser's poetics by virtue of 'unpretentious devices of native satire and allegory that were adopted by English Protestant authors', which some identify with Puritan doctrine.

[16] Knapp J., "Spenser the Priest", *Representations* 81 (Winter 2003) 62. See Mallette R., *Spenser and the Discourses of Reformation England* (Lincoln: 1997).

[17] King J.N., "Spenser's Religion", in Hadfield A. (ed.), *The Cambridge Companion to Spenser* (Cambridge: 2001) 208. For an account of the reception history of Spenser's religion, see King's survey "Religion", in Es B. van (ed.), *A Critical Companion to Spenser Studies* (New York: 2006) 58–75. See also King J.N., *Spenser's Poetry and the Reformation Tradition* (Princeton: 1990).

[18] Gross K., *Spenserian Poetics: Idolatry, Iconoclasm and Magic* (Ithaca: 1985) 29.

own worst enemy'.[19] Noting disparaging marginalia in an early edition of the *Faerie Queene*, Stephen Orgel argues, 'Vices and virtues, villains and heroes often do look the same in the poem, and this is certainly part of its moral structure; but our Puritan reader also provides a good index to the degree to which Roman Catholicism remained an indispensable and genuinely troubling element in Protestant poetics, as in the Elizabethan religious imagination generally'.[20] My approach neither pinpoints Spenser's religious identity nor identifies his poetics strictly with a specific set, however broadly construed, of Reformation doctrines.[21] *The Faerie Queene* exists in a landscape described by Regina Schwartz and Deborah Shuger, one in which literary compensations replace lost sacramental forms in the wake of the Reformation. Shuger describes Renaissance poetry as the only medium capable of absorbing the energy and function of confession.[22] Schwartz investigates the literary return of the Eucharist in Milton and Herbert as an index of 'a persistent nostalgia for material presence' that articulates a 'hunger' for prohibited modes of sacramentality.[23] Spenser's hunger was not for a specific sacrament but for the corporeal and affective resources

[19] Kane S., *Spenser's Moral Allegory* (Toronto: 1989) 31.

[20] Orgel S., "Margins of Truth", in A. Murphy (ed.), *The Renaissance Text* (Manchester: 2000) 104. Orgel is not alone in associating a quasi-Catholic affiliation with the poetics of *The Faerie Queene*. Darryl Gless, in attempting to correlate Spenser's poetics and the wide array of Reformation doctrines, explores a series of theological struggles common to Protestants and post-Tridentine Catholics. See Gless D., *Interpretation and Theology in Spenser* (Cambridge: 1994). Harold Weatherby explains the apparently Catholic resonances in the poem with reference to the remnants of Augustinian theology, Greek and Latin patristic authors, and Greek Orthodox liturgy. See Weatherby H., *Mirrors of Celestial Grace* (Toronto: 1994).

[21] For a more literal examination of specific sacraments in Spenser's *Faerie Queene*, see *Reformation* 6 (2002) 103–178 for a special section, "Spenser's Theology".

[22] Shuger D., "'Gums of Glutinous Heat' and the Stream of Consciousness: The Theology of Milton's *Maske*", *Representations* 60 (1997) 16. 'By silencing confession', Shuger argues, 'the Reformation may have intensified, although it did not create, the felt disjunction between one's public identity and the unspeakably complex and strange inner creature known only to oneself [...] In post-Reformation England [...] the intimate movements of thought, desire, and flesh disclose themselves *only* in poetry, which thus functions – I think for the first time – as the primary cultural language of inwardness'.

[23] Schwartz R., "Real Hunger: Milton's Version of the Eucharist", *Religion and Literature* 31,3 (1999) 1–2. See also idem, "From Ritual to Poetry: Herbert's Mystical Eucharist", in Kessler M. – Shepherd Ch. (eds.), *Mystics: Presence and Aporia* (Chicago: 2003) 138–160. Schwartz also examines the lingering presence of the Mass and sacrificial theories of Christ's death in "Tragedy and the Mass", *Literature and Theology* 19,2 (2005) 139–158 and "*Othello* and the Horizon of Justice", ed. Schwartz R. (ed.), *Transcendence* (New York: 2004) 81–104.

adumbrated by the suffering, bleeding body of Christ. His challenge at the opening of *The Faerie Queene* was to articulate pain as an integral part of Holiness, succumbing neither to the temptations of violence endemic to epic-romance nor to narratives of militant Christian defense nor reducing suffering to a passive, aversive, or negative state. To do so, Spenser dramatizes the ramifications of the neutralization of the suffering of Christ in the wake of Reformation iconoclasm while championing pain as an index of the texture of lived experience and the ground of a sociality rooted in sympathy.

The tension between suffering and violence appears early in "The Legend of Holiness", as Spenser introduces his hero, the Redcrosse Knight, 'pricking on the plaine'. Among other figures that establish the active, even carnal, nature of Redcrosse is the horse that we see not only 'pricking' on the plain but also 'chid[ing] his foming bitt' and 'disdayning to the curbe to yield' (1.1.1). For John Calvin, the unruly horse describes the relationship between human passion and divine will: 'When [God] seeth that we be dull vpon the spurre, and that we be ouerslowe and restie: he muste needes pricke vs so much the more roughly: according as we commonly say, A rough horse must have a rough ryder'.[24] Calvin justifies human suffering as the necessary if painful goading of erring humanity; God as rough rider must break the disobedient steed. It is perhaps no surprise that Calvin makes this remark in the midst of a massive exegesis of *The Book of Job*. Suffering is merely the furnace in which the purity of the soul is tested, as in the case of gold; it is nothing in itself other than the display of obedience or disobedience. Regarding Job, the important thing for Calvin is God's function as 'our buckler and shielde, our wall and trench, our rampyre and bulwarke, our towre and fortresse'.[25] Calvin's conception leaves room not for the experience of pain but only for militant defense against depravity. Although Calvin wrote 159 sermons on *The Book of Job* and though Job may have suffered silently and stoically at first, his later ravings provoke condemnation: 'For Job raungeth out of his boundes and useth such excessive and outrageous talke, that in manie poyntes he seemeth a desperate person. And specially he so chafeth, as it seemth that we would even resist God'.[26] That even Job is a poor

[24] John Calvin, *Sermons on Job* (Edinburg: 1993) 27.
[25] Calvin, *Sermons on Job* 20.
[26] Calvin, *Sermons on Job* 1.

example suggests Calvin's hostility to representing bodies experiencing pain, bodies that should instead demonstrate obedience.[27]

If the suffering Job was eminently fallible and if the suffering Christ was increasingly unavailable, how might the experience of suffering be conveyed in a poem concerned with Holiness? This is precisely the question Spenser raises with the figure of the fallible Redcrosse, who is not merely a triumphant Christian hero caught in a Calvinist dialectic of masculine violence and victimization but rather a subject learning to experience pain. Redcrosse may be the martial man, a 'iolly knight [...] one for knightly giusts and fierce encounters fitt', but he is also a bearer of pain. His armor, 'wherein old dints of deepe woundes did remaine,/ The cruell markes of many' a bloody fielde' (1.1.1.) itself marks more than a contrast between experience and naïveté. Redcrosse must grow into the armor he wears, learning to endure and experience pain – his own and other people's. That is, he must not become hardened to it, as the Latin verb *indurare* might suggest; rather, he must bear up in the experience of pain in time. Redcrosse is, after all, named for the symbol he bears:

> And on his brest a bloodie Crosse he bore,
>
> The deare remembrance of his dying Lord,
> For whose sweete sake that glorious badge he wore,
> And dead as liuing euer him ador'd: (1.1.2).

Redcrosse pays homage to Christ as a crusading knight who defeats the opponents of Holiness wearing the traditional armaments of the patron of the Order of the Garter, Saint George. He is the hero of Christian epic: a martial saint. But his shield is not merely an abstract sign of Holiness. Rather, it reintroduces the suffering and salvific body of Christ in a way that was problematic for Orgel's Puritan annotator of *The Faerie Queene*, who tersely remarks in the margins of this passage, 'This is not the way to adore him'.[28]

The encounter with Fradubio represents another attempt to reintroduce the texture of suffering to a landscape denuded of corporeal and

---

[27] Thomas More, who found value in the suffering of Christ, saw Job differently: 'Now it is true [Tobias and Job] bore their calamities bravely and patiently, but neither of them, so far as I know, was exactly jumping with joy or clapping his hands out of happiness' (*The Sadness of Christ* [New York: 1993] 41–42).

[28] Orgel, "Margins of Truth" 103.

affective experience by heroic iconoclastic violence. Redcrosse has at this point shifted his allegiance from the pure Una to the duplicitous Duessa, with whom he makes a 'fair seemely pleasaunce'. In a clear echo of Una and Redcrosse's initial adventure in the wandering wood, the two seek respite from the sun, thus shifting from epic action to romance pleasure, from pricking on the plain to cooling in the shade. Here, Redcrosse endeavors to fashion an object of beauty, making for Duessa a garland. To fashion beauty, however, is to commit violence; as Redcrosse plucks branches from a tree, 'drops of gory bloud' pour forth from the 'rifte' of the wound (1.2.30). Redcrosse's attempt to adorn his lady with a beautiful thing of his own making turns out to be the forceful fashioning of another person's body and constitutes a form of violence with shocking consequences. Redcrosse's response to the 'piteous yelling voice' makes this clear: 'Astond he stood, and vp his heare did houe,/ And with that suddein horror could no member moue' (1.2.31). Redcrosse's horror closely resembles another scene of heroic masculinity's dis-identification with suffering: that of Aeneas faced with the voice of his slain companion and compatriot, Polydorus, whose blood pours from a myrtle tree Aeneas rends in order to consecrate an altar for the sake of a new Trojan settlement named after him. Redcrosse's initial paralysis embodies the shock of masculinity faced with a materiality that is neither docile nor silent; he faces instead the threat of the voice of another person's pain, which summons the hearer into a state of compassionate witness and prevents the gesture of heroic, nation-building self-assertion.

Redcrosse's paralysis derives from a particularly masculine lack of receptivity to pain; he experiences the pain of others as an obstacle or an assault. Just prior to this incident, Redcrosse wins the hand of Duessa from the Saracen knight in a battle that exposes the consequences of heroic violence. Redcrosse, 'prickte with pride/ and hope' (1.2.14), does not notice, as the narrator does, the consequence of his violent pricking, which (even prior to the battle) devolves on another body. In this case, his horse 'spurred fast' begins to bleed: 'adowne his coursers side/ The red bloud trickling staind the way, as he did ride' (1.2.14). Like the dwarf who bears Una's material 'needments', the horse, here, bears the suffering flesh on which the aggressive and sexual impulses of Redcrosse's 'pricking' depend. Though this moment foregrounds the suffering bodies on which masculinity depends and against which it exercises itself, the battle itself reveals the way a dedication to violence renders masculine subjects incapable of conceiving of suffering and the veritable outsourcing of pain (as labor) to the bodies of others. Redcrosse and Sans Foy fall on each with extraordinary vigor; they are

> daunted with theyr forces hideous,
>
> Their steeds doe stagger, and amazed stand,
> And eke themselues too rudely rigorous,
> Astonied with the stroke of their owne hand (1.2.15).

The two, like 'rams', pound one another, producing repeated concussive shocks and resulting bewilderment. These men, '[a]stonied both, stand sencelesse as a blocke' (1.2.16). Paralyzed, 'vnmoued as a rocke' the two hold 'idely,/ The broken reliques of their former cruelty' (1.2.16) violence incites idolatry as epic masculinity leaves 'reliques' of cruelty in its wake.

Despite the obliterating nature of violence, markers of suffering – such as the blood of Redcrosse's horse and the blood and voice of Fradubio – stain the landscape of "The Legend of Holiness". Fradubio insists upon his experience of pain, and in contrast to the shock of masculine violence, which produces stony insensibility, he assures Redcrosse of an intense if vegetative sensibility: 'For though a tree I seme, yet cold and heat me paines' (1.2.33). Redcrosse gets over his initial surprise once the 'dreadfull passion/ was ouerpast, and manhood well awake' (1.2.32), suggesting at first that masculinity is incompatible with the experience of either pain or compassion. He attempts to contain the potentially overwhelming experience of that suffering, trading the experience of pain for the experience of comfort by encouraging Fradubio to express himself in a cathartic narrative: 'He oft finds med'cine, who his griefe imparts;/ But double griefs afflict concealing harts' (1.2.34). Redcrosse uses a familiar language of suffering as that which can be purged from the body, cured as a disease, or conceived of in the logic of economy. To imagine a calculus in which pain is a quantity to be doubled or canceled would be to denude pain of the qualitative, experiential intensity that grounds Fradubio's capacity for both sensation and sentience.

Built into the narrative of Fradubio's fall – and the failure of masculinity – are the seductions of beautiful appearance, which produce violence and occlude suffering. Duessa, with her 'forged beauty' (1.2.36), entices Fradubio to battle another knight and win her hand. By virtue of her 'hellish science', Duessa then casts a 'foggy mist' over Fraelissa's beauty, which is not just dimmed but replaced with a 'foule vgly forme' (1.2.38). Fradubio's response is not just to shun but to destroy the seemingly grotesque Fraelissa. Without Duessa's restraint he 'would haue kild her' (1.2.39). Yet Fradubio discovers Duessa to be what Fraelissa seemed: a foul, deformed hag:

> Her neather partes misshapen, monstruous,
> Were hidd in water, that I could not see,
> But they did seeme more foule and hideous,
> Then womans shape man would beleeue to bee (1.2.41).

One might read the scene as a manifestation of Duessa's sinful carnality or of Spenser's misogyny or of both. But an odd interplay of seeing and seeming ambiguates the scene. The spectacularly gruesome genitalia of the hag Duessa were 'hidd' so that Fradubio 'could not see', yet they also 'seeme' to him plain in all their horror. Does Fradubio see Duessa as she is in a moment of revelation? Or does he see the manifestation of a woman's body as grotesque depravity? That this scene is constructed retrospectively suggests that Fradubio's 'vision' is a projection that compensates for the vulnerability that compromises heroic masculinity by shifting the burden of suffering to a figure of demonized, feminine materiality.

It is all too easy to dismiss Duessa as morally culpable or as the projection of a misogynistic culture. But what are we to make of the displacement of Fradubio's love, Fraelissa, who slips in and out of a narrative concerning the conflict between violent masculine subjectivities and the feminine materiality in which such subjectivities are rooted? We see in that displacement the emergence of sentimentality, which responds to beauty instead of pain. Just before Redcrosse encounters Fradubio, he allies himself to Duessa, having won her in combat and having experienced great pity for her (fabricated) tale of dispossession and exile:

> He in great passion al this while did dwell,
> More busying his quicke eies, her face to view,
> Then his dull eares, to heare what shee did tell,
> And said, 'Faire lady, hart of flint would rew
> The vndeserued woes and sorrowes, which ye shew (1.2.26).

To be sure, this is another instance of Duessa's duplicity, as she manipulates the compassion of a knight eager to rescue suffering damsels. Yet the real shock comes from the masculine psychology produced by the mingling of beauty and the *appearance* of suffering. Duessa is more attractive for not only having been 'won' in battle but for seeming to have suffered; her visual appearance alone consumes his attention, while his 'ears are dull' to the actual (dubious) tale. Masculinity of Redcrosse's variety seeks out feminine beauty either to win as a trophy through the exercise of force or to defend from the highly arousing violence of others. The suggestion of sympathy with masculine suffering, however, paralyzes Redcrosse. Fradubio's voice produces stony, insensate paralysis, as Redcrosse's hair literally bristles in defensive horror.

Redcrosse's failure to learn from Fradubio has less to do with moral turpitude than with an inability to genuinely and compassionately respond to the suffering of others, a problem especially keen for male, heroic subjects for whom identification with abject masculinity is all too real a possibility. Feminine objects of desire are easily rendered sentimental objects of pity, making suffering valid only when subsumed under the expression of the beautiful. Despite Redcrosse's failure to free Fradubio and Fraelissa, the episode closes with contrition:

> When all this speech the liuing tree had spent,
> The bleeding bough did thrust into the ground,
> That from the blood he might be innocent,
> And with fresh clay did close the wooden wound (1.2.44):

However naïve, Redcrosse's gesture is one of reparation and repair, as violated organic matter returns to nurturing earth. A previously implacable, silent tree gains a voice, a history, and, perhaps, a projected future. One might say that Redcrosse fashions, in this act of reparation, a living idol, as if bodies reduced by violence to stock matter may be returned to organic fecundity.

Redcrosse is, of course, distracted from real suffering and the possibility of reparation by a closing display of false suffering from Duessa. It is no surprise that Spenser might associate duplicitous suffering with Duessa. The surprise comes as Duessa becomes a figure of real suffering and a site of compassion in 'The Legend of Holiness' while the virtuous Una comes to exemplify sentimentality in which the alliance of compassion and beauty distracts from real suffering. Immediately following Duessa's false suffering, Una appears as an object of sympathy in the first eruption in *The Faerie Queene* of a tremulous narrative 'I':

> Nought is there vnder heau'ns wide hollownesse,
> That moues more deare compassion of mind,
> Then beautie brought t'vnworthie wretchednesse
> Through enuies snares or fortunes freakes vnkind:
> I, whether lately through her brightnes blynd,
> Or through alleageance and fast fealty,

Which I do owe vnto all womankynd,
Feele my hart perst with so great agony,
When such I see, that all for pitty I could die (1.3.1).

The obtrusive narrator affirms the dangerous link between compassion and beauty already present in the legend. Then, in a gesture that exceeds any moralizing rhetoric, the narrator identifies himself as an 'I' through an experience of painful sympathy with the suffering of Una. This suffering identification presents simultaneously the first narrative intervention in the body of the poem *and* a threat to the narrator's existence. The very writing of *The Faerie Queene* seems to be threatened by this sympathy: the narrator nearly 'steepe[s]' its 'lines with teares' (1.3.2). Such sentiments find extreme articulation in 'The Legend of Friendship'; there, the narrator's 'softened heart' makes him 'wish' his narrative 'neuer had bene writ' (4.1.1).

Of course, there may be something more than a little disingenuous about a work whose narrator plunges women into distress over and over again only to bemoan their constant peril. One might wonder, then, if this is not, rather, some variety of veiled sadism, in which a taste for the distress of vulnerable, beautiful women finds shelter in a histrionic display of sympathy. Yet the events of the canto depart nervously from this moment of heart-piercing compassion. The suffering Una is also the beautiful Una, whose beauty enables mastery. Having lost the protection of her knight-errant through Duessa's machinations, Una encounters a lion who desires 'to haue attonce deuourd her tender corse'. As these rhymes confirm, that desire is transformed by beauty, as Una 'his bloody rage aswaged with remorse' (1.3.5). Beauty 'maister[s] the most strong' just as 'simple truth' can 'subdue auenging wrong' (1.3.6).

Where beauty is involved, we come to learn, compassion becomes a degraded form of sentimentality that masks violence. Una's relationship to the lion succinctly demonstrates the displacement of violence from beauty. Una may continue on – vulnerable, humble, beautiful and true in her seemingly innocent wanderings *because* the lion provides not only protection but also enviable offensive capabilities of which she remains blissfully unaware. Indeed, as Una and the lion come to the home of the Catholic idolaters Abessa, Corecca, and Kirkrapine, the narrative emphasizes her weariness and need of shelter, as if to justify the lion's violence. Upon hearing nothing from the cottage of the idolaters, the lion rips open the home to allow Una entrance, thus terrifying the occupants, who huddle in the corner 'nigh dead with feare, and faint astonishment' (1.3.13). Having terrified her hosts, Una belatedly requests lodging for the night and then lies down to lament the loss of the Redcrosse Knight.[29] This is the consistent pattern of events; Una's suffering and weariness come to the fore in a narrative in which expressions of beautiful suffering are juxtaposed with outbursts of violence. The next idolater astonished by Una's lion is Kirkrapine (church rapine): the lion 'Vnder his Lordly foot him proudly hath supprest' (1.3.19). We return to the same discourse used to describe the proud beast that submitted himself to the weak Una, though the violence of lordly pride operates in her service as she weeps in a corner for her lost lord, oblivious to the ongoing slaughter:

> His bleeding hart is in the vengers hand,
> Who streight him rent in thousand peeces small,
> And quite dismembred hath: the thirsty land
> Dronke vp his life; his corse left on the strand (1.3.20).

The target of iconoclastic violence is not merely greed or the luscious trappings of Catholic worship. Rather, violence is directed against a familiar signifier of devotional adoration: the bleeding heart. Suffering, too, becomes the target of violence. Una sleeps through this dismemberment, waking the next morning to continue her search. Beauty proceeds ignorant of pain as violence, beauty's restless and disavowed unconscious, exerts gruesome force.

Beauty, posing as truth, becomes in Spenser's analysis the idolatry enabling and inciting iconoclastic violence, as is clear in the scene of Una's rescue at the hands of 'A rude, mishapen, monstrous rablement' of fauns and satyrs (1.6.8). Compassion for the beautifully suffering Una drives the action. As the troop comes upon the maiden they are captivated by her appearance:

> All stand amazed at so vncouth sight,
> And gin to pittie her vnhappie state,
> All stand astonied at her beautie bright,
> In their rude eyes vnworthy of so wofull plight (1.6.9).

[29] It is notable, as well, that in marking time in this canto, reference is made to the constellation Cassiopeia, thus suggesting the narrative of Andromeda, the damsel saved by Perseus, which provides a model for the legend of St. George. Thus, Una's vulnerability is stressed immediately following and immediately prior to extraordinary acts of violence committed on her behalf.

The repetition of 'amazed' intensifies our sense that Una's beauty – later referred to as 'beauty sovereign' – is at the heart of the problem here, as opposed to the extent to which these rude savages display the errors of primitive idolatry. Idolatrous beauty encourages sentimentality, in which one's sympathy ('compassion of her tender youth') becomes a source of pleasure. To be utterly absorbed in one's pity for others is, to be sure, a species of idolatry, one that encourages the representation of gorgeous and overwhelming spectacles of suffering of the variety Una experiences. As postures of suffering beauty incite idolatry, iconoclastic violence becomes all the more necessary. Beauty and violence are, for Spenser, sides of the same coin.

That retribution might be the secret heart of suffering Friedrich Nietzsche argues in *On the Genealogy of Morals*, where he claims that Judeo-Christian values come to be rooted in a slave mentality characterized by an inversion of values that valorizes weakness and suffering. The consequence is the 'submerged hatred, the vengefulness of the impotent' that produces a dangerous form of *ressentiment* lodged within an apparently meek exterior.[30] More recently Wendy Brown has parlayed Nietzsche's notion of *ressentiment* into the idea of a 'wounded attachment' whereby an identity or an entire community comes to be defined by the memory of past suffering, which lodges an intense *ressentiment* at the heart of those identities and communities, serving only to perpetuate violence and animosity.[31] While Brown refers to identity politics in the contemporary world of a liberal politics of toleration and multiculturalism, we might argue that the virulent zeal of iconoclasm conceals itself within the wounded attachment to Protestant obedience. Una demonstrates this in as much as she represents an early modern ethos depicted in William Tyndale's *The Obedience of a Christian Man* (1528), which advises believers to 'despise not the chastising of the Lord, neither faint when thou art rebuked by him. For whom the Lord loveth him he chasteneth: yes and he scourgeth every son whom he receiveth. [...] If ye be not under correction (whereof all are partakers) then are ye bastards and not sons'.[32] For Tyndale, as for Calvin, suffering is the sign of obedience to the will of God. One questions God no more than one questions the physician who causes pain to cure the

[30] Friedrich Nietzsche, *Basic Writings of Nietzsche* (transl. W. Kaufman) (New York: 2000) 473.
[31] Brown W., *States of Injury* (Princeton: 1995) 52–76.
[32] William Tyndale, *The Obedience of a Christian Man* (New York: 2000) 11.

patient, an analogy that reveals his attitude to the body: 'The surgeon lanceth and cutteth out the dead flesh, searcheth the wounds, thrusteth in tents, seareth, burneth, seweth, stitcheth and layeth corsies to draw out the corruption, and last of all layeth to healing plasters and maketh whole'.[33] While Tyndale aims at the health of the body, the violence of the methods reveals that though the body should not be 'killed' it should 'be tame'.[34] The only healthy body is a punished body. For all that the works of Nietzsche and Brown may, in their skepticism about suffering, make the project of attending to its experiential dimensions more difficult, they are themselves a product of intense suspicion about suffering consequent to the iconoclastic zeal of Tyndale and others.

Indeed, the dialectic of violence central to Tyndale has serious ramifications for a poetic project such as Spenser's. A consequence of the valorization of stern, divine, masculine violence is that, despite exhortations to suffer patiently without seeking revenge or relief, a veritable armory of retributive fantasies lurks behind the placid surface of obedient Christianity. Though Christians should follow 'the peaceable doctrine of Christ' and 'obey and suffer', they can hope that God will 'take vengeance of his enemies and shooteth arrows with heads dipped in deadly poison at them and poureth his plagues from heaven down upon them and sendeth the murrain and pestilence among them, and sinketh the cities of them and maketh the earth swallow, and compasseth them in their wiles and taken them in their own traps and snares, and casteth them into the pits which they digged for other men, and sendeth them a dazing in the head and utterly destroyeth them with their own subtle counsel'.[35] The logical end of Tyndale and Una's vision of Protestant truth is that it must utterly denude the body of its capacity for suffering or sympathy, both of which constitute idolatry. Tyndale's ultimate target is, not surprisingly followers of the Catholic faith, whose disobedience manifests itself, interestingly enough, as addiction to both pain and the imagination. Not only are Catholics all too wedded to penance 'after the example of Baal's priests which (3 Kings 18) cut themselves to please their God'. Like Calvin, Tyndale stresses the extent to which idolaters rely on 'the maliciousness of their own imaginations or inventions' and the visions of the crazed who 'do things which they

[33] Tyndale, *The Obedience of a Christian Man* 58.
[34] Tyndale, *The Obedience of a Christian Man* 133.
[35] Tyndale, *The Obedience of a Christian Man* 30.

of Bedlam may see that [...] are but madness'.[36] Imagination comes to be intimately associated with the suffering body, and as the imagination becomes the locus of idolatrous error, it becomes the primary route to the suffering body and to compassion for the pain of others.

Against a Spenserian poetics dedicated to conveying the enigmatic, lived experience of the flesh, whose texture is pain, and the enigmatic workings of sympathy, which is the basis of social life in *The Faerie Queene*, we see juxtaposed the transformation of the Redcrosse Knight into the ideal allegorical body of Protestant theology. Already, as Arthur rescues the Redcrosse Knight and hauls his body up from the dungeon of Orgoglio, Redcrosse is constituted as the abject, alien, suffering body of pre-Reformation theology. Hearing the woes of Redcrosse through an iron door, Arthur, like Polydorus and Redcrosse before him, experiences disorientation:

Which when that Champion heard, with percing point
  Of pitty deare his hart was thrilled sore,
  And trembling horrour ran through euery ioynt,
  For ruth of gentle knight so fowle forlore (1.8.39):

The danger of compassion inheres in a threat to the inviolable masculinity of subjectivity, a masculinity threatened by the conflation of sufferer and witness. Heroic masculinity responds, as Arthur does, with defensive violence: 'He rent that yron dore,/ With furious force, and indignation fell' (1.8.39). While Arthur spares neither 'long paines' nor 'labors manifold' to draw Redcrosse from the dark pit of his prison, he remains unable to contemplate the spectacle of suffering masculinity and abstracts the scene, reading suffering in a crudely allegorical way:

This daies ensample hath this lesson deare
Deepe written in my heart with yron pen,
That blisse may not abide in state of mortall men (1.8.44).

Despite that carnal figure of words and lessons written 'in [the] heart with yron pen', Arthur avoids the distasteful suffering of the Redcrosse Knight hauled up from the dungeon just as so much post-Reformation theology avoids the suffering Christ. The body is replaced with the moral lesson it teaches, allowing Arthur to avoid an encounter with the pain of another.

---

[36] Tyndale, *The Obedience of a Christian Man* 27; 45.

The peril of identifying with suffering flesh, as in the narrative commentary on Una's suffering, is not, of course, limited to the narrator or to heroic knights. Even Una, who engineers the rescue of the Redcrosse Knight, must be purged of pain. Despite her resolve to wander patiently in search of him, an overpowering and physical grief overpowers her. Coming upon Redcrosse's abandoned arms and hearing some report of her lord from the dwarf, Una collapses, her very body seeming to flicker in and out of appearance: 'Yet might her pitteous hart be seene to pant and quake' (1.7.20). Indeed, later the dwarf must bring Una back from a deathlike swoon and make the 'flitted life' return to 'her natiue prison' (1.7.21). When she meets Arthur, she speaks in 'bleeding words' and must be convinced by him to exorcise her dark and troublesome passion, bringing her to the rule of right reason. In an oddly pat exchange, we see again pain rendered manageable by articulation, as Arthur encourages Una to narrate her grief despite her inclination not to:

> But griefe (quoth she) does greater grow displaid,
> If then it find not helpe, and breeds despaire.
> Despaire breeds not (quoth he) where faith is staid.
> No faith so fast (quoth she) but flesh does paire.
> Flesh may empaire (quoth he) but reason can repaire (1.7.41).

Conceived as a prison, Una's troublesome body, not only in spite of but in opposition to her pain, must be ruled by reason, which is what Arthur offers in the form of this advice. The excessive, repetitive speech tags in this dialogue ('quoth he', 'quoth she') are particularly of note. As William Flesch points out in a recent article, the lack of typographic conventions for the quotation of reported speech lends extra function and interest to speech tags.[37] Here they serve to emphasize the stifling regularity and marked predictability of the nuggets of wisdom that follow. Spenser stresses in this little dialogue the way in which Una and Arthur bring the bleeding words of pain into a safer economy, one that depends on semantic, prosodic, and formal structures to discipline Una's wayward and unreliable body. Likewise the rhyming repetition – 'paire', 'empaire' and 'repaire' acts to render pain reasonable. For Una, the body is a prison that suffering renders feeble and unreliable. But just

[37] Flesch W., "The Poetics of Speech Tags", in Rasmussen M.D. (ed.), *Renaissance Literature and Its Formal Engagements* (New York: 2002) 159–184.

at the moment Una finally gains a body through suffering Redcrosse's loss, Arthur draws her back to the ineffable realms of truth, reason, and light. He seeks out the dark wound of Una's suffering, convinces her to 'disclose the breach', and brings it to light in order to exorcise it, all the while acting the part of Tyndale's physician.

The surgical precision with which Arthur excises Una's grief offers considerable contrast to the canto's singular moment of visceral compassion, which comes as Duessa throws aside her rich garments to mourn Orgoglio:

> Such percing griefe her stubborne hart did wound,
> That she could not endure that dolefull stound,
> But leauing all behind her, fled away (1.8.25):

It is not danger or capture Duessa flees but a 'stound', which is the doleful reverberation of Orgoglio's passing. If earlier Duessa feigned suffering to ensnare the Redcrosse Knight and distract him from the tale of Fradubio and Fraelissa, here she casts aside objects of beauty and power, losing the opportunity to escape as grief pierces her stubborn, recalcitrant heart. We might remember the efforts of Duessa to save her previous consort Sans Foy, nearly slain by Redcrosse. Duessa distracts Redcrosse and conceals Sans Foy's body to prevent 'his thirsty blade/ To bathe in blood of faithlesse enimy' (1.5.15). As Redcrosse's wounds are tended and '*Duessa* wept full bitterly' (1.5.17), the narrator interrupts to comment on the lure of false grief:

> As when a wearie traueiler that strayes
> By muddy shore of broad seuen-mouthed *Nile*,
>
> Vnweeting of the perillous wandering wayes,
>
> Doth meete a cruell craftie Crocodile,
> Which in false griefe hyding his harmefull guile,
> Doth weepe full sore, and sheddeth tender teares:
> The foolish man, that pitties all this while
> His mournefull plight, is swallowed vp vnwares,
> Forgetfull of his owne, that mindes anothers cares (1.5.18).

The stanza's opening suggests a moralizing comparison that oddly misses its mark. What does the simile refer to? Who is the crocodile? Duessa's grief is not, in fact, false, even if she often is. Furthermore, Duessa is, at this moment, powerless to harm anyone. She is, rather, overly concerned with the harm that has befallen Sans Foy. Redcrosse is not even privy to her grief – no less victim to it. Indeed, it is far too late for the knight of Holiness, who has already been taken in and who cannot, for the moment, think of anything but killing infidels. It seems unlikely that this warning would be addressed to the reader, as Spenser goes on to narrate Duessa's great labor to bring Sans Foy back to life. Tortured by grief, she descends into the underworld, into the ancient realm of 'grisly Night'. Duessa elicits sympathy from the dread Night:

> Her feeling speaches some compassion mou'd
>
> In hart, and chaunge in that great mothers face:
> Yet pitty in her hart was neuer prou'd
> Till then: for euermore she hated, neuer lou'd (1.5.24).

Despite the warning to beware crocodiles and their false tears, the narrative gives us no reason to doubt Duessa's pain. Her grieving display performs the miraculous feat of drawing feelings of compassion from the previously inaccessible heart of Night. Pain wells up from a dark cosmogony attended by Duessa, whose compassion brings life to a mortally wounded body. In one of the many ironies of the *Faerie Queene*, Duessa briefly becomes the locus of genuine sympathy in "The Legend of Holiness", as if her material duplicity were the only place for suffering and compassion to lodge given the denuded, excoriated body of Protestant theology.

Like her compassion for Sans Foy, Duessa's oddly touching grief for Orgoglio is also dismissed upon her defeat. Duessa is, on Una's insistence, stripped to reveal 'her misshaped parts'. Fradubio's misogynistic fantasy is at last fulfilled in the revelation of the nether parts of 'a loathly, wrinckled hag, ill fauoured, old' (1.8.46). She is, as has been much noted, a monstrous mix of bestial pieces. Her disgusting appearance, minutely anatomized, reveals the monstrosity of flesh and alludes to earlier instances of gross carnality: breasts 'lyke bladders lacking wind', from which 'filthy matter' wells, and 'skin as rough, as maple rind' (1.8.47). Duessa bears the burden of female matter, a burden made more palpable in the experience of pain. Whereas Arthur could dig into Una's pain and, with emphatic reason, scourge any taint of suffering physicality, Duessa combines features from the monster Error (in her grossly productive genitalia), the wood of Error (in her rough skin), and Orgoglio (in his bladder-like body).[38] Duessa

[38] That this is maple rind reminds us of the opening catalogue of trees, of course, and the characteristic of the maple that is 'seldom inward sound'.

embodies the taint of sinful matter and thus is subject to violence; she can be stripped, demonized and cast out. That is her function in "The Legend of Holiness". After crude flesh has been banished, the heroes may enjoy the spoils of Orgoglio's castle: 'Where store they fownd of al, that dainty was and rare' (1.8.50). Marking the transition from the moment of Redcrosse's greatest physical need, the sustenance offered to him comes as a banquet replete with choice foods, thus enforcing the distinction between the gross substances associated with Duessa and the ethereal beauties associated with Una.

Arthur's moralizing commentary, along with the stripping of Duessa, marks the beginning of the reclamation of the Redcrosse Knight and his transformation into the allegorical body of Protestant theology. In the House of Holiness, his 'dainty corse' is arrayed in ashes and sackcloth. He fasts and prays constantly. His wounds swell up and 'the superfluous flesh' is treated to hot pincers, the 'iron whip' of Penance, the sharp 'prick' of Remorse, the stinging salt water of Repentance, all of which are allegorical operations that aim at rendering the dark matter of the body obedient. In the dungeon of Orgoglio and the House of Holiness alike, we find those 'curious and problematic texts' described by Shuger in which the collision of Protestant Passion narrative and martyr discourse display 'their ambivalent fascination with revenge, torture, and the dialectics of male violence and victimization'.[39] These acts of purification strikingly intermingle a Catholic rhetoric penance with the discourse of torture common to accounts of martyrdom so effectively deployed by English Protestants. Moreover, they anticipate a phenomenon Walter Benjamin associates with baroque aesthetics, when 'martyrdom prepares the body for emblematic purposes'.[40] As Julia Reinhard Lupton emphasizes, 'Baroque martyrology [...] did not use emblems to represent torture so much as it used the disarticulating apparatus of torture to carve up the body into material for emblems'.[41] The violence inflicted in the House of Holiness, that veritable factory of bodily obedience, runs counter to devotional practices of suffering rooted in the *imitatio Christi* that predate the Reformation. In his study of voluntary flagellation, Niklaus Largier discusses practices of self-mortification stretching from early Christianity through the Counter-Reformation in which pain served not just to mortify the flesh but to

[39] Shuger, *Renaissance Bible* 12.
[40] Benjamin W., *Origins of German Tragic Drama* (London: 1977) 217.
[41] Lupton J.R., *Afterlives of the Saints* (Stanford: 1996) 42.

enliven it, awakening thoughts, feelings, and the imagination, making 'real pain and suffering into the foundation of an imaginary unity with Christ'.[42] In place of 'the connection of pain with the absolute affirmation of life embodied by Christ as God-man', the House of Holiness delivers the emblematic body of Protestant theology. At the end of his scourging, Redcrosse encounters Contemplation, who represents the result of such discipline:

> There they doe finde that godly aged Sire,
> With snowy lockes adowne his shoulders shed,
> As hoary frost with spangles doth attire
> The mossy braunches of an Oke halfe ded.
> Each bone might through his body well be red,
> And euery sinew seene through his long fast:
> For nought he car'd his carcas long vnfed;
> His mind was full of spirituall repast,
> And pyn'd his flesh, to keepe his body low and chast (1.10.48).

The bones and connecting sinews read clearly as if the body were a holy X-ray. Contemplation presents the ideal body of the burgeoning science of anatomy, a discipline that, however important to the history of medicine, demonstrates the consequence of ideologies that render the body a source of evidence or knowledge communicated visually: ocular proof requires dissection. Contemplation is no more than the carcass of a half-dead tree, a starved and obedient Fradubio. Suffering sentience, replaced by discipline, leaves behind the palest form of allegory.

The representatives of truth, goodness, and beauty must purge themselves of pain and its representative physicality, creating Reformed bodies. The burden of pain must therefore be outsourced, lodging in the bodies of the enemies of Protestant truth. At the close of "The Legend of Holiness", the dragon is at once the goading engine of heroic violence and the recipient of this burden of experiencing and expressing pain. The dragon, struck once,

> cryde, as raging seas are wont to rore,
> When wintry storme his wrathful wreck does threat,
> The rolling billowes beat the ragged shore,
> As they the earth would shoulder from her seat,
> And greedy gulfe does gape, as he would eat
> His neighbour element in his reuenge (1.11.21).

[42] Largier N., *In Praise of the Whip* (New York: 2007) 64.

Pain becomes a deafening and unintelligible noise as its catastrophe threatens to engulf its surroundings in 'a gushing riuer of blacke gory blood' (1.11.22). Yet even the dragon's fire causes temporary harm to a Redcrosse increasingly impassive, impervious, or miraculously restored in the face of pain. As Redcrosse sheds his searing armor as if it were a troublesome layer of flesh, the narrative shifts from his experience of pain to the memory of heroic labor:

> Not that great Champion of the antique world,
> Whom famous Poetes verse so much doth vaunt,
> And hath for twelue huge labours high extold,
> So many furies and sharpe fits did haunt,
> When him the poysoned garment did enchaunt
> With *Centaures* blood, and bloody verses charmd,
> As did this knight twelue thousand dolours daunt,
> Whom fyrie steele now burnt, that erst him armd,
> That erst him goodly armd, now most of all him harmd (1.11.27).

Little trace remains of the shock of sympathy that briefly passes between Redcrosse and Arthur in the dungeon of Orgoglio. Instead, the comparison between Redcrosse and Hercules highlights competition: a quantification of the violence (twelve thousand dolors, like twelve labors) withstood by the warriors. The pain of Hercules' temporally extensive labors is compressed here into the annihilating instantaneity of fiery violence. The medieval and early modern association of Christ with Hercules further indicates an occlusion of Christian suffering by heroic violence.

The suspended, suffering Redcrosse in Orgoglio's dungeon has no place here, where the martial comes to the fore in the exercise of righteous violence.

The defeat of the dragon is the defeat of the idolatry constituted by experiences of suffering and sympathy. These experiences are replaced by the virtuous violence of a martial Christianity, for which the fall into sinful, suffering flesh constitutes the wounding incursion of the past on the present that justifies righteous combat. The wounded past is redeemed by present violence. Yet if the *telos* of the Book of Holiness was never in question, the aftermath of the fight, featuring, as it does, the body of the victor and the vanquished, raises questions about the idolatry of violence. While the court celebrates Redcrosse's victory, a crowd – 'the raskall many ran,/Heaped together in rude rablement' – surrounds the victor and all admire him with 'gaping wonderment' (1.12.9). It seems even citizens of Una's righteous kingdom constitute a naïve and unsophisticated rabble prone to idealizing and idolizing a Christian conqueror. Their 'gaping wonderment' smacks of the same stupefaction produced by the violent beauty of Una unveiled.

If Redcrosse himself spurs a potentially idolatrous following, the body of the dragon, marked by violence, inspires fascination. When we hear the crowd is dismayed with 'ydle fear' we must take the word 'idle' seriously. In one sense, the dragon is dead and the people's fear unwarranted. The aftermath of the battle's spectacular violence fascinates these spectators, even though the object of fascination is an immobile corpse:

> Some feard, and fledd; some feard and well it faynd;
> One that would wiser seeme, than all the rest,
> Warnd him not to touch, for yet perhaps remaynd
> Some lingring life within his hollow brest,
> Or in his wombe might lurke some hidden nest
> Of many Dragonnettes, his fruitfull seede;
> Another saide, that in his eyes did rest
> Yet sparckling fyre, and badd thereof take heed;
> Another said, he saw him moue his eyes indeed.
>
> One mother, whenas her foolehardy chyld
> Did come too neare, and with his talants play
> Halfe dead through feare, her litle babe reuyld,
> And to her gossibs gan in counsell say;
> How can I tell, but that his talants may
> Yet scratch my sonne, or rend his tender hand.
> So diuersely them selues in vaine they fray;
> Whiles some more bold, to measure him nigh stand,
> To proue how many acres he did spred of land (1.12.10–11).

"The Legend of Holiness" begins by asking what it is to experience suffering. It closes by asking how we witness and respond to violence. Thomas A. Prendergast suggests that the 'idolatrous seductions of violence' are a central concern for *Beowulf*, noting that, like much heroic poetry, the poem 'unfolds as an idolatrous memorialization of the pleasures of violence, a pleasure compulsively repeated in the very language of the text'.[43] A core concern for *Beowulf* is the potentially unstoppable cycle of retribution aided by compulsive iterations or memories of violence. Indeed, as René Girard argues, 'Vengeance [...] is

[43] Prendergast T.A., "'Wanton Recollection': The Idolatrous Pleasures of *Beowulf*", *New Literary History* 30 (1999) 130.

an interminable, infinitely repetitive process'.[44] Spenser's rabble believes that at any moment the beast could spring back to life and spawn new dangers, as if a host of offspring lay in wait to pour forth from its body. Even the admittedly hysterical mother of Spenser's passage recognizes a real, if not a literal, threat. The community that assembles here at the close of the legend comes together in victory, and their unity is marked most by a fascination with spectacular violence and its gory aftermath. The very attempt to 'measure' the dragon, to quantify its body, runs counter to the way bodies are experienced (how they suffer and live) or imagined (this is, after all a dragon) in the way anatomy creates knowledge through the disarticulation of bodies; to see their physical truth, they must be cut apart. Contemplation, then, is not merely a spiritual state to attain but a worldview requiring the sacrifice of imagination and lived experience for the rigor of moral discipline.

In the Old English devotional poem "The Dream of the Rood", the rood in question is that tree hewn into the cross on which Christ was crucified. Like Fradubio, it bleeds and speaks, which frightens the narrator of the poem. The rapturous glory provoked by the tree, bedecked with treasure and witnessed by hosts of angels, is inseparable from the suffering that marks it, rendering stock, hewn matter a living, speaking tree. While the poem imagines Christ as a hero and in the terms of Anglo-Saxon warrior culture, such militancy is never isolated from suffering. Fradubio reminds Redcrosse of the centrality of an active, engaged experience of pain, one so thoroughly alienated in the wake of the Reformation that suffering appears as if in a dream or in the remnants of mythic and literary inheritance, where it is the task of the imagination to return to the body its sense of lived experience through pain, emblematized in the flow of blood from a speaking tree. No trees bleed or speak in the landscape of Contemplation, and all the dragons have been slain, for the iconoclastic fervor of Reformation iconoclasm wills the reduction of complexity of thought, feeling, and imagination to a state of passive, obedient witness in the face of extreme violence. Such violence is hypnotic, whether in the form of the beautiful or the grotesque, in the delicacy of Una's progress or in the convulsions of the dragon's death and its morbid aftermath. If there is not merely a critique of violence in "The Legend of Holiness", which there surely is, then there is also, in the experience of lived embodiment so centrally

[44] Girard R., *Violence and the Sacred* (Baltimore: 1977) 14.

embedded in Spenser's poetics, a form of resistance. The familiar features of *The Faerie Queene*, those very features that seem to render Spenser difficult, obscure, nostalgic, or conservative, are the stylistic correlatives of an alternative Spenserian modernity – the nearly hypnotic rhymes of the Spenserian stanza, the shudderingly visceral style, the willfully antiquated language, the patterns of repetition, variation, and dilation. We might construe such features as a response to the willful excision of history 'at the heart of the Edwardine reform', including 'the necessity of destroying, of cutting, hammering, and scraping, or melting into a deserved oblivion the monuments of popery, so that the doctrines they embodied might be forgotten'.[45] Spenser may have written as 'a generation was growing up which had known nothing else, which believed the Pope to be Antichrist, the Mass a mummery, which did not look back to the Catholic past as their own, but another country, another world'.[46] At the same time, that other country, that other world lingered in traces of pre-Reformation corporeal habits and ethical sensibilities that comprise the substance and experience of Spenserian holiness. Faced with the alienating violence of Protestant iconoclasm, Spenser locates in fairyland and in the fabric of poetry a world in which what it means to suffer, to sympathize, or to socialize – even the capacity to experience ourselves, each other, and the world around us – might be excavated from the fantastic archaeology of national and religious history in order to be imagined anew.

[45] Duffy E., *The Stripping of the Altars* (Yale: 1992) 480.
[46] Duffy, *The Stripping of the Altars* 593.

Selective Bibliography

ASTON M., *England's Iconoclasts* (Oxford: 1988).

BELLAMY E., "The Broken Branch and the 'Liuing Well': Spenser's Fradubio and Romance Error in *The Faerie Queene*", *Renaissance Papers* (1985) 1–12.

BENJAMIN W., *Origins of German Tragic Drama* (London: 1977).

BROWN W., *States of Injury* (Princeton: 1995).

CALVIN JOHN, *Sermons on Job* (Edinburg: 1993).

CHENEY D., *Spenser's Images of Nature: Wild Man and Shepherd in 'The Faerie Queene'* (New Haven: 1966).

DUFFY E., *The Stripping of the Altars* (Yale: 1992).

FLESCH W., "The Poetics of Speech Tags", in Rasmussen M.D. (ed.), *Renaissance Literature and Its Formal Engagements* (New York: 2002).

GIRARD R., *Violence and the Sacred* (Baltimore: 1977).

GLESS D., *Interpretation and Theology in Spenser* (Cambridge: 1994).

GROSS K., *Spenserian Poetics: Idolatry, Iconoclasm and Magic* (Ithaca: 1985).

HUME A., *Edmund Spenser: Protestant Poet* (Cambridge: 1984).

HOUGH G., *The First Commentary on 'The Faerie Queene'* (privately published, 1964).

KANE S., *Spenser's Moral Allegory* (Toronto: 1989).

KENNEDY W., "Rhetoric, Allegory, and Dramatic Modality in Spenser's Fradubio Episode", *English Literary Renaissance* 3 (1973) 351–368.

——, "Fraubido", in Hamilton A.C. (ed.), *The Spenser Encyclopedia* (Toronto: 1990).

KING J.N., "Spenser's Religion", in Hadfied A. (ed.), *The Cambridge Companion to Spenser* (Cambridge: 2001) 200–217.

——, "Religion", in Es B. van (ed.), *A Critical Companion to Spenser Studies* (New York: 2006).

——, *Spenser's Poetry and the Reformation Tradition* (Princeton: 1990).

——, *English Reformation Literature: The Tudor Origins of the Protestant Tradition* (Princeton: 1982).

KNAPP J., "Spenser the Priest", *Representations* 81 (Winter 2003) 61–78.

LARGIER N., *In Praise of the Whip* (New York: 2007).

LEWIS C.S., *The Problem of Pain* (New York: 2000).

LUPTON J.R., *Afterlives of the Saints* (Stanford: 1996).

LUXON T., "'Not I, But Christ': Allegory and the Puritan Self", *English Literary History* 60 (1993) 899–937.

MALLETTE R., *Spenser and the Discourses of Reformation England* (Lincoln: 1997).

MORE T., *The Sadness of Christ* (New York: 1993).

NEILL K., "The Degradation of the Red Cross Knight", *English Literary History* 19 (1952) 1013–1032.

NIETZSCHE FRIEDRICH, *Basic Writings of Nietzsche* (transl. Walter Kaufman) (New York: 2000).

ORANGE L.E., "Sensual Beauty in Book I of *The Faerie Queene*", *Journal of English and Germanic Philology* 61 (1962) 555–561.

ORGEL S., "Margins of Truth", in Murphy A. (ed.), *The Renaissance Text* (Manchester: 2000) 91–107.

PHILLIPS J., *The Reformation of Images* (Berkeley: 1973).

PRENDERGAST T.A., "Wanton Recollection': The Idolatrous Pleasures of *Beowulf*", *New Literary History* 30 (1999) 129–141.

QULLIGAN M., *The Language of Allegory* (Ithaca: 1978).

SCARRY E., *The Body in Pain* (Oxford: 1985).

SCHWARTZ R., "Real Hunger: Milton's Version of the Eucharist", *Religion and Literature* 31,3 (1999) 1–18.

——, "Tragedy and the Mass", *Literature and Theology* 19,2 (2005) 139–158.

——, "*Othello* and the Horizon of Justice", Schwartz R. (ed.), *Transcendence: Philosophy, Literature and Theology Approach the Beyond* (New York: 2004) 81–105.
——, "From Ritual to Poetry: Herbert's Mystical Eucharist", in Kessler M. – Shepherd Ch. (eds.), *Mystics: Presence and Aporia* (Chicago: 2003) 138–161.
Scott S.C., "From Polydorus to Fradubio: The History of a Topos", *Spenser Studies* 7 (1986) 27–57.
Shroeder J.W., "Spenser's Erotic Drama: The Orgoglio Episode", *English Literary History* 29 (1962) 140–159.
Shuger D., *The Renaissance Bible* (Berkeley: 1994).
——, "Gums of Glutinous Heat' and the Stream of Consciousness: The Theology of Milton's *Maske*", *Representations* 60 (1997) 1–21.
Spenser Edward, *The Faerie Queene* (ed. A.C. Hamilton, 2nd ed.) (London: 2007).
Tyndale William, *The Obedience of a Christian Man* (New York: 2000).
Weatherby H., *Mirrors of Celestial Grace* (Toronto: 1994).

BODIES IN PAIN AND THE TRANSCENDENTAL ORGANIZATION OF HISTORY IN JOOST VAN DEN VONDEL

Frans Willem Korsten

> For we are in need of pleasure only when we are in pain because of the absence of pleasure, and when we are no in pain, then we no longer need pleasure.
>
> And this is why we say that pleasure is the starting point and goal of living blessedly.
>
> – Epicurus, *Letter to Pythocles*

Introduction

I want to start by proposing that we take seriously the fact that pain is related etymologically to Latin *poena* (punishment, fine, indemnification, or sorrow) and that the Latin *poena* in turn goes back to Greek *poinè*, which could also mean retaliation or compensation. If we do so, pain becomes, firstly, not something you have, but something you get in return for, or as a consequence of something. It is, therefore, always related to a history. Secondly, you suffer pain for a reason. In this respect, and by implication, the notion of pain may be related to notions of justice. Consequently, in the light of *poena* and *poinè*, pain can be defined within the frames of history and justice as either something that is inflicted on you for a justified reason, because of things that happened in the past, or as form of payment, as a matter of justice, in relation to the future. With regard to these two possibilities, so I will argue in what follows, the Christian conceptualization of pain acquires new meanings in relation to the physical body of subjects and in relation to a more elusive politico-cultural body that not only transcends history, but also directs its course (it should be noted that I am not referring to divine transcendence here, but to that what transcends the particularity of a historical situation). In Christianity the infliction of bodily pain is considered to be necessary for the just organization of history, or the production of just history. That is to say: bodily pain is used to fuel the propelling force of society's politico-theological organization through time. It is this dimension of pain that is investigated in several plays by Joost van den Vondel, Holland's most famous seventeenth-century playwright, who lived from 1587 to 1679.

What may have caused Vondel's concern with the relation between bodily inflicted pain and the realization of a somehow 'just' history? First of all, he lived in a country that had seen many bodies in pain in its recent history. Seemingly endless atrocities had taken place in the context of an uprising against the king and a violent suppression of that revolt. Additionally, the Low Countries experienced several forms of civil strife or violent social tensions. Ultimately the Northern Low Countries waged a full-scale war against the mighty empire of Spain. This had all happened in the name of different forms of Christianity. What was at stake has often been described as a particular social, political, cultural, or, indeed, religious conflict in which the States of the Low Countries fought for their freedom. As such, the entire conflict can be located in a specific historical moment, and the pain it embodied can remain restricted to its own era. My hunch, however, is that Vondel, who was enormously troubled by the incessant violence and its historical recurrence, traced a more fundamental problem in the construction of Europe's politico-cultural 'house'. It was a problem that transcended the historicity of particular circumstances and that concerned the *necessity* of a historically particular pain for the realization of the one righteous history. Such a history could acquire its transcendental quality only when the particularity of bodily pain could be transposed to a general politico-cultural body, as if the politico-cultural body of a society was in pain through time, in order to preserve its shape and direction. In addition to addressing the pains of his time, then, Vondel was very much concerned with this latter form of pain as well.

In what follows I will take a closer look at three plays in which Vondel explores the question of whether, in order to realize a 'right' kind of history, bodily pain is necessary for the transposition of pain to a politico-cultural body.[1] The first play, *Gysbreght van Aemstel*, was written by a middle-aged Vondel at the peak of his career in 1637. It was

[1] The texts can be found in Vondel's *Collected Works*, edited by J.F.M. Sterck *et al.*, but also online at www.dbnl.org/letterkunde/goudeneeuw. For my readings of the plays I made use of my previous work in *Vondel belicht: voorstellingen van soevereiniteit* (Hilversum: 2006), which will be published in English in the course of 2009.

written for the opening of the first official city theatre of Amsterdam. The second play, *Leeuwendalers*, was written in 1647 to be performed as part of the festivities surrounding the signing of Europe's first collective peace treaty, that of West Phalen, in 1648. The third was written at a very high age, when Vondel's texts had come to play only a marginal role in the society of the Dutch republic. His *Noah* was never performed and went unnoticed in 1667. In their own peculiar way, these are radical plays that contain highly disconcerting elements for Christians of any denomination. In fact they embody powerful arguments against the dynamics of pain I described above.

Martyrdom, Rape and Just History

One Christian view of the relation between pain and just history is famously captured by the dictum that 'the blood of martyrs is the seed of the church', which must be one of the more wrongly attributed quotes in the history of modern scholarship. Tertullian, who is always referred to as the author of this dictum, actually states that 'semen est sanguis christianorum',[2] rather than 'sanguis martyrum semen christianorum'. Still, the latter phrase is so well known and important that it was even included in the testament of the late Pope John Paul II. And it must be said: although Tertullian's actual statement may be slightly different ('blood is seed for Christians') he is indeed referring, at this moment in his text, to the blood of martyrs. In fact he is discussing the struggle of the church against the pagans as a just war that eventually will be won because the blood of martyrs is like seed.

The dictum *semen est sanguis Christianorum* is a wonderful combination of metaphor, synecdoche and metonymy (for those who may be misguided by the arrangement of words in the Latin: although 'semen' comes first, 'blood' is the subject of the verb). Through synecdoche the blood of martyrs stands for the martyrs themselves. Through metonymy the martyrs who stand at the origin of the church shift into the glorious church that will be established later. Synecdoche comes in again where these martyrs are already part of the young church and, as such, represent the whole. By extension, the entire church can be

---

[2] Tertullian, *Apologeticum*, ed. Oehler F., rev. Glover T.R., <www.tertullian.org/latin/apologeticus.htm> L.13, accessed 15 January 2008.

seen as a martyr, and that is a clear message to the faithful. Finally, strengthened by a metonymical shift that connects seed and blood or blood and seed, and built upon the synecdoche that the blood is part of the martyrs, a simile is established that likens martyrs to human seed. They will have off-spring. The more Christian blood is shed, the more off-spring, and the more populous and powerful the church will become, so Tertullian wants it.

Hidden behind the density of synecdoche, metaphor and metonymy, there is one new conceptualization of pain, and possibly two. Pain is not just inflicted upon the body. It is something that will in time prove to be productive, or it is a means of *buying something back*, as Tertullian explicitly states in the immediate context of the quote.[3] To be sure, the etymological meaning of *poena* and *poinè* already implies some kind of compensation, but there the pain is meant to compensate others. That is to say: pain is a form of payment. In the case of Christianity, however, if pain is inflicted because of one's faith, it is an investment from which the 'owner' of the pain can profit over time, and this does not just hold for the individual self, but also for an entire community. This option is distinctly different from that put forward by Giorgio Agamben in his *Homo sacer*, who holds that the sufferer is somehow needed to establish a community. The second new Christian conceptualization of pain is established when pain is projected *through time* from particular bodies to a more general politico-cultural body, thus producing the truth of the Christian faith, and buying the faithful the ultimate, future victory of the Christian church – or, even more generally, of the Christian *civitas*.

Apart from history, there is also justice at stake. Discussing the power of martyrs in relation to the law, the legal theorist and lawyer Robert Cover puts it succinctly:

> Law is the projection of an imagined future upon reality. Martyrs require that any future they possess will be on the terms of the law to which they are committed (God's law). And the miracle of the suffering of the

[3] Tertullian states: 'ubi accessit, pati exoptat, ut totam dei gratiam redimat, ut omnem veniam ab eo compensatione sanguinis sui expediat?' (*Apologeticum* L, 15). Alexander Souter translates this as: 'who when he has joined us, does not eagerly desire to suffer, that he may buy back the whole favour of God, that he may procure all indulgence from him by the payment of his own blood ?' (Tertullian, *Tertullian's Defence of the Christians against the Heathen*, trl. A. Souter <www.tertullian.org/articles/mayor_apologeticum/mayor_apologeticum_07translation.htm> accessed 15 January 2008.

> martyrs is their insistence on the law to which they are committed, even in the face of world-destroying pain.[4]

In relation to history and Christian martyrs, pain is that which is needed to ground and fuel the projection of the future history and world of the *civitas dei* as a reality, and it is meant to start it, and then continue it, as the only true and righteous 'nation'. Hence, pain is not so much related to the destruction of language or a world, as Elaine Scarry argues in her famous study *The Body in Pain*, but to the production of a new body, a new world and a new language. In this context, it is not hard to see how Tertullian's remark about martyrs ultimately goes back to the martyr of martyrs, Christ himself, who, through his pain, also produced, or bought us, the ultimately new and just history. What is remarkable here, is that the foundation of that new order is not realized through violence, a mechanism that Walter Benjamin explored so intensely in his *Zur Kritik der Gewalt*, but that a new order is built upon the very subject that underwent violence and was in pain (which was, of course, what disturbed Nietzsche so much).

Both martyrdom and Tertullian's dictum are pivotal to Vondel's *Gysbreght van Aemstel*. The play deals with events that had occured in the actual history of Amsterdam. The major protagonist of the play, Gijsbreght van Aemstel, is based on a historical figure with the same name, who lived in the thirteenth century and was one of the most powerful vassals under count Floris V. The latter was a perhaps cunning, but also power-hungry figure who wanted to centralize his administration and expand his possessions. As a consequence, he wanted no real power underneath him. He deliberately ignored the rights of his major vassals, and even raped the wife of one of them: Machteld, the wife of Geeraerdt van Velsen. The latter then rose against his lord, with the help of his father in law, Herman van Woerden, and with the uncle of Machteld, Gijsbreght. The three captured Floris, with the intention of either delivering him to the English king, who was to judge him as a peer, or to the States of Holland, who were to judge him as the ultimate sovereign body. But Floris was immensely popular with the common folk, who marched against Geeraerdt's castle when they heard of Floris' capture. The three lords then tried to flee with their victim, but got stuck in a fen – where Geeraerdt decided to kill Floris

[4] Cover R., *Narrative, Violence, and the Law: The Essays of Robert Cover*, ed. Minow M. *et al.* (Ann Arbor: 1997) 207.

on the spot. This became the root of long-lasting tensions, some of which resulted in the siege of Amsterdam, Gijsbreght's city. This siege is where the play starts – on Christmas eve.

At the beginning of the play we are informed that the siege has unexpectedly been lifted. For no clear reason the troops from neighbouring counties and cities have left the stage, and Gijsbreght sighs with relief that God, in his justice, has finally shown mercy to the people of his beleaguered citadel. To anyone familiar with the battle of Troy, the signs are telling. Of course, the troops did not really leave; a small group of enemy soldiers is hiding just outside the city in a ship with firewood – and firewood is what the citizens of the city are in dire need of in the midst of winter. The ship is hauled inside the walls, and during the night the band of soldiers escapes and opens the gates, and the enemy troops pour in. A ruthless battle ensues, in which almost the entire city goes up in flames. The enemy troops slaughter whomever they meet, and rape the women, even nuns. Finally Aemstel has to retreat to the last remaining stronghold: his castle. At first Gijsbreght shows every desire to become a martyr in a struggle for justice, but he is then called back by his wife who tells him to flee the city with all remaining survivors. This is what he eventually decides to do. The play ends with his safe escape to a land of milk and honey elsewhere.

The play is one of the most frequently studied plays by Vondel. As Johan Koppenol states, almost nothing is what is seems in *Gysbreght*.[5] Whereas the opening sentence refers to the justice of God and the protection by God, this is followed by a complete subversion of divine justice and protection in the rest of the play. With the exception of Koppenol, most scholars have seen this as an example of God's sovereignty and inscrutability. Jan Konst, in a study on *fortuna, fatum* and *providentia dei* in the Dutch tragedies between 1600 and 1720, puts God's actions with regard to Gijsbreght's city under the heading of 'The Meaningfulness of Divine Rule' ('Zinvolheid van het Godsbestuur'). Others explain how God's behaviour is understandable in the light of Amsterdam's future.[6] The city had to be destroyed in order to rise

[5] Koppenol J., "Nodeloze onrust: Het 'roomse karakter' van Vondels *Gysbreght van Aemstel*", *Nederlandse letterkunde* 4,4 (1999) 313–329.

[6] Konst J.W.H., *Fortuna, Fatum en Providentia Dei in de Nederlandse tragedie 1600–1720* (Hilversum: 2003); Maljaars A., "'Niet min Godvruchtelijck als dapper': Gijsbrecht van Aemstel verdedigd tegen zijn critici", *De zeventiende eeuw* 17,2 (2001) 138–163; Smit W.A.P., *Van Pascha tot Noah: een verkenning van Vondels drama's naar continuiteit en ontwikkel-*

gloriously from its ashes. This, of course, leaves the question of why it had to be destroyed in the first place. In relation to this question, others state that the play contains a warning, a kind of collective 'memento mori', to the powerful and glorious Amsterdam of 1638.[7]

It is surprising that, although some scholars have mentioned one of the rapes in the play, none of them so far has pointed out that rape may be *the* central theme of the play. Hence the infliction of pain is a central theme.[8] That theme is introduced at the start of the play, in Gijsbreght's very first monologue, when he describes how Floris raped his niece. At the beginning of the third act, Gijsbrecht's wife Badeloch has a short nap, in which she has a dream. In that dream her niece Machteld appears. She does not appear as a spirit from heaven, however, but as a distinctly earthly woman. Badeloch sees the pained woman she has known, mutilating herself because of the pain inflicted upon her. She speaks with a hoarse voice and is very much concerned about the fate of her daughter, Klaeris, who is abbess of the cloister outside the city walls. She fears that history will repeat itself and advises everybody to flee.

Gijsbreght immediately dismisses the dream as a chimera: 'It is nothing but deceit imagined by the brain' (l. 824).[9] Yet Gysbreght's illusion that the city is safe is instantly broken by someone who runs in and shouts that the enemies have entered in the city. Meanwhile the question is why the text should emphasize that Machteld did not appear as a heavenly spirit, but as the raped and pained woman she was, and somehow still is. She very much resembles the city of Amsterdam, that

---

ing in hun grondmotief en structuur, vols. I, II, III (Zwolle: 1956–1962); Smits-Veldt M.B., "Inleiding", *Joost van den Vondel, Gysbreght van Aemstel* (Amsterdam: 1994).

[7] Koppenol, "Nodeloze onrust"; Parente J.A., "The Theatricality of History in the Dutch Golden Age: Joost van den Vondel's *Gysbreght van Aemstel*", in Hermans Th – Salverda T. (eds.), *From Revolt to Riches: Culture and History of the Low Countries 1500–1700 – International and Interdisciplinary Perspectives* (London: 1993) 255–267.

[8] Smits-Veldt, in her important new edition of the play, does not mention any of the rapes in her summary of the play. Studies that do not address the issue of rape are Knuvelder G.P., *Handboek tot de geschiedenis der Nederlandse letterkunde*, vol. 2 ('s-Hertogenbosch: 1971) 338–342; Smit W.A.P., *Van Pascha tot Noah: een verkenning van Vondels drama's naar continuïteit en ontwikkeling in hun grondmotief en structuur* (Zwolle: 1956–1962) vol. I; Stipriaan R. van, "Gysbreght van Aemstel als tragische held", *De zeventiende eeuw* 12 (1996) 359–377. The remarkable silence on this topic may be caused by the fact that rape is a matter of 'inscription and erasure', as Higgins and Silver have it (Higgins L.A. – Silver B.R. [eds.], *Rape and Representation* [New York: 1991] 2). Once inscribed it remains hard to speak about it.

[9] ''t Is louter ydelheid, die zich het brein verbeeld.' (l. 824).

is compared by the chorus to a virgin woman after the first act, and is described there, in a highly ambiguous context, as a virgin who is raped:

> To the honour of God, who on his throne
> Is seated, so high and lordly;
> From where he could see, how full of desire,
> The county of Sparen vied for of Amstel's crown.
> How revenge with swords and spears
> Wanted to trim the tower-crown from the head
> Of the beautiful and renowned city,
> And wanted to wrest away by violence of hordes
> The citadel's girdle from her loins
> And plunder her jewel and treasure
> And violate the honourable and faithful
> Like the rapist of the lady of Velzen (*Gysbreght*, l. 417–428).[10]

The desire to sing of God's glory is evoked in the first line, yet gives way to a detailed description of God's high throne as an excellent vantage point for observing, without intervening, the rape of the city virgin of Amsterdam, explicitly compared here to Machteld van Velzen.

Politically, rape is intrinsic to some conceptualizations of sovereignty.[11] Many conceptualizations of sovereignty since Jean Bodin provide an implicit or explicit motivation for rape of individual women, but more prominently of metaphorical women such as cities, counties, nations, or of Justitia herself. The key characteristic of the ultimate sovereign is that he may act at will, and enforce at will. This is explicitly addressed in the play. In the opening monologue Gijsbreght describes Floris V as such a kind of sovereign. His rape of Machteld is a symbolic act to demonstrate and inscribe his supreme power. Machteld is the wife, the daughter and the niece of Floris' major vassals. It is this act that

---

[10] 'Tot lof van God, die op zijn' troon/ Gezeten is, zo hoog en heerlijck;/ Van waar hy zien kon, hoe begeerlijck/ Het Sparen stack na Aemstels kroon./ Hoe wraeck met zwaerden en met speeren/ De torenkroon van 't hoofd wou scheeren/ Der schoone en wijd vermaerde stad,/ En rucken door geweld van benden/ Der vesten gordel van haer lenden/ En plondren haer kleenood en schat;/ En schenden d'edele en getrouwe/ Gelijck de schender Velzens vrouwe' (*Gysbreght*, l. 417–428).

[11] The starting point of considering rape as a distinctly political act was Brownmiller S., *Against Our Will: Men, Women and Rape* (New York: 1975). For studies of the theme of rape in literature, see Saunders C., *Rape and Ravishment in the Literature of Medieval England* (Cambridge: 2001) and Wolfthal D., *Images of Rape: The 'Heroic' Tradition and its Alternatives* (Cambridge: 1999).

Gijsbreght describes as the motivating factor of what ensued later. It all started

> With Floris' lustful breast, and the shameful embracing
> And raping of my niece, that beautiful flower from Velzen;
> The insult against the nobility, the infliction of its Right,
> Which he had sworn on with his own mouth (*Gysbreght*, l. 113–116).[12]

Two kinds of infliction are addressed here, and shift into each other. The rape of Machteld shifts into the rape of the rights of the nobility – rights that Floris with his own mouth had sworn to uphold. Consequently the rape acts politically in two ways. It is a symbol of Floris' sovereignty, but also provides the noblemen with a reason for rising against him. In other words: rape is the engine propelling the history that develops in the play. Yet that development is not so much a development, but rather a repetition.

Machteld, in Badeloch's dream, advises everyone to flee. She fears the repetition, that, as it turns out, will indeed take place. Gijsbreght's sister Kristijn is pulled out of a church by her hair by Witte of Haemstede, a bastard son of Floris, who enters the cloister of Klaeris a little later, smothered with blood (l. 1416).[13] In the cloister, he first kills the bishop who had sought refuge there, and when Klaeris faints on the bishop's corpse, he rapes her. Then, however, she awakens, and moans:[14]

> my bridegroom, see how I suffer here below,
> And how I am violated. O pure virgin Mary!

[12] 'Uit Floris geile borst, en 't schandelijck omhelzen,/ En schennen van mijn nicht, die schoone bloem van Velzen;/ 't Verongelijcken van den adel, in zijn Recht,/ Bezworen met zijn' mond' (*Gysbreght*, l. 113–116).

[13] Parente states that Vondel's concept of history is cyclical, and hence pessimistic (Parente, "The Theatricality of History" 256). Although I agree that repetition is an important element in Vondel's plays, I question whether it is appropriate to refer to repetitions as cyclical. Rather, Vondel concerns himself with repetition and difference, as both *Gysbreght* and *Leeuwendalers* demonstrate.

[14] Smits-Veldt shows how the play is further complicated when we consider how the way in which Gozewijn is slaughtered resembles the pagan slaughtering of the white sacrificial ox (Smits-Veldt M.B., "Vondels *Gysbreght van Aemstel* onder de loep: twee gevallen van tekstinterpretatie", *Spektator* 17,5 [1988] 380–396). Things become even more complex if we consider that the actor playing Gozewijn was Willem Ruyters, a notorious figure (and drunkard) – also drawn by Rembrandt, see Dudok van Heel S.A.C., "Willem Bartel(omeu)sz Ruyters (1587–1639) Rembrandt's bisschop Gosewijn", *Amstelodammer* 66 (1979) 83–86.

> O Clara, do you behold this? Lady Machteld, see your child (*Gysbreght*, l. 1477–1479).[15]

Klaeris is suffering and calls upon Christ, her spiritual bridegroom, the virgin Mary, Saint Clara, and her mother. This apostrophe is a felicitous one, here, for it allows Klaeris not just to be the rapist's victim, but also to remain a subject whose infliction and pain is acknowledged by the ones she loves.

Note that Klaeris does not call upon on God – who was described by the chorus after the first act as a neutral onlooker who does not intervene when innocent people are raped and slaughtered. This is emphasized once more when, after the third act, the chorus describes the slaughter of the children of Bethlehem, apostrophizing the biblical figure of Rachel, whose tomb lies next to the road to Bethlehem. Her ghost now roams the fields to see what is happening. The chorus asks her to stop crying for her dead, slaughtered children because:

> Your children die like martyrs
> And firstlings of the seed
> That is beginning to grow from your blood
> And that will flower gloriously in honour of God
> And that no cruelty will destroy (*Gysbreght*, l. 946–950).[16]

This is very similar to Tertullian's dictum, yet with a significant twist. Here it is Rachel's blood that will feed the seed. That seed is not human semen but the seed of flowers. Instead of Tertullian's more economic imagery of investment and success, we have an imagery that emphasizes joy and glory. Nevertheless, here, too, the pain inflicted on particular bodies will be transformed into a force that transcends historical particularity, that 'will not perish'. However, instead of continuing cruelty, this force will be able to resist cruelty, and this is another crucial difference with Tertullian, who needs new blood to form new seed.

We may conclude that the play at least addresses Christianity's remarkable conceptualization of pain and suffering as inflicted in particular circumstances, and then, transcendentally, geared productively towards a glorious future. This is not the same as the pain and suffering

[15] 'mijn bruidegom, zie neder hoe ick lije,/ En hoemen my schoffeert. o zuivre maeghd Marije!/ O Klaere, aenschouwtghe dit? vrouw Machtelt, zie uw kind' (*Gysbreght*, l. 1477–79).

[16] 'Uw kinders sterven martelaeren,/ En eerstelingen van het zaed,/ Dat uit uw bloed begint te groeien,/ En heerlijck tot Gods eer zal bloeien,/ En door geen wreedheid en vergaet' (*Gysbreght*, l. 946–950).

that are somehow fitting for fallen humanity, whose existence on earth cannot be other than painful. That pain corresponds to the punitive aspect of *poena*. In contrast, the pain and suffering of Christians is productive and will not just be a kind of investment with revenues in the future, but will also *direct* history to the ultimate victory of the church. In other words, the infliction of pain is aimed at a distinct historical goal that is considered to be *just*.

It is remarkable, however, that the play does not endorse this option, since Gijsbreght and his wife Badeloch do not offer themselves as willing martyrs. They have ample opportunity to do so but they *refuse*. They even refuse to accept the repetitive pain of history, that is caused by the politico-cultural body in pain, and that continues to re-fuel history. They flee elsewhere to start a new life. What does this mean in relation to Vondel's ideas on the transcendental transformation of pain? Let me turn to the second play, *Leeuwendalers*, and focus more specifically on the element of pain and justice.

Eternal Debt and Pain, or an End to the Suffering

The plot of *Leeuwendalers* is based on a dynamic of violence and pain. The play is an allegory depicting the struggle between the northern and southern Low Countries. Because they have kept fighting amongst themselves, the gods have become angered. In the name of the gods a high-priestess called Velleede has therefore punished the inhabitants of *Leeuwendaal* (*Lionvalley*, allegorically indicating the area of both the northern and southern Low Countries). Each year, a youngster from the North or South must be chosen by lot as a sacrifice. He is tied to a tree, after which Wildeman (Wild Man) comes to shoot an arrow through his heart. This has continued for twenty years.

The play takes place on the day the lots are drawn. Hageroos (Rosebush), a beautiful orphan girl, is so troubled by the annual sacrifice that she is hunting a white stag, which she wants to offer as a replacement. By contrast, Adelaert (Noble Nature), the adopted son of the lord of the South, does not care much about the impending sacrifice, since he is hunting Hageroos instead. Nevertheless, as one might have expected, he is eventually chosen as this year's scapegoat. He is tied to the tree and Wildeman appears. But then Hageroos jumps before him and refuses to go away. When Wildeman decides to shoot an arrow through both hearts then, the god Pan suddenly intervenes. He orders that enough blood has been spilled, or rather, he wants no more spilling of his own blood. Pan disappears, leaving the puzzled onlookers behind. Hageroos' old foster-mother reveals that Hageroos is the grandchild of Pan, that is to say that she is his own blood.

Pain plays a role explicitly when the gathered community complains and wails in fear of the required sacrifice, and the lord of the country addresses them as follows:

> You pious citizens, may Pan spare you for a long time
> And hoist your happiness to the top in the course of the years.
> It pains us to see you in such a woeful state.
> The cows are eating grass and clover in the fields;
> You are eating your own heart, crushed as if by hoops
> Of steel [...] (*Leeuwendalers*, l. 477–482).[17]

Here it appears as if the citizens are in pain because they are paining themselves: 'eating their own heart'. In part this is surely the case; after all, it is they who fight each other incessantly. Yet, as often happens in his plays, these lines are complicated by Vondel's use of metaphor. First, there is a contrast with the natural lives of cows that are not, apparently, troubled by pain. But there is also a shift from the particular to the transcendental: cows are contrasted with the one heart of the politico-cultural body. The artificiality of the citizens' position is emphasized by the claim that they are eating their own heart. Moreover, it is as if the heart is being tormented by hoops that keep it together painfully and forcefully. Who is the agent that has tied the hoops around the heart, thus transposing the pain of a particular situation to a pain that acts through time?

It is of interest, in this light, that the pain and suffering produced by the conflict in Leeuwendaal do not accord with what the gods want. Nevertheless, they seem to add to the pain and suffering by means of the annual sacrifice which they have decreed. At the beginning of the play, Hageroos' foster-mother, who fled Leeuwendaal because of the incessant wars, and who now has returned, asks why these lands have to suffer so much. One of the characters, a blind common crier, answers her as follows:

---

[17] 'Ghy vrome burgers, lang moet vader Pan u spaeren,/ En haelen uw geluck in top met uwe jaeren:/ Ons jammert u te zien zoo jammerlijck gestelt. De koeien eten gras en klaver, langs het velt;/ Ghy eet uw eigen hart, beknelt gelijck met hoepen/ Van stael' (*Leeuwendalers*, l. 477–482).

> We are celebrating this day, this feast, not in honour of any man
> Nor thoughtlessly, but because of a verdict, yes, to appease the gods,
> And to offer them a man, in order to prevent greater evil.
> Already the quarrels in Leeuwendaal had risen highly
> And the earth had drunk the blood of the field gods,
> When Velleede advised us by word of her own mouth
> To present to this Wildeman, whom father Pan had sent us,
> A young man, chosen arbitrarily by lot,
> As a target of God's anger and as a form of repentance
> (*Leeuwendalers*, l. 48–56).[18]

The argument appears confused, partly because so many different gods are in play at the same time. First there are 'the gods' in general; then there are the 'field gods', a clear sign that we are dealing with classical gods, and this is affirmed when Pan enters the field. But then, in the final line we meet a distinctly Christian God, with a capital G. The sacrifice and the pain which it brings operate differently in relation to these different Gods. In relation to the gods of line 49, the sacrifice is meant as a payment in advance, a form of barter: suffering serves to present even heavier burdens. Then with Pan, the element of arbitrariness comes in: it does not matter what particular young man is sacrificed. But with the Christian God, the sacrifice and pain become a form of retribution, a repaying of a debt.

The latter element is crucial in the Christian context. It is not for nothing that Christianity has been described as a system that operates through eternal debt. In his study on violence, Slavoj Žižek describes the difference between the Jewish God and the Christian one as follows:

> Usually, it is Judaism which is conceived as the religion of the superego and of man's subordination to a jealous, mighty and severe God, in contrast to the God of mercy and love who is Christian. However, it is precisely through not demanding from us the price for our sins, through paying this price for us himself, that the Christian God of mercy established himself as the supreme superego agency: 'I paid the highest price for your sins, and you are thus indebted to me *for ever*.'[19]

---

[18] 'Wy vieren dezen dagh, dit feest, geen' mensch ter eere,/ Noch reuckloos, maer door last, ja Godtheên tot een' zoen,/ En offren haer een' man, om erger te verhoên./ Het Leeuwendaelsch krackeel was reede hoogh geloopen,/ En d'aerde had het bloet der Ackergoôn gezopen,/ Wanneer Velleede ons riedt met haren eigen mont,/ Voor dezen Wildeman, dien vader Pan ons zondt,/ Een' Jongelingk, by keure en lotinge uitgekoren,/ Te stellen, tot een wit en boete van Godts toren' (*Leeuwendalers*, l. 48–56).

[19] Žižek S., *Violence: Six Sideways Reflections* (London: 2008).

In other words, the suffering and the pain of Christ were so inconceivably great that human beings will have to repay for ever. Consequently, they will be in pain for ever.

Vondel, however, again offers a radical alternative through his play. The blind common crier also suggests that the system of retribution could come to an end, although he does not understand as yet how this could be the case. People have asked the high-priestess Velleede,

> But she can only comfort us with ambiguous riddles
> That Pan will cure the prolonged suffering
> When the wild bow will aim at his heart (*Leeuwendalers*, l. 68–70).[20]

At the end of the play, this riddle will be solved. Hageroos will prove to be the daughter of the son of Pan, and therefore made of his known flesh and blood. She is, metonymically, his own heart. But there is also the shift from the particular human body to the larger body of the transcendental god, whose name, tellingly, is *Pan*, and whom the orator in the preface has described as all-transcending. When Wildeman aims at the heart of this particular human being, he also aims at the heart of all. He who embodies 'all' then decides that the suffering must stop. In this way, Pan does exactly the opposite of the Christian God. He does not install a system of eternal debt and eternal pain, but of life's exuberance. In this way, the play can end on a description of a country that knows nothing but prosperity and fullness: 'The cows are giving milk and cream,/ It is all butter to the bottom. Everyone sings of PEACE and HARMONY, PEACE and HARMONY.'[21]

Does this mean that Vondel is implying that the politico-cultural body can do without pain? Does it mean that he therefore rejects the wilful infliction of pain on particular bodies as the fuel of a transcendental history? Let me turn, finally, to Vondel's very last play. Although he published some translations afterwards, *Noah* can be considered as Vondel's artistic testament. In it we will again meet a joyful world without sacrifice, but this time that world will be destroyed. As we will see, *Noah* presents how the Christian organization of history is distinctly

[20] 'Maer zy vertroost ons slechts met dubbelzinnigheden,/ Dat Pan genezen zal de langgeproefde smart,/ Wanneer de wilde boogh hem micke naer zijn hart' (*Leeuwendalers*, l. 68–70).

[21] 'De koeien geven melck en room./ Het is al boter tot den boôm./ Men zingt al PAIS en VRE.
PAIS en VRE' (*Leeuwendalers*, l. 2018–2021).

political and how, in relation to this, God's violence is the opposite of divine violence. Let me turn to the organization of history first.

Pain, Memory and Joy

Noah is subtitled *or the ruin of the first world*,[22] and indeed, ruined this world is. Consider this description, which is given by the arch-shepherd, one of the last to see a world disappear:

> You comfort yourself, but to no avail, if you think that high mountains
> Will allow you to escape this curse, in a little wood, an oak tree,
> But by a storm and the strong current, these are being
> Destroyed, and torn away from their roots and soil.
> The towers are collapsing, pressed together as dust and cement.
> Thousands of dead corpses, animals, cattle, are floating there,
> And drowned people, going, swirling, from here to there,
> And major buildings, and roofs, farms, houses.
> The resistance of dams, dikes and sluices does not count.
> The mother is trying to save her off spring, the father his son,
> But it is all too late, for one can only hear one sound
> Of wailing, spread all over the eddying of the waters.
> Now the music of wedding parties is silent, this rejoicing, laughing, roaring,
> Is rapidly being de-formed into a dreadful, icy moaning.
> The drowning bride, dies in the tired arm of her bride groom.
> The last left-over, a horde of deadly ghosts,
> scrambling on the mountains, panting heavily, tries, whilst climbing,
> to save its soul, but the grim ocean
> fuelled by revenge, horrifies the pale moon,
> who sees the waves, like a bladder full of wind, surge.
> The highest mountain top sinks in the water for more than fifteen ells.
> Thus, everything that lived on the ground of the earth sinks.
> The crying turns into silence, as soon as this all utters its final breath (*Noah*, l. 1032–1054).[23]

[22] Joost van den Vondel, *Noah, of ondergang der eerste weerelt* (1667).

[23] 'Gy troost u, och vergeefs, en waent op hooge bergen/ Dien vloek t'ontvlughten, in bosschaedje en eiken boom:/ Maer och die worden door den storm, en sterken stroom/ Verdelght, en afgerukt van hunnen gront en wortel./ De torens storten in, geplet aen gruis en mortel./ Daer drijven duizenden van dooden, dieren, vee/ En drenkelingen heene, in 't ronde, in 't lang en breê,/ De hooftgebouwen en de daeken, hoven, huizen./ Hier gelt geen wederstant van dammen, dijken, sluizen./ De moeder pooght haer vrucht, de vader zijnen zoon/ Te redden, och te spa, men hoort al eenen toon/ Van jammeren, gespreit op 't zwalpen van de wateren./ Nu zwijght de bruilofts-galm, dat juichen, lachen, schateren/ Wort snel misschapen in een ysselijk gekarm./

This passage does not present a fixed visual perspective: we move from the close-up of a bride dying in the arms of her bridegroom to a panorama of the drowning world seen from the moon. Past and present fold and unfold, turning the sounds of roaring laughter into that of roaring waves. Life and death intertwine, from the panting sounds of the last souls still alive to their ultimate end in silence. The highest mountains are described in relation to elements that suggest a typically Dutch, flat and low-lying landscape, with dams and dikes and sluices. Meanwhile, in the end, this is the representation of a massive destruction, an entire world in pain, hopelessly struggling upward to preserve the last tiny particle of life. Meanwhile also, please note that it is not just human kind that is being punished and in pain. It is an entire world in pain – a world in which 'everything that lived on the ground of the earth' is destroyed. Before our eyes, happiness is being de-formed or 'mis-shaped', as the original text has it, into misery.

Of course, when the play informs us that 'everything that lived on the ground of the earth' was destroyed, we know this is not the case. There's also this huge boat, crammed full with a small family of human beings and the entire collection of living beings on the planet, preferably in the form of two representatives, male and female. Throughout European history, this boat has been seen as a symbol for the Church; accordingly, the fresh start after the flood must be understood spiritually. Such a spiritual reading is explicitly affirmed, but also complicated, at the end of the play, when the disobedient souls are addressed 'that taunted God's goodness/when the ark was built'. The ark is described as

> A prefiguration of the church, in which you will save
> Those entrusted to you, as in a free citadel,
> Through the water, the prefigured bath as the only means of
> Grace that can wash the stain from the soul (*Noah*, l. 1579–1583).[24]

De bruit verdronken, sterft in 's bruigoms moeden arm./ Het uiterste overschot, een drom van dootsche schimmen,/ Aen 't klautren op 't geberght, pooght hygende, onder 't klimmen,/ Haer ziel te bergen: maer de grimmige oceaen,/ Gedreven van de wraek, verschrikt de bleeke maen,/ Die ziet de golven, als een blaes vol wint, opzwellen./ De hooghste berghkruin zinkt in 't water vijftien ellen./ Aldus verzinkt het al wat op den aerdtboôm leeft./ 't Geschrey wort stom, zoo dra het al dien dootsnik geeft' (*Noah*, l. 1032–1054).

[24] 'Godts goetheit tergende, toen d'ark wert toebereit;/ Een voorbeelt van de kerk, waerin gy uw vertrouden,/ Als in een' vryburgh, door het water zult behouden,/ Het afgebeelde badt en eenigh middel van/ Genade, die de smet der ziele afwasschen kan' (*Noah*, l. 1579–1583).

The play suggests that the freshness of the new world is deceptive: the world has not been washed clean once and for all. On the contrary, it needs the recurrent water of baptism to wash it clean time and again.

One reason for this repetition is that the new world will not start without memory. One need only think, here, of the possibility of a new world without a memory of the flood. That flood would then be literally a matter of pre-history: something irretrievably lost in an unknown and unknowable past. However, as the description makes clear, the pain of the ruined world can still be felt, and *must* still be felt. On the hand, then, the pain can be located in history as produced by, and the result of a particular event. As such, it is the object of what has been called 'common' memory, from which a collective memory can arise. Yet from that moment on, the pain is taken up, as in a boat, by a politico-cultural body. It then becomes the object of what has been called *deep* memory. This pain is not the object of a narration from an external point in time from which one remembers, but can still be sensed as an active pain.[25] The pain of past destruction may fuel the production of a distinct kind of history only insofar as it is still felt and still presents itself – as a pain not just different from past suffering but propelled away from it, while preserving itself as the same.

Paramount in trauma studies has been the way in which painful traumatization results in a kind of freezing, both of traumatized subject and of history, as if subjects remain caught in history.[26] Partly in contrast, painful infliction, in the Christian context, serves to move history, turning it into just history and directing it towards a just end. Therefore, throughout its development, that history has to be kept in check, and pushed towards its end. This is where people indeed remain caught in a history that has a transcendental force. Yet we have seen that Vondel also appears to go against this way of dealing with pain, in relation to the justness of transcendental history. In order to put this in sharper focus, we will have to move back in time, to the way in which Vondel represents history before the flood.

Urania is queen of the world in which Noah is the prophet of doom. The queen carries the name of the muse of astronomy, and by

---

[25] On these different kinds of memory, see Alphen E. van, *Art in Mind: How Contemporary Images Shape Thought* (Chicago: 2005) 170.

[26] Alphen E. van, *Caught by History: Holocaust Effects in Contemporary Art, Literature and Theory* (Stanford: 1997).

implication she represents the *kosmos*. *Kosmos* means a total system in a state of harmonious order, as opposed to *kaos*. The connotations of ornamentation in *kosmos* also indicate that this is a pleasurable, beautiful system. The world that queen Urania rules is such a system: full of love, beauty and a certain peace. As her classical name, Urania, indicates, the world before the flood is a pagan one, in which Christianity is embodied by the figure of Noah. However, the first voice that speaks in the play marks *a difference within*. Apollion, also known as Lucifer – the figure of evil within Christianity – speaks first, and describes this world as completely harmonious. The reason for this harmony is

> That since heaven's revenge drove the first father
> From Eden, with a sword of lightning rays, this
> World remained unharmed by curses belched forth.
> Here the sweet taste finds everything that man lusts to find:
> Pleasure-grounds, grassy banks, brooks, wells, everywhere.
> The fruits are dripping from the branches into the mouth
> And melt on the tongue. The birds are singing and warbling.
> The dancing, the playing, the unending banqueting,
> The marrying: the entire year is pregnant with it.
> One binds no souls to whatever kinds of laws, to no force
> Of Enochs example, to no commands or interdictions (*Noah*, l. 65–75).[27]

The reason that this world is so harmonious, then, is that no more divine curses have been 'belched forth'. In Apollion's eyes, God is the evil one, whose curses ended the first harmonious state of being in paradise, which was not a world yet. Since then, there have been no more curses, and as a result this first world – and the implication of the term 'world' is that history has become possible – is in a state of harmony.[28] This is also because the life-world is not bound to any kind of law, not even a divine law. Urania's world is far from lawless, yet it

---

[27] 'Want sedert 's hemels wraek den eersten vader dreef/ Uit Eden, met een zwaert van blixemstralen, bleef/ Dees weerelt ongeschent van uitgebraekte vloeken./Hier vint de snoeplust al wat 's menschen lust loopt zoeken,/ Lusthoven, beemden, beek en bronnen in het ront./ De vruchten druppen van de takken in den mont,/ En smilten op de tong. de vogels quinkeleeren./ Het dansen, speelen, het gedurigh banketteeren,/ En bruiloften gaet hier het gansche jaer in zwang./ Men bint de zielen aen geen wetten, en bedwang/ Van Enochs voorbeelt, of geboden en verboden' (*Noah*, l. 65–75).

[28] The editorial gloss in Vondel's *Collected Works* offers a different view. Commenting on the phrase 'curses belched forth', it explains that 'the devils [...] have not been able to cause much disaster, that is to say: material damage'. The editors apparently had difficulty in accepting the implications of the words 'belches forth'. That is to say, they could not accept the idea that the viewpoint of the devil is presented here *in its own right*.

is not ruled by an absolute sovereign. If they do anything at all, Urania and her husband Achiman 'let be', or take care that everything stays as it is. But before elaborating on the different kinds of sovereignty that are at stake, and the differences in modalities of history, let me first focus on the 'difference within' embodied by Apollion.

Apollion's words resonate strongly with the description that Adam gives in another play by Vondel, *Adam Expelled* (1664), which Vondel saw as forming a trilogy with *Lucifer* and *Noah*. In *Adam Expelled*, although it is Adam who is speaking, the reference to the Apollion passage is remarkable. One could, of course, argue that, there, an as yet uncorrupted Adam speaks, whereas here the devil is speaking. Yet this would not do justice to both the complex nature of speaking subjects and of the artistic text. The aesthetic power of the Apollion passage resides in the fact that it is so ambiguously tempting. Through the devil's eyes, one sees an environment that somehow is paradise. With regard to that paradise, the text in the *Bible* cannot be the only, not even the dominant source of the description. In Genesis, paradise is certainly a rich garden, yet it is made for man to work in. Appetite, desire, pleasure, joy, let alone lust do not play a role. Through Adam we hear another cultural voice, from classical times: a pagan voice that describes the *aurea aetas*. Considered from the viewpoint of Christianity, therefore, two 'Others' are in play here: a pagan classical one, and a devilish one from within.

Both in *Adam Expelled* and in *Noah*, it is these others that describe a world ruled by pleasure. Urania also makes this explicit when she describes the state of human beings in her world as follows:

> In this way the body did not feel pain: and the mind remained at peace,
> While between cradle and grave, free from sorrow,
> One would make use of everything that befalls man during his life (*Noah*, l. 818–820).[29]

Time is remarkable 'solid' here: the mind 'remains' at peace, and there is a solid block of time 'between cradle and grave'. It is also worth nothing that the voice of Epicurus is clearly audible, who described *hèdonè* in part as the absence of pain, and who claimed that the good life is ultimately based upon the feeling of well-being. Let me immediately add

[29] 'Zoo voelde 't lijf geen smart: zoo bleef de geest gerust:/ Terwijl men, tusschen wiegh en graf, bevrijt voor treuren, Gebruikte al wat den mensche in 't leven magh gebeuren' (*Noah*, l. 818–820).

that for Epicurus this well-being, or pleasure, is not related to irrational passions or the hunt for pleasure. A state of well-being is only possible if people act moderately and wisely, avoiding excesses. Pleasure and virtue can only go hand in hand if people relate passions to time, that is to say to consequences. Passions in themselves are not wrong, but should be tempered by calculations.

In the classical era, Cicero, especially in his *De finibus bonorum et malorum*, was one of the writers who attacked Epicurus for his contention that *honestas* and *voluptas* can mutually reinforce each other. But of course there is more at stake than this relatively simple conflation of the two concepts, as was proven by the even more vehement attacks from Christian church fathers, who would successfully remove Epicureanism from the politico-cultural stage for more than a thousand years.[30]

In Vondel's *Noah*, the demonization of Epicurus is literalized in the character of the devil Apollion, who describes a world in which *hèdonè* is realized. One could argue that this demonization also extends to Urania, yet she presents *kosmos*, and consequently harmony. As we saw, Apollion's words resonate with Adam's. How can we understand this puzzling, disturbing, destabilizing ambiguity? Let me return to Vondel's treatment of history, and the forces that propel it while simultaneously causing it to repeat itself.

The Destructive Frame of History

A major problem that Christianity built into the societies of Europe was that it could not think politics. It did do a lot of politics, of course, in the form of the institution of the Church or in the form of papal policies, but principally Christianity hollowed out the domain of politics proper. Human beings were not, and could not be, autonomous actors in charge of their own history. As a result, Christian societies, in their many shapes, were constantly thrown into a state of schizophrenia, in

[30] The first to rehabilitate Epicurus was Lorenzo Valla (1407–1457) with his *De voluptate*. He was earlier than Pierre Gassendi (1592–1655) with his *De Vita et Moribus Epicuri*, who is more often referred to. To D.S. Hutchinson the restoration of Epicureanism has not been really successful until today, due to the relentless attacks on it. In his introduction to Epicurus' texts, he asks the reader 'to ignore two thousand years of negative prejudice'. See Hutchinson D.S., "Introduction", in *The Epicurus Reader: Selected Writings and Testimonia*, trl. and ed. Inwood B. – Gerson L.P. (Indianapolis, Cambridge: 1994) xv.

the modern sense of that word. By characterizing this state as a form of schizophrenia, I mean to define it as a type of illness, one that would propel European societies into modernity, not directly but relatively unpredictably, in a typically schizophrenic way.

That Christianity should assume that human beings could not be considered as, even thought of as, autonomous actors is the result of something else: the conceptualization of God in Judaism, Christianity and Islam alike. As the texts of the *Tanach*, *Bible* and *Qur'an* show in all clarity, there is never one, stable God. The so-called one God bristles and sometimes roars because of his internal differences. One particular kinds of split is that between a destructive and violent God on the one hand, and a loving and caring God on the other; between a God who is completely good but who nevertheless made and allows evil; between a God who is both outside and inside human history. In Christianity these splits were multiplied by the Trinity, as a result of which God was simultaenously abstract, absolute spirit, and human body. Furthermore, Christianity complicated things considerably by presenting a God that became human in order to save humankind, which he himself had created, and then killed himself in the form of a Son, who turned the abstract God into a father. The mother, meanwhile, was, and remained, a constant threat to the so-called unity of the Trinity.

Still, this God could have allowed for some kind of autonomous politics, if he had not interfered with human history. But he does interfere, for a principal and specific reason: God's sovereignty in the three monotheistic religions is absolute. He is able to do, allows himself to do, and must be allowed to do anything. This is also the major reason why Christianity cannot think politics, at least not in a conceptually clear way. It is also the reason why this God must be violent and must produce pain. If he refrained from producing violence and pain, he would not be absolutely sovereign. However, in the *Tanach* and the *Bible*, the show of force has transcendental consequences: it produces history, and a particularly painful one at that. One example of this is the way in which God hurls humanity into toilsome and troublesome history by driving it out of paradise; another is the episode with which I started: the flood. God does not simply cause pain in order to demonstrate his absolute sovereignty, but in order to produce a particular, distinct and just kind of history.

This is emphasized at the end of the fourth act of Vondel's *Noah*, when the chorus describes the form and meaning of the rainbow. By default, the rainbow is understood as sign of God's bond with mankind, or as the promise that he will never send a flood again; that he will, in other words, refrain from destroying. Yet Vondel uses the rainbow to indicate the frame within which human history will be caught:

> [God] puts a sign in the clouds,
> The rainbow, for all peoples,
> Bended in the middle of the frame
> Of the world, where it descends and rises
> before the eye; a bow made up of many colours
> that most of all die out in blue and red.
> The blue indicates the flood of this world
> The red a fire and a world in ashes,
> Two verdicts, one now finished,
> The other one to be pronounced later,
> When humanity will perish
> And will stand for the final judgement (*Noah*, l. 1443–1455).[31]

As is often the case with Vondel, he twists the average order or shape of things, in the form of a typically baroque 'insanity of vision'.[32] Normally we tend to say that the rainbow rises and descends, with Vondel it first descends and then rises. Or perhaps more accurately, it is split up, considered both from its top and from its bottom. Seen in this way, it indeed emphasizes better how human history is caught within a frame. One end of that frame indicates, tellingly, not paradise, but the flood – hence destruction. The other end indicates, tellingly, not heaven, but a world in ashes. It is, indeed a history of sameness.

However, like many thinkers and artists of his time, Vondel was both fascinated and abhorred by atrocities committed in a century of religiously fuelled wars, and puzzled by the question of how to make history in an autonomous and relatively harmonious way. Clearly, Vondel's work does not contribute to the powerful surge in materialist

[31] 'En zet een teken aen de wolken,/ Den regenboogh voor alle volken,/ Gebogen midden in de lijst/ Der weerelt, daer hy daelt en rijst/ Op 't oogh; een' boogh uit veele verven,/ Die meest in blaeu en root versterven./ Het blaeu bediet den weereltvloet;/ Het root een' brant en weereltgloet,/ Twee oordeelen, een nu gestreeken, Het ander namaels uit te spreeken, Wanneer het menschdom zal vergaen, En voor de jongste vierschaer staen' (*Noah*, l. 1443–1455).

[32] On the insanity of vision in the baroque, see Buci-Glucksmann C., *La folie du voir: De l'esthétique baroque* (Paris: 1986); Buci-Glucksmann C., *Le baroque littéraire: theorie et pratiques* (Paris: 1990); Bal M., *Quoting Caravagio: Contemporary Art, Preposterous History* (Chicago – London: 1999) and Grootenboer H., *The Rhetoric of Perspective: Realism and Illusionism in Seventeenth-Century Dutch Still-Life Painting* (Chicago: 2005). For the relation between baroque and Vondel, see Kramer W., *Vondel als barokkunstenaar* (Antwerp: 1946).

philosophy in the seventeenth century, although it does define itself in relation to that philosophy.[33] In relation to this materialism and the autonomous potency of human history and life, Vondel's explorations introduce yet another type of European schizophrenia, as may have become clear from the examples taken from *Noah*: the split between the classical world and Christianity (in themselves consisting of many different cultural strains). In classical antiquity and Christianity, questions surrounding the grounds of politics and its legitimate sphere of action are posed differently and lead to mutually exclusive answers. They also lead to different historical paths, or different forms of history.

In the world that precedes the flood there is no history in the sense we moderns, or early moderns, would understand it: it exists in time, not through time, in a state of well-being. That does not mean, of course, that there is no violence, and hence no pain. Remarkably, the violence at stake is the kind described by Walter Benjamin as sovereign and divine. In a notoriously dense consideration of different forms of sovereign violence that provoked close readings by, amongst others, Jacques Derrida, Hent de Vries and Slavoj Žižek, Benjamin introduces his ideas on divine violence.[34] Such violence is violent without following a strategy, without implementation, without intention, without obeying an order, that grounds or preserves it. It is like violence caused by a God passing by, or a volcano erupting, or a mob raging through the streets. The pain which such violence provokes could be described as somehow *natural*. Such pain is part of nature, affecting bodies, but it does not stand in the service of founding a cultural order.

In Vondel's plays God is distinctly counter-natural, that is to say: cultural. As a result, he only *seems* to be the source of a divine violence. He intervenes, in fact, as a distinctly political figure. He wants to have it his specific way, in order to reorganize the polity and start a distinct history. The lustful, swarming world has to be changed, by means of a purposefully painful act, into a bio-politically organized world, a world of oppositions, in which life is not just contained within an artificial boat, but also disciplined. The expansive world of abundance is now

---

[33] Blom H.W., *Morality and Causality in Politics: The Rise of Materialism in Dutch Seventeenth Century Political Thought* (Utrecht: 1995).

[34] Derrida J., "Force of Law: The 'Mystical Foundation of Authority'", in Anidjar A. (ed.), *Acts of Religion* (New York – London: 2002) 228–298; Vries H. de, *Religion and Violence: Philosophical Perspectives from Kant to Derrida* (Baltimore – London: 2002); Žižek S., *Violence: Six Sideways Reflections*.

given direction: the rainbow frames the world between destruction by water and destruction by fire. The arc indicates how the position of mankind has changed accordingly: it has become responsible for what happens to life. Hence, both the domain and the definition of politics have changed. Humankind will have to produce the world, and not 'anew', since the former world was precisely *not* a world of production, but of joy, pleasurable reproduction and natural pain. As a result history changes, that is to say, it comes into being in the modern sense. We enter a world in which *hédoné* or *voluptas* and natural pain are far out of sight, and in which modernity becomes possible: a world in which the infliction of pain and the violation of all life is not just the order of the day, but is needed in order to produce that world and propel it towards its end.

Vondel does not simply show us another possibility, nor does he present us with a golden age whose loss we can mourn nostalgically. *Noah* presents on the hand an absolute sovereign who reigns through the show of force and the production of pain, and on the other hand a kind of sovereignty that does not have to prove its power by violation, but that will, principally, let life be. In relation to this, the play presents two radically different conceptualizations of history, one of which is almost inconceivable to us moderns: a world that exists *in time*, and does not move *through time* from beginning to end like the world after the flood. Within this latter, teleological version of history, the infliction of pain does not so much function to keep human beings 'caught in history', as traumatized subjects who cannot shake off the pain of history, but as schizophrenic ones, being pained, chasing themselves, and life with it, through a history that somehow remains the same, in order to be relieved from pain in the end. That is to say: when, or if, they find the ultimate profit of salvation.

Selective Bibliography

AGAMBEN G., *Homo Sacer: Sovereign Power and Bare Life*, trl. Heller-Roazen D. (Stanford: 1998).

ALPHEN E. VAN, *Caught by History: Holocaust Effects in Contemporary Art, Literature and Theory* (Stanford: 1997).

BROWNMILLER S., *Against Our Will: Men, Women and Rape* (New York: 1975).

BENJAMIN W., "Critique of Violence", in idem, *Selected Writings*, vol. I, 1913–1926 Cambridge MA – London: 2004) 236–252.

BLOM H.W., *Morality and Causality in Politics: The Rise of Materialism in Dutch Seventeenth Century Political Thought* (Utrecht: 1995).

COVER R., *Narrative, Violence, and the Law: The Essays of Robert Cover*, ed. Minow M. *et al.* (Ann Arbor: 1997).

DERRIDA J., "Force of Law: The 'Mystical Foundation of Authority'", in Anidjar A. (ed.), *Acts of Religion* (New York – London: 2002) 228–298.

HIGGINS L.A. – Silver B.R. (eds.), *Rape and Representation* (New York: 1991).

HUTCHINSON D.S., "Introduction", in Inwood B. – Gerson L.P. (eds. and trsl.), *The Epicurus Reader: Selected Writings and Testimonia* (Indianapolis – Cambridge: 1994) i–xv.

KIRSCH J., *God Against the Gods: The History of the War Between Monotheism and Polytheism* (New York – London: 2004).

KNUVELDER G.P., *Handboek tot de geschiedenis der Nederlandse letterkunde*, vol. II ('s-Hertogenbosch: 1971).

KOPPENOL J., "Nodeloze onrust: Het 'roomse karakter' van Vondels *Gysbreght van Aemstel*", *Nederlandse letterkunde* 4,4 (1999) 313–329.

KORSTEN F.W., *Vondel belicht: voorstellingen van soevereiniteit* (Hilversum: 2006).

KONST J.W.H., *Fortuna, Fatum en Providentia Dei in de Nederlandse tragedie 1600–1720* (Hilversum: 2003).

KRAMER W., *Vondel als barokkunstenaar* (Antwerpen: 1946).

MALJAARS A., "'Niet min Godvruchtelijck als dapper': Gijsbrecht van Aemstel verdedigd tegen zijn critici", *De zeventiende eeuw* 17,2 (2001) 138–163.

PARENTE J.A., "The Theatricality of History in the Dutch Golden Age: Joost van den Vondel's *Gysbreght van Aemstel*", in Hermans Th. – Salverda T. (eds.), *From Revolt to Riches: Culture and History of the Low Countries 1500–1700 – International and Interdisciplinary Perspectives* (London: 1993) 255–267.

SAUNDERS C., *Rape and Ravishment in the Literature of Medieval England* (Cambridge: 2001).

SCARRY E., *The Body in Pain: The Making and Unmaking of the World* (Oxford – New York: 1985).

SMIT W.A.P., *Van Pascha tot Noah: een verkenning van Vondels drama's naar continuïteit en ontwikkeling in hun grondmotief en structuur*, vols. I–III (Zwolle: 1956–1962).

SMITS-VELDT M.B., "Vondels *Gysbreght van Aemstel* onder de loep: twee gevallen van tekstinterpretatie", *Spektator* 17,5 (1988) 380–396.

——, "Inleiding", in Joost van den Vondel, *Gysbreght van Aemstel* (Amsterdam: 1994).

STIPRIAAN R. VAN, "Gysbreght van Aemstel als tragische held", *De zeventiende eeuw* 12 (1996) 359–377.

VONDEL JOOST VAN DEN, *De werken van Vondel: Volledige en geïllustreerde tekstuitgave in tien delen*, ed. Sterck J.F.M. – Moller H.W.E. – De Vooys C.G.N. – De Klerk C.R. (Amsterdam: 1927–1937).

VRIES H. DE, *Religion and Violence: Philosophical Perspectives from Kant to Derrida* (Baltimore – London: 2002).

WOLFTHAL D. *Images of Rape: The 'Heroic' Tradition and its Alternatives* (Cambridge: 1999).

ŽIŽEK S., *Violence: Six Sideways Reflections* (London: 2008).

SCHMERZ HAT NICHTS GUTES: SPINOZAS BEGRIFF VON *TRISTITIA* UND *DOLOR*

Anne Tilkorn

Dieser Aufsatz eröffnet zwei Blickrichtungen, die eine präsentiert Spinozas Umfeld und möchte Spinozas Standpunkt zum Schmerz als einen beschreiben, der sich von den zeitgenössischen, kultur- und religionsgeschichtlichen Auffassungen wie auch von denen seines direkten philosophischen Vorgängers Descartes abhebt. Ein zweiter, kurzer Blick möchte die gezeigte Besonderheit mit der Moderne verbinden und Spinoza als eine Quelle der Inspiration[1] für aktuelle Tendenzen in der Forschung sichtbar machen.[2]

‚Schmerz' in der antiken Philosophie

Die antike Philosophie verhandelt das Problem des Schmerzes im Zusammenhang der Theorie des glücklichen oder guten Lebens. Schmerz erscheint darin als das Ergebnis einer Disharmonie im Leben, er tritt auf, sobald die Natur einer Sache zerstört wird. Erst durch das Reetablieren der ursprünglichen Harmonie kann das Gefühl von Freude den Schmerz ablösen. Platon vergleicht den Schmerz mit Gefühlen von Hunger und Durst, die auch dann aufhören, wenn der physische Zustand wieder im Lot ist.[3] Aristoteles sieht eine unmittelbare Verbindung zwischen ethischen Handlungen und dem Gefühl von Lust und

---

[1] Dass Spinozas radikal neuer ethischer Ansatz – den Menschen schlicht als natürliches Ding zu klassifizieren – eine Provokation und Irritation für das traditionelle und moderne Denken bedeutet, betont bereits Manfred Walter. Für ihn ist diese Radikalität der Beginn der Moderne. Walther M., „Freiheit und Notwendigkeit: Die Umgestaltung der praktischen Philosophie durch Spinoza als Irritation und Provokation des ethischen und politischen Denkens in der Neuzeit", in Balibar E. – Seidel H. – Walther M. (Hrsg.), *Freiheit und Notwendigkeit. Ethische und politische Aspekte bei Spinoza und in der Geschichte des (Anti-)Spinozismus* (Würzburg: 1994) 12.

[2] Ich danke Haim Mahlev herzlich für seine konstruktiven Anmerkungen und die stetige Diskussion.

[3] Plato, *Philebos*, hrsg. von W.F. Otto – E. Grassi – G. Plamböck (Hamburg: 1959) 31d and 42c/d.

Unlust. Da wir von Kindheit an unsere Handlungen mit dem Maßstab der Freude oder der Unlust messen, müsse die ethische Diskussion diesem Rechnung tragen. Im Mittelpunkt seiner Überlegungen steht die Gefahr, die vom freudigen Affekt ausgeht, denn er kann zu extremem und damit schlechtem Verhalten verleiten.[4] Auch die stoische Philosophie sieht eine Verknüpfung zwischen Gefühlen und Moralität; der Weise wird als jemand charakterisiert, der keine übertriebenen Gefühle hat. Ihr System umfasst vier Grundgefühle: Schmerz (*lype*), Angst (*phobos*), Begierde (*epithymia*) und Freude (*hedone*). Mitleid (*eleos*), Neid (*phthonos*) und Eifersucht (*zelos*) sind Unterarten des Schmerzes.[5] Er steht der Vernunft entgegen und setzt mit der Annahme der Gegenwart von etwas Schlechtem ein.[6] Es ist offensichtlich, dass diese Gedankengänge sich nicht mit physischem Schmerz auseinandersetzen, sondern mit Schmerzen, die die geistige Seite des Menschen beeinträchtigen. Ob Schmerz grundsätzlich als etwas ausschließlich Physisches verstanden werden kann, ist – wie ich später zeigen möchte – eine wichtige Frage in Spinozas Philosophie. Hier bleibt festzuhalten, dass Schmerz als etwas thematisiert wird, dass uns aus der Balance bringt. Zwischen geistigem und physischem Schmerz wird nicht eindeutig differenziert.

Schmerz in religiösen Kontexten

Wenn Gott gut ist, warum lässt er Leid und Schmerz zu – jede Religion muss mit dieser Frage umgehen. Die Antwort des Alten Testaments lautet, erst mit dem Sündenfall ist das Leid in die Welt getreten. Diese Genese begreift den Schmerz als Strafe. Hätte Adam den Apfel nicht gegessen, gäbe es kein Leiden. Hiob stellt dabei einen zugespitzten Fall dar, denn er leidet, obwohl er nichts Schlechtes getan hat. Hier hat das Leiden die Funktion eines Glaubenstests. Die Schlüsselinterpretation des Leidens in der Christlichen Theologie sieht in ihm ein Zeichen dafür, dass wir der Auferstehung bedürfen. Das Neue Testament und seine Darstellung Jesu Schmerzen beim Erleiden des Kreuzestods betont diese Auffassung. Jesus leidet bis zum Ende und jeder Mensch, der auf

[4] Aristoteles, *Nikomachische Ethik*, hrsg. und übers. von F. Dirlmeier (Stuttgart: 1969), II, 1104 b 27.

[5] Boeri M.D. – Vigo A.G., „Die Affektenlehre der Stoa", in Engstler A. – Schnepf R. (Hrsg.), *Affekte und Ethik. Spinozas Lehre im Kontext* (Hildesheim: 2002) 55–56.

[6] Boeri – Vigo, „Die Affektenlehre der Stoa" 56.

Erden zu leiden hat, ist durch sein Leiden mit Christus und dessen Leiden verbunden. Bezeichnenderweise ist das apostolische Schreiben von Papst Johannes Paul II. aus dem Jahr 1984 mit dem Titel *Salvifici Doloris* – „Über den Sinn des menschlichen Leidens" überschrieben. Die „heilbringende Kraft des Leidens" sowie die „Entdeckung des Sinnes des Leidens" werden darin als Kern des Christentums und der Christusnachfolge ausgemacht. In der Frühen Neuzeit stand vor allem das innere Nacherleben seines Lebens und Sterbens im Fokus.[7] Die Reformation schließlich bricht mit der Auffassung, Schmerzen könnten reinigend und befreiend sein. Man knüpft an die Geschichte Hiobs an und begreift den Schmerz als eine Prüfung Gottes. Im Aushalten des Leids könne die eigene Kraft und Stärke des Glaubens zu Tage treten.[8] Einerseits verweist das Leiden immer auf die Erbsünde, andererseits auf die Möglichkeit der Erlösung im Jenseits.[9]

Das jüdische Denken betrachtet das Leiden einer nicht schuldig gewordenen Person als ein unverstehbares Mysterium. Es ist etwas Schlimmes, das nicht verstanden werden kann und dem Einzelnen steht es frei, sich zu beklagen und zu jammern – wie Hiob. Der Rebellion gegen den Schmerz sind keine Grenzen gesetzt und sich selbst Schmerzen zuzufügen ergibt keinen Sinn – anders als bei christlichen Vorstellungen wie der Askese oder der Selbstkasteiung.[10]

Im Islam dagegen herrscht die Ansicht vor, mit Not müsse ohne zu klagen umgegangen werden. Schmerzen seien gottgegeben und müssten ertragen werden, auch wenn sie nicht verstehbar seien. Der Einzelne solle aber sein eigenes Leiden nicht verherrlichen, vielmehr stammten

[7] Langemeyer G., Art. „Nachfolge Christi", in *Lexikon der katholischen Dogmatik* (Freiburg: 1987) 384. Einige Interpretationen betonen, dass die christliche Religion hier eine Relation vom individuellen Schmerz zum Leiden Christi aufmacht, so dass der Einzelne im Schmerz Christus und seinem Schmerz begegne. Vgl. Varone F., *Ce Dieu censé aimer la souffrance* (Paris: 1986) 220; Le Breton D., *Schmerz. Eine Kulturgeschichte* (Zürich – Berlin: 2003) 103. Max Scheler hingegen sieht in seinem Buch *Vom Sinn des Leidens* in der Möglichkeit, aus dem Schmerz ein Gebet zu machen, ein charakteristisches Merkmal der griechisch-orthodoxen Kirche. Im Mittelalter sind in der bildenden Kunst die Wundmale Christi, die drastischen Todesarten biblischer Gestalten und der christlichen Märtyrer die einzigen Darstellungen körperlicher Verletzungen. Vgl. Blume E. – Hürlimann A. – Schnalke T. – Tydarellis D. (Hrsg.), *Schmerz. Kunst und Wissenschaft* (Begleitbuch zur Ausstellung, Berlin: 2007) 115.

[8] Le Breton, *Schmerz* 106.

[9] Roselyne Rey analysiert differenziert die Parallelität einer entstehenden wissenschaftlichen Medizin, die die Leiden der Menschen verringern möchte zu einer bzw. den verschiedenen Theologien, die versuchen, dem Leid einen Sinn zu geben. Rey R., *The History of Pain* (Cambridge, London: 1995) 85 ff.

[10] Le Breton, *Schmerz* 98.

auch die Mittel, die zur Heilung nützen, von Gott. Die Möglichkeit zur Bekämpfung der Schmerzen und Krankheiten sollen ausgeschöpft und erweitert werden.[11]

Descartes' mechanistische Erklärung

Descartes stellt die philosophische Position dar, von der Spinoza sich direkt absetzt. Oben[12] wurde bereits die Radikalität Spinozas betont, den Menschen nicht als „einen Staat im Staat"[13], d.h. nicht als Krone der Schöpfung oder als außerhalb der natürlichen Ordnung zu beschreiben und dies seinen philosophischen Kollegen vorzuwerfen. Auch Descartes begeht diesen Fehler, er begreift den Menschen als von den übrigen Lebewesen oder Naturphänomenen grundsätzlich unterschieden.[14] Manifest wird dies bei ihm nun besonders in der Diskussion um den Schmerz. Schmerz ist für Descartes eine Empfindung, die es nur dann geben kann, wenn Leib und Seele als eine verbundene Einheit auftreten.[15] Dies sei beim Menschen der Fall, bei den Tieren allerdings nicht, denn die Tiere besitzen laut Descartes keine Seele. Seine Schlussfolgerung musste also lauten, dass Tiere keine Schmerzen haben. Im religiösen christlichen Kontext würde dies tatsächlich Sinn ergeben, da Tiere ja keine Sünden begangen haben und deshalb auch nicht mit Schmerzen bestraft werden müssten. Bis heute wird die Diskussion um den Geist der Tiere und damit indirekt auch um die Schmerzempfindung der Tiere fortgeführt, wobei Descartes mit seiner Position stets eine Provokation bleibt.[16]

---

[11] Le Breton, *Schmerz* 108–109.

[12] S. Anm. 1.

[13] Baruch Spinoza, *Ethik in geometrischer Ordnung dargestellt*, übersetzt von W. Bartuschat (Hamburg: 2006) III, Vorwort.

[14] Spinoza, *Ethik* III, Vorwort. Einen direkten Vorwurf macht Spinoza Descartes im Vorwort zu seiner Affektenlehre: „Natürlich weiß ich, daß der berühmte Descartes, wenngleich auch er glaubte, daß der Geist über seine Handlungen eine unbedingte Macht habe, sich immerhin bemüht hat, menschliche Affekte durch ihre ersten Ursachen zu erklären und in eins damit den Weg aufzuzeigen, auf dem der Geist eine unbedingte Herrschaft über seine Affekte haben könne. Er hat aber, wenigstens meiner Ansicht nach, dabei nichts weiter dargetan als die Gewandtheit seines großen Geistes, wie ich an geeigneter Stelle zeigen möchte".

[15] Vgl. Wild M., *Die anthropologische Differenz. Der Geist der Tiere in der frühen Neuzeit bei Montaigne, Descartes und Hume* (Berlin – New York: 2006), Kapitel III, 2.

[16] S. z.B. den Sammelband Perler D. – Wild M. (Hrsg.), *Der Geist der Tiere. Philosophische Texte zu einer aktuellen Diskussion* (Frankfurt a.M.: 2005).

Gehen wir, um die beiden Grundbegriffe Leib bzw. Körper und Seele und ihre Verbindung zu klären, einen Schritt zurück – zu Descartes' Substanzbegriff. In dem Buch *Principia philosophiae* (1644) definiert Descartes ‚Substanz' als *causa sui*, d.h. als etwas, das unabhängig von irgendetwas anderem existiert. Er listet drei Substanzen auf: Gott, die Seele („res cogitans") und den Körper („res extensa"). Descartes räumt zwar ein, dass Seele und Körper in ihrer Existenz von Gott abhängen, dennoch setzt er den Begriff der Substanz auch hier an.

Die Konsequenz seiner Substanzentheorie ist, dass die *res extensa* unabhängig von der *res cogitans* existiert. Seine sehr persönliche Zweifelsstrategie führt in den *Meditationes de Prima Philosophia* (1641) erneut zur Konfrontion der zwei Welten und thematisiert dabei das Phänomen des Schmerzes. Von seiner konkreten Situation ausgehend versucht Descartes nacheinander an der Existenz der Dinge, die ihn umgeben, und schließlich auch an seinem eigenen Körper und seinen eigenen Empfindungen zu zweifeln:

> Später haben aber allmählich vielerlei Erfahrungen das ungeteilte Zutrauen zu den Sinnesempfindungen erschüttert. Bisweilen erschienen Türme, die von ferne rund aussahen, von nahem viereckig, und mächtige Statuen, die dort oben standen, nahmen sich von unten gesehen gar nicht groß aus, und noch in unzähligen anderen derartigen Fällen merkte ich, wie trügerisch das Urteil der äußeren Sinnesempfindungen war; ja nicht bloß der äußeren, auch das der inneren Sinneseindrücke! Womit kann ich wohl vertrauter sein als mit meinem Schmerz? Und doch hörte ich gelegentlich von Leuten, denen man ein Bein oder einen Arm abgenommen hatte, sie empfänden scheinbar zuweilen Schmerz in dem fehlenden Körperteil. So schien es mir denn nicht mehr so gewiss, dass ein Glied mich schmerzte, selbst wenn ich den Schmerz in ihm fühlte.[17]

Er leitet daraus nicht die Nicht-Existenz des Körpers oder seiner Schmerzen ab, sondern kommt zu dem Ergebnis, dass es einzig Gott sein kann, der garantiert, dass wir von unseren Empfindungen nicht betrogen werden, dass nicht nur unsere Seele, an deren Tätigkeit des Zweifelns wir am Ende gar nicht zweifeln können, sondern auch unser Körper und seine vagen Empfindungen existieren. Hier beschreibt Descartes

[17] René Descartes, *Meditationen*, hrsg. von J. Timmermann, dreisprachige Ausgabe (Göttingen: 2004) 212; übersetzt und hrsg. von G. Schmidt (Stuttgart: 1986), „Meditatio Sexta".

nun unseren Körper wie auch den der Tiere als eine Maschine: „So kann ich auch den menschlichen Körper als eine Art Maschine ansehen, die aus Knochen, Nerven, Muskeln, Adern, Blut und Haut zusammengepasst ist und auch geistlos all die Bewegungen ausführt, wie sie jetzt unwillkürlich, also ohne den Geist, ablaufen".[18]

Aber wo findet die Verbindung zwischen dieser Körper-Maschine und der rationalen Seele statt?

> In ganz ähnlicher Weise lehrt die Physik, dass, wenn ich Schmerzen im Fuß empfinde, dies durch Vermittlung der im Fuß verbreiteten Nerven geschieht, die sich von da wie Schnüre bis in das Gehirn erstrecken. Werden sie nun im Fuß angezogen, so ziehen sie auch an den innern Teilen des Gehirns, mit denen sie in Verbindung stehen (von wo sie ausgehen und wo sie enden). Dort erregen sie eine gewisse Bewegung, die von der Natur dazu bestimmt ist, den Geist mit der Empfindung des gleichsam im Fuß lokalisierten Schmerzes zu affizieren.[19]

Für Descartes liegt die Verbindung zwischen Körper und Seele im Gehirn und nicht bloß irgendwo im Gehirn, sondern er lokalisiert die Zirbeldrüse als den exakten Ort, an dem der Übergang stattfindet.[20] An genau diesem Punkt konnte Spinoza seinem philosophischen Kollegen nicht mehr folgen.

Spinoza zur Einheit von Körper und Geist

Es ist offensichtlich, dass Descartes' Argument sich im Kreis dreht: Er fragt nach der Verbindung der Substanz der Extension mit der Substanz der Seele und lokalisiert diese wieder in der Substanz der Extension – die Zirbeldrüse ist etwas Physisches, Ausgedehntes.

Spinoza stimmt Descartes darin zu, dass etwas Ausgedehntes, der Körper, sich grundsätzlich von etwas Nicht-Ausgedehntem, der Seele oder dem Denken, unterscheidet.[21] Aber diese Grundverschiedenheit

---

[18] Descartes, *Meditationen*, Nr. 232, 201 f.

[19] Descartes, *Meditationen*, Nr. 98.

[20] „Nachdem ich mir aber die Sache sorgfältig untersucht habe, bin ich mir gewiß, erkannt zu haben, daß der Körperteil, über den die Seele ihre Funktionen unmittelbar ausübt, keineswegs das Herz ist, noch auch das ganze Gehirn, sondern nur der innerste von dessen Teilen, welches eine gewisse sehr kleine Drüse ist, die inmitten der Hirnsubstanz liegt". Descartes, *Die Leidenschaften der Seele*, Erster Teil, Artikel 31.

[21] Spinoza *Ethik* I, def 2: „Z.B. heißt ein Körper endlich, weil wir stets einen anderen begreifen, der größer ist. So wird ein Gedanke von einem anderen Gedanken begrenzt.

löst Spinoza nicht auf. Er sieht, dass sich beide nicht irgendwo im Raum treffen können, da die Räumlichkeit eine Eigenschaft ist, die nur dem Körper zukommt. Ein Gedanke ist nicht ausgedehnt, das Gehirn jedoch sehr wohl. Spinozas Lösung des Körper-Geist-Problems, also des Problems, wie beide zueinander kommen, ist radikal. Er behauptet, „[d]ie Ordnung und Verbindung der Ideen ist dieselbe wie die Ordnung und Verbindung der Dinge".[22] Obwohl Körper und Geist so verschieden sind, dass sie sich nicht berühren oder in Wechselwirkung treten können, schreibt Spinoza ihnen eine vollständige Simultaneität bzw. analoge Struktur zu. Am Beispiel des Menschen können wir veranschaulichen, was Spinoza damit meinen kann. Am einzelnen Menschen wird deutlich, dass dieser nicht in zwei Teile auseinanderklafft; vielmehr bildet seine Gedanken- und Ideenwelt mit seinem Körper eine Einheit, befindet sich letzterer auch in Raum und Zeit. Wieder müssen wir zur Definition der Substanz zurückgehen, um zu verstehen, wie Spinoza den Gedanken dieser prinzipiellen Gleichheit von Körper und Geist begründet. Descartes hatte das Argument der Unabhängigkeit von Anderem ausgearbeitet: den Begriff der *causa sui*. Spinozas Theorie des Absoluten radikalisiert Descartes dahingehend, dass er nicht mehr drei unterschiedliche selbständige Substanzen akzeptiert, sondern nur noch eine einzige. *Extensio* und *cogitatio* hängen – Descartes hatte es eigentlich bereits zugegeben – von der absoluten *causa sui*, von Gott ab, sie sind jetzt Attribute der einen Substanz. Gott hat eine unendliche Anzahl von Attributen, unser Wissen von dieser unendlichen Menge ist jedoch beschränkt: nur diese beiden sind uns bekannt. Das alte Problem von Einheit und Vielheit löst Spinoza durch seine völlig neue Konzeption des Ausdrucks. Die eine Substanz manifestiert sich auf bestimmte Art und Weise, wobei erst durch die Formen des Ausdrucks die Verschiedenheit der Dinge zum Vorschein kommt. Die Substanz ist wesentlich eine sich ausdrückende Substanz, d.h. „hinter" dem präsent gewordenen gibt es nicht noch etwas Verborgenes oder Transzendentes.

Der Schlüssel zu Spinozas Theorie von Körper und Geist ist, dass die Substanz sich nur ein einziges Mal ausdrückt, aber innerhalb aller ihrer Attribute. Ein Attribut eröffnet Erkennbarkeiten der Substanz, es ist eine Weise, wie sich das Wesen der Substanz manifestiert. Das

---

Dagegen wird ein Körper nicht von einem Gedanken begrenzt, noch ein Gedanke von einem Körper".

[22] Spinoza, *Ethik* II, p7.

Sichausdrücken in verschiedenen Attributen bedeutet, dass ein und derselbe Ausdruck zur selben Zeit in allen Attributen präsent ist. Da wir nur die Attribute Ausdehnung und Denken kennen, beschränkt sich unsere Rede über das Sich-Ausdrücken der Substanz auf den Ausdruck als physisches oder als geistiges Phänomen.

Die konkreten ausgedehnten oder geistigen Einzeldinge wie Bäume, Häuser, Körper, Ideen, Begriffe oder Gefühle, die innerhalb der beiden Attribute manifest werden, nennt Spinoza Modifikationen oder Modi der Attribute. Spinozas Philosophie des Ausdrucks denkt an dieser Stelle vollkommen anti-aristotelisch, denn das geformte Einzelding wird nicht durch etwas der Form Externes bestimmt, sondern die Form selbst ist es, die sich bestimmt.[23] Die Form des Attributs Ausgedehntsein wird durch einen bestimmten ausgedehnten Gegenstand lediglich eingeschränkt – „omnis determinatio est negatio". Die Ausdehnung selbst bleibt in jedem ausgedehnten Ding dieselbe. Demnach ist ein individueller Mensch einmal eine Modifikation, die innerhalb der Sphäre der *extensio* stattfindet – als unser Körper – und einmal in der Sphäre der *cogitatio* – als die Idee unseres Körpers.

Dem Rechnung tragend, dass eine Verbindung von Körper und Geist nicht innerhalb eines der beiden Attribute stattfinden kann, sowie der am Phänomen des Menschen offensichtlichen Tatsache, dass beiden gleichwohl etwas Gemeinsames zukommt, lautet Spinozas Antwort, dass nur der Begriff einer Substanz, die sich selbst nur ein einziges mal, jedoch auf unterschiedliche Arten ausdrückt, diese gegenläufigen Argumente vereinen kann. So sind Körper und Geist zwei Perspektiven auf ein einmaliges Sich-Ausdrücken, zwei Erscheinungen ein und derselben Aktion.[24] Tatsächlich sind sie derselbe Ausdruck der einen, derselben Substanz, die Unterschiede gibt es erst innerhalb der Sphären, in denen der Ausdruck manifest wird.[25] Die beiden Sphären sind

[23] Peter Reisinger spricht konsequenterweise vom Modus als dem Ausdruck des Ausdrucks. Vgl. Reisinger P., „Modelle des Absoluten", in Löw R. (Hrsg.), *Oikeiosis. Festschrift für Robert Spaemann* (Weinheim: 1987) 229.

[24] Die Attribute sind die Möglichkeiten, wie die Substanz aufgefasst werden kann: s. Spinoza, *Ethik* IIp7s.

[25] Spinoza, *Ethik* III, p2s: „Dies läßt sich noch klarer aus dem in Anmerkung zu Lehrsatz 7 des 2. Teils Gesagten verstehen, daß nämlich der Geist und der Körper ein und dasselbe Ding sind, das bald unter dem Attribute Denken, bald unter dem Attribut Ausdehnung begriffen wird. Das macht es, daß die Ordnung oder Verknüpfung von Dingen ein und dieselbe ist, ob nun die Natur unter diesem oder unter jenem Attribut begriffen wird, und folglich daß die Ordnung der Aktivitäten und des Erleidens

absolut parallel[26]. Es kann keine Modifikation gedacht werden, die nur innerhalb eines der beiden Attribute stattfindet und nicht gleichzeitig im anderen.

Entsprechend zu jedem physischen Objekt existiert auch eine Idee dieses Objekts. Das Wort ‚parallel' ist vielleicht noch zu schwach, um zu betonen, dass es keinerlei Kontakt zur anderen Seite, zur anderen Sphäre gibt. Jedes Attribut ist absolut, jedes für sich.[27] So verhindert Spinoza logische Fehler wie den einer Descarteschen Zirbeldrüse.

Spinozas Theorie des Schmerzes

Die Folgen dieser zugespitzten Substanztheorie für Spinozas Verständnis von physischem Schmerz sind zunächst, dass es für jedes physische Ereignis unbedingt ein geistiges Äquivalent geben muss, ein Ereignis im Reich der Ideen. Hier soll nicht tiefer in Spinozas Theorie des Bewusstseins und in die Diskussion darüber, ob und in wieweit er damit unbewusste Ideen im Sinne Sigmund Freuds antizipiert, vorgedrungen werden;[28] was wir jetzt festhalten wollen, ist die Übereinstimmung, die er für Körper und Ideen ermittelt. Unsere Seele ist darin nichts anderes als die Idee unseres Körpers.[29] Im Gegensatz zu Empfindungen, die uns etwas über externe Gegenstände mitteilen, stehen wir mittels der Gefühle selbst im Fokus. Das Gefühl des Schmerzes ist insofern im Rahmen von Spinozas Affekttheorie, nicht im Rahmen seiner

---

unseres Körpers mit der Ordnung der Aktivitäten und des Erleidens des Geistes von Natur aus zugleich ist".

[26] Barbara Handwerker Küchenhoff weist zurecht auf die Problematik der Begriffs ‚parallel' hin: Wenn jeder Seite eine selbständige Existenz zukommt, können sie nicht in einem parallelen Verhältnis zueinander stehen. Handwerker Küchenhoff B., *Spinozas Theorie der Affekte. Kohärenz und Konflikt* (Würzburg: 2006) 40.

[27] Stefan Büttner begreift die Attribute als absolute Geschlossenheiten; ihre Formen des Ausdrucks legten das Wesen der Substanz offen (*explicare*). Die Attribute seien „Erscheinungen, Reflexionen der Substanz, die gegeneinander entpositionalisiert sind". Vgl. Büttner S., „Spinozas Attribut der Ausdehnung und Kants Form der Anschauung – ein systematisch orientierter Vergleich", in Piarek H. – Walther M. (Hrsg.), *Kontexte – Spinoza und die Geschichte der Philosophie* (Wroclaw: 2001) 114.

[28] Da Spinoza dem Körper sehr viel Aufmerksamkeit widmet und immer wieder betont, dass wir nicht ahnen, was unser Körper alles kann, muss er automatisch auch Ideen annehmen, die diesen unbekannten Körperfunktionen entsprechen – noch nicht bekannte und insofern unbewusste Ideen.

[29] Der Körper ist das *Objekt der Idee*, die den menschlichen Geist ausmacht. Der Körper selbst hat natürlich keine Ideen. Vgl. Spinoza, *Ethik* II, p13.

Epistemologie mit den drei verschiedenen Erkenntnisgattungen[30] zu untersuchen. Nicht die Wahrheit über die Außen-, sondern die der Innenwelt ist zu verhandeln. Dennoch sind unsere Gefühle nicht ohne ein Außen, ohne das Affiziertwerden von Gegenständen zu verstehen. Spinoza beschreibt die ganze Wirklichkeit – Innen- und Außenwelt – als vom *conatus* bestimmt.[31] Jedes Einzelding ist bestimmt von einem Streben, das sich auf das Ding selbst bezieht.[32] Die Natur oder das Wesen jedes Menschen ist genau dieses Streben. Es kann entweder glücken oder aber frustriert und eingeschränkt werden. Von vorneherein sieht Spinoza den Menschen dabei als Teil der Welt. Sein *conatus* ist nichts Unverbundenes, für sich Stehendes, sondern steht in grundsätzlichem Bezug zu seiner Umgebung. Ist das Streben erfolgreich, so weckt es in uns ein positives Gefühl, bleibt unser Streben hingegen unerfüllt, entstehen negative Gefühle. Im dritten Buch der Ethik („Von dem Ursprung und der Natur der Affekte") gibt Spinoza einen Überblick über die Abstufungen dieser beiden Gefühlstendenzen. Lehrsatz 11 betont erneut die Deckungsgleichheit von Körper und Geist: „Was auch immer die Wirkungsmacht unseres Körpers vermehrt oder vermindert, fördert oder hemmt, dessen Idee vermehrt oder vermindert, fördert

[30] Spinoza, *Ethik* II, p40, Anm. 2. Die Erkenntnis, die wir mittels der Wahrnehmung erlangen, ist verstümmelt und verworren. Sie entspricht nicht der Ordnung des Verstandes. Wahrnehmen und Erinnern vergleicht Spinoza mit den Worten anderer, es seien Zeichen, aus denen wir Erkenntnis schöpfen, die jedoch keine verlässliche Erkenntnis liefern. Wahrnehmungen, Erinnerung und Hören oder Lesen bezeichnet er als „Erkenntnis erster Gattung, Meinung oder Vorstellung". Von ihr grenzt er die „Erkenntnis zweiter Gattung, die Vernunfterkenntnis" ab: Jetzt ist die erste Ebene, die vom individuellen, konkreten Kontakt zu Einzeldingen oder Vorstellungen bestimmt war, überschritten, hin zu allgemeinen Zusammenhängen. Gemeinbegriffe und adäquate Ideen der Eigenschaften von Dingen, sind offenbar nichts, was die Sinne am Gegenstand ablesen können, sondern etwas, das die Vernunft hervorbringen muss.

[31] Spinoza, *Ethik* II, p6: „Unaquaeque res, quantum in se est, in suo esse perseverare conatur". Die Übersetzung dieses Satzes ist immer bereits eine Interpretation. So übersetzt Wolfgang Bartuschat: „Jedes Ding strebt gemäß der ihm eigenen Natur, in seinem Sein zu verharren", hingegen formuliert Jakob Stern: „Jedes Ding strebt, soviel an ihm liegt, in seinem Sein zu verharren". Der Terminus *conatus* bleibt in meinen Augen besser unübersetzt, da sonst schnell falsche Assoziationen, z.B. die einer Intention oder auch eines teleologischen Ziels, geweckt werden. Zu diesem Problem äußert sich auch Ursula Renz: „Zwischen ontologischer Notwendigkeit und zufälliger Semantik", in Landweer H. (Hrsg.), *Gefühle – Struktur und Funktion* (Berlin: 2007) 41.

[32] Hans Blumenberg beschreibt ausführlich, die Entwicklung dieses Verständnisses von Selbsterhaltung, das kein externes Ziel außerhalb seiner Selbst enthält. Blumenberg H., „Selbsterhaltung und Beharrung. Zur Konsitution der neuzeitlichen Rationalität", in Ebeling H. (Hrsg.), *Subjektivität und Selbsterhaltung* (Frankfurt a.M.: 1996) 144–145.

oder hemmt unseres Geistes Macht des Denkens".[33] Anschließend, im Beweis des Lehrsatzes, differenziert er zwischen Affekten, die aus einer Ausweitung unserer Kraft („potentiam agendi") resultieren und solchen, die das Ergebnis ihrer Verringerung sind: handelt es sich um die Steigerung der Geisteskraft, nennt er dieses Gefühl *laetita* (Freude), handelt es sich um ihre Abnahme so spricht er von *tristitia* (Trauer). Einen Affekt, der sich auf die Zunahme des Tätigkeitsvermögens von Körper *und* Geist bezieht, bezeichnet er mit den Begriffen *titillatio* (Lust) oder *hilaritas* (Heiterkeit), den analogen, negativen Affekt mit *dolor* (Schmerz) oder *melancholia* (Schwermut). Die Unterscheidung zwischen den Begriffen Lust und Heiterkeit hat denselben Hintergrund wie die Differenz zwischen Schmerz und Schwermut: Lust wie Schmerz beziehen sich auf einen bestimmten Teil des Körpers beziehungsweise des Geistes, während die Heiterkeit und die Schwermut sich beide jeweils auf den ganzen Körper und den ganzen Geist beziehen.

Das vierte Buch der Ethik („Von menschlicher Knechtschaft") kommt auf diese Definitionen zurück und zieht die Schlussfolgerung, dass Freude gut und Trauer unmittelbar schlecht sei.[34] Hier wendet er das Kriterium der Vergrößerung oder Verkleinerung unseres Strebens in einer Analyse ganz unterschiedlicher Affekte an. Sich rückbeziehend auf seine Definition der Begriffe Heiterkeit und Schwermut, wird sein Argument detaillierter. Weil der Affekt der Heiterkeit nicht auf einen bestimmten Teil des Körpers fixiert ist, stellt er kein asymmetrisches Verhältnis im Modus Mensch dar und das bedeutet, dass dieser Affekt „immer gut" ist. Analog gilt für die Schwermut, die wiederum alle Teile des Körpers betrifft, dass sie aus diesem Grund „immer schlecht" ist.[35] Interessant ist dabei weniger, dass etwas Schlechtes, das alle Teile des Körpers affiziert, immer schlecht ist, sondern vielmehr, dass auch etwas Gutes, das aber nur einen Teil von uns betrifft, leicht negative Folgen haben kann. Das Ungleichgewicht ist gefährlich, der *conatus* kann nicht so zur Geltung kommen wie ohne diese einseitige Belastung. Generell gilt, dass je mehr Teile eines Menschen einbezogen sind, die Chancen für ein Gelingen des Strebens desto besser stehen.

---

[33] Spinoza, *Ethik* III, p11.

[34] Spinoza, *Ethik* V, p41: „Freude ist nicht unmittelbar schlecht, sondern gut; Trauer andererseits ist unmittelbar schlecht".

[35] Spinoza, *Ethik* IV, p42: „Heiterkeit kann kein Übermaß haben, sondern ist immer gut; Schwermut andererseits ist immer schlecht".

An dieser Stelle lohnt es, einen Bogen zurück zur antiken Philosophie zu denken. Dieses Gleichgewicht hatte auch sie vor Augen – das heißt, die Gefühle wurden insbesondere von den Stoikern nicht grundsätzlich verurteilt, aber sie müssen in einem ausgewogenen Verhältnis stehen. Genauso ist für Spinoza die Lust nichts Gutes mehr, wenn sie als exzessive Lust auftritt, denn dann ist sie auf einen bestimmten Teil unseres Körpers fixiert und schwächt unser Tätigkeitsvermögen. Im Rahmen dieser Überlegungen vervollständigt Spinoza seine Interpretation des Schmerzes folgendermaßen: Manchmal kann Schmerz tatsächlich ein Gutes haben, nämlich genau dann, wenn er auf eine mögliche Gefahr, die in exzessiver Lust liegen kann, aufmerksam macht. In diesem Fall funktioniert er wie ein Alarm und verhindert Schlimmeres.[36] Dies ist allerdings die einzige positive Funktion, die der Schmerz laut Spinozas *Ethik* haben kann.[37] Da Schmerz prinzipiell immer eine Minderung unserer Fähigkeiten ist, hat er schlicht nichts Positives an sich.

Angesichts dieser Auffassung wird offensichtlich, dass Spinoza sich selbst grundsätzlich gegen die christliche Religion stellt, die im Leiden Christi eine Hilfe für jeden Christen sieht, sein eigenes Leid zu ertragen. Während dort Jesu Schmerzen eine Quelle und ein Grundpfeiler des Glaubens ist, verweigert Spinoza ihm jegliche Positivität. Ausdrücklich heißt es bei ihm im vierten Teil der *Ethik*:

> Fürwahr, nur ein finsterer und trübsinniger Aberglaub verbietet, sich zu erfreuen. [...] Keine Gottheit, noch sonst irgendwer, der nicht neidisch ist, erfreut sich meiner Ohnmacht oder meines Unglücks, noch rechnet er Tränen, Schluchzen, Furcht und anderes dieser Art, die Zeichen eines ohnmächtigen Gemüts sind, zu Tugend.[38]

Schmerz verstehen

Für Spinoza steht es außer Frage, dass Schmerzen oder jegliche Einschränkung und Zerstörung unseres Körpers,[39] von uns nicht gewollt

---

[36] Spinoza, *Ethik* IV, p43: „Lust kann ein Übermaß haben und schlecht sein, während Schmerz insofern gut sein kann, als die Lust oder Freude schlecht ist".

[37] Fast ironisch ist eine Nebenbemerkung am Ende des vierten Teils zu lesen, wo er noch eine positive Eigenschaft des Schmerzes beschreibt: Der Schmerz werde gut genannt, insofern er anzeige, dass der verletzte Teil noch nicht abgestorben sei. Vgl. Spinoza, *Ethik* IV, p58sch.

[38] Spinoza, *Ethik* IV, p45sch.

[39] Spinoza, *Ethik* III, p10: „Eine Idee, die die Existenz unseres Körpers ausschließt, kann es nicht in unserem Geist geben, sondern ist ihm entgegengesetzt".

sein kann, denn der Körper ist nicht bloß Gefäß oder Hülle unserer Seele. Seine Ablehnung von asketischen Praktiken oder von Akten der Selbstkasteiung und -verstümmelung überschneidet sich mit der jüdischen Denktradition. Die Übereinstimmung der Ordnungen von Körper und Geist schließt Vorgänge, die eine der beiden negieren oder übergehen, von vorneherein aus. Die Analogizität beider Seiten ist aber kein Dualismus. Eine Person ist die Einheit ihrer beiden Seiten. Unsere Überlegungen haben bis jetzt einen wichtigen Punkt ausgeklammert, der auch für die Argumentation hinsichtlich der Schmerzempfindung von Relevanz sein wird. Als bloßer Modus der Substanz scheinen wir ihrem Ausdrucksverhalten ausgeliefert und zur Passivität verdammt. Doch Spinoza eröffnet uns einen Weg der Aktivität: über das Erkennen.

Im Folgenden möchte ich nun genauer auf die Rolle, die die Erkenntnis für Spinoza spielt, eingehen. Spinozas Theorie ist eine Theorie der Immanenz:[40] Die Substanz ist nichts Transzendentes oder Jenseitiges, ihr Ausdruck ist total. Es gibt keine versteckte, mystische Wahrheit einer anderen Welt. Vielmehr hängt unser Unwissen damit zusammen, dass unsere Kapazitäten nicht unendlich sind und wir nicht die Details einer jeden Kausalkette in Gänze nachvollziehen können. Prinzipiell ist die Welt erkennbar.[41] Vorhin war bereits die Unterscheidung zwischen Epistemologie und Affektenlehre angedeutet worden. Jene handelt von den Erkenntnisarten, die uns zur Verfügung stehen, diese von den Gefühlen, die dem *conatus* gemäß in uns entstehen und die uns auch motivieren, bestimmte Dinge zu tun und andere zu lassen.[42] Noch-mal: Epistemologie, Erkenntnistheorie, handelt davon, wie wir verlässliche Kenntnis von der Welt, von kausalen Vorgängen in ihr haben können. Es geht um die intersubjektive Welt außer uns. Gefühle dagegen sind unsere ureigene Innenperspektive, spiegeln unser Streben mit seinen Widrigkeiten und seinen gelingenden Momenten wider. Die Frage nach der Erkennbarkeit von Gefühlen erübrigt sich, wenn damit gemeint sein soll, wie wir Wissen über unsere Gefühle erlangen können. Die Gefühle sind als solche bereits Nachrichten oder Wissen über uns, denn

---

[40] Sara Hornäk gibt einen klaren Überblick über frühere Begriffe von Immanenz und beschreibt wie Deleuze/Guattari den ihrigen erweitern. Ebenso überzeugend ist ihr Vergleich mit der Immanenz, die sie in den Gemälden von Johannes Vermeer, erkennt. Vgl. Hornäk S., *Spinoza und Vermeer. Immanenz in Philosophie und Malerei* (Würzburg: 2004).

[41] Dieselbe Idee ist auch im wachsenden Gewicht der mathematischen Wissenschaft bereits vor Spinoza zu finden.

[42] *Ethik* III, p2. Anm.: „Denn ein jeder handhabt alles von seiner Affektivität her".

nur weil wir Gefühle haben, wissen wir, wie es uns geht. Wenn Spinoza den *conatus* mit unserem Wesen gleichsetzt, dann sind die Gefühle, die gleichursprünglich mit dem Streben entstehen, unmittelbare Einblicke in unser Wesen, in dieses gelingende oder eingeschränkte Streben nach Selbsterhaltung. Auf die Frage „Wie geht's?" antworten unsere Gefühle und ich kann sagen, ob ich fröhlich bin oder eifersüchtig oder wütend. Dieses Wissen ist als ein unmittelbares, nicht begrifflich abgeleitetes, ein zur ersten Erkenntnisart zu zählendes Wissen. Wozu nun eine Affektenlehre, wenn klar ist, das die Einsicht in unseren Zustand immer schon gewährleistet ist? Spinoza bleibt nicht bei der Erklärung, was ein Gefühl ist, stehen, sondern er liefert eine Genese der Gefühle und möchte ihre Verursachtheit sichtbar machen. Er möchte die erste Erkenntnisart verlassen und will die Gefühle in ihrer Kausalgeschichte erklären, darlegen, wie sie entstehen wie es auch das Anliegen Descartes' in der *Passion de l'âme* gewesen war.[43] Der nächste Schritt liegt nahe und zielt darauf ab, die Erkenntnis dieser Verursachung zu verwenden. Schließlich lässt die Einsicht in die Genese Schlüsse im Sinne von Ratschlägen zu. Die Erkenntnis der Gefühle, genauer die Erkenntnis ihrer Entstehung, kippt am Ende um in praktische Philosophie, plötzlich geht es um unser Handeln in der Welt und wie wir auf unsere Gefühle und unser Streben Einfluss nehmen können.

Wie hängen mithin Erkenntnis und Schmerzempfindung zusammen? Die Definition des Schmerzes weist ihn als eine Minderung unseres Strebens aus, das uns körperlich wie geistig betrifft. Dabei bleibt unser Streben lebendig, ein negatives Streben oder eine Pause im Streben kann nicht gedacht werden, wenn die ganze Wirklichkeit mit dem *conatus* selbst identifiziert wird. Ein Begreifen der Genese des Schmerzes bedeutet nun wiederum, dass beide Seiten miteinbezogen werden müssen, die körperlichen Aspekte und die geistigen. Betrachten wir ein Beispiel des französischen Philosophen Alain. Sein Buch *Die Pflicht glücklich zu sein* beginnt mit der Geschichte eines weinenden Babys. Das Kindermädchen stellt diverse psychologische Hypothesen auf, z.B. ob das Kind denselben Charakter wie sein ständig aufgebrachter Vater hat.

---

[43] Linus Gemmeke sieht weitere Gemeinsamkeiten in den Affekttheorien Spinozas und Descartes. Auch hinsichtlich ihrer Einschätzung der Erkenntnis überwiegen in seinen Augen die Gemeinsamkeiten. Vgl. *Ethik contra Moral. Ein Vergleich der Affektenlehren Descartes' und Spinozas* (Berlin: 2003).

Sie sucht nach Erklärungen, bis sie plötzlich die Nadel, „die wirkliche Ursache des ganzen Aufruhrs, entdeckt hat".[44]

An Alains Beispiel lassen sich zwei Argumente, die letztlich auf Spinozas Theorie des Menschen zurückgehen, ablesen: Erstens, Erkenntnis ist immer Erkenntnis von Ursachen.[45] Zweitens müssen kausale Zusammenhänge innerhalb einer Sphäre nachvollzogen werden, Erklärungen können nicht zwischen den Attributen hin und her springen. Der Mensch ist zwar eine Einheit, eine Person und unser Körper und unser Denken existieren nicht ohne einander.[46] Doch die beiden Seiten dieser Einheit dürfen nicht verwechselt werden, wenn wir nach Erklärungen suchen. Schmerz zu verstehen heißt dann für Spinoza: wir müssen ihn zweimal verstehen, einmal als physischen und einmal als geistigen. Wir dürfen jedoch nicht überkreuz denken. Wenn wir also physische Schmerzen haben, müssen wir uns auf die Suche nach physischen Ursachen, nach der Nadel, machen. Hier wird auch die Kritik Spinozas am Christentum überdeutlich, denn die Erklärungen, Schmerz und Leid seien eine Strafe, bleiben nicht innerhalb ihrer Ursachenketten, sie gehen überkreuz und wollen einen physischen Schmerz mit Kategorien, die der Sphäre des Denkens entstammen, erklären. Eine Krankheit oder ein Erdbeben haben mit Begriffen wie dem der Strafe oder der Schuld nichts zu tun.

Die Lücke, die es zwischen der Erkenntnis und dem praktischen Handeln gibt, wurde bereits angedeutet. Wissen ist nichts, was uns automatisch weiterhilft. Wie kann Erkenntnis über die Ursachen des Schmerzes nun praktisch werden in dem Sinne, dass der Schmerz gelindert werden kann und unsere Selbsterhaltung stärker vollzogen werden kann? Wie kippt das Erkennen hier in die Praxis um, wenn die Sache sich komplizierter gestaltet als das Entfernen einer Nadel? Was nützt die Erkenntnis, wenn die diagnostizierte Krankheit unheilbar ist? Ein Einwand wäre, dass es sich bei einer solchen Diagnose offenbar um das Kundtun von Unwissen handelt, nicht um Wissen. Aber Spinoza würde

---

[44] Alain, *Die Pflicht glücklich zu sein*. Aus dem Franz. übersetzt von A. Fabri (Frankfurt a.M.: 1975; uspr. Paris, Edition Gallimard: 1928) 7.

[45] Auch Rainer Wiehl betont den Zusammenhang von Erkenntnis und Kausalität, in beiderlei Richtung. Wiehl R., „Spinoza und das psychophysische Problem", in Hammacher K. – Reimers-Tovote I. –Walther M. (Hrsg.), *Zur Aktualität der Ethik Spinozas* (Würzburg: 2000) 184.

[46] Ich danke Inja Stracenski ganz herzlich dafür, den Horizont meines Verständnisses von Spinoza bedeutend vergrößert zu haben – auch mittels der Diskussion via Email.

entgegnen, dass auch dieses Erkennen praktisch werden und befreiend wirken kann. Er reklamiert eine dritte Funktion von Erkenntnis, die nicht beim Erkennen kalter Fakten bleibt, sondern die als affektiv wirksame Erkenntnis in der Praxis Wirkungen zeitigt.[47] Dabei ist nun zu beachten, dass Erkenntnis nur dann wirksam werden kann, wenn sie selbst einen Affekt mit sich bringt: „Ein Affekt kann nicht anders gehemmt oder aufgehoben werden als durch einen Affekt, der dem zu hemmenden Affekt entgegengesetzt ist und der stärker als dieser ist".[48] Erkenntnis muss selbst Gefühle erzeugen. Wie dies gelingen kann, zeigt Spinoza in seiner Affektenlehre. Hier schreibt er, dass die Erkenntnis des Guten und Schlechten selbst als Affekt der Freude oder Trauer manifest wird.[49] Was ist damit gemeint? Er argumentiert, dass nicht jede Erkenntnis Freude generiert, sondern nur die, die erkennt, was für unser Streben hilfreich ist. Spinoza biegt seinen Gedanken schließlich wieder zum Anfang zurück, wenn er sagt, am nützlichsten für das Streben ist das Denken selbst. Mit anderen Worten, wir selbst sind am meisten wir selbst, wenn wir denken. Die Produktivität des Denkens ist so reine Aktivität, reines Streben. Die größte Selbststeigerung und damit auch die größte Freude erfahren wir im Erkennen selbst, das Erkennen ist gewissermaßen immer gut. Der Kategorische Imperativ Spinozas würde also lauten „Erkenne das Gute!" und das Gefühl der Freude würde sich daraus sofort mit ergeben.

Führen wir uns das Beispiel des gebrochenen Arms vor Augen. Die Erklärungen, die den Unfall auf der Treppe nachvollziehen, etwa das offene Schuhband als Ursache des Stolperns, nützen zur Linderung und Heilung wenig. Gefragt ist jetzt medizinisches Wissen über das

[47] „Insofern der Geist einsieht, daß alle Dinge notwendig sind, hat er eine größere Macht über die Affekte, anders formuliert, erleidet er weniger von ihnen." Spinoza, *Ethik* V, p6. Anmerkung: „Je mehr diese Erkenntnis – daß Dinge notwendig sind – sich auf Einzeldinge erstreckt, die wir deutlicher und lebhafter vorstellen, umso größer ist die mit ihr verbundene Macht des Geistes über die Affekte, was auch die Erfahrung selbst bestätigt. Wir sehen nämlich, daß die Trauer, irgendein Gut verloren zu haben, gemildert wird, sobald der Mensch, der es verloren hat, sich klar macht, daß dieses Gut auf keine Weise erhalten werden konnte. In ähnlicher Weise sehen wir, daß niemand ein Kleinkind bemitleidet, weil es nicht sprechen, laufen oder vernünftig denken kann und so viele Jahre nahezu ohne Selbstbewußtsein verbringt. Würden hingegen die meisten von uns als Erwachsene geboren und nur der eine oder andere als Kind, dann würde jeder die Kinder bemitleiden, weil er dann das, was Kindheit ist, nicht als einen natürlichen und notwendigen Sachverhalt, sondern als einen Fehler oder ein Gebrechen der Natur ansähe".

[48] Spinoza, *Ethik* IV, p7.

[49] Spinoza, *Ethik* IV, p8.

Zusammenwachsen von Knochen. Das Wissen des Arztes, eigentlich eine Erkenntnis, die zu den „kalten Fakten", hier Vorgänge des Körpers betreffend, zählt als angewandtes Wissen zur Erkenntnis des Guten insofern der Heilungsprozess eingeleitet wird, und der verletzte Mensch sein eigenes Streben besser fort zu setzen vermag. Auch als sein eigenes kann dieses ärztliche Wissen für den Verletzten in einem bestimmten Sinn zur Heilung beitragen. Nämlich insofern als der Patient, der über die Vorgänge und ärztlichen Maßnahmen in seinem Körper eingeweiht ist, nicht so leicht von ihnen überwältigt wird. Je mehr wir wissen, desto mehr können wir entspannen, behauptet ja Spinoza. Hier kann nun der Bogen in die andere Richtung geschlagen und die Relevanz des spinozanischen Denkens für moderne Interpretationen von Schmerz angedeutet werden, in denen mittels empirischer Studien die Notwendigkeit der Einbezogenheit von Patienten in die ärztlichen Entscheidungen und medizinischen Anwendungen aufgezeigt wird. Menschen, die mit ihren Schmerzen ohne jegliche Erklärung allein gelassen werden, leiden unter größeren Schmerzen als diejenigen, die genau informiert worden waren, zeigte bereits 1964 eine Studie über postoperative Schmerzen.[50] Der Wissenskontext, in dem Empfindungen gemacht werden, beeinflusst offenbar die Intensität mit der sie wahrgenommen werden. Dieser Umgang der Patienten mit Wissen demonstriert die Kraft, die Spinoza dem Erkennen zutraut. Nicht zu vernachlässigen ist dabei die Irrelevanz eines Schlussfolgerns, das die absolut geschlossenen Sphären miteinander vermischt. Ein bloßes Trösten kann das Wissen über die körperlichen Gegebenheiten nicht ersetzen.

Entscheidend für Spinozas Sicht auf den Zusammenhang von Schmerz und Erkenntnis bleibt mithin, dass das Wissen sich affektiv bemerkbar machen kann. Die Erkenntnis des Guten entspricht dem Affekt der Freude genauso wie der Geist dem Körper entspricht, schreibt er.[51] Entsprechung heißt, Wissen und Affekt sind zwei verschiedene Perspektiven, die eine kann nicht auf die andere reduziert werden und beide berühren sich nicht. Aber wir können wechseln! Wir müssen nicht

[50] Egbert L.D. – Battit G.E. et alii, „Reduction of postoperative pain by encouragement and instructions of patients: a study of doctor patient rapport", *New English Journal of Medicine*, 270 (1964) 825–827, zitiert nach Le Breton, *Schmerz* 76. Le Breton schlussfolgert, die Vorenthaltung von Sinn und die Verweigerung ihm gegenüber wirke keineswegs als Schutz des Individuums. Ein Schmerz, dem eine Ursache, eine Bedeutung zugeordnet wurde, lasse sich besser ertragen als ein Schmerz, der ohne Sinn belassen worden sei und den der Betroffene nicht begriffen habe.

[51] Vgl. Anm. 47.

bei der Perspektive des Erkennens bleiben, sondern können auch die affektive Sichtweise einnehmen.

Die genaue Analyse, worauf es bei der Erkenntnis dessen, was gut ist, ankommt, liefert Spinoza in den beiden letzten Büchern der *Ethik*. Das echte, affektiv gewordene Wissen, das die Lücke zwischen dem kalten Erkennen und dem warmen Gefühl zu schließen vermag, können wir erlangen, wenn wir unsere Affektstruktur vollständig erkannt haben. Dazu gehört die Einsicht in die Notwendigkeit der Einsicht.

Wenn ein Affekt sich auf viele und verschiedene Ursachen bezieht, die der Geist zusammen mit dem Affekt selbst betrachtet, ist er weniger schädlich; wir leiden weniger durch ihn und geraten gegenüber jeder einzelnen seiner Ursachen nicht so leicht in Affekte, als dies bei einem anderen gleichgroßen Affekt der Fall ist, der sich nur auf eine einzige oder auf nicht so viele Ursachen bezieht.[52]

> Beweis: Ein Affekt ist nur insofern schlecht oder schädlich, als er den Geist hindert, denken zu können (nach LS 26. und 27. des 4. Teils); mithin ist der Affekt, der den Geist dazu bestimmt, viele Objekte zugleich zu betrachten, weniger schädlich als ein anderer gleichgroßer Affekt, der den Geist in der Betrachtung nur eines oder einiger weniger Objekte derart festhält, dass er an andere Objekte nicht denken kann.[53]

Das Einordnen des Schmerzes in ein Wissen um seine Ursachen kann den Schmerz kontrollierbarer, eingegrenzter machen. Gleichzeitig kann das Denken Perspektiven eröffnen, die die Fixierung auf das eine schmerzende Körperteil lösen. Die Ideen ermöglichen sich selbst mehr Gedankengänge als die eine unbestimmte Angst, die mit dem Schmerz auftritt. Das meint Spinoza, wenn er sagt, je mehr Ideen wir denken, desto weniger können wir von einer einzigen bestimmt werden. Je mehr Wissen wir haben, desto weniger werden wir von einer einzelnen Sache gebannt. Spinoza nannte sein Buch *Ethik*, denn sein Anliegen ist das gute Leben. Und die Erkenntnis ist es, die es besser – affektiv besser – gestalten kann.

---

[52] Spinoza, *Ethik* EV, p9.

[53] Ebd.

Auswahlbibliographie

ALAIN, *Die Pflicht glücklich zu sein*, aus dem Frz. übersetzt von A. Fabri (Frankfurt a.M.: 1975; urspr. Paris: 1928).

ARISTOTELES, *Nikomachische Ethik*, hrsg. und übersetzt von F. Dirlmeier (Stuttgart: 1969).

BLUME E., HÜRLIMANN A., SCHNALKE T., TYRADELLIS D. (Hrsg.), *Schmerz. Kunst und Wissenschaft*, Begleitbuch zur Ausstellung (Berlin: 2007).

BLUMENBERG H., „Selbsterhaltung und Beharrung. Zur Konstitution der neuzeitlichen Rationalität", in Ebeling H. (Hrsg.) *Subjektivität und Selbsterhaltung* (Frankfurt a.M.: 1996) 144–208.

BOERI M.D., VIGO A.G., „Die Affektenlehre der Stoa", in Engstler A., Schnepf R. (Hrsg.), *Affekte und Ethik. Spinozas Lehre im Kontext* (Hildesheim: 2002) 32–60.

BÜTTNER S., „Spinozas Attribut der Ausdehnung und Kants Form der Anschauung – ein systematisch orientierter Vergleich", in Piarek H. – Walther M. (Hrsg.), *Kontexte – Spinoza und die Geschichte der Philosophie* (Wroclaw: 2001) 109–125.

CARMASSI P., *Divina Officia. Liturgie und Frömmigkeit im Mittelalter* (Wolfenbüttel: 2004).

DESCARTES RENÉ, *Meditationes de Prima Philosophia*, übersetzt und hrsg. von G. Schmidt (Stuttgart: 1986).

——, *Die Leidenschaften der Seele.* Übersetzt und hrsg. von K. Hammacher (Hamburg: 1984).

GEMMEKE L., *Ethik contra Moral. Ein Vergleich der Affektenlehren Descartes' und Spinozas* (Berlin: 2003).

GIANCOTTI E., „The Theory of the Affects in the Strategy of Spinoza's Ethics" in Yovel Y. (Hrsg.), *Desire and Affect. Spinoza as a Psychologist* (New York: 1999) 129–139.

HANDWERKER KÜCHENHOFF B., *Spinozas Theorie der Affekte. Köhärenz und Konflikt* (Würzburg: 2006).

HORNÄK S., *Spinoza und Vermeer. Immanenz in Philosophie und Malerei* (Würzburg: 2004).

LANGEMEYER G., Art. „Leid", in *Lexikon der katholischen Dogmatik* (Freiburg: 1987) 346–347.

LE BRETON D., *Schmerz. Eine Kulturgeschichte* (Zürich – Berlin: 2003).

PLATO, *Philebos*, hrsg. von W.F. Otto – E. Grassi – G. Plamböck. (Hamburg: 1959).

REISINGER P., „Modelle des Absoluten", in Löw R. (Hrsg.), *Oikeiosis. Festschrift für Robert Spaemann* (Weinheim: 1987) 225–249.

RENZ U., „Zwischen ontologischer Notwendigkeit und zufälliger Semantik. Zu Spinozas Theorie der menschlichen Affecte", in Landweer H. (Hrsg.), *Gefühle – Struktur und Funktion* (Berlin: 2007) 35–57.

ROMBACH H., *Substanz, System, Struktur: Die Ontologie des Funktionalismus und der philosophische Hintergrund der modernen Wissenschaft* (Freiburg i. Br.: ^{2}1981).

SPINOZA BARUCH, *Ethik in geometrischer Ordnung dargestellt* (Hamburg: 2006).

WALTHER M., *Metaphysik als Anti-Theologie. Die Philosophie Spinozas im Zusammenhang der religionsphilosophischen Problematik* (Hamburg: 1971).

——, „Freiheit und Notwendigkeit: Die Umgestaltung der praktischen Philosophie durch Spinoza als Irritation und Provokation des ethischen und politischen Denkens in der Neuzeit", in Balibar E. – Seidel H. – Walther M. (Hrsg.), *Freiheit und Notwendigkeit. Ethische und politische Aspekte bei Spinoza und in der Geschichte des (Anti)Spinozismus* (Würzburg: 1994) 11–23.

WIEHL R., „Spinoza und das psychophysische Problem", in Hammacher K. – Reimerstovote I. – Walther M. (Hrsg.), *Zur Aktualität der Ethik Spinozas* (Würzburg: 2000) 173–197.

WILD M., *Die anthropologische Differenz. Der Geist der Tiere in der frühen Neuzeit bei Montaigne, Descartes und Hume* (Berlin – New York: 2006).

Yoshida K., *Vernunft und Affektivität. Untersuchungen zu Spinozas Theorie der Politik* (Würzburg: 2004).

Yovel Y. (Hrsg.), *Spinoza on Knowledge and the Human Mind* (Leiden: 1994).

IMAGINING PHYSICAL PAIN IN A SIXTEENTH-CENTURY HUNGARIAN POISONING TRIAL[1]

Emese Bálint

In 1572, the court of Klausenburg (Kolozsvár), royal free town and *civitas primaria*[2] of the Transylvanian principality, investigated an unusual case of poisoning.[3] On the Saturday before St. Martin's day[4] the elderly Margit, wife of Albert Kalmár, accused her son-in-law, the barber Bálint Borbély, of murder. This case was shaped by the characteristics of local legal practice: the town lacked a public prosecutor, and litigation therefore started after an accusation by a private person. In this case it was the victim's closest female relative to accuse Bálint Borbély of murder. He repudiated the accusation and brought fourteen witnesses to testify in his favor. A total number of thirty witnesses presented the following story: Margit's daughter Orsolya, still in childbed in her husband's house, drank some wine sent to her during a friendly gathering. That wine affected her immediately and she soon showed symptoms usually associated with poisoning. Witness testimonies revolved around the wine she drank: the accusation stated that the wine contained poison deliberately used by the barber, while the defense maintained that the woman was killed by the wine, not by the barber (or poison). The testimonies contain vivid descriptions of Orsolya's pain. During her long agony she told visitors, the future witnesses, about the nature of

[1] I thank the editors, Karl Enenkel and Jan Frans Dijkhuizen, as well as Giulia Calvi, Thomas V. Cohen, Anu Korhonen and the conference participants in Leiden for valuable comments on earlier drafts.

[2] In the second half of the sixteenth century, Klausenburg (Kolozsvár) developed into an important commercial and artisan center of approximately 8000 Hungarian and German inhabitants.

[3] D.J.A.N. Cluj (Romanian National Archives, Cluj County), Fond Primăria Oraşului Cluj-Napoca, Protocoale de judecată (hereinafter: Prot.Jud.) Doc II. 6/1572–1575, fol. 111–115.

[4] In the multiethnic setting of Klausenburg, court proceedings were registered in Hungarian. Although the town was Protestant, official documents often specify dates with reference to certain saints' days, both in Latin or Hungarian headings of the protocols (*sabato ante Martini; szent György nap előtt hétfőn* – the Monday before Saint George).

her pain experience, and as deponents gave testimony in court, some referred to imaginary objects within the body.

These narratives form an excellent starting point for analyzing discourses of pain, bodily perceptions and medical knowledge of the late sixteenth century. My analysis will focus on the witnesses' interpretations of pain, and on the blend of medical and legal conceptions in the trial. The conceptions of pain put forward during the trial were based on the sensations of the sufferer, on the readings of her feelings by witnesses, and on the emotional responses of those in intimate contact with the sufferer. Most witnesses deposing in the trial are almost anonymous to us; they appear without any traces of age, family or economic circumstances, and only give short descriptions of their stories. Yet their depositions offer a glimpse of local medical lay knowledge, and the individual narratives add up to a cultural discourse formed around the sick woman's bed. Her pain experience had contributed to the formation of discourse communities (and in a similar manner, pain communities) that later transmitted several meanings of illness behaviour by their mediation and by their verbal testimonies.[5] This article looks at bodily experience as a product of cultural settings and social relations, and will explore several influences that created an understanding of pain in this early modern community.[6] To illustrate the nature of popular knowledge visible in the witnesses' depositions, I will use a contemporary remedy book for simple folk, the *Ars Medica* compiled in the 1570s.[7]

My analysis argues that there was two-way traffic between lay and learned medical concepts; a pluralism and fluid interchange of ideas and information that was an important general feature of early modern European culture, from religion to health. Contemporary letters and

[5] Porter R., "The Patient's View: Doing Medical History from Below", *Theory and Society* 14,2 (1985), especially 176; and Condrau F., "The Patient's View Meets the Clinical Gaze", *Social History of Medicine* 20,3 (2007) 525–540.

[6] Gowing L., *Common Bodies: Women, Touch and Power in Sixteenth-Century England* (Yale: 2003); Howard S., "Imagining the Pain and Peril of Seventeenth-Century Childbirth: Travail and Deliverance in the Making of an Early Modern World", *Social History of Medicine* 16,3 (2003) 367–382.

[7] *Ars Medica* is considered the first Transylvanian overview of medical practice from the early 1570s, collected and translated into Hungarian by György Lencsés (1530–1593) a non-practicing physician. It has survived in three manuscript copies and was published in 1947 as *Egy 16. századi orvosi könyv* [A medical book of the sixteenth century] (ed. Varjas B.), (Kolozsvár: 1947). Parts of the *Ars Medica* have been identified as translations from Jean Fernel's *Universa Medicina.*

diaries show an eclectic openness among the elite towards all manners of medical knowledge, a willingness to resort to popular healers and remedies. Likewise, what seems to be popular knowledge was in fact increasingly exposed to the ministrations of educated practitioners, and to the impositions of elite medicine.[8]

Understanding the meanings of illness always calls for explanations that search for causes and expound a truth about the order of the world and the body of the sick person. European medical knowledge of the early modern period mainly rested on theories of humouralism and environmentalism.[9] Accordingly, explanations of the causes of disease were based on the concepts of pollution and impurity. Lay and learned people alike understood health as the proper balance of the four humours, and saw disease as arising from imbalance. This could be further influenced and affected by the environment (for example, the condition of the air or water, an especially hot or wet summer, or unfavorable conjunctions of the planets). By stressing the strong influence of the environment, these theories could easily coexist with other systemic beliefs: sudden and inexplicable changes in the human condition could be explained by human agency: an enemy could cause physical harm by means of lethal substances or objects. Representations of the human body extended from one-sex models (featuring, for example, menstruating men) to significantly different male and female anatomies, often exceeding in their somatic range the essential differences between human and animal.[10] Similarly, bodies were perceived as permeable via many open orifices and via the skin, rather than encapsulated by the skin and defended from the outside.[11] As we

[8] Porter R., "The People's Health in Georgian England", in Harris T. (ed.), *Popular Culture in England, c. 1500–1850* (New York: 1995) 124–142.

[9] Lindemann M., *Medicine and Society in Early Modern Europe* (Cambridge: 1999); Nutton V., "Humouralism", in Bynum W.F. – Porter R. (eds.), *Companion Encyclopedia of the History of Medicine*, vol. I (London – New York: 1993) 281–291.

[10] Medieval and early modern conceptions of the body were based on the principle that men and women were fundamentally similar: bodies only had one sex, and the female reproductive organs were seen as an inverted form of the male genitalia. See Gowing, *Common Bodies* 17–19.

[11] Pomata G., "Menstruating Men: Similarity and Difference of the Sexes in Early Modern Medicine", in Finucci V. – Brownlee K. (eds.), *Generation and Degeneration: Tropes of Reproduction in Literature and History from Antiquity to Early Modern Europe* (Durham: 2001); Kivistö S., "G.F. von Franckenau's Satyra Sexta (1674)", in Korhonen A. – Lowe K. (eds.), *The Trouble with Ribs: Women, Men and Gender in Early Modern Europe* (Helsinki: 2007) 82–102; Duden B., *The Woman Beneath the Skin: A Doctor's Patients in Eighteenth-Century Germany* (Cambridge, MA – London: 1998).

will see, the sixteenth-century trial narratives discussed in this article were informed by these complex models of the human body and by a composite repertoire of knowledge.

Poison or Wine? Possible Causes of Death in Witness Testimonies

In 1572 the judicial court of Klausenburg was in fact the low council of the town, with its six German and six Hungarian senators, headed by a Hungarian judge.[12] These wealthy burghers – merchants or artisans – were all literate to a certain degree but had received no formal education in medicine (or in law, for that matter), and did not have a court-appointed expert on hand to perform postmortem dissection to state the exact cause of the woman's death. In criminal cases the *peritus* view came from barbers who had cared for the wounded, or from midwives testifying in trials of infanticide.[13] In cases of poisoning, legal tradition concentrated on witness descriptions of the symptoms, and other indicators of guilt. Evidence of poisoning was rather vaguely defined and very close to sorcery; poisoning was seen as similar to witchcraft techniques for administering malefic substances (*megétetés*) to a victim. The attention of doctors and judges usually concentrated on three points of the examination. They first looked for external signs of poisoning, such as swelling, skin color, or the degree of corpse decay (poisoned corpses were believed to remain intact either for abnormally short or extremely long periods). Equally important were the victims' laments and accusations during sickness. As a second set of evidence, experts investigated the immediate environment of the poison victim. Suspects were expected to have handled, sent, and bought poison, or to have collected poisonous herbs or contacted suspected sorcerers, or to have been alone in the kitchen on the first day of illness. A third method

[12] By the 1450s, Kolozsvár's Hungarians outnumbered Germans but did not yet dominate political and commercial life. Supported by the central government, Hungarians soon arranged for a parity principle, and shared the seats of the high council (*centumviri*), with 50 Hungarian and 50 Saxon councilors. Councillors elected the judge (*judex primarius*) and the senate of twelve (low council) whose first senator was the second judge (*judex regius*), the king's representative. Hungarian and German judges took yearly turns: if the first judge was Hungarian, the second judge was Saxon, and vice versa. This system could not always prevent conflicts between Hungarians and Germans.

[13] Pakó L., "Kényszer vagy erkölcsi romlottság? Csecsemőgyilkosságok Kolozsvárt a 16. század utolsó évtizedében" [Pressure or immorality? Infanticides in Kolozsvár of the late sixteenth century], *Korunk* 3 (2005) 84–93.

of collecting evidence was the investigation of suspicious substances around the victim by administering them to animals, and observing the effect.[14] As our case unfolds, we will see how several arguments added such small details to form a narrative against the suspected barber. In the testimonies, the victim moaned with pain as her body was swollen and troubled with convulsive movements, her stomach ached, and in addition, she blamed her husband for her sickness. The barber's medical knowledge, which had qualified him as a *peritus* in other criminal cases, incriminated him when he was brought to court as an *imputatus*.

When Margit, the plaintiff's mother-in-law, appeared in court to accuse Bálint the barber, witnesses constructed two narratives to present the history of illness. The defense pursued a different line of argumentation that absolved the barber from poisoning but used arguments that formed a different universe. The two versions dovetailed in their avowal that the victim had already been ill and in bed when the barber gave her a sort of medicinal wine, they all said, wormwood wine, a bitter-tasting curative liquid made of different herbs and spices, and named after one component wormwood (*Artemisia absinthium*), best known as the primary ingredient in absinthe. Incidentally, wormwood wine is not completely unfamiliar to modern readers: the closest in taste and in composition is vermouth. Widely used to help problems of the stomach and of the whole digestive system, wormwood wine was also given to women in order to hasten childbirth and expel afterbirth.[15]

In this particular case, however, wine did not cure. After the sick woman had drunk of the wormwood wine, her condition suddenly changed for the worse, and she soon died. The idea of the critical turning point was a familiar element in contemporary understandings of disease processes: after Orsolya went into a 'crisis', she failed to come out cured.[16] In discussing what followed the turning point, the two

[14] Katona G., *Bizonyítási eszközök a XVIII–XIX. században. A kriminalisztika magyarországi előzményei* [Legal evidence in the eighteenth and nineteenth centuries. The advance of criminology in Hungary] (Budapest: 1977) 324–333.

[15] Wine, like oil, was the basis of many liquid medicines, used since antiquity, for cleansing wounds, and of various laxatives and emetics. Most ingredients came from plants, some from animals, and few from minerals. Siraisi N., *Medieval & early Renaissance Medicine: An Introduction to Knowledge and Practice* (Chicago: 1990) 148.

[16] Crisis was part of the medical prognosis, and given that not all illnesses were curable, a physician needed to ensure that he was not to blame if his patient died. Methods for predicting a crisis through calculations were also available to practitioners. See Kusukawa S., "Medicine in Western Europe in 1500", in Elmer P. (ed.), *The Healing Arts: Health, Disease and Society in Europe 1500–1800* (Manchester: 2004) 1–26.

parties offered conflicting narratives. The accusation claimed that the wine contained poison, without stating what the killing substance was. Strong flavours in the wine could have concealed the taste of poison in it – if any was to be found in the cup. Also, curing with wormwood wine required caution, especially in inexpert hands. It could cause intoxication and provoke symptoms very much like those described by witnesses in this trial: stomach pain, spasms, hallucination, and loss of consciousness. Not even practitioners had absolute control over the amount or concentration in which medicines were administered; their dosage was largely intuitive.[17] Wormwood overdose, to use the modern term, could cause the death of the patient. Yet is it unlikely that the witnesses had this in mind when accusing the barber of poisoning. They all referred to a premeditated action, and according to one witness, the barber responded to this allegation with the following words: 'I have never poisoned anyone.'[18]

The defendant's witnesses offered a completely different interpretation of the turning point, and stated that the non-natural substance of wine had caused an imbalance within the victim's body, which eventually led to her death. In medical theory, non-naturals did not form part of the body's internal workings. They included the surroundings (air), exercise (walks, riding, massages and sex), ingested substances (food, drink, medicine), those things that are eliminated or retained (secretions and excretions), and the passions of the soul (emotional states: anger, grief and envy). Diagnosis in these testimonies ignored the pain and other physical symptoms that were so important for the accusation, and stressed the physical constitution of the woman.[19] According to one of the witnesses for the defense, the victim had been of a weak nature, already suffering from other conditions when the turning point occurred:

> Márton Kalmár declares that Orsolya, the daughter of Albert Kalmár's wife had already been ill. He [the witness] heard it from herself that the moment she drank the wormwood wine that was brought to her by

---

[17] Siraisi, *Medieval & Early Renaissance Medicine* 148.

[18] Prot.Jud. Doc II. 6/1572–1575, fol. 114.

[19] A healthy body had a good complexion – that is, a good balance of humours and arrangement of the parts of the body. A diseased body did not have a good balance – in fact, it had an imbalance caused by a deficiency in or an excess of one or more of the humours. Elmer, *The Healing Arts* 8.

> the apprentice, it became cold in her stomach, and that has caused her death.[20]

In this deposition one can recognize the idea of healing by opposition. For example, in the case of an illness that caused excessive heat, a medicine was administered with a strong cold property.[21] Similarly, warming up the stomach by drinking fluids of hot qualities was one of the healing procedures often practiced by medical professionals and lay people alike. Wine, in general, was reserved for the old, as the progressive decline in their natural heat required a supplementary source of warmth to overcome the coldness that accompanies old age. The benefits of drinking wine ran as follows:

> Wine assists nutrition, digestion and the generation of blood. It distributes the digested humours, speedily nourishes, makes the heart happy, eliminates windiness, encourages urination, increases the natural warmth, fattens convalescents, reawakens the appetite, activates sweat, assists sleep, clears the blood when it is turbid, opens obstructions, takes nutrition to all parts of the body, thins the coarse humours, improves skin color and helps to discharge all excrements.[22]

Likewise, the general model of the sexes believed women's bodies to be wetter and colder, essentially the inverse of the male body; therefore administering wine to a sick woman was expected to manifest its healing properties. Accordingly, cold and moist distemperature would have been corrected with a hot and dry regimen that also included hot herbs in the wine.[23] Despite all beneficial attributes of the wormwood wine, it did not heal the sick woman: she had drunk some, and instead of restoring the balance of humours and degrees, the wine 'became cold in her stomach, and caused her death.' This interpretation eventually pointed to the failure of wine: the liquid within the body had become poisonous, killing instead of nourishing.

---

[20] Prot.Jud. Doc II. 6/1572–1575, fol. 112.

[21] Elmer, *The Healing Arts* 10.

[22] Camporesi P. citing Baldassare Pisanelli's *Trattato della natura de' cibi e del bere* (1587), in *The Anatomy of the Senses: Natural Symbols in Medieval and Early Modern Italy* (Polity: 1994) 80.

[23] Evaluation of food and nutrition was also firmly rooted in humoral physiognomy. See Albala K., *Eating in the Renaissance* (Ewing, NJ: 2002).

Pain Symbols in Witness Narratives

Two important and pervasive ways of conceptualizing illness and disease are through metaphor and visual imagery. Individuals who have experienced illness and pain often revert to metaphorical discourse to conceptualize and articulate to themselves and to others their experience.[24] The following section will discuss the characteristic features of three witness narratives that represent pain through metaphors. Unusual as some of the images are, they must have been understood by the community since a metaphor can only be effective if it relies at least in part on pre-established knowledge and belief systems. I will rely on the Transylvanian *Ars Medica* to decipher diverse layers of the sick body's perception. Three of the witnesses during the trial in 1572 reported that the sick woman localized pain in her stomach and articulated her painful experience in terms of objects inside her stomach. In her explanation, the ingested wine turned into an object, which in the witnesses' subsequent individual narrations was associated with commonplace objects from everyday life. In their testimonies, this entity within the body took up the form of a square object, a cannonball, and a piece of meat. As a basic characteristic, these disease metaphors refer to imbalance and disorder; the image of an object within the digestive tract surely stood for a blockage that obstructed the natural, healthy flow of bodily fluids. A healthy stomach was deemed especially important. In different medical systems informed by humouralism, the stomach was associated with roots of a tree, but it could also be described in architectural terms, as the kitchen of the household.[25] The purity of the stomach required that harmful liquids and any blocking objects be eliminated.

By medico-legal definition, the physical pain caused by poison was believed to be of three kinds: sharp, or convulsive, or numbing.[26] There is no trace of numbing pain in these narratives, while sharp ache and strong convulsions can be linked to the images of the square object

[24] Lupton D., *Medicine as Culture: Illness, Disease and the Body in Western Societies* (London: 2003) 54–83.

[25] The body was also perceived as a house, a fortress, an edifice, a cell, a cage box, or a coffer. These various architectural metaphors form a coherent system in the French surgeon Henri de Mondeville's treatise on the human body (1306–1320). See Lupton, citing Pouchelle's study of de Mondeville's work, in "Representations of Medicine, Illness and Disease" 59–60.

[26] Katona, *Bizonyítási eszközök* 328.

and the cannonball in the stomach. The first metaphor referred to a square object hurting from the inside: the wine felt 'in her stomach like a square object, and if she got rid of it she would be cured immediately'.[27] It is easy to imagine that razor-like edges and pointy corners of the square object inside the body could have inflicted sharp pain, maybe similar to 'arrows of flatulence and needles of pain caused by bile'.[28] In some cultures, these sharp objects inside the body can take up diverse shapes, from a stone or a crystal to fragments of bones, or even leaves, all capable of causing a cutting pain.

The second witness who reported the victim's words to the judges likened the nature of pain to a canonball inside the stomach. Put simply, the witness claimed that the dying woman 'felt it immediately; [the wine] stopped in her stomach just like a cannonball'.[29] The first mental representations of a cannonball are obvious: its weight and a strong sensation of coldness. The sensation of coldness in the stomach can be associated with previous images of the wine turning cold after ingestion, and the pure weight of the cannonball can be linked to the hardness of the stomach and the impossibility of digestion. Descriptions of bodily pain through sensations of cold and weight seem universal, sometimes understood in gendered terms: often, stomach pains were said to be much worse than labor pains.[30]

The next metaphor used by a witness to describe the woman's unbearable pain once again combines the imaginary with the physical-anatomical. The third witness who described the victim's upset stomach used the image of a piece of meat that acted like a fatal blockage inside the woman's body: the wine she drank 'stopped in her stomach just like a piece of meat'.[31] This image, again, invites a multi-layered interpretation. Very different from the two previous imaginary objects within the body, meat can be seen as a non-natural substance causing indigestion, and becoming rotten very quickly, disturbing the purity of the stomach. In similar cases of stomach ache, the function of medicine was to restore the balance that had been disturbed, and the principle of medication rested either on the idea of opposition, or on the idea of facilitating blocked passages to flow. It was widely believed that

---

27 Prot.Jud. Doc II. 6/1572–1575, fol. 112.
28 Lupton, "Representations of Medicine, Illness and Disease" 60.
29 Prot.Jud. Doc II. 6/1572–1575, fol. 111.
30 Siraisi N., *Medieval & Early Renaissance Medicine* 41.
31 Prot.Jud. Doc II. 6/1572–1575, fol. 112.

removal of the object would effect rapid cure. In practice, the removal of the object, therefore the reduction of pain, could be produced in two ways: by massage or by purgation. The former is closer to magical beliefs, as it is supposed to act directly on the body, and help remove the object causing the problem.[32] The alternative method of taking purgatives was also widely employed in the sixteenth century, and it was aimed at removing putrid matter in order to keep the body's passages open. And it was, of course, often the best thing to do if one had eaten spoiled food.

The uneasy, or even painful feeling caused by a piece of meat inside the female belly suggests a gendered experience. The *Ars Medica* uses the image of a piece of meat inside the uterus to describe molar pregnancy, when a mass of abnormal tissues (what modern medicine calls a hydatidiform mole or *Mola hydatidosa*) [33] fills the womb, and causes fatigue, unexplained weight loss, increased heart rate, heat intolerance, sweating, irritability, anxiety, muscle weakness, and thyroid enlargement:

> *Mola* is almost like a piece of meat that grows in the uterus, and occasionally takes up definite forms. Often this is a hideous creature covered with skin or membrane; inside mingle some soft and lose flesh, interspersed by tiny veins but lacking bones, inner parts, limbs and bowels. This creature extracts life through veins, grows like a plant, and fills the womb like a fetus of eight months. At times it attaches to the uterus so much that women are forced to carry it for four or even five years, sometimes for their whole lives. At times it attaches loosely to the uterus and falls out on the third or fourth month, so it cannot grow further.[34]

This varied range of pain metaphors points to a human body that was fragile, and imperfectly protected against the outside world. The

[32] In a different case I found that massage was used to cure digestive problems; the person who performed the cure was the household servant.

[33] "Hydatidiform mole", *Medical Encyclopedia*, National Library of Medicine <http://www.nlm.nih.gov/medlineplus/ency/article/000909.htm> accessed 9 May 2008.

[34] *Ars Medica* 336: 'Ez szinte olyan, mint egy összesült darab hús, mely a madrának üregében terem, ki néha mutat valami formát. Ez gyakorta rút darab állat, és bőrrel vagy hártyával körül vétetve vagyon, és belől abban lágy összezavarodott hús vagyon, ki sok apró erecskékkel meghintetett, de csontok, belső részek, tagok, és belek nélkül vagyon. Ez magának éltetést az erek által szív, és szinte úgy növekedik, mint a plánták, annyira megteríti penig a hasat, mint a nyolc holnapi gyermek. Néha ez igen odaragad a madrához, hogy némely asszonyállatok kényszeríttetnek ezt elviselni négy avagy öt esztendeig is, néha penig ugyan teljes életekben ott viselik madrájokban. Néha penig oly kevéssé ragad a madrához, hogy harmad- vagy negyedholnapra kiesik onnét, és szinte megnövekedésére nem mehet'.

environment invaded the body in mineral, vegetable, and animal form. Within this system, the mouth was the opening that controlled what went into the body. Similarly, controlling the traffic between the inside and the outside, the doctor, or the ill person, could immediately respond to any kind of uneasiness. With apparent certitude, by regulating the non-natural substances 'one could restore the body to health or, more importantly, prevent the natural balance of a body from tipping over into imbalance'.[35] All these images imply a subsequent need to conceptualize the human body as ordered, reasoned, pure, and clean. Metaphors worked to 'naturalize' discourses of illness and disease, in this way 'turning that which is problematic into obvious'.[36]

Pain and Proof in Court

So far, we have seen many voices reflected in the testimonies constructed around two competing narratives. In urban and rural cultures alike, illness and the healing process took place within the community, and people surrounding the sick person in life made constant reference to diagnosis, healing and convalescence. Memories and retellings that ended up in court had previously confronted other versions, had shared knowledge and gossip, and finally were structured into legal records. In this sense, social relations created communication systems and information networks, through which messages were sent and phenomena compared.[37] Mediation, however, was not a one-way process or a mere filtering down of facts. The way information was selected and adapted to fit the legal testimony represented only the end point in a journey that combined multi-layered symbols and understandings of pain. The individual illness experience was transmitted orally to different members of the community, who in turn further transmitted information; thus the judicial search for explanations and proofs in somebody's disease leads to a new aspect of the modern historical analysis.

The nature of the victim's social environment is only indirectly recorded in the legal documents of this case but surely, overt expressions

[35] Nutton, "Humouralism" 289.

[36] Lupton, "Representations of Medicine, Illness and Disease" 58.

[37] Bar-On Y., "Neighbours and Gossip in Early Modern Gynaecology", in Blécourt W. de – Usborne C. (eds.), *Cultural Approaches to the History of Medicine* (Basingstoke – New York: 2004) 36–55.

of pain invited help and care. In this particular case, bystanders had been capable only of offering moral support and relief, while the only person whom they had expected to interfere with the sickness did nothing, and let his wife die. As a medical practitioner, the barber took care of the sick and the wounded, and according to trial records of other cases from the town, he had been the person of first recourse when urgent medical help was needed.[38] In some of the witness accounts, he was depicted as indifferent and passive, while others told of his verbal violence and hostile attitude towards his wife. Either way, his behavior indicated guilt.

Fact-finding, in this case of poisoning, brought together medical and legal argumentations, and both were shaped by an individual experience further transmitted through collective and public discourses. No medico-legal expertise was used in the tribunal of Klausenburg at the end of the sixteenth century; as a consequence, causality and facts were not arranged in coherent theories or frameworks typical of criminal investigation in later centuries. The legal facts on which the accusation rested, described the physical evidence of the victim's agony: painful convulsions, extreme thirst, and swelling. Aggravating proof of the barber's guilt centered on the laments and accusations of the dying woman. According to sixteenth-century legal standards, familiarity with healing practices, or access to eventually poisonous substances also pointed to guilt. All these were aggravated by circumstantial evidence: exceptional cruelty as a husband, and negligence as a practitioner.

Compared to other poison trials, our Klausenburg case lacks two important elements, both related to the absence of a medical expert in the court. First, no suspected poison, either powder or liquid, was produced in court to demonstrate with certainty the causality between

[38] The early modern medical marketplace comprised a variety of healers of distinct ranks and with different skills. Medical practitioners in the court of the Transylvanian prince and king of Poland István Báthory were *balneatores, barbitonsores, tonsores, chirurgi, doctores*, and *medici*. See Veress E., *Fontes Rerum Hungaricarum III: Báthory István lengyel király udvari számadás- könyveinek Magyar- és Erdélyországi adalékai (1576–1586)* (Budapest: 1918). On a local level, the picture was even more colourful, with medicine women, ointment women or dilettante tooth-pullers, and one characteristic of healing was that it was not separated from domestic work. Managing and treating sickness often remained largely in the hands of the sufferers themselves. In this typical setting, often referred to by historians as 'bedside medicine', the patient exercised most power and autonomy, while the intervention of doctors was only one (sometimes the last) weapon in the therapeutic arsenal. See Jewson N.D., "Medical Knowledge and Patronage System in Eighteenth-Century England", *Sociology* 8,3 (1974) 369–385.

the barber's agency and his wife's death. A validation at once legal and medical would have required that the suspicious substance be given to animals: cats, kittens, dogs, pigs, or even pigeons.[39] Second, there was no inspection of the corpse, or dissection of organs.[40] Instead, the court heard a set of witnesses ready to offer other types of explanation and refute legal facts.[41] While the legal facts of this case placed pain at the centre of their argumentation, those offering medical explanation had never looked for such proof. In fact, pain was a diagnostic tool in medicine but recognition of direct causality was rarely the case, and medicine was based on systems of interpretation of the body that lacked a vocabulary for facts. Different expressions – for example *res, particularia, experimenta* or *sensibilia* – were used to cover more or less the semantic field of what we call today 'fact' when we refer to causality.[42]

Consider the following testimony of a woman on the accuser's side. Her words depict the agony of the dying woman and indifference shown by her husband; all these were facts intended to demonstrate the barber's guilt in poisoning his wife:

> Orsolya, the wife of Imre Szőcs, declares that she once went to see the wife of Bálint the barber in her sickness, and when she got there, sickness hit [Bálint's wife] so badly that [the witness] feared death. The husband was washing hair, and [the witness] called out to him saying that his wife was dying. He said: but that is her fate. Again, the woman had more severe tremors, and started breathing heavily, and [the witness] asked him to see to his wife because she would die. There was no other man around the house but [the barber] himself and the one whose hair he washed. He said: I am not going, I am not leaving this no matter how hard she moans. When sickness left, [the ill woman] asked for water; as she spoke, sickness hit her again, but did not last as long as it had for the first time. Then [the witness] asked why is that condition on her. She said that her husband sent her wormwood wine to drink, and she must die because of that.[...][43]

---

[39] Cohen T.V., "The Lady Lives, the Pigeon Dies", in *Love and Death in Renaissance Italy* (Chicago: 2004) 173–197.

[40] Burney I., "A Poisoning of No Substance: The Trials of Medico-Legal Proof in Mid-Victorian England", *Journal of British Studies* 38 (1999) 59–92.

[41] On facts and the law, see Shapiro B., *A Culture of Fact: England, 1550–1720* (Ithaca NY – London: 1999).

[42] Crisciani C., "Fatti, teorie, 'narratio' e i malati a corte. Note su empirismo in medicina nel tardo medioevo", *Quaderni Storici* 108,3 (2001) 695–717.

[43] Prot.Jud. Doc II. 6/1572–1575, fol. 114: 'Orsolya kis Szőcs Imréné azt vallja, hogy egykor ment volt Borbély Bálintné(t) látogatni betegségében, azonban hogy oda jutott volna, a betegség elütötte volna, és hogy ott lelné elijed, hogy meghal. Az ura fejet

This account – in unison with the other declarations – described pain in the most prosaic way, reminding the judges of details like repeated convulsions and moaning but without specifying empirical proof, as if witnesses had never looked under the covers to look for signs of poisoning, as if they had never touched the agonized body. Seemingly, observers took the sufferer's sensation-based diagnosis for granted, and this gave the sick woman the authority to determine how to interpret bodily states: when she was ill and when she felt well. This contrasts sharply with women's power and authority over other women's bodies in certain spheres of knowledge like proof of pregnancy. Not extensively studied, the practices of touch must have given women a sense of authority in the neighborhood and household as 'women pushed and nudged each other, shared beds, touched each other's breasts, or felt bellies'.[44] In this case of poisoning, however, authority was left to a man in the house, the husband (whose presence perhaps might have inhibited female touching), who was a healer with the knowledge to help the sufferer, but had caused damage as well. Witnesses used Bálint's reluctance to help his suffering wife as proof of his guilt. In addition, the victim had repeatedly announced her death in a formula that took on a prophetic power and became a legal tool in the hands of the accuser. To say 'because of you I die' would have had little power if the victim recovered but took on weight if she did indeed die.

Those witnesses in 1572 who claimed that the dying women accused her husband of her sudden sickness also tried to show that the husband was heartless, indifferent to suffering, not taking his wife to the doctor outside the town, and showing a hostile attitude by insulting the sick woman. Some of the barber's cruelty was social and psychological: he did not come help a wife in distress and seek remedy. In contrast, he had been caring for other's hygiene and health. Professional negligence, however, was not the only accusation against the barber. One woman quoting Bálint's words in the court, reported how he had scolded his wife for what he saw as an unjust accusation:

---

mos volt, és ő hí(v)á hogy odamenne, mert meghalna felesége. Mond hogy de ugyan törvénye a(z) neki. Esmét jobban kezd verekedni, hortyogni, az Istenért kéri, hogy hozzá látna, mert meghal. Egyéb ember penig nem volt a háznál, hanem őmaga és akinek fejét mossa volt. Mond, hogy én nem megyek, ezt el nem hagyom ám nyegjen. Mikor elhatta volna a betegség, innia kér és hogy szólni akar volt, esmét elüti a betegség, de nem tart annyira rajta, mint először. Azután megkérdi, miből vagyon őrajta a nyavalya. Azt mondta, hogy az ura küldött irmes bort innia, az miatt kell meghalni'.

[44] Gowing, *Common Bodies* 6. See also 40–51.

> Klára, the widow of István Tót declares that she heard the deceased wife of Bálint Borbély telling him in the face: you gave me the wormwood wine which is making me die. Bálint Borbély scolded her and told: you are a liar, you colic bitchy soul, because I have never poisoned anyone, you meager bitchy soul. She [the witness] further declares that the [dying woman's] mother took her to the doctor in Makó, and stayed there with her, but the doctor said that he could not help because it was so much spread on her.[45]

In her deposition, the witness did not use extravagantly expressive words or well-constructed language often found in late medieval religious writings on bodily pain or pain of the soul.[46] This poisoning case, indeed, gives us little talk about pain. We have symptoms, not of pain, but of a bodily condition. The witness, a burgher woman, described suffering in plain words that were able to communicate an extraordinary sensation. But like other witnesses, her interest in the court was in the shape of the ailment, not in the anguish. Unlike religious writings on the painful experiences of saints, or on their miraculous healings, this fragment describes an actual situation: the general distress of a woman, her convulsions and the subsequent fatigue, and finally the vocal expression of pain. The sufferer's sensation-based bodily knowledge mingled with the visual diagnosis of witnesses, thus removing the locus of interpretive authority from the person feeling the sensation to the outside observers. The case presented here offers a picture of individual sensation and visualized knowledge at the same time. The female body was presented in relations to illness and pain, and witnesses narrated their visual experience of the woman's pain. The sufferer's mediated view in the depositions overcomes, or at least complements shortcomings of the official record. Once we go beyond the voices of practitioners, we are offered a different perspective on sickness and illness behavior.

---

[45] Prot.Jud. Doc II. 6/1572–1575, fol. 114: 'Klára néhai Tót Istvánné azt vallja, hogy hallotta Borbély Bálintné szemébe mondta az uránák ezt, hogy te adattat énnekem az irmes bort kitűl meg kell halnom. Borbély Bálint szidta, és azt mondta: hazudsz kólikás kurva lélek, mert egyébkort sem étettem én senkit meg, szegényből lett kurva lélek. Azt is vallja, hogy a makai orvoshoz vitte volt az anyja, ott is vele volt, az orvos is azt mondta, hogy nem használhat neki, mert igen el hatotta'.

[46] Cohen E., "The Animated pain of the Body", *The American Historical Review* 105,1 (2000) 36–68.

Conclusion

The aim of this paper was not to decide whether the barber really poisoned his wife.[47] Rather, I have explored the intersections between legal practice and early modern medicine by analyzing depositions by a number of witnesses. In addition to accusing the barber or testifying to his credibility, witnesses related the dying woman's pain in a manner that required accuracy for the judges' ear but still remained highly subjective, offering clues about cultural and social arrangements of the early modern period. It is certainly true that the plausibility of their testimonies to the interrogators and to themselves depended on shared knowledge, but the process by which witnesses described the woman's pain is far more complex than a mere recapitulation of cultural stereotypes.

When deponents stressed the writhing, pain and agony of the sufferer, it was above all on her body that the drama focused, as if it became a blank sheet, with pain and suffering written clearly upon it. Their vocabulary reflected an extraordinary fluidity of repertoires and systems of classification that straddled the distinction between medical knowledge and popular beliefs. Understandings of pain and of the workings of the body relied on a system that integrated theoretical, learned, and popular medicine: humoralism, which stressed the importance of the inner balance, environmentalism, which referred to the ingested non-natural substance of the wine, and a less systematic set of beliefs close to sorcery, in which human agency could affect one's health. This healing culture was distinct in the sense that did not see a sharp demarcation between the inside of the body and the outside world.

Perhaps the most important feature of this culture can be located in the verbalization of pain. Metaphors used to describe pain referred to unusual objects inside the human body. The images of a square object and a canon ball inside the aching stomach were taken from outside the medical repertoire, while the image of a piece of meat

[47] The transcript does not contain the outcome of the trial. Twenty years later Bálint Borbély was still living in Klausenburg, and several trial transcripts of the early 1590s recorded his witness depositions as a barber. Prot.Jud. Doc II.8/1590–1594, fol. 44; 84; 388; 404; 462; 470; 472. He was also a registered burgher in the *Regestrum* of 1593. Fond Primaria Municipiului Cluj, Socoteli, Pach. 5/XX–XXI (1593), fol. 1–95. Indirectly we know of his remarriage as his wife Marta was a complainant in 1593, and witnessed in another trial in 1594. Prot.Jud. Doc II.8/1590–1594, fol. 366; 466. Trial records of 1590–1594 by courtesy of László Pakó (unpublished transcripts).

can indicate familiarity with the medical discourses of the time. The parallel occurrence of these captivating images shaped by individual and communal experience, once again, blurs any clear-cut distinctions between popular and learned medicine.

Selective Bibliography

Albala K., *Eating in the Renaissance* (Ewing, NJ: 2002).

Bar-On Y., "Neighbours and Gossip in Early Modern Gynaecology", in Blécourt W. de – Usborne C. (eds.), *Cultural Approaches to the History of Medicine* (Basingstoke – New York: 2004) 36–55.

Camporesi P., *The Anatomy of the Senses. Natural Symbols in Medieval and Early Modern Italy* (Cambridge: 1994).

Cohen E., "The Animated Pain of the Body", *The American Historical Review* 105,1 (2000) 36–68.

Cohen T.V., *Love and Death in Renaissance Italy* (Chicago: 2004).

Condrau F., "The Patient's View Meets the Clinical Gaze", *Social History of Medicine* 20,3 (2007) 525–540.

Crisciani C., "Fatti, teorie, 'narratio' e i malati a corte. Note su empirismo in medicina nel tardo medioevo", *Quaderni Storici* 108,3 (2001) 695–717.

Duden B., *The Woman Beneath the Skin: A Doctor's Patients in Eighteenth-Century Germany* (Cambridge, MA – London: 1998).

Elmer P. (ed.), *The Healing Arts. Health, Disease and Society in Europe 1500–1800* (Manchester: 2004).

Gowing L., *Common Bodies: Women, Touch and Power in Sixteenth-Century England* (New Haven – London: 2003).

Howard S., "Imagining the Pain and Peril of Seventeenth-Century Childbirth: Travail and Deliverance in the Making of an Early Modern World", *Social History of Medicine* 16,3 (2003) 367–382.

Katona G., *Bizonyítási eszközök a XVIII–XIX. században. A kriminalisztika magyarországi előzményei* [Legal evidence in the eighteenth and nineteenth centuries. The advance of criminology in Hungary] (Budapest: 1977) 324–333.

Kivistö S., "G.F. von Franckenau's Satyra Sexta (1674)", in Korhonen A. – Lowe K. (eds.), in *The Trouble with Ribs: Women, Men and Gender in Early Modern Europe.* Studies across Disciplines in the Humanities and Social Sciences 2 (Helsinki: 2007) 82–102.

Kusukawa S., "Medicine in Western Europe in 1500", in Elmer P. (ed.), *The Healing Arts. Health, Disease and Society in Europe 1500–1800* (Manchester: 2004) 1–26.

Lindemann M., *Medicine and Society in Early Modern Europe* (Cambridge: 1999).

Lupton D., *Medicine as Culture: Illness, Disease and the Body in Western Societies* (London: 2003).

Nutton V., "Humouralism", in Bynum W.F. – Porter R. (eds.), *Companion Encyclopedia of the History of Medicine*, vol. I (London – New York: 1993) 281–291.

Pakó L., "Kényszer vagy erkölcsi romlottság? Csecsemőgyilkosságok Kolozsvárt a 16. század utolsó évtizedében" [Pressure or immorality? Infanticides in Kolozsvár of the late sixteenth century], *Korunk* 3 (2005) 84–93.

Pomata G., "Menstruating Men: Similarity and Difference of the Sexes in Early Modern Medicine", in Finucci V. – Brownlee K. (eds.), *Generation and Degeneration: Tropes of Reproduction in Literature and History from Antiquity to Early Modern Europe* (Durham: 2001).

Porter R., "The Patient's View: Doing Medical History from Below", *Theory and Society* 14,2 (1985) 175–198.

——, "The People's Health in Georgian England", in Harris T. (ed.), *Popular Culture in England, c. 1500–1850* (New York: 1995) 124–142.

Shapiro B., *A Culture of Fact: England, 1550–1720* (Ithaca NY – London: 1999).

Siraisi N., *Medieval & Early Renaissance Medicine: An Introduction to Knowledge and Practice* (Chicago: 1990).

VARJAS B. (ed.), *Egy 16. századi orvosi könyv* [A medical book of the sixteenth century], (Kolozsvár: 1947).

VERESS E., *Fontes Rerum Hungaricarum III: Báthory István lengyel király udvari számadáskönyveinek Magyar- és Erdélyországi adalékai (1576–1586)* (Budapest: 1918).

SEVERING WHAT WAS JOINED TOGETHER: DEBATES ABOUT PAIN IN THE SEVENTEENTH-CENTURY DUTCH REPUBLIC

Lia van Gemert

Introduction

In the seventeenth-century Dutch Republic, physical pain was written about by a wide range of authors operating in a variety of discourses. In this article I will look at reflections on pain in a number of Dutch medical, literary, historiographical, judicial and philosophical texts. I will show that Dutch writers approached pain both from a practical, medical and an ethical perspective, and that the two approaches were often connected. Although the French philosopher René Descartes lived and worked in the Republic during this time, his famous mechanistic understanding of pain does not inform the texts that I will consider. This is not to say that Cartesian views of pain were not discussed at all by Dutch writers of this era; the texts that I have selected for this article are intended as a starting point for further research into conceptions of pain in the seventeenth-century Dutch Republic.

I will start with the views on pain put forward by the Dutch physician Johan van Beverwijck (1594–1647), and then move on to a number of literary texts from the period. Like Van Beverwijck, literary writers interpreted pain as a sign that both body and mind were in need of purification. Pain also formed a starting point for ethical discussions: I will look at a number of Dutch commentaries of the seventeenth century that were highly critical of the infliction of pain in torture and judicial punishment, and advocated moderation. I will end with a brief discussion of René Descartes' revolutionary ideas about the perception of pain.

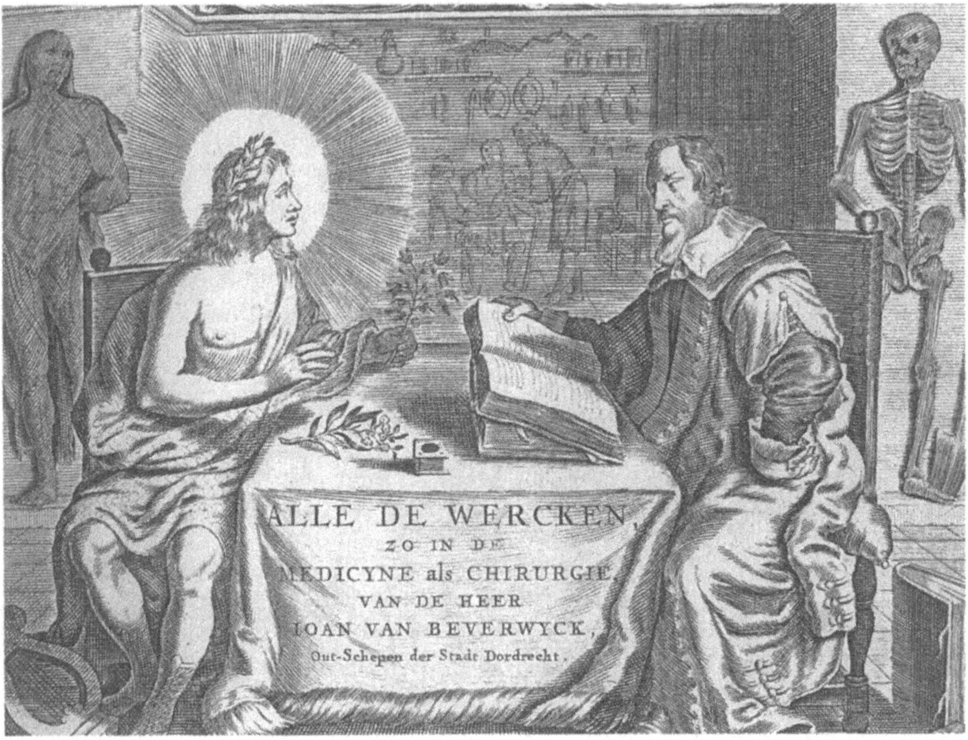

Fig. 1. Johan van Beverwijck discusses his books on health with Apollo. Title page of Johan van Beverwijck, *Wercken der genees-konste, bestaende in den Schat der gesontheyt, Schat der ongesontheyt, Heel-konste* (Amsterdam, Jan Jacobsz. Schipper: 1664). Private copy.

Johan van Beverwijck: A Progressive Physician

The writings of the Dordrecht physician John van Beverwijck form a fascinating entry point for mapping the understandings of pain in the early modern Dutch Republic. Although he worked as the local 'city doctor' and surgeon, and was not affiliated with a university, he did belong to the intellectual vanguard of Dutch medical culture. Van Beverwijck had studied at several European universities and had graduated at Padua, one of the centres of anatomical scholarship. He was the first Dutch physician to acknowledge Harvey's ideas on the circulation of the blood and expanded on them in a surgical treatise on bladder and renal stones (*De calculo renum & vesicae liber singularis*, 1638; translated into Dutch as *Steen-stuck*). He also wrote a famous trilogy: *Schat der gesontheyt* (1636), *Schat der ongesontheyt* (1639) and *Heel-konste* (1645) (*Treasure of Health, Treasure of Illness* and *Surgery*). This first complete medical encyclopedia in Dutch, often reprinted, offered a systematic survey of conditions of health, as well as the causes and treatments of all known diseases. It was based on the classical galenic doctrine of the four humours, which was supplemented with the ideas of Harvey.[1]

Van Beverwijck's customary method was to compare a range of existing sources, mostly medical theories from antiquity to his own day, with his own observations and experiences. Hij had a pronounced interest in discovering general patterns of health and illness, and especially in issues of urology (kidneys, bladder and urinary passages). He also enjoyed taking part in current medical debates: he corresponded with William Harvey and René Descartes about the circulation of the blood, and with Anna Maria van Schurman about the question of whether God had pre-determined each human life span.[2] Van Beverwijck also made use of the writings of other physicians, such as botanical studies, surgeon's books, treatises on specific diseases such as scurvy and the plague, and practical medical surveys. Moreover, he had clearly studied also non-

---

1 Gemert L. van, "Johan van Beverwijck"; in Bynum W.F. – Bynum H. (eds.), *Dictionary of Medical Biography* (Westport – London: 2007) vol. I, 203–204. Quotations are taken from Johan van Beverwijck, *Wercken der genees-konste, bestaende in den Schat der gesontheyt, Schat der ongesontheyt, Heel-konste* [...]. (Amsterdam, Jan Jacobsz. Schipper: 1664; private copy). For an anthology, translated into modern Dutch, see Johan van Beverwijck, *Schat der gezondheid*, ed. L. van Gemert (Amsterdam: 1992).

2 This correspondence was published under the title *The Verge of Our Lives* (*Pael-steen onsens levens*). See: "Aenhangsel van brieven", in Van Beverwijck, *Wercken der genees-konste*, 232–235; 204–213; 192–201.

medical sources, such as the Bible, travel accounts and historiographical works, for any insights into illness, recovery and death. He would finally compare all of these materials with his own experiences, and describe his own medical remedies whenever he felt this was relevant. In this way, he did indeed compile the 'treasure' of the encyclopedia's title: a richly informative book that offers a mixture of theory and practice, and that, beside its serious medical content, contains a light touch. Van Beverwijck's work was made all the more attractive by the poems of his friend and fellow townsman Jacob Cats, who offered summaries in verse of the many topics that Van Beverwijck touched upon. Cats also time and again recommended Van Beverwijck's works, for example in the proem to *Steen-stuck (Treatise on bladder and renal stones)*:

> Learn, Citizens, Holland's Citizens, learn
> From what is being offered here
> By one who places all he knows
> Always in the service of your well-being.[3]

According to Van Beverwijck, humanity suffers pain as a result of the Fall; in this way he reiterates the Christian notion that pain is one of God's ways of punishing humanity for its sins. For Van Beverwijck, the fact that pain can be extremely fierce and cruel is an indication that it is indeed a divine matter. As a result, 'humans do not have the power to go against Nature', he once remarked.[4] This is also why pain is so often associated with death, and experienced as a punishment worse than death. The only real solution for excessive, uncontrollable pain is the end of all sensation in death, but, in Van Beverwijck's own experience, this is a solution that people shy away from: 'I have often seen that very old, infirm people who had called for death because of their unbearable pain, still had a strong desire to live once they approached death'.[5]

---

[3] 'Leert, Burgers, Hollands Burgers, leert
Het geen' u weder wert vereert
Van een, die al wat dat hy weet,
Gedurigh in u dienst besteet', in Van Beverwijck, *Treasure of Illness* II, 228.

[4] 'De Menschen en hebben oock de macht, noch de kracht niet, om tegens de Nature in te gaen', in Van Beverwijck, *Heel-konste* 143.

[5] '[...] alsoo ick dickwils gesien hebbe, dat oock stock-oude en daer by gebreckelicke lieden, die uyt onverduldigheyt van pijn dickwils om de doot geroepen hadden, de selve beginnende te genaken, noch met groote begeerte na het leven joockten [...]', in Van Beverwijck, *Treasure of Health* 3.

Even though pain is God's punishment for sin, this does not mean that lifelong, unrelieved suffering is inevitable, since God is also merciful: 'God does not punish without healing'.[6] This entails an opportunity, or rather an obligation, for the physician to employ his expertise, yet in order to do so, he first has to arrive at a scientific understanding of how pain works. This brings us to the field of philosophy. Van Beverwijck expounds his basic understanding of pain in *Heel-konste* (*Surgery*):

> All pain consists in the severing of what was put together, and this is its most likely cause. Likewise, the medicine that takes pain away by a countering force does effectively alleviate the pain, but cannot be seen as removing the pain since it only softens it, while the cause remains present. Such a medicine is either moderate, and appropriate to the composition of our body, or warm in the first degree, and composed of fine matter.[7]

Van Beverwijck is clearly indebted to Aristotle, although he does not refer to him in this passage – unlike in some of his other writings. Aristotle argues for a unity between body and mind (in spite of their different natures), and Van Beverwijck subscribes to this idea, for example in the following passage from the *Treasure of Health:*

> Our Soul and Body differ a great deal from each other, and are therefore tied together by the innate heat of the body [...], as Aristotle argues in Book 2, Chapter 4 of his *Book of the Soul.*[8]

This remark helps to clarify the passage on pain quoted above: body and soul are tied together by body heat; pain is caused by a disconnection between them, and this pain can only be alleviated by an appropriate medicine that either corresponds to the balance between the elements in our body, or has a certain temperature. The pain is then eased, but the cause of the breach between body and soul is not removed. Since Van Beverwijck believed that the soul is immutable, and

---

[6] 'Dat Godt niet en slaet, of hy salft wederom'. Van Beverwijck, *Treasure of Illness* I 101.

[7] 'Alle pijn bestaet in 't ontdoen van 't gene te samen gevoeght is, ende dat is de naeste oorsaeck; gelijck het middel, 't welck die wech neemt door tegenstrijdende kracht, de pijn recht stilt, maer even wel niet pijn-versachtend genoemt werdt, dan alleen 't gene, de oorsaeck blijvende, de pijn alleen versoet, ende versacht. Soodanigh middel is ofte gematight, ende ons lichaem gelijck; ofte werm in den eersten graed ende fijn van stoffe', in Van Beverwijck, *Surgery* 21. With thanks to Jeroen Jansen.

[8] 'Also ons Ziele en Lichaem van malkanderen veel verschillen, en derhalven door de ingeboren wermte met eenen bandt aen malkanderen gehecht zijn [...] gelijck Aristoteles betuyght in sijn 2. Boeck van de Ziele op het 4. Capittel [...]', in Van Beverwijck, *Treasure of Health* 21.

that it sets the body in motion as its instrument (as long as body and soul are connected), it is plausible to assume that he locates the causes of the severing of body and soul in the body.[9] It is worth investigating whether he is consistent on this point throughout his medical works. For the purposes of this article, the most important point is that for Van Beverwijck, pain can be fought by means of interventions in the body. This brings us to Van Beverwijck's ideas about concrete medical remedies for pain.

It is clear that Van Beverwijck was very much interested in the alleviation of pain; pain is even included as a separate entry in the index to his encyclopedia. He developed his own surgical techniques for removing bladder and renal stones, which he described in *De calculo renum & vesicae liber singularis* (*Steen-stuck*; 1638). Central to Van Beverwijck's methods was an attempt to keep the cut as small as possible and to minimize the infliction of pain.[10] In *Surgery* he warns against touching the nerves while opening a vein for blood-letting: it causes severe pain and may even lead to death. In general, nerves are very sensitive, he states: a heavy wound for instance, 'usually affects nervous parts, and causes great pain there, those parts being very sensitive, and that pain in its turn causes a great influx of fluids: thus the afflicted part must inevitably swell, and if that does not happen, it gives signs that the fluids have gone inside, and reach more vital parts, where they cause much more harm'.[11] Van Beverwijck gives short shrift to any illusions of invulnerability or immunity, or to any medical remedies that promise anything like it. As the various wounds on the titlepage of *Surgery* also suggest, all tales about magical ointments, incantations and rituals have no basis in reality.[12] Incidentally, this view of magic as powerless and illusory is frequently encountered in seventeenth-century Dutch texts.

The preparation of medicines is, of course, an important part of analgesics. Van Beverwijck offers elaborate prescriptions for specific ailments –

[9] 'Want de Ziele en kan niet beschadigt werden, maer blijft altijt even de selve, en onveranderlick, soo lang de mensche leeft, en doet de eygen wercken, als sy maer het eygen Werck-tuygh [lichaam] en heeft', in Van Beverwijck, *Treasure of Health* 25.

[10] Van Beverwijck, *Treasure of Illness* II 228–287, esp. 285–287.

[11] Van Beverwijck, *Surgery* 63; 133: 'Want alsoo een sware Wonde, gemeenlick zenuwachtige Deelen raeckt, in de welcke, als seer gevoelick zijnde, sy nootwendigh groote pijn verweckt, ende die wederom groote toevloeying van vochtigheyt: soo moet dan van oock het gequetste Deel noodtsaeckelick opswellen, ende sulcks niet geschiedende, geeft te kennen, dat die vloet sijnen loop na binnen, ende voornamer Deelen genomen heeft; waer hy veel meerder schade doet'.

[12] Van Beverwijck, *Surgery* 127.

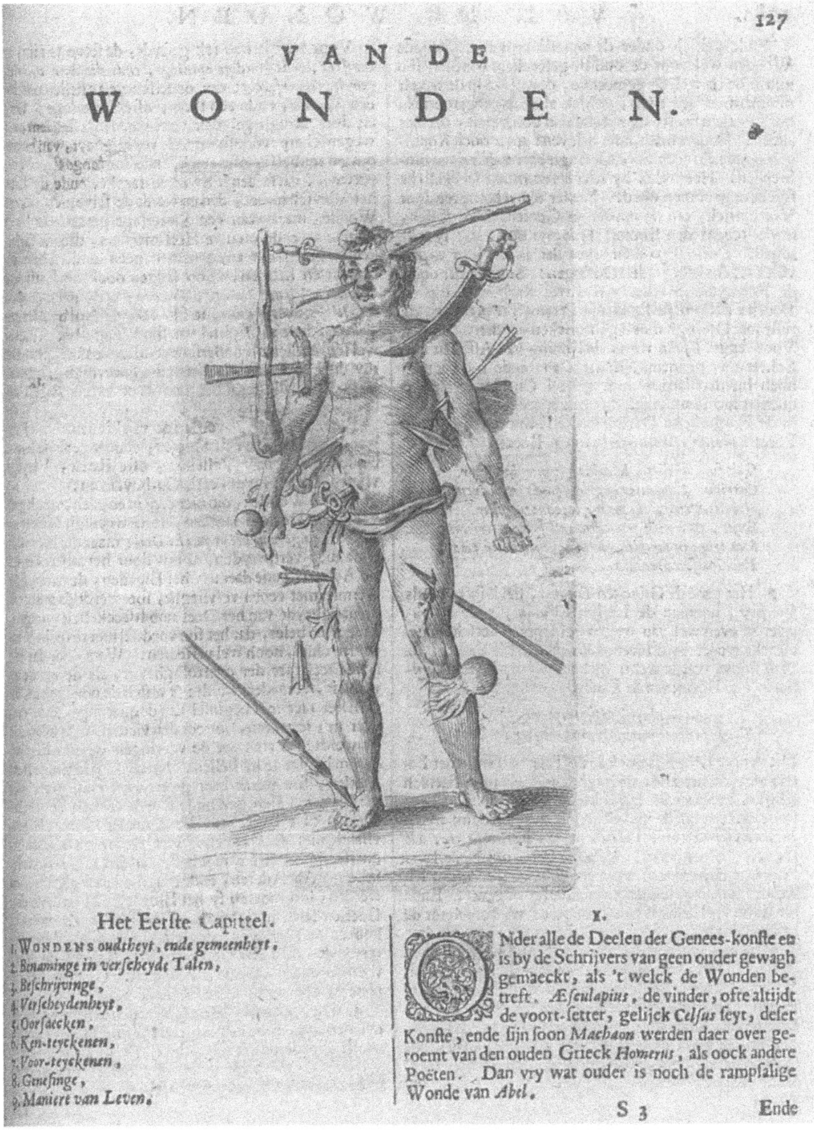

127

VAN DE

WONDEN.

Het Eerste Capittel.

1. WONDENS *oudtheyt, ende gemeenheyt,*
2. *Benaminge in verscheyde Talen,*
3. *Beschrijvinge,*
4. *Verschèydenheyt,*
5. *Oorsaecken,*
6. *Ken-teyckenen,*
7. *Voor-teyckenen,*
8. *Genesinge,*
9. *Maniere van Leven.*

I.

ONder alle de Deelen der Genees-konste en is by de Schrijvers van geen ouder gewagh gemaeckt, als 't welck de Wonden betreft. *Æsculapius*, de vinder, ofte altijdt de voort-setter, gelijck *Celsus* seyt, deser Konste, ende sijn soon *Machaon* werden daer over geroemt van den ouden Grieck *Homerus*, als oock andere Poëten. Dan vry wat ouder is noch de rampsalige Wonde van *Abel*.

S 3 Ende

Fig. 2. First page of the book on wounds in *Heel-konste*. In: Johan van Beverwijck, *Wercken der genees-konste bestaende in den Schat der gesontheyt, Schat der ongesontheyt, Heel-konste* (Amsterdam, Jan Jacobsz. Schipper: 1664) 127. Private copy.

always based on a basic Galenic system, with four degrees to indicate the potency of a particular medicine, and detailing the wet, dry, cold or hot qualities of the remedy (always opposed to those of the ailment). He also frequently informs the reader where he gets his ingredients, for example in the vicinity of Dordrecht. Such topographical details point to Van Beverwijck's views on the ideal geographical origins of medical ingredients. In his treatise *Introduction to Dutch Medicines* (*Inleydinge tot de Hollantsche genees-middelen*) he argues that, thanks to God's providence, every region in the world contains the remedies for the ailments that are specific to it. Jacob Cats summarized this view as follows: 'Although sickness and pain may strike us,/ The entire country is a medicine'.[13] This principle applies everywhere: in Greenland, sailors find scurvy grass and sorrel as a remedy for scurvy (it was unknown, of course, that this was related to the vitamin C content of both plants). Holland itself has a plentiful supply of medicinal herbs, such as daisies, dandelions and eyebright ('Ogentroost' in Dutch, a cure for eye conditions). Van Beverwijck remarks that indigenous medicines are to be preferred over exotic ones, since much more is known about their effects, and the chances of being deceived when purchasing them, therefore, are also lower. Moreover, they are considerably cheaper than medicines from abroad – the Dutch business sense never fails to show.

The mix of anecdotes and explanatory comments and the supporting literary passages result in a medical manual that is at the same time aimed at a general, cultivated bourgeois readership. The basic moral of Van Beverwijck's encyclopedia is evident on every page: illness and pain can to a certain extent be avoided by living prudently and simply. If pain still strikes, it forms a sign that both body and soul are in need of purification. The well trained doctor guides the patient reliably through this process.

[13] 'Dan, al treft ons sieckt' en pijn,/ Gantsch het Lant is medicijn', in Van Beverwijck, *Treasure of Illness* I 101–124 (quotation Cats 106); see also Gemert L. van, "Johan van Beverwijck als 'instituut'", in *De zeventiende eeuw* 8 (1992) 99–106, esp. 102 and Cooper A., "The Indigenous versus the Exotic: Debating Natural Origins in Early Modern Europe", *Landscape Research* 28 (2003) I, 51–60.

Pain as a Moral Incentive

Just as Van Beverwijck's medical trilogy has a number of literary aspects, seventeenth-century Dutch literature itself is frequently informed by medical discourse. Many texts refer to the Galenic system: humoral theory served as a template for characterization on the basis of the four human types (choleric, sanguine, phlegmatic and melancholic), and there are frequent allusions to the properties of matter (hot, cold, wet, dry). Literary texts also frequently reiterate the idea that illness and pain are a punishment from God, and that a well trained doctor is not only a welcome guide in the purification of the body, but also in fostering the understanding that the healing process requires a change in lifestyle. An example of this moralizing approach is Jan Luyken's emblem *The Doctor*. Luyken describes pain as a 'hellish venom' – this not only describes a physical observation, but also adds a moral dimension to the 'venom' of pain. The ultimate physician is God himself, while the earthly physician is his temporary representative; the diseased body has to suffer in order to obtain eternal life:

> The Doctor
> God is the medicine for deadly hellish venom.
>
> When Life is feeble and diseased,
> One takes a vile and bitter Drink,
> So that the Body can be cured.
> Why then not endure some temporary bitterness
> So as to be healthy in eternity?[14]

In addition to this metaphysical connection between the worldly and the divine, seventeenth-century literary writers devote ample attention to the physical dimension of pain, for example Jan Six van Chandelier in his 1656 Spa poems, in which he describes a trip to a health resort in Belgium (then part of the Southern Netherlands). The Spa waters

---

[14] 'DE DOCTER
God is de medicyn, voor doodlik hels fenijn.

Is 't Leeven machteloos en kranck
Men neemd een vieze of bit're Dranck,
Of 't Lichaam, weeder mocht geneesen:
Waarom dan voor een korten tydt,
Niet aangevaard wat bitterheid,
Om eeuwiglyck gesond te weesen', in Jan Luyken, *Spiegel van het menselyk* bedryf (Amsterdam, Johannes en Caspaares Luiken: 1694). Facsimile edition ed. by L. de Vries (Amsterdam – Brussels: 1984).

De Docter.
God is de Medecyn, Voor doodlik hels fenyn.

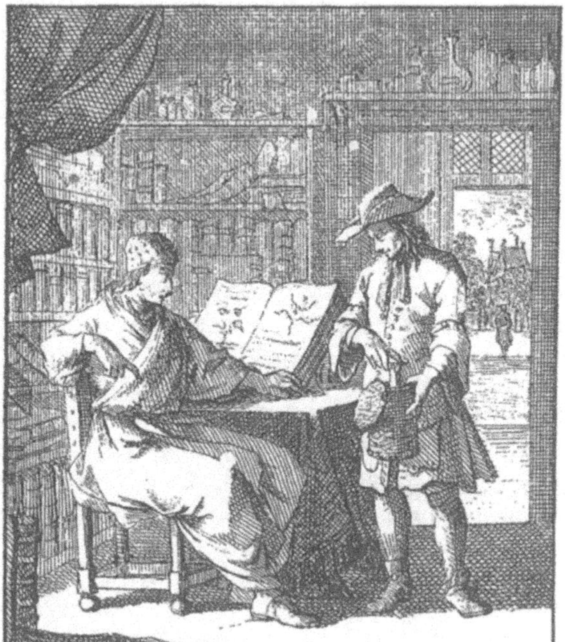

Is't Leeven machteloos en kranck
Men neemd een viese of bit're Dranck,
Of't Lichaam weeder mocht geneesen:
Waarom dan voor een korten tydt,
Niet aangevaard wat bitterheid,
Om eeuwiglyck gesond te weesen.

Fig. 3. Jan Luyken, "De docter". From Jan Luyken, *Spiegel van het menselyk bedryf* (Amsterdam, Johannes en Caspaares Luiken: 1694), pages not numbered. Private copy.

purify the entire body and free it of painful cramps: 'Delicious, freely given water that flows into the stomach, from which the body is nourished, creeps imperceptibly through the body from the head to the feet to cleanse it of dirt and tormenting spams'.[15]

In their descriptions of pain sensation, writers often draw on the characteristics of a specific disease: scurvy is described as 'tearing', while the pain caused by bladder and renal stones is characterised as 'hardened', 'stony', 'sharp' and 'stinging'. Even though stones did not always have to be surgically removed, and could be evacuated spontaneously, they did, of course, remain painful. In 1627, Constantijn Huygens wrote an ingenious poem for the funeral of Elisabeth Bax, who had suffered more pain in getting rid of stones than in giving birth. Bax herself speaks in the poem and describes the stone as her last infant:

> I have given birth to four children and a stone,
> But the last childbed was the toughest,
> And the last child's cries were the loudest,
> even though it was dumb as a stone.[16]

The dead Elizabeth complains that she would rather be in her stony grave than suffer from her stones any longer.

Death had relieved Elisabeth Bax of her pain, but what could one do if death did not arrive while at the same time there was no adequate remedy for pain? Huygens also offered an answer to this question. He urged his readers to reflect upon their moral sins, for instance in his poem *Ooghen-troost* (1647).[17] The title, literally 'eye comfort', refers both to the analgesic plant eyebright that was used to cure eye conditions and to the poem's aim of providing moral support for the visually handicapped.[18] Huygens – who suffered from a painful eye condition

---

[15] 'Maar kostlik kostloos sap, dat vloeijende, in de kooken
Des boesems, en dan daar, waar 't lichaam werd gestooken,
Van 't hoofd, tot in den teen, onvoelik gaat doorkruipen,
En suiveren van vuil, en martelende stuipen', in Jan Six van Chandelier, *Gedichten*, ed. A.E. Jacobs (Assen – Maastricht: 1991), vol. I 163–164.

[16] 'Vier Kinderen en een' Steen gebeurde 't mij te baren;
Maer 't laatste kinderbedd' was 'tswaerste wedervaren,
En 't laeste kind riep luydt, all was het stom als steen', in Constantijn Huygens, *De gedichten*, ed. J.A. Worp (Groningen: 1893), vol. II 179.

[17] Huygens Constantijn, *Ooghen-troost*, ed. Zwaan F.L. (Groningen: 1984).

[18] Van Beverwijck also frequently refers to eyebright as an ingredient in medicines for eye conditions. On the distinction between surface and depth, external appearance and inward truth in this poem, see Pieters J. – Gosseye L., "Blindheid en inzicht. De

himself – wrote *Ooghen-troost* for a female friend who was in danger of becoming blind in one eye.

The poem also voices the notion that blindness is a punishment from God, a purifying scourge that will lead to spiritual insight. Huygens formulates this insight in a satirical and moralizing manner: many individuals are blind in a figurative sense since they greatly overrate themselves. A long list of these metaphorically blind (the miserly, the prodigal, the wrathful) serves to illustrate not only that mental blindness is worse than physical blindness, but also to demonstrate the limitations imposed on the human will. Only those who are fully aware of this are properly pious Christians; only they will 'see God'. Suffering can only be conquered by subjecting oneself to God's power.[19]

In Christian discourse, blindness often serves as a metaphor for human stubbornness towards God. A well known biblical example is Samson, who neglected his duties as a man of God because of his love of Delilah. His punishment was a painful blinding – his eyes were cut out.[20] Once he had become blind, Samson came to understand his sins and God restored his immense physical strength. Samson destroyed the Philistine temple, dying with those he killed (Judges 13–16). This Old Testamental episode leads us to the moral question of whether humans (as opposed to God) can legitimately inflict pain on others. In the seventeenth-century Dutch Republic, the answer to this question was dependent on context. It seems that in Old Testamental narratives the infliction of pain is justified, certainly if the victims are God's enemies.[21]

---

retoriek van het lezen in Constantijn Huygens' *Ooghen-troost*", *Tijdschrift voor Nederlandse taal- en letterkunde* 123,3 (2007) 208–225.

[19] 'Blind en onblind is een, de vrome sullen God sien', Huygens Constantijn, *Ooghen-troost* 148, l. 1002.

[20] The pain of Samson's blinding makes logical sense: it forms an atonement for his sins. Van Beverwijck remarks that he will not discuss Samson's case as his love story is well known enough (Van Beverwijck, *Treasure of health* 45).

[21] This can be observed, for example, in two Dutch tragedies about Samson: Abraham de Koning's *Simson's tragedy* (Amsterdam, Abraham de Koning: 1618) and Joost van den Vondel's *Samson or Sacred Revenge* (Amsterdam, weduwe Abraham de Wees: 1660), included in *De werken van Joost van den Vondel* (Amsterdam: 1936), IX 173–239. See Gemert L. van, "Schuld en boete bij Vondel en De Koning", forthcoming; and: Gemert L. van, "De krachtpatser en de hoer. Liefde en wraak op het zeventiende-eeuwse toneel", in Bots Hans – Gemert Lia van (eds.), *Schelmen en prekers. Genres en de transmissie van cultuur in vroegmodern Europa* (Nijmegen: 1999) 15–37. The text of Van den Vondel's play is also online at <http://www.dbnl.org/tekst/vond001dewe09_01/vond001dewe09_01_0001.htm>.

The Pain of Torture – Victims and Perpetrators

How did Dutch writers view the infliction of pain during judicial punishment and torture – as opposed to the pain of illness? Contemporary debates about the use of the rack provide a particularly useful starting point for answering this question. Even in the tolerant Dutch Republic, the rack was frequently used, although its application was bound to strict rules and regulations. A suspect could only be tortured on the rack if there were at least two depositions from reliable witnesses, or from one eye witness. The rack could only be used a limited number of times, and the torture could only be repeated if new evidence of guilt arose.

In spite of these regulations, the temptation to inflict the pains of the rack with little or no restraint could be strong, especially if political issues – often intermixed with religious ones – were at stake. The year 1575 witnessed a notorious episode of excessive torture during the aftermath of the alleged betrayal of the Northern Quarter (the peninsular area north of the IJ). In this year Spanish troops attempted to take back this part of Holland, which had been held by Protestant rebels since 1572. This attempt failed, yet there were suspicions that Catholic peasants had been about to betray the area to the Spanish, and a special committee was installed to investigate the matter. This committee far exceeded its competence: several prisoners were savagely tortured and died. One of the accused survived his ordeal and took legal action against the judges. The Northern Quarter episode forms the subject of a fascinating monograph by Henk van Nierop.[22]

One of the important historical accounts of these horrendous events is Pieter Corneliszoon Hooft's detailed description, based on the judicial documents, in his magisterial work on the beginnings of the Dutch Revolt against Spain, *De Nederlandsche Historien* (*The History of the Netherlands* I, 1642).[23] Hooft relates, for instance, how one prisoner was

[22] See Nierop H. van, *Het verraad van het Noorderkwartier. Oorlog, terreur en recht in de Nederlandse Opstand* (Amsterdam: 1999). An English translation of this excellent study will appear in 2009: *Treason in Holland: War, Terror and the Rule of Law in the Revolt of the Netherlands* (Princeton U.P.).

[23] I quote from the recent anthology in modern Dutch: P.C. Hooft, *Nederlandse Historiën. Een keuze uit het grote verhaal van de Nederlandse Opstand*, ed. F. van Gestel – E. Grootes – J. de Jongste (Amsterdam: 2007) 168–173. In the 1642 edition of *Nederlandsche Historien* Hooft's account can be found in chapter X 422–425. For a complete overview of the historiographical tradition, see van Nierop, *Het verraad* 253–273.

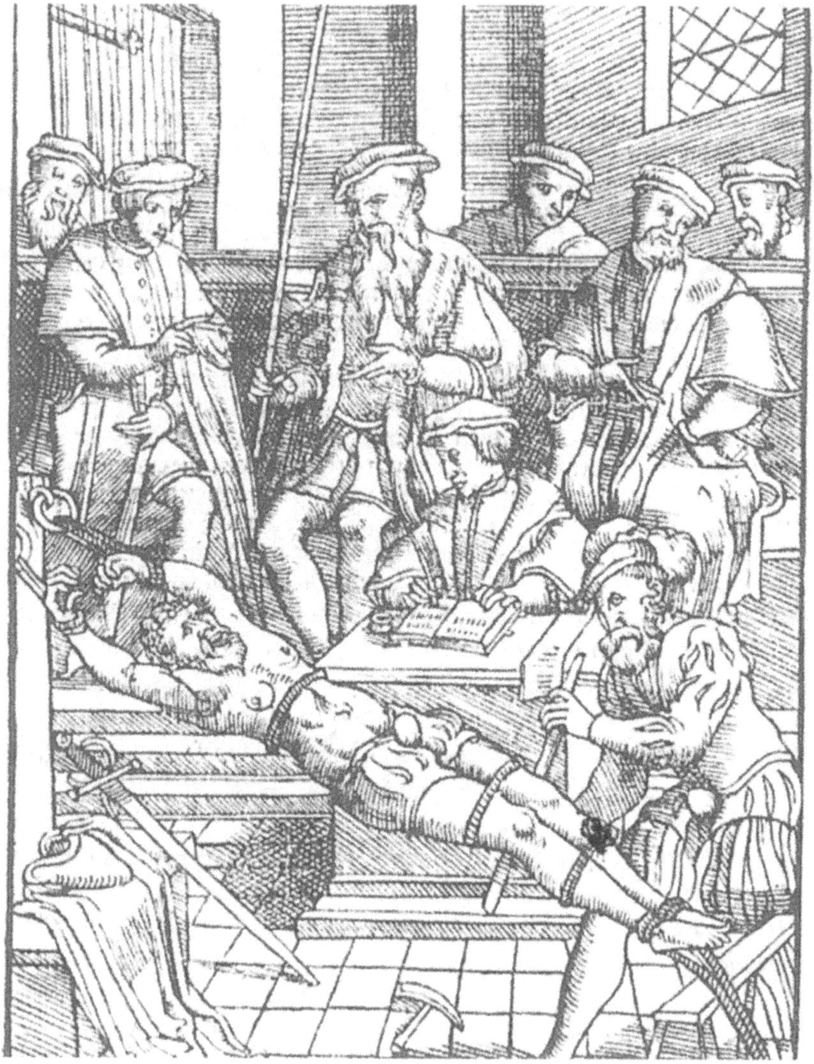

Fig. 4. Arnold Nicolai (?), Prisoner on the rack. From Joos de Damhouder, *Practycke ende handbouck in criminele zaeken* (Leuven, Wouters – Bathen: 1555) 56. Copy of Amsterdam University Library.

suspended from a ladder, with his arms twisted behind his back, and a two hundred-pound weight hanging from his big toe; another was covered in pieces of linen that were doused with brandy and set on fire so that his skin and soles were singed. This was only the beginning: one of the prisoners was tortured 22 or 23 times, Hooft states, not only by the usual means of the whip and the rack, but also by burning sulphur and candles on his shaven skin. Meanwhile, he was given only salted herring to eat, and nothing to drink. Then came digger wasps, who left their sting deep inside the prisoner's navel, and after that a heated stone bell with a a rat inside it was placed on his belly, so that the animal tried to escape by biting its way into the prisoner's body. The prisoner's penis was covered in cream and sucked on by a calf; his groins were blown up by means of a cane that been inserted into his penis and beaten with branches. Small wonder that this prisoner confessed the crimes he had been accused of. He was sentenced to death but revoked his confession on the scaffold and professed his innocence until the executioner strangled him.

This was too much even for seventeenth-century writers who had lived through the Spanish-Dutch war. Hooft notes that the events on which he reported brought tears to his eyes and stiffened his fingers and that he is aware that his readers feel pain and grief too. His only reason for going into so much detail was a didactic one: eventually the judges were made to suffer for their crimes, and for Hooft, the episode reveals how the power of reason and justice eventually triumph over cruelty and inhumanity.

Another contemporary source that offers a detailed description of the Northern Quarter episode, and condemns the excessive violence, is Daniel Jonktys' *De pyn-bank wedersproken en bematigt* (*The Rack Disputed and Tempered*), which first appeared in 1650, and was frequently reprinted. Joachim Oudaan wrote an accompanying poem. Both writers follow Hooft's description; Oudaan's poem is an interrogation by Justice, addressed to the rack. Justice's questions are in italics:[24]

---

[24] Daniel Jonktys, *De pyn-bank wedersproken en bematigt* (Rotterdam, Joannes Naeranus: 1651; private copy). This edition also contains the poem by Oudaan: 'Op de tijtel-print, van de wedersproke pyn-bank, in-gestelt door den achtbaren, hoog-geleerden heere Daniel Jonktys, artzeny-geleerde, oud-schepen der stede Rotterdam', 2v–3v (see the appendix to this article). Jonktys' tract is an adaptation of the Latin *Tribunal reformatum, in quo sanioris et tutioris justitiae via, judici Christiano in processu criminali commonstratur, rejecta et fugata tortura, cujus iniquitatem, multiplicem fallaciam, atque illicitum inter Christianos usum, libera et necessaria dissertatione* (1624) by Joannes Grevius. Grevius does not refer to the

Rack, report on your instruments of affliction:
[...]
One [suspect] was tied to a ladder,
Many hundreds of pounds hanging
From the thumbs of his feet,
Where no bath of sweat can be staunched.
The gang of torturers greedily drinks the blood
And get thirstier the more blood is shed.
The windlass pulls at the limbs,
The midriff is no longer covered by skin.
Jugs full of brandy poured into strips of linen
Scorch the flesh from the head down to the footsoles.
Candles, pitch and coals burn armpits and soles,
And each limb is pulled loose.
Crushing and stretching the elbows to a yard's length
Do not stop until the torturer is tired of it.
What else? Sulphur smoke,
Insects planted on the navel
Bore their sting into it.
They pour boiling oil,
Or tie split canes
Onto the exposed muscles.
Go on! They put hot dishes
On the flesh of the belly,
And heat them further with a fire from above;
The rat inside, suffocating in the heat,
Bites and rips with teeth and claws
Deeply into the belly underneath the stone jar.
This is not all! Must I add
What they gave a calf to suck on,
Where they inserted thin canes?
What bodily member they blew up in this manner?
Or what (who would not become enraged!)
the entire body was suspended from?
Does the pain lessen after the unwinding?
In order to banish sleep,
The rod comes down on the flesh,
They offer only salted herring as food,
And no drink, no matter how much this is begged for,
The heart so dry, the mouth so hoarse.
What evidence did they find?
High treason, but only on flimsy grounds.
Greed for your possessions

---

events in the Northern Quarter; for his information about this episode, Jonktys relied on Hooft and a second historical source by Pieter Bor Christiaensz.

(Poor people, without intercessors)
Was the only guilt, and the only cause
Of the blood that was shed.

Jonktys was both a physician and sheriff, and in the 231–page tract that follows Oudaan's poem, he pleads for the abolishing of the rack, or at least for a limiting of its use, since it cannot guarantee a fair judicial process. According to both Jonktys and Oudaan, the rack is ineffective as a judicial instrument, since it does not prove or disprove innocence; it is also unreasonable, and even inhuman, because of the excessive pain that is causes. Jonktys emphasizes that judges and other authorities are duty-bound to use their power responsibly, and they should realize that only God knows the truth about a criminal case, and that judgment ultimately belongs only to Him.

The seventeenth-century Dutch Republic saw another example of excessive violence – this time it occurred after the judicial process had been completed. In 1672, the brothers Johan and Cornelis de Witt were lynched by a frenzied crowd. This murder was the result of a deep-running political conflict between republicans and Orangists. Yet the lynching of the De Witt brothers has been remembered especially as a savage slaughter in which the brothers' bodies were horrendously mutilated. Among the bewildered bystanders was Joachim Oudaan, who had written the proem to Jonktys' *The Rack*. This time, he recorded his experiences in a diary, but felt inadequate to the task: 'in short, the frenzy has been so extreme that I am unable to express it adequately with the pen, or even with the mouth'.[25] In spite of this, he did write a tragedy on the De Witt murder, *Fratricide in The Hague or Frenzied Mirth*, only six months after it took place. This play does not present the lynching directly but in a report written for the De Witt family.[26]

In the case of the Northern Quarter episode, it is worth asking why the authorities condoned the excesses committed by the judicial committee. Van Nierop offers some plausible explanations for their behaviour.[27]

[25] 'Int kort de dolheijd is zoo groot geweest, dat ik niet magtig genoeg ben, die genoegzaam uit te drukken, met de penne, zelfs niet met de mond', in Joachim Oudaan, *Haagsche Broeder-Moord of Dolle Blydschap Treurspel*, ed. Werkgroep Utrechtse neerlandici (Utrecht: 1982) 139.

[26] Oudaan, *Haagsche Broeder-Moord of Dolle Blydschap* 108–118. This fiercely anti-Orangist play was not printed until 1712, at the beginning of the Second Stadtholderless Era.

[27] Van Nierop, *Het verraad*, esp. 166–178.

The atrocities served in part to show the prisoners' dishonourableness (and hence to show that they could not be entrusted with the rebels' cause), while the fact that the war was not going well for the Protestant rebels may also have been a factor. In addition, the judges would lose face if none of the prisoners confessed. That the judges often drank heavily during the proceedings, and frequently kept away from the actual tortures may indicate that they did realize how morally objectionable their behaviour was. We have already seen that Hooft, Jonktys and Oudaan also stressed the importance of a clean conscience.[28]

In addition to judges, torturers formed a second group involved in the judicial process. They had a reputation for being in league with the devil, since they operated in a shadowy zone between life and death; they were also often seen as having no honour, since they tortured defenceless, potentially innocent people. Torturers were frequently foreigners and often formed a more or less closed, socially marginalized group; the job was passed on from father to son. How did these professionals view the suffering that they inflicted? In the case of the Northern Quarter, we have one fascinating, if perhaps not entirely reliable, testimony from Stijn Jansdaughter, the wife of the torturer Jacob Michielsz. This 22-year-old Luxembourger (officially a countryman since Luxembourg was one of the provinces of the Netherlands) had the usual reputation for cruelty, yet his wife claimed that Michielsz was a sensitive soul: during the trials, he would come home tired and in a bad mood, the skin of his hands peeling off as a result of the manual force needed in stretching and torturing. He would often cry out of pity for his victims and say: 'I cannot torture them any longer, yet I have to do it, otherwise I will be fired'.[29]

In the case of the De Witt episode, there is a similar testimony, whose reliability is also uncertain, but whose symbolic significance is

---

[28] This view had been expressed before, during the trial of pensionary of state Johan van Oldenbarnevelt, who was accused of high treason and was executed in 1619. Joost van den Vondel, the most famous Dutch poet of the period, wrote a bitter complaint against the judges, the *Geuse Vesper of Siecken-troost voor de Vierentwintigh* ('Evening prayer of a "Geus" or "comfort" for the 24 judges'). God will punish you, he predicts, and until then a worm will gnaw your heart; your conscience will torment you. Vondel Joost van den, *Geuse Vesper of Siecken-troost voor de Vierentwintigh*, in: *De werken van Joost van den Vondel* (Amsterdam: 1929) III 339–340. Also on: http://www.dbnl.org/tekst/vond001dewe03_01/vond001dewe03_01_0050.htm

[29] '[...] ick en can die gevangens niet langer pijnigen; nochtans moet ick sulcx doen oft ick worde geslagen'. See Van Nierop, *Het verraad* 167–170; quotation on 169.

nevertheless considerable. In 1673, De Witt's torturer, the inexperienced Jan Christiaens/Corstyaense, wrote a note to De Witt's widow, Maria van Berckel; it was included in the 1712 edition of Oudaans tragedy *Fratricide in The Hague*. Christiaens was consumed by remorse, and begs Van Berckel for forgiveness. He confesses to having tortured De Witt out of fear (probably of losing his job), even though the latter was innocent, and claims that he wants never to torment anyone in this manner again. De Witt maintained his innocence and even summoned his judges to God's tribunal. In the midst of his tortures he exclaimed: 'O God, now I feel that You are a mighty God, since now I have ceased to feel pain'.[30] These two men, then, do not conform to the stereotype of the cruel and insensitive torturer: they did their job, but their conscience troubled them. It is not unlikely that some members of the crowed that murdered De Witt also later felt ashamed about their behaviour.

In 1623 Constantijn Huygens wrote a character sketch in verse entitled *A Torturer*.[31] It is an example of the classical genre of the *charactère*, one of whose first practitioners was the Greek writer Theophrastus (371–287 BC). As in the other poems by his hand that I have discussed so far, Huygens bombards his reader with a range of ingenuous leaps of thought, couched in subtle, deliberately arcane language that is both serious and comic in effect. Surprisingly, Huygens initially avoids any associations with cruelty, and emphasizes the technical skills which a torturer needs to carry out his work. He presents the torturer as a respectable killer, trained according to the traditions of his profession. The torturer has to operate in a cool-headed manner: some hesitation is allowed since any sign of technical failure will elicit fury from the crowds present at an execution. In other words, a sense of professional duty is paramount. This also applies to judicial torture in the service of truth-finding: untruth must be 'pierced through and through' by

---

[30] 'O Godt, nu gevoel ick dat ghy een groot godt syt want nu gevoel ick geen pyn meer [...]'. Oudaan, *Haagsche Broeder-Moord* 119. The note is listed under no. 11411a in J.A.N. Knuttel's catalogue of pamphlets. For Christiaens see Panhuysen L., *De Ware Vrijheid. De levens van Johan en Cornelis de Witt* (Amsterdam – Antwerpen: 2005) 452; 501 n. 129. Panhuysen assumes that the note is genuine.

[31] Constantijn Huygens, "Een Beul", *Zes zedeprinten* ed. Werkgroep van Utrechtse neerlandici (Utrecht: 1976²) 80–91. Also at: www.let.leidenuniv.nl/Dutch/Huygens/HUYG23.html#CH1623038 and www.fransmensonides.nl/beul_hoofd.htm (with a translation in modern Dutch).

'beating and whipping' it, and by 'squeezing it with ropes, tongs and branches'.[32]

If the poem at first suggests that a torturer's job is a purely technical affair, in the final 8 of the 54 stanzas of the poem, Huygens suddenly addresses the ethical dimension of his subject: a vengeful torturer commits a moral error and is unjust. Ultimately, the torturer represents every human being: only very few are able to withstand the torment of their conscience, and the pain of remorse is worse than bodily pain.

Beyond Pain

'O God, now I feel that You are a mighty God, since now I have ceased to feel pain' – according to his torturer, Cornelis de Witt spoke these words on the rack.[33] They suggest that De Witt had gone beyond pain, and that his faith in God had enabled him to do so. This may also apply to the torture victims in the Northern Quarter episode, who frequently professed their faith in God. The question of whether it is physically possible not to experience pain was investigated in the seventeenth century by René Descartes in his *Traité de l'homme*, which he probably wrote in 1633–1634, but whose publication he postponed since he feared persecution.[34] It eventually appeared at Leiden in 1662, twelve years after his death, in a Latin translation. The original French manuscript was published in Paris in 1664.

In the *Traité de l'homme* Descartes expounded the revolutionary view that the soul is immaterial, and that the body is a machine created by God. Descartes saw body and soul as two separate substances that function independently yet are also connected internally. He realized that this was a paradoxical view of the relation between body and mind,

---

[32] 'Soo boort hy door en door en door der logenen beklem;/ En legt sy [de waarheid] diep en dwers, en kan sy qualick rijsen,/ Slaet, geesselt nijptse 'r uyt met Touw en Tangh en Rijsen [...]', in Huygens, "Een Beul" 84, vs. 42–44.

[33] 'O Godt, nu gevoel ick dat ghy een groot godt syt want nu gevoel ick geen pyn meer [...]', in Oudaan, *Haagsche Broeder-Moord* 119.

[34] For the issues discussed here, see especially Verbeek Th., "Een Ziel in een Lichaam", in idem, *De wereld van Descartes. Essays over Descartes en zijn tijdgenoten* (Amsterdam: 1996) 101–117; idem, "Crisis te Utrecht: 1641–1642", in Koops W. – Dorsman L. – Verbeek Th. (eds.) *Née Cartésienne – Cartesiaansch Gebooren. Descartes en de Utrechtse Academie 1636–2005* (Assen: 2005) 22–38; Gijn J. van, "Descartes en de geneeskunde", in ibidem 83–101. The date of *Traité de l'homme* has been inferred from a letter to Mersenne from 1646. See Van Gijn, "Descartes en de geneeskunde" 85.

but explained the connection between the two as a divinely ordained fact. The link between body and mind serves to enable humans to respond adequately to real-life situations. Man is a machine but not an automaton; he can adapt to his surroundings. The machine is set in motion when the body transmits signals via the nervous system to the pineal gland.[35] The pineal gland, in turn, stimulates muscular movement. The drawing of the kneeling boy by the fire illustrates Descartes' argument:

> Thus, if fire *A* is near foot *B*, the particles of this fire (which move very quickly, as you know) have force enough to displace the area of skin that they touch; and thus pulling the little thread *cc*, which you can see to be attached there, they simultaneously open the entrance to the pore [or conduit] *de* where this thread terminates [in the brain]: just as pulling on one end of a cord, one simultaneously rings a bell which hangs at the opposite end. Now the entrance of the pore or small conduit *de*, being thus opened, the animal spirits from cavity *F* enter and are carried through it – part into the muscles that serve to withdraw this foot from the fire, part into those that serve to advance the hands and bend the whole body to protect it.[36]

Descartes referred to this process as automatic movement (he did not yet use the word 'reflex').

Descartes approached pain from a purely analytical, philosophical perspective, and was uninterested in the ethical dimension of pain. He posited a direct relation between bodily damage and physical pain, and assumed that pain can be stopped by removing its cause or by manipulating the reception of pain signals by the brain. Cutting nerves seemed a theoretical option, but in practice this turned out to cause new pain (we saw earlier that Van Beverwijck warns against touching the nerves directly), and Descartes' theory could not account for this new pain (just as it could not explain the workings of emotional pain).

The question of whether seventeenth-century Dutch writers knew about and made use of Descartes's views on pain is an open one. Descartes's theory of pain sensation was not published during his lifetime, but he may have discussed it informally, for example in a circular

---

[35] Zie Verbeek, "Een Ziel in een Lichaam" 109–110 and Van Gijn, "Descartes en de geneeskunde" 92–93.

[36] Translation from René Descartes, *Treatise of man.* French text with translation and commentary by Th. St. Hall (Cambridge MA: 1972) 34–35 (in the French original 26–28).

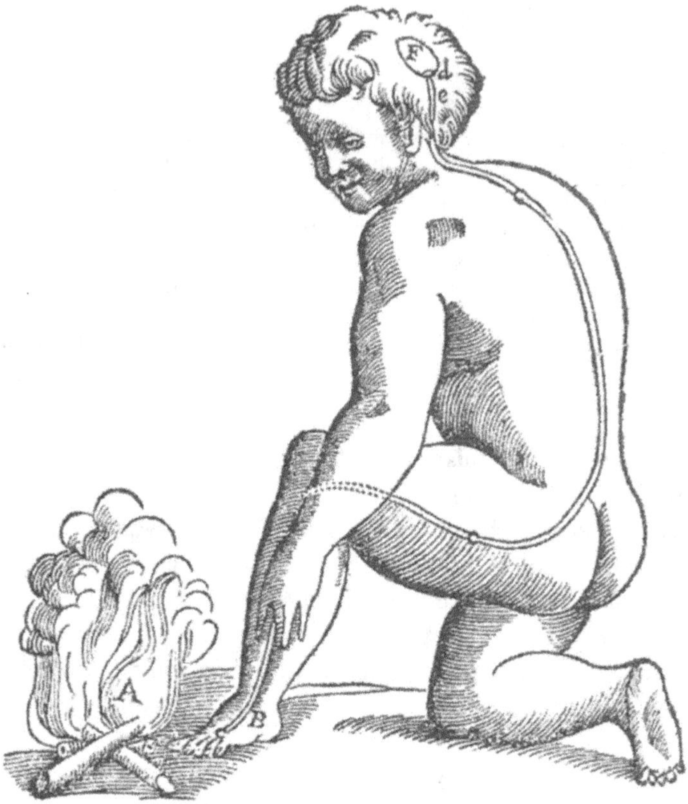

Fig. 5. Gerard van Gutschoven, The perception of pain according to Descartes. From René Descartes, *Traité de l'homme* (Paris, Claude Clerselier: 1664) 27. Copy of Amsterdam University Library.

letter. Van Beverwijck and Huygens corresponded with Descartes, yet it seems that they did not discuss Descartes' ideas about pain.[37]

Conclusion

According to his torturer, Cornelis de Witt spoke the following words on the rack: 'O God, now I feel that You are a mighty God, since now I have ceased to feel pain'.[38] They suggest that De Witt had gone beyond pain, and that his faith in God had enabled him to do so. This may also apply to the tortured victims in the Northern Quarter episode, who frequently professed their faith in God. In investigating the possibility of eliminating the physical sensation of pain altogether, Descartes seems to have occupied an isolated position within seventeenth-century Dutch pain discourses. Descartes approaches pain from an amoral, purely analytical perspective, whereas the dominant medical, literary, historiographical and judicial conceptions of pain proceeded from Galenic and Christian models. In the Galenic approach, pain is a sign that the balance between the four humours has been disturbed, while in Christian conceptions, pain could be seen as a punishment for the Fall, and therefore a necessary part of each human life. Yet this punishment does not mean that human beings are entirely powerless to do anything about their pain. Both in the Galenic and Christian approach, pain serves as a sign that both body and mind are in need of purification. Dutch writers of the seventeenth century often combine the two frameworks: there is often a seamless transition from descriptions of physical pain to moral lessons about the change in moral behaviour that is necessary to alleviate the pain. God can inflict pain, and in some cases man has the right to inflict pain on his fellow human beings, provided this is done in the service of God, and is aimed at purification. Yet early modern Dutch writers roundly condemn the infliction of pain without restraint and out of self-interest, and see this as a form of arrogating an authority that belongs only to God.

---

[37] See for example the "Aenhangsel" [Appendix] in Van Beverwijck, *Wercken der genees-konste* 204–205, followed by letters to and by Descartes from 1637, 205–213.

[38] 'O Godt, nu gevoel ick dat ghy een groot godt syt want nu gevoel ick geen pyn meer [...]'. Joachim Oudaan, *Haagsche Broeder-Moord* 119. The situation is comparable to that of Samson in Vondel's play *Samson*, referred to earlier in this article: 'I have conquered my blindness, my sorrow; strike me further if you wish', Samson says to his warder (''k Heb mijne blintheit, mijn verdriet/ Verwonnen. wiltge, sla me stijver' [*Samson* 1077–1078]).

Apppendix

Joachim Oudaan: "Op de tijtel-print, van de wedersproke pyn-bank, in-gestelt door den achtbaren, hoog-geleerden heere Daniel Jonktys, artzeny-geleerde, oud-schepen der stede Rotterdam", in Daniel Jonktys, *De pyn-bank wedersproken en bematigt* (Rotterdam, Joannes Naeranus: 1651) fol. 2v–3v.

[...]
Pijn-bank, meldt uw' teyster-stukken.
[...]
Aan een ladder, vast gebonden,
Bindtm'er een; veel honderd ponden
Aan de duymen van zijn voet,
Daar geen zweet bat is te stulpen.
Dorstig wordt, in bloed te gulpen,
't Pijnders-rot na meerder bloed.
't Wind-as moet de leden trekken,
Dat de huyd geen rif kan dekken.
Brandewijn, met kannen vol,
Weg-geplengt in lijnwaat strooken,
Hoofd-waard af, om 't vleesch te schrooken,
Brandt tot onder 't voeten-hol:
Teffens kaarssen, pek, en kolen,
Koken oxelen, en zolen,
Dat geen lid een lid en bindt:
Weer aan 't trekken, en aan 't knellen,
Elle-bogen tot een elle,
Tot de beul zig beu bevindt.
Wat al meer? Een smook van zwavel:
Torren plant men op de navel,
Die 'r een angel trekken uyt:
Ziedend' oly doet men gieten,
Of men bindt gesplete rieten
Op de spieren zonder huyt.
Vaar al voort. Gebakke testen
Doet m' op 't weeke buyk-vleesch vesten.
Vuyr daar boven, en een rat,
Die door hitt' in naar benauwen
Bijt en rijt, met tand en klauwen,
Diep ter buyk in, onder 't vat.
Dat's 't noch al niet. Zal ik tuygen
Wat m' een zog-kalf dede zuygen?
Waar men schibbens hout in dreef?
Welk een lid men op dee blazen?
Of waar aan (wie zouw niet razen!)

't Gansche lichaam hangen bleef?
Suft de weedom na 't ontspannen?
Om de slaap voorts weg te bannen,
Girst de garde door het vleesch;
Geeft men pekel-haring t'eten;
Laaft geen dronk (hoe zeer bekreten)
't Hart zoo droog, de mond zoo heesch.
Wat wierd hier door uyt-gevonden?
Land-verraad, op losse gronden.
'k Acht verlekk'ring op uw' goed,
(Arme menschen, zonder voorspraak)
Was alleen de schuld, en oorzaak
Van het zoo geplengde bloed [...].

Selective Bibliography

Beverwijck Johan van, *Wercken der genees-konste, bestaende in den Schat der gesontheyt, Schat der ongesontheyt, Heel-konste* [...] (Amsterdam, Jan Jacobsz. Schipper: 1664).

——, *Schat der* gezondheid, ed. L. van Gemert (Amsterdam: 1992).

Cooper A., "The Indigenous versus the Exotic: debating natural origins in early modern Europe", *Landscape Research* 28 (2003) I, 51–60.

Descartes René, *Treatise of man.* French text with translation and commentary by Th.St. Hall (Cambridge MA: 1972).

Gemert L. van, "De krachtpatser en de hoer. Liefde en wraak op het zeventiende-eeuwse toneel", in Bots H. – Gemert L. van (eds.), *Schelmen en prekers. Genres en de transmissie van cultuur in vroegmodern Europa* (Nijmegen: 1999) 15–37.

——, "Johan van Beverwijck als 'instituut'", *De zeventiende eeuw* 8 (1992) 99–106.

——, "Johan van Beverwijck", in Bynum W.F. – Bynum H. (eds.), *Dictionary of Medical Biography* (Westport – London: 2007) I 203–204.

——, "Schuld en boete bij Vondel en De Koning" (forthcoming).

Gijn Jan van, "Descartes en de geneeskunde", in Koops W. – Dorsman L. – Verbeek Th. (eds.), *Née Cartésiennne – Cartesiaansch Gebooren. Descartes en de Utrechtse Academie 1636–2005* (Assen: 2005) 83–101.

Hooft P.C., *Nederlandse Historiën. Een keuze uit het grote verhaal van de Nederlandse Opstand*, ed. F. van Gestel – E. Grootes – J. de Jongste (Amsterdam: 2007).

Huygens Constantijn, *De gedichten*, ed. J.A. Worp, 9 vols. (Groningen: 1893).

——, "Een Beul", in *Zes zedeprinten*, ed. Werkgroep van Utrechtse neerlandici (Utrecht: 1976[2]) 80–91. Also at: www.let.leidenuniv.nl/Dutch/Huygens/HUYG23.html#CH1623038 and www.fransmensonides.nl/beul_hoofd.htm.

——, *Ooghen-troost*, ed. F.L. Zwaan (Groningen: 1984).

——, *Mijn leven verteld aan mijn kinderen*, ed. F.R.E. Blom, 2 vols. (Amsterdam: 2003).

Jonktys Daniel, *De pyn-bank wedersproken en bematigt* (Rotterdam: Ioannes Naeranus, 1651, private copy).

Koning Abraham de, *Simsons Treur-spel* (Amsterdam, Abraham de Koningh: 1618).

Luyken Jan, *Spiegel van het menselyk bedryf* (Amsterdam, Johannes and Caspaares Luiken: 1694) facsimile edition by L. de Vries (Amsterdam – Brussel: 1984).

Nierop H. van, *Het verraad van het Noorderkwartier. Oorlog, terreur en recht in de Nederlandse Opstand* (Amsterdam: 1999).

Oudaan Joachim, *Haagsche Broeder-Moord of Dolle Blydschap Treurspel*, ed. Werkgroep Utrechtse neerlandici (Utrecht: 1982).

Panhuysen L., *De Ware Vrijheid. De levens van Johan en Cornelis de Witt* (Amsterdam – Antwerpen: 2005).

Pieters J. – Gosseye L., "Blindheid en inzicht. De retoriek van het lezen in Constantijn Huygens' *Ooghen-troost*", *Tijdschrift voor Nederlandse taal- en letterkunde* 123,3 (2007) 208–225.

Six van Chandelier Jan, *Gedichten*, ed. A.E. Jacobs (Assen – Maastricht: 1991).

Verbeek Th., "Een Ziel in een Lichaam", in idem, *De wereld van Descartes. Essays over Descartes en zijn tijdgenoten* (Amsterdam: 1996) 101–117.

——, "Crisis te Utrecht: 1641–1642", in Koops W. – Dorsman L. – Verbeek Th. (eds.), *Née Cartésiennne – Cartesiaansch Gebooren. Descartes en de Utrechtse Academie 1636–2005* (Assen: 2005) 22–38.

Vondel Joost van den, *Geuse Vesper of Siecken-troost voor de Vierentwintigh* submitted in: *De werken van Joost van den Vondel* (Amsterdam: 1929) III 339–340. Also at: www.dbnl.org/tekst/vond001dewe03_01/vond001dewe03_01_0050.htm.

——, *Samson of Heilige Wraeck* (t'Amsterdam: weduwe Abraham de Wees, 1660); submitted in: *De werken van Joost van den Vondel* (Amsterdam 1936) IX 173–239. Also at: www.dbnl.org/tekst/vond001dewe09_01/vond001dewe09_01_0001.htm.

SEEING, FEELING, JUDGING: PAIN IN THE EARLY MODERN IMAGINATION

Stephen Pender

Individual experience is central to what Lucinda Beier has called 'the social history of suffering',[1] a phrase which captures theories and practices associated with hygiene and therapeutics, surgery and lay healing, the gibbet and the clinic, as well as sites of devotion and worship. Perhaps because its records, and its vocabularies, are uneven or confused, confected or vague, too few scholars have explored the experience of pain in the past – surely central to a social history of suffering. Such a history for early modernity might be characterised as an ensemble of feelings in search of a language: the multiple, variegated meanings of grief, of suffering, and of pain suggest a roiling, disarticulate period of ill-feeling. To cite one of many examples: in *The Benefite of Affliction* (1616), Charles Richardson offered the term "affliction" as an entrepot for suffering as wide-ranging as imprisonment, shipwreck, the death of a friend, spouse, or child, death in childbirth, violent death, and numerous forms of 'inward fear & horror of conscience'.[2] From a seventeenth-century English doctor who treated apostumes and the pox, palsy and melancholy[3] to the women who menstruated from their ears in early eighteenth-century Germany,[4] the term "pain" maps a varied, sometimes fantastic collection of misery. Of course, all forms of suffering were mediated by a sufferer's felt and imagined sensations.

'I judge myself only by actual sensation, not by reasoning', Montaigne wrote in 1588; those who depend on reason, or on medical 'persuasions and counsels', are susceptible to false prognostications, vain diagnoses,

---

[1] McCray Beier L., *Sufferers and Healers: The Experience of Illness in Seventeenth-Century England* (London – New York: 1987) 3.

[2] Charles Richardson, *The Benefite of Affliction* (London: 1616) 15–23, *passim.*

[3] *A Seventeenth-Century Doctor and His Patients: John Symcotts, 1592?–1662*, Poynter F.N.L. – Bishop, W.J. (eds.), in *The Publications of the Bedfordshire Historical Society*, vol. 31 (Streatley: 1951) 25–26.

[4] Duden B., *The Woman Beneath the Skin: A Doctor's Patients in Eighteenth-Century Germany*, trl. Th. Dunlap (Cambridge, Mass.: 1991).

ignorant practitioners.[5] But what is sensation? How is it related to pain? How does the imagination localise, adjust, and register suffering? Here, I explore several disparate early modern nociceptive instances – from Montaigne's experience of pain through Descartes' famous podiatric excursion in the sixth meditation to late seventeenth-century animadversions on vitalism and suffering – in order to suggest that pain finds its history in speculative anatomies, that the imagination is central to early modern conceptions of suffering, and that there seems to be a shift, between 1580 and 1680, from the dominant conception of pain as a sensation related to touch to various interventions that suggest pain is a threat to vitality itself. I present an essayist concerned with the variable fates of his body, a philosopher exploring the ways in which pain speaks to inwardness, and an unorthodox physician probing the viscera for chains of causation. Despite their dissimilarity, each nociceptive instance speaks to a particular conception of embodiment, pain, and expression: from the psycho-physiology of Montaigne, for whom the expression of pain is crucial, through Descartes, for whom pain signifies inwardness, to the physician Everard Maynwaring, to whom pain speaks of the labyrinthine nature of causality in the human body.

Exploring these instances, I shall leave aside what I have mentioned briefly, the discourse of affliction, in which affective or physical pain was an occasion to sift one's spiritual inventory, to test one's faith, to embrace and exemplify tolerance, patience, and humility. Affliction, perseverance, and recovery were seen as benefactions by Roman Catholics and the reformed; relapse signified obduracy.[6] '[A]ffliction is not evil', writes John Donne, 'it is rather evil to have none'.[7] Of course, afflictions were treated: physicians of the body (surgeons, apothecaries, doctors) and of the soul (philosophers, theologians, rhetors) prescribed analgesics and cordials, diversions and distractions, in order to assuage physical, affective, and spiritual suffering. Although the 'avoidance of pain' was

---

[5] *The Complete Essays of Montaigne*, trl. D.M. Frame (Stanford U.P.: 1958) 840. Further references to this text are included in parenthesis.

[6] *The Sermons of John Donne*, Simpson E.M. – Potter G.R. (eds.), 10 vols. (Berkeley – Los Angeles: 1953–1962), vol. III 67; Harley D., "The Theology of Affliction and the Experience of Sickness in the Godly Family, 1650–1714: The Henrys and the Newcomes", in Grell O.P. – Cunningham A. (eds.), *Religio Medici: Medicine and Religion in Seventeenth-Century England* (Aldershot: 1996) 277, comments that 'afflictions, whether of mind, body or estate, were sent by God as a correction for sin, for the good of the sinner'.

[7] *Sermons* 3.67.

'integrated into surgical pathology and therapeutics', and surgeons accepted pain as an indication of the feasibility of an operation,[8] I am interested in pain as it was imagined by sufferers and physicians in their delicate, probative excursions into the body. As conceptions of pain shift from the psycho-physiological through the mechanistic to the vital, the relationship between suffering, feeling, and expression invites interrogation: is there a "direct relationship" between the ways in which pain is borne, the ways in which it was felt along the pulses, and nociceptive expression, as Rosalind Rey argues?[9] Past representations of pain probably depict normative rather than actual behaviour. Still, we might ask if changing conceptions of pain – from a sense moored to touch to an attack on the organism itself – occasion new forms of expression, keeping in mind that there is rarely expressive adequation for feeling. Even by the late eighteenth century, as one physician insists, language had 'not yet been adjusted with any degree of exactness to our inward feelings'.[10] Pain is distinct among "inward feelings" and perceptual states because it has no object; instead, as Elaine Scarry argues, the imagination is pain's 'intentional object'.[11] Pain affects, even colonises the imagination but appealing to the imagination also remedied pain. As we shall see, somatic and noetic suffering were treated imaginatively in early modernity: images were thought lenitive, cordial, healing, and they were used to divert and distract, to inspire passions contrary to those occasioned, for example, by pain. Since antiquity, pain, fear, and the imagination have been intimate: pain limns imaginary anatomies, fear fleshes them out.

In antiquity, pleasure and pain are the 'supreme genera of the emotions', and it seems that all emotions were a variable admixture of both.[12] Laughter, for example, was pleasured combined with

---

[8] Wear A., *Knowledge and Practice in English Medicine, 1550–1680* (Cambridge: 2000) 246; see also Siraisi N.G., *Medieval and Early Renaissance Medicine: an Introduction to Knowledge and Practice* (Chicago: 1990) 171–172, and Thomas K., *Religion and the Decline of Magic* (London: 1971) 3–24.

[9] *The History of Pain*, trl. L.E. Wallace, J.A. and S.W. Cadden (Cambridge, Mass.: 1998 [1993]) 4; 50–88. Further citations will appear in parenthesis in the text.

[10] Thomas Beddoes, *Hygiea*, 3 vols. (Bristol: 1802–1803) 2.78, quoted in Porter R., "Western Medicine and Pain: Historical Perspectives", in Hinnells J.R. – Porter R. (eds.), *Religion, Health, and Suffering* (London – New York: 1999) 367.

[11] *The Body in Pain: the Making and Unmaking of the World* (New York – Oxford: 1985) 164.

[12] Frede D., "Mixed Feelings in Aristotle's *Rhetoric*", in Rorty A.O. (ed.), *Essays on Aristotle's* Rhetoric (Berkeley: 1996) 259.

malice (*Philebus* 48a ff.). For Plato, pain itself was medicalised: pain is the disintegration of somatic equilibrium, just as pleasure is its restoration (*Philebus*, 31d; 32a–b). At least in the *Rhetoric*, Aristotle follows Plato closely; pleasure is a movement of the soul, a settling down (*katastasis*) into its natural state, while pain is the opposite (1369b 33–35). Like fear, pain is found in the faculty of desire and, according to Aristotle, all passions are *logoi enhuloi*, 'emattered accounts',[13] a term which suggests that affections have corresponding material states and actions, that all affections are common to the psyche and to the body (*De anima* 436a 7–8). Neither a dualist nor a physicalist, Aristotle argues that somatic states, like pain, necessarily involve actualisation or alteration, either of which is sufficient to occasion feeling.[14] While it offers a different conception of pleasure than the *Rhetoric*, in the *Nichomachean Ethics* Aristotle mentions pain in passing. Although few who succeeded him adhered to his position, Aristotle argues that pain upsets and destroys the nature of the person who feels it (1119a 23). But, with the possible exception of the Hippocratic *Places in Man* (*De locis in homine*), even ancient physicians were relatively uninterested in the effects of pain; overall, they consider pain merely a symptom of disease, something that might be cured along with distemper, not a sensation which impugns the whole person. As a consequence, ancient medicine is rather poor in the rhetoric of pain.[15]

A resplendent language of pain emerges in Hellenistic philosophy and rhetoric, drawing generously from various schools of peripatetic and Stoic thought. Most writers dismiss the notion that pain might be eliminated altogether; instead, they classify pain among the 'indifferents,' those things over which we have little or no control, which we should endure nobly. To Seneca, the populariser of pragmatic Stoicism, pain is a matter of opinion: pain is slight, Seneca argues, 'if opinion has added nothing to it'. We suffer 'according to opinion'.[16] Nor are the wise

[13] 126a 10–11; 403a 19–25. All references to Aristotle are from *The Complete Works of Aristotle*, ed. J. Barnes, 2 vols. (Princeton: 1995 [1984]) and will be included in parenthesis in the text.

[14] See Everson S., "Psychology", in Barnes J. (ed.), *The Cambridge Companion to Aristotle* (Cambridge: 1995) 168–194, esp. 184 ff.

[15] See Horden P., "Pain in Hippocratic Medicine", in Hinnells – Porter (eds.), *Religion, Health, and Suffering*, 295–315 and references.

[16] Seneca, *Ad Lucilium Epistulae Morales*, trl. R.M. Gunmere (Cambridge, Mass.: 1953) 78,13 (p. 189). The entire letter is a treatise on consolation. See also, for example, Meric Causabon, *Treatise of Enthusiasme* (1655), who argues that the experience of

free from pain, although they suffer and react rationally and decorously. Cicero amplifies this popular Stoic notion in books two and three of the *Tusculan Disputations*, which treat *dolor* and *aegritudo*, and concludes that sorrow or grief arises 'not by nature but by judgement, by false belief, by a sort of summons to pain, when we decide we should feel it'. Distress is a function of our perception of our situation rather than how bad it might be in actuality. Pain is evil, Cicero concedes, but it pales compared to disgrace; no one is immune from pain, but those who steel themselves with philosophical mediation, who recognise pain's indifference, are insusceptible to distress.[17] This notion persists at least until Descartes.[18] Although I cannot do justice to the rich constellation of terms for and views of pain in this period, overall what emerges is a broad commitment to what Sextus Empiricus called *ataraxia* and *metriopatheia*: tranquillity or 'freedom from disturbance' and, 'in the case of things unavoidable', 'moderation in affection'.[19] These doctrines explicitly counter Aristotle's notion that pain is deeply debilitating, and render clear the relationships between nociception and expression: physical and emotional pain should be borne with equanimity and moderation, sensibilities and dispositions which subvent the consistency and wholeness of self.

Drawing on Cicero's discussions of pain, in which virtue, magnanimity, endurance, and courage appear as balms,[20] Augustine too insists that the wise either avoid pain, if possible, or accept it voluntarily, with dignity. For Augustine, who wrote about human bodies more than any other patristic author, pain arises from abjection; at its foundation, it is physical, occasioned by illness and need, but it is also a question of will.[21] After the fall, when creation was afflicted, bodies were no longer

pain depends on attitudes and dispositions: 'where the will is obstinately bent, [...] the sense, if not altogether taken away, yet is nothing near so great, or so sharp as it is in others, where no such preparation [pain was but opinion] is made'; ed. P.J. Korshin (Gainesville: 1970) 75; 77–78.

[17] *Tusculan Disputations*, trl. J.E. King (London: 1966 [1927]) III, 82–83; III, 54 (cf. IV, 60); II, 30; III, 25.

[18] Letter to Elisabeth, 18 May 1645, in *The Correspondence Between Princess Elisabeth of Bohemia and René Descartes*, ed. and trl. L. Shapiro (Chicago – London: 2007) 85–88.

[19] Sextus Empiricus, *Outlines of Scepticism*, ed. J. Annas – J. Barnes (Cambridge: 1994) I, 29–30; see Hankinson R.J., *The Sceptics* (London – New York 1994) 286–292.

[20] *De finibus*, trl. H. Rackham (Cambridge, Mass.: 1967) II, 95.

[21] See Lössl J., "Dolor (dolere)", in Mayer C. (ed.), *Augustinus-Lexikon*, II.3/ 4 (Basel: 1999) 582–591. For Augustine on the human body, see Miles M.R., "Corpus", in ibid., II.1/ 2 (1996) 6–19.

in a 'condition' to serve even the debased will: they become sick, age, and die, which they should not 'if our nature were in every way and in all its parts obedient to our will'. Physical pain is an evil, part of the constellation of suffering that results from original sin. While he argues that we must not speak too much about *dolor*, pain is always also fear and *dolor animi*. It is felt in the soul: the 'pain of the flesh is nothing but a distress of the soul arising from the flesh, and a kind of disagreement with what the body is suffering'. Desire is felt by 'the man himself' – 'the flesh' as the whole man, body and soul, in Augustine's formulation – or by 'some part of the soul'.[22] So, too, pain, which we suffer wholly. Pain is a sign of depravity that obscures 'the whole human reality'.[23] Augustine's thought about pain developed in relation to the work of Julian of Aeclanum who argued, in contrast, that pain is a 'good teacher', that neither physical nor emotional pain is inherently evil, and that sensibility determined one's experience of pain which, if borne well, can be of singular assistance. Only one's attitude toward pain can be considered evil.[24] As Cicero insists, the right disposition towards pain has precepts and rules which forbid weakness.[25]

Conflicting views of pain evident in this debate persist, but the notion that pain affects the whole person is largely dormant in the middle ages. Although a detailed map of pain in the period would be highly variegated, and include martyrs and mystics, physicians and monks, scholars have argued that, overall, physical pain 'baffled the neat taxonomies of scholastic medicine', with the result that 'medical writing on pain is sporadic and far less consistent than theological discourse'.[26] Drawing on Augustine, most authorities considered sin the origin of pain; pain was a problem more for theologians than medical practitioners. While medieval physicians speculated about the treatment and causes of pain – Avicenna, for example, insists that 'all causes of pain belong to two kinds: the sudden alteration of complexion [...] and the solution of

---

[22] Augustine, *The City of God Against the Pagans*, ed. and trl. R.W. Dyson (Cambridge: 1998) XIV, 15 (612–613).

[23] Lössl, "Dolor (dolere)" 586.

[24] See Lössl J., "Julian of Aeclanum on Pain", *Journal of Early Christian Studies* 10,2 (2002) (203–243) 208–209.

[25] *De finibus*, II, 94.

[26] Cohen E., "The Animated Pain of the Body", *American Historical Review* 105,1 (2000) (36–68) 49.

continuity'[27] – normative attitudes towards suffering, frequently determined by impassivity, are found in the work of theologians, poets, and visual artists. Peter Lombard, for example, thought that 'the soul feels pains, some of them through the instrument of the body (*instrumentum corporis*), some not'.[28] In his lengthy treatment of pain in the *Summa theologiae*, Aquinas distinguishes interior from exterior nociception: while the latter is moored to the haptic, interior pain, or sorrow, is 'more profound', for evil is apprehended more clearly by interior perception than external sense.[29] For Aquinas, pain tests autonomy: just as pleasure both causes and indicates courses of action, so pain affects our will. For example, intense pain can interrupt or prevent learning, and pain intensifies if 'hurtful things' are 'pent up within us'. If sorrow is released, Aquinas argues, anticipating a number of early modern claims, the 'soul's energies are turned to things outside itself, and interior pain is lessened'. Sorrow is 'assuaged by [...] expressing it in tears or sobs or even words' (139). We desire separation from sorrowful things, Aquinas argues, because we desire unity of self (119).

The expression if not the experience of pain in the middle ages was determined by pain's purpose and the sufferer's status: martyrs embraced and expressed pain differently from those who sought the assistance of saints, mystics tended to agree with Julian of Aeclanum, and the elite inclined towards impassivity. As Esther Cohen has argued, the shift

---

[27] *Liber canonis in medicina philosophi* (Venice: 1564), quoted in Cohen, "Animated Pain" 47–48. And it seems medieval Italian surgeons used anaesthesia; see Jones I.B., "Popular Medical Knowledge in Fourteenth-Century English Literature", *Bulletin of the Institute of the History of Medicine* 5 (1937) (405–451 and 538–588) 573–574. The 'solution of continuity' is, according to Aristotle, 'the disruption of parts naturally conjoined is not pain, but a cause of pain' (145b 12–14). In *On the Affected Parts*, Galen comments that pain is a solution of continuity of parts either from distemper or incisions, fractures, tension, and the like (trl. R. Siegel [Basle: 1976] 47–48 [2.5]). In *A Physical Dictionary* (London: 1657), the term is defined as 'a division of such parts as naturally ought to be united'. An earlier dictionary defines 'solutio continuitatis' as 'a dissolving of that which necessarily belongeth to another' (Christopher Wirtzung [augmented by Jacob Mason], *Praxis Medicinae Universalis; or A Generall Practise of Physicke* [London, Edmund Bollifant: 1598], third index). The term was taken up by various writers to describe schisms and unproductive separations; see, for example, Donne, *Essays in Divinity*, ed. E.M. Simpson (Oxford: 1952) (50–51) 10–11, where it describes a church 'wounded by schismes', and Francis Bacon, *The Works of Francis Bacon*, ed. J. Spedding et al. (London: 1857–1874) IV, 373, where it describes artificial divisions in the arts and sciences. For other instances, see Rey, *History of Pain* 63 ff.

[28] Cohen, "Animated Pain" 43.

[29] *Summa Theologiae*, 61 vols., *Pleasure* (1a2ae. 31–39), trl. E. D'Arcy (London: 1964) 83; 103; 105.

from the chivalric code to the overt search for suffering, from 'denial of pain to its validation and expression, was a momentous change in the history of European sensibilities, affecting fields as disparate as mysticism and law, medicine and theology'.[30] This shift in sensibilities has been characterised, famously, as the "civilising process", which came to fruition in early modernity. Briefly, in the sixteenth century, not only the elite but the middling sorts increasingly repressed their passions in order to emulate court culture; according to Norbert Elias, forms of restraint progressively underwrote social participation and success in the polity. Scholars have criticised Elias' Blochian portrayal of emotional life in the middle ages, and the instances of nociception I examine should further nuance his thesis for early modernity, for sufferers were not only enjoined to embrace pain and bear it decorously, they were also urged to present a 'mortification by example', in Donne's words, and display, often for devotional purposes, their sickness and suffering, agues and agonies.[31]

Although contemporary investigations of pain pose similar questions – what is the relationship between feeling and expression? how might we imagine pain?[32] – the early modern period was intensely concerned with representing, evaluating, and utilising pain. From prolonged, intense war, public execution, and inquisitions through the nociceptive store of Montaigne's *Essais* and medical *historia* to the growing obligation to detail mental and physical affliction in autobiography and pathography, the sixteenth and seventeenth centuries knew well the vales of pain and sorrow. Examining the records of an early seventeenth-century physician, for example, Michael MacDonald concludes that there is 'plenty of evidence that Englishmen were more aware of mental suffering

[30] Cohen E., "The Expression of Pain in the Later Middle Ages: Deliverance, Acceptance, and Infamy", in Egmond F. – Zwijnenberg R. (eds.), *Bodily Extremities: Preoccupations with the Human Body in Early Modern European Culture* (Aldershot: 2003) (195–219) 217–218. Although Daniel du Moulin has argued that the 'attention that medieval medical textbooks have given to the management of pain, as well as the interest [...] in the problem of surgical anaesthesia, does not make it plausible that pain *perception* was less acute than today'; see his "A Historical-Phenomenological Study of Bodily Pain in Western Man", *Bulletin of the History of Medicine* 48 (1974) (540–570) 561, emphasis his, 569.

[31] Elias N., *The Civilising Process: the History of Manners and State Formation and Civilisation*, trl. E. Jephcott, 2 vols. (Oxford: 1994). For criticism, see, for example, Rosenwein B.H., "Controlling Paradigms", in eadem (ed.), *Anger's Past: The Social Uses of an Emotion in the Middle Ages* (Ithaca: 1998) 233–247; esp. 237–240.

[32] See, for example, Aydede M. (ed.), *Pain: New Essays on Its Nature and the Methodology of Its Study* (Cambridge, Mass.: 2005).

after 1580 than they ever had been before; and only a small amount of the anguish they were discovering was madness'.[33] As Keith Thomas argues, those in the period who lived past age thirty-five 'could anticipate a lifetime of intermittent pain'.[34] While it seems that early modern physicians were not overly concerned with analgesia, an attitude which might have changed because popular, "quack" practitioners promised gentle remedies, the seventeenth-century witnessed an increase in the number of university theses on pain.[35] In one sense, the period 1580 to 1680 might be seen to revisit and revivify the distinction between Augustinian notions of pain, absorbed by most later Christian traditions, which place it in the soul, and Aristotelian conceptions, which suggest that pain is at once somatic and noetic. In this rich cosmos of pain, I focus on three nociceptive moments, all of which treat pain differently: Montaigne is generally seen to be among the first to fully explore pain autobiographically, Descartes treats pain as one of the measures of embodiment, and Maynwaring explores pain as an attack on the 'vital force' of the body in the first vernacular treatise on the subject in England. I begin with Montaigne.

For Montaigne, pain involves knowledge, sensation, and cozenage; it calls into crisis moderation and temperance, regimen and habit, and does so, in part, via the imagination. 'I test myself in the thickest of pain', Montaigne writes, 'and have always found that I was capable of speaking, thinking, and answering as sanely as at any other time, but not as steadily, being troubled and distracted' (577). Pain does not entirely derange, but renders speaking and thinking labile, unsteady, disordered. As he argues in the "Apology for Raymond Sebond", illness imprints 'characters' on things, which appear otherwise than they might to the healthy; appearances are affected by 'disordered states' (453). Illness and pain vex judgement, too: although we do not 'feel' them, fevers, apoplexies, even severe colds 'prostrate' cognition (424). We cannot even discern the gravity of our own afflictions: what we think is a simple ailment, a cold or a sprain, masks something severe (642). Still, when most stricken, Montaigne is able to 'broach subjects

---

[33] MacDonald M., *Mystical Bedlam: Madness, Anxiety, and Healing in Seventeenth-Century England* (Cambridge: 1981) 149.

[34] Thomas, *Religion and the Decline of Magic* 6.

[35] Porter, "Wester Medicine and Pain" 375–376 and Du Moulin, "Bodily Pain in Western Man" 550.

as remote as possible from his condition', but only with a paroxysm of sudden effort; sustained engagement is inconceivable (577). Pain clearly assaults the intellect, the senses, the passions and the body, but it is the imagination that concerns Montaigne: when confronted with an array of symptoms and indications that presage illness, he argues for a shift of resources, a redeployment of energies, away from prolepsis toward immediacy. Against the anticipation of pain, against the uncertainty of diagnosis and prognosis, Montaigne recommends several forms of prophylaxis: bridling the imagination, keeping case histories, and experimenting with prevarication.

Psychological pain, Montaigne avers, afflicts him much less than it does others; he is insensible to 'accidents' that do not approach 'head-on'. But 'really essential and bodily sufferings', he continues, 'I feel very keenly'. He also keenly feels the approach of sickness: when he is healthy, he conceives illness 'in imagination so unendurable that in truth I had more fear of them than I have found pain in them' (575). The anticipation of illness commonly inspires acute anxiety: many things 'seem to us greater in imagination than in reality', he writes. 'I have spent a good part of my life in perfect and entire health; [...] [this] state [...] made me find the thought of illnesses so horrible that when I came to experience them I found their pains mild and easy compared with my fears' (268; cf. 39).

The imagination is central to the experience of pain and illness; at least physicians recognise as much. 'Why do doctors work on the credulity of their patient beforehand with so many false promises of cure', Montaigne asks, 'if not so that the effect of the imagination may make up for the imposture of their decoction?' (73). The 'effect of the imagination' is astringent, cordial, compensatory, but it is also debilitating, wayward, antinomian. Because the imagination might turn 'even your health into a fever' (802), it must be assuaged, flattered, fooled: 'I treat my imagination as gently as I can, and would relieve it, if I could, of all trouble and conflict. We must help it and flatter it, and fool it if we can' (836). Once set in motion, Montaigne argues – and he clearly has the imagination in mind – the soul is 'lost in itself' unless it is directed to an object or an action (14). But intense fear is worrisome, and perhaps even trumps pain. He concludes that the faculties of the soul, 'as we employ them', trouble us as much as they serve us (575) and he cautions against prolepsis:

> Do not expect me to go and amuse myself testing my pulse and my urine so as to take some bothersome precaution; I shall be in plenty of time when I feel the pain, without prolonging it by pain of fear. He who fears he will suffer, already suffers from his fear. [...] Besides, the ignorance and uncertainty of those who presume to explain the workings of Nature and her inner processes, and all the false prognostications of their art, should make us know that she has utterly unknown ways of her own. [...] Except for old age, [...] in all other ailments I see few signs of the future on which to base our divination (840).

In response to the uncertainty of symptomatology, Montaigne settles on sensation: 'I judge myself only by actual sensation, not by reasoning. [...] Look at those who do otherwise, and depend on so many different persuasions and counsels: how often imagination oppresses them, without the help of the body!' (840). Montaigne distrusts the 'vague field' ('champ vague') of the imagination (21); we suffer its waywardness as we do the passions (cf. 69).[36] A few years later, Thomas Wright offers a similar, typical view: 'the imagination putteth greene spectacles before the eyes of our wit, to make it see nothing but greene, that is, serving for the consideration of the Passion'. In thrall to the imagination, deliberation and judgement are impaired: the wit is vexed by 'the vehemency of the imagination', which occasions 'false representation', in turn the cause of a 'false conceit' in the mind. The imagination's power rests in representing reasons that favour the passion 'very intensively, with more shew and appearance than they are indeed'. Because of that power, those in 'greate paine, or exceeding pleasure, can scarce speake, see, heare, or thinke of any thing, which concerneth not their passion'.[37] Like intense pleasure, pain assaults sense and cognition.

But the imagination is also a source of healing; phantasms function remedially, as Descartes will suggest at the end of *The Passions of the Soul*[38] and as one early seventeenth-century medical writer advises,

> The Physitian therefore that will cure these spirituall sicknesses ["rightly termed the passions of the soule"], must invent and devise some spirituall pageant to fortifie and help the imaginative facultie, which is corrupted

[36] See P. Norton G.P., "Image and Introspective Imagination in Montaigne's *Essais*", *PMLA* 88,2 (1973) 281–288 and, especially, Lyons J.D., *Before Imagination: Embodied Thought from Montaigne to Rousseau* (Stanford: 2005) 32–60.

[37] Thomas Wright, *The Passions of the Minde in Generall* (London, Valentine Simmes: 1604 [second edition]; ed. T. Sloane [Urbana: 1971]) 51–52; see also 34.

[38] See, for example, *The Passions of the Soul*, trl. S.H. Voss (Indianapolis – Cambridge: 1989) 211; 133–134.

> and depraved; yea, hee must endeavour to deceive and imprint another conceit, whether it be wise or foolish, in the Patients braine, thereby to put out all former phantasies.[39]

These tactical appeals to the imagination would have been known from various classical treatments, especially the *Tusculan Disputations*. By the sixteenth century, it seems such remedies – devising images and 'pageants' to distract one who suffers from 'a tumultuous troubled soul' – fell within the purview of physicians as well as rhetoricians and moral philosophers, all of whom drew on the Stoic and Aristotelian traditions of identifying passion, judgement, and the imagination.[40] Montaigne offers the same cure: love remedies grief, he argues, and variation 'solaces, dissolves, dissipates' while the imagination, over time, furnishes us with other business, breaking up our initial sensations, whatever their strength (634–635). It should be no surprise, then, that in his library, following his own prescriptions, Montaigne not only felt able to read and write, but to heal.

Healing involves a form of self-reflexive exemplarity, in which one's past experience of illness serves as a key to future episodes. Excoriating medicine for its diagnostic and nosological uncertainty, Montaigne proposes his own experience of illness as remedy. If medicine is based on 'examples and experience' – 'so is my opinion', Montaigne adds – then what better example, what better experience than his own? (579; cf. 827). Montaigne writes his own medical case history (*historia*):

> For lack of a natural memory I make one of paper, and as some new symptom occurs in my disease, I write it down. Whence it comes that at the present moment, when I have passed through virtually every sort of experience (*estant quasi passé par tout sorte d'exemples*), if some grave stroke threatens me, by glancing through these little notes, disconnected like the Sibyl's leaves, I never fail to find grounds for comfort in some favourable prognostic from my past experience (837–838).

Distilled into unsewn leaves, the records of Montaigne's symptoms offer comfort in their familiarity. He not only writes his own medical history, he not only consults and deliberates about his case, he writes his own *consilium* as well. If he judges himself solely by sensation, the disconnected leaves of his own casebook – the *Essays* themselves, and

---

[39] William Vaughan, *Approved Directions for Health, Both Naturall and Artificiall: Derived from the Best Physitians as well Moderne as Auncient*, fourth edition (London, T. Snodham: 1612) 90.

[40] See my "Rhetoric, Grief, and the Therapeutic Imagination in Early Modern Europe" (forthcoming, 2008).

"Of Experience" in particular, might be thought of as a lengthy *historia* and *consilium* – offer a flexible remedy and a thorough admonition to the strictures of learned medicine. His own 'science' of self-description, his study of self (273), is an antidote to the debilitating uncertainty of an art which proposes universal solutions to particular problems; we should, he argues, become our own physicians, circulate in ourselves, as he puts it, dissecting, recording, sifting our symptoms. His scepticism about medicine is checked by the potential exemplarity of his own experience of illness; the potency of exemplarity, in turn, is a result of the infirmity of reason. Famously rejecting reason's universalising claims, he also dismisses method in the arts and sciences, including medicine (581; cf. 827). Even as his Pyrrhonism wanes in the final essays, he nevertheless presents his experience of 'bodily health [...] pure, not at all corrupted by art or theorizing' (826). Both reason or 'theorizing' and experience are protean (815); with respect to medicine, experience is 'on its own dunghill' and 'reason yields it [sc. experience] the whole field' (826).

However imperfect, the instrument used to prise significant moments from the flow of experience, especially the experience of pain, is the example. Examples are lame (*cloche*), they are 'hazy mirror[s], reflecting all things in all ways' (834), but – and here, perhaps, he has the Aristotelian *paradeigma* in mind – they are serviceable.[41] Although Montaigne is a diligent *venator*, he hunts for particulars, for traces, signs and clues, rather than causes; he detects along the axis of particularity the impossibility of total knowledge, unless that knowledge is articulated autologically.[42] He is his own example. Montaigne thus engages in a critique of medicine by using particulars – physicians he has known, the "poor patient", his own experience – to assail its normativity. He moves quite freely between the general, theoretical aspects of medicine he excoriates and the particularity of individual pathologies, examples, and experiences of illness, impugning the universalism of medical

[41] The *paradeigma* is 'a variety of induction which brings out the meaning of a thing by comparing it with one or more other things which are like it *but clearer or better known*'. See Else G.F., *Aristotle's* Poetics: *The Argument* (Cambridge, Mass.: 1957) 19 (emphasis in the original). On exemplarity in Montaigne, see Lyons J.D., *Exemplum: The Rhetoric of Example in Early Modern France and Italy* (Princeton: 1989) 118–153.

[42] Lyons J.D., "Circe's Drink and Sorbonnic Wine: Montaigne's Paradox of Experience", in Gelley A. (ed.), *Unruly Examples: On the Rhetoric of Exemplarity* (Stanford: 1995) 86–103.

theory with the tractable experience of his own embodiment.[43] In effect, Montaigne uses the non-naturals – air, food and drink, evacuation and repletion, exercise and rest, sleep and waking, the passions of the soul – as a template for self-knowledge, arguing that participatory, useful, and therapeutic knowledge of the self issues from the body.[44] In this, like others in the sixteenth century, he follows Celsus, whom he cites as a critic of medicine (596). In *De medicina*, Celsus writes that a healthy man, 'who is both vigorous and his own master, should be under no obligatory rules, and have no need either for a physician or an ointment-healer [*iatrolepta*]'.[45] One who is 'his own master' might, then, compile a record of his own symptoms: the causal regress that characterises learned medicine – and, Montaigne adds, what 'I say of medicine may be applied generally to all knowledge' (362; cf. 396) – is halted by applying the astringent remedy of particular, somatic experience to the empty generalities of medical thought. For Montaigne, the noumenal and the phenomenal rarely meet – most rarely, perhaps, in the experience of illness.[46]

He also impugns physicians. They must know 'too many details, considerations, and circumstances', the 'patient's constitution, his temperament, his humours, his inclinations, his actions, his very thoughts and fancies', to make their practice certain: how shall a physician 'find the proper symptom of the disease, each disease being capable of an infinite number of symptoms?' The 'very promises of medicine are incredible'. Whereas surgery is 'more certain, because it sees and feels

---

[43] As Jean Starobinski has shown, the essay "Of Experience" is organized around the non-naturals ("The Body's Moment", *Yale French Studies* 63 (1983) 273–305) and, as Timothy Hampton argues, 'the body emerges [throughout the *Essays*] as the material signifier of the condition of the soul' (*Writing from History: The Rhetoric of Exemplarity in Renaissance Literature* [Ithaca and London: 1990] 171). Montaigne is well aware of the 'grands débats' about dietetics in the sixteenth century; see Céard J., "La Culture du Corps: Montaigne et la Diététique de son Temps", in Tetel M. – Mallary Masters G. (eds.), *Le Parcours des* Essais *de Montaigne 1588–1988* (Paris: 1989) 83–96; esp. 86–87.

[44] Starobinski, "The Body's Moment" 276.

[45] Celsus, *De Medicina*, trl. W.G. Spencer, 3 vols. (Cambridge: 1971) I, 1. Elyot writes in *The Castell of Helth* (London: 1536), paraphrasing Celsus, that a 'man that is hole and well at ease, and is at libertie, ought not to bynde hym selfe to rules, or nede a phisition' (281).

[46] Yet Montaigne's particular ailment (bladder stone) offers little to "guess about". Although nature has 'utterly unknown ways of her own', with a simple illness we 'are freed from the worry into which other diseases cast us by the uncertainty of their causes and conditions and progress'. Mitigating his earlier scepticism, Montaigne asserts that, with the stone, 'the senses reveal to us what it is, and where it is' (839–840). Illness in general, however, offers no such certainty (838–839).

what it is doing', physicians have no '*speculum matricis* to reveal to them our brain, our lungs, our liver' (586–587). Indeed, for Montaigne the exploration of symptoms, of that which begins 'inside' and is only accessible to sensation, is the problem of pain in early modernity: how does one convey sensation? how does one speak about pain inside oneself? To emphasise his point, he offers an anecdote about visiting his physicians: many a time, he writes, 'when safe and free from these dangerous attacks [of the stone], I have taken pleasure in communicating their symptoms to the doctors as if they were just beginning inside me. I suffered the doom of their horrible conclusions most comfortably, and remained that much more obliged to God for his grace and better informed of the vanity of this art' (840). Montaigne prevaricates in order to discredit the feigned sagacity of his physicians, but he also suggests that his own mendacity is matched only by his physicians': they, too, play on the imagination, they accept his false conveyances, they prescribe terribly.

In the end, although it threatens the whole person, nociception depends on the disposition of the soul: there is no 'reason, prescription, or might' that has power against the soul's inclinations. Of the many 'thousands of attitudes at its disposal', Montaigne recommends a disposition conducive to preservation; then 'we shall be not only sheltered from all harm, but even gratified and flattered [...] by ills and pains' (39). Against what might be called an extreme, limiting case – the vehement pain that saints embrace, afflicting the body with 'atrocious and appropriate torments', welcome in their severity (681) – Montaigne suggests that 'there are diseases, as there are wounds, that are medicinal and salutary' (837). The soul's disposition is altered by pain and sickness; in fact, there are pains, he argues, that might not even be ours because they are unavailable to sensation. Passions which 'touch [only] the rind of us cannot be called ours', he writes. 'To make them ours, the whole man must be involved; and the pains which the foot or the hand feel while we are asleep are not ours' (271). What we 'feel' while we are asleep, because it does not involve the 'whole man,' is not ours. Sensation, here, is crucial, and it is related to touch: 'I leave aside the sense of touch, whose operations are closer, more vivid and substantial, which, so many times, by the effect of the pain it brings to the body, overthrows all those beautiful Stoical resolutions' (448). Pain affects resolve: Stoical resolution does not mean that we do not suffer pain, but that we are not distracted by it. With Montaigne, then, resolution means cozening the imagination, lying to doctors, assuaging fear that might offer more grief than any illness; it means engaging evaluative, moral questions about conduct, cognition, and regimen; and it means, I would argue, engaging rhetorical therapy. If the 'body finds relief in complaining, let it do so. If it thinks that the pain evaporates somewhat [...] for crying out more violently, or if that distracts its torment, let it shout right out' (577).

The evanescence of pain evident in Montaigne – the ways in which it spurs evaluation, not only of the passions but of states and dispositions of the soul – is transformed into probative inwardness and mechanism in one of his readers, Descartes. For Descartes pain, too, evokes the imagination. In the sixth meditation, Descartes begins by suggesting the salient difference between imagination and pure understanding: we can think of a pentagon without imagining it, but if we apply the 'mind's eye' to its five sides and its area, we must apply some 'peculiar effort of mind which is not required for understanding'.[47] Imagination, he asserts, is not a necessary constituent of his essence; it depends on something 'distinct from [him]self', and it points to his composite nature. When the mind understands, it turns towards itself; when it imagines, it turns towards the body and 'looks at something in the body' which conforms to intellection. He concludes that 'it may be this very body that enables me to imagine corporeal things'.

As Dennis Sepper has shown, like most early moderns he draws much of his account of the imagination from Aristotle's *De anima*.[48] Thinking about the soul in this period exhibits what Katherine Park calls 'an impulse to favour simpler and more physiological explanations for organic phenomena'. Philip Melanchthon is typical: 'if anyone wants to enquire into the faculties and actions of the soul, he must know the organs and parts of the body'. Physiology, broadly defined, becomes the principal means for explaining organic function, and more and more commentators enlist anatomy in their explorations.[49] In part, these efforts build on Aristotle's conception of the physiological bases of

[47] *The Philosophical Writings of Descartes*, ed. J. Cottingham, R. Stoothoff, D. Murdoch, and A. Kenny, 3 vols. (Cambridge: 1985–1991) II, 52. All further references are included in parenthesis in the text.

[48] Sepper D., *Descartes' Imagination: Proportion, Images, and the Activity of Thinking* (Berkeley – Los Angeles: 1996) 13–35, *passim*.

[49] Park K., "The Organic Soul", in Schmitt Ch. et al. (eds.), *The Cambridge History of Renaissance Philosophy* (Cambridge: 1988) 477; 479 (quoting Melanchthon's *Liber de anima*); 481–482.

thinking: the correspondence between mental dispositions and somatic states is clear in *De anima* and in other texts of the *Parva naturalia*, which investigate 'affections that are common to the soul and body' (in *De sensu*, 436a, or *De memoria*, 453a 14 ff., for example), as well as in the pseudo-Aristotelian *Physiognomica* (805a 1 ff.), which suggests, with some resonance for scholars of the history of pain, that there is a fundamental correspondence between mental dispositions and bodily states. In the *Regulae*, imagination is a 'truly cognitive power', akin to *ingenium*, and Descartes draws on traditional scholastic and early modern terminology to suggest as much.[50] But in the *Meditations*, imagination remains more or less a matter of survival, its sophistication emptied out with sure purpose: exploring the ways in which pain funds the preservation of the mind/body composite in a world of uneven sentience.

The realm of Descartes' composite is replete with sensation: heat and cold, hunger and thirst, pleasure and pain. The vivid perception of the senses, and especially of these pleasure and pain, to which he returns repeatedly, occasions questions in the mediator not dissimilar to Augustine's: why should 'that curious sensation of pain give rise to a particular distress of mind'? What is the necessary connection between hunger and food, between 'the sensation of something causing pain and the mental apprehension of distress that arises from that sensation?' (II, 52–53), Descartes asks, invoking the question that opens this paper: what is the relationship between the sensation and apprehension of pain? Does it have a bearing on expression? In a sense, the answers to these questions suggest a dweller in thrall to its dwelling: we have apprehensions of distress because we wish, quite simply, to preserve health and avoid pain. Like Aristotle, Descartes claims that the 'whole self can be affected by various beneficial or harmful things with which it comes in contact' (II, 56–57).

'There is nothing that my own nature teaches me more vividly than that I have a body, and that when I feel pain there is something wrong with the body' (II, 56). For what can be more internal than pain, he asks? (II, 53). Pain tests the limits, and the province, of inward sensation: it offers a way into the phenomenology of experience, it is a prime constituent in his investigation of mind/ body intrication and, with Descartes' thick description and redescription of traditional moral philosophical fields, it funds the emergence of a self-regarding subject,

[50] Sepper, *Descartes' Imagination* 33; 85–85.

one who is poised to underwrite traditional algetic therapies with a new, physiological foundation. Famously, in the sixth mediation, he writes:

> Nature also teaches me, by these sensations of pain, hunger, thirst and so on, that I am not merely present in my body as a sailor is present in a ship, but that I am very closely joined and, as it were, intermingled with it, so that I and the body form a unit. If this were not so, I, who am but a thinking thing, would not feel pain when the body was hurt, but would perceive the damage purely by the intellect, just as a sailor perceives by sight if anything in his ship is broken. Similarly, when the body needed food or drink, I should have an explicit understanding of the fact, instead of having confused sensations of hunger and thirst. For these sensations of hunger, thirst, pain and so on are nothing but confused modes of thinking which arise from the union and, as it were, intermingling of the mind with the body (II, 56).

Self-separation might occasion perfect perception but, with the union of mind and body, 'confused modes of thinking' reign. For the most part, passions, including the experience of pain, rely on confused ideas, whereas reason, of course, traffics only in 'clear and distinct' thought. Like passions, 'confused thoughts' are those which involve the body; as Descartes suggests, in 'many cases the grasp of the senses is very obscure and confused', they provide 'very obscure information' (II, 55; 58). Yet the senses, including and perhaps especially pain, offer information 'conducive to the preservation' of health, by discerning what is harmful or beneficial to the composite of mind and body (II, 60; 57). Still, although this system is the best available, designed by a benevolent God, by our very nature as composite things, and by the fact that 'a given motion in the brain must always produce the same sensation in the mind' (II, 61), there is frequent misprision. We are thirsty when we should not be, for example in certain kinds of sickness; but we are only occasionally rather than continuously misled, at least for the health and preservation of the body. The confused thought that is pain depends on a particular mechanism, in which the nerves convey sensation to the mind, in which the animal spirits are activated ("moved" is the most common term).[51] But this mechanism is flawed for two reasons: in terms of locating sensation, its medium (the strings and spirits that enable nervous impulses) is overly taxed, since sensory and motor functions occupy the same nerve; and its responses are determined by habit

---

[51] See Sutton J., *Philosophy and Memory Traces: Descartes to Connectionism* (Cambridge: 1998) 23–49.

(II, 61–61), since animal spirits are prone to assume the same paths or configurations when confronted with similar sensations, which of course opens the possibility of unlearning them.[52]

As a result, pain is an example of a thought that can be clear without being distinct, for 'people commonly confuse [the perception of intense pain] with an obscure judgement they make concerning the nature of something which they think exists in the painful spot and which they suppose to resemble the sensation of pain; but in fact it is the sensation alone which they perceive clearly' (I, 208). Montaigne's 'I judge myself only by actual sensation, not by reasoning' becomes, for Descartes, confused, confected: because we are bodies, and because we imagine, we cannot have a distinct thought about pain.[53] As Arnauld and Nicole put it in the Port Royal *Logic*, 'pain is only in the Sense'.[54] Pain may be called a 'clear idea', because it strikes us so sensibly, 'but yet it is confus'd, because [the idea] represents *Pain* to us, as being in the Hand, when indeed it lies in the Sence' (97). We may endure wounds without any sense of pain, they argue, citing Descartes' phantom limb example and the fact that we have, from childhood, habitually 'imagin'd' pain in certain ways (102, 100). And they draw on Augustine to argue that 'pain [is] nothing but a certain sadness of the Mind wherewith it was afflicted for the sufferings of the Body, to which it was join'd by God' (103).[55] Sorrow is mediated by images, as we have learned from Montaigne, and Augustine confirms Arnauld and Nicole's insight again: when I am healthy and I pronounce the word 'pain', he writes in the *Confessions* (X, 15), I must have the *image* of pain in my memory, since this pain is not present to me. This image is surely a confused thought.

In a sense, for Descartes pain is both aesthetic and anaesthetic: much like Montaigne, Descartes' intervention balances Stoic and Neostoic

[52] As he will suggest in *The Passions of the Soul*, the animal spirits are, in the end, joined with certain kinds of volition, not with the flesh (§ 44).

[53] It might be that such sensing is accomplished by the *imaginatio-phantasia*, as Sepper suggests, a complex faculty which involves itself in all activities of the human being, except pure intellection. In this sense, "sensation" is cognition applying itself with and to the imagination. This notion reappears in the remedy Descartes' suggests in the final articles of the *Passions of the Soul* where, in some sense, the question concerns the intensity of sensation, the quality or duration of titillation, epitomised on the one hand by pain and on the other by visiting the theatre.

[54] Antoine Arnauld – Pierre Nicole, *Logic; or, the Art of Thinking* (London, T.B.: 1693) 101; further references included in parenthesis in the text.

[55] See also *The Leibniz-Arnauld Correspondence*, ed. and trl. H.T. Mason (Manchester: 1967) 87; 78–79.

concerns with the psycho-physiological tradition of early modern self-care manuals. But where Montaigne valorises pain as a test not only of cognition (are these pains mine?) but of temperance, moderation, and care, Descartes insists that pain is a confused thought that teaches us our bodies, as it were: there is a physiological foundation of sensation, he attests, but one susceptible to the interventions of the will. In the end, though, he proposes much the same remedies for pain as Montaigne or, for that matter, Seneca: in effect, in *The Passions of the Soul* and in his letters to Princess Elisabeth in the mid-1640s, Descartes calls for temperance, for 'a settled disposition', as the bulwark against superabundant feeling (III, 265–267). In the absence of a tempered soul, other techniques are to hand: griefs as well as other passions are militated by the 'presence of agreeable objects' which aid the mind 'by chasing from it all the passions which partake of sadness' (III, 297). In fact, the customary recommendation of physicians, to free one's mind from all 'sad thoughts' (III, 250), is a panacea: when faced with daily frustration, we should 'so far as possible [...] distract our imagination and senses' from our cares and consider them prudently with the intellect alone' (III, 249). Some remedies against excessive passion are difficult, Descartes concludes in a 1646 letter, but it is 'enough in general to have imagined circumstances more distressing than one's own and to be prepared to bear them' (III, 287). In Descartes' phenomenology of nociceptive experience, thick description funds an evaluative, self-regarding subject, one who is poised to render the traditional cures and therapies with a new, physiological foundation for his or her thinking.

My final "nociceptive instance" is the publication of the Helmontian physician Everard Maynwaring's *Pains Afflicting Humane Bodies* in 1682. Maynwaring was a prolific physician and polemicist, publishing no less than thirty books and pamphlets on subjects ranging from scurvy, hygiene and regimen, longevity and venereal disease to medical history, medical ethics, and chemical medicine between 1663 and 1699. From the mid-1660s, drawing largely on the work of Johannes Baptista van Helmont, whom he endorses frequently, he was a staunch and vocal advocate for chemical medicine and a searing critic of orthodox Galenism. 'Chymistry makes a man an exact Naturalist', Maynwaring avers, 'and this is the foundation for a Physitian to stand upon'.[56] He was also a nascent vitalist.

[56] Everard Maynwaring, *Medicus Absolutus* (London, Printed for the booksellers: 1668) 32.

Drawing on wide philosophical and medical reading, Maynwaring suggests that pain indicates a crisis in vitality: it is not, as the Galenists claim, *ubi est dolor, ibi est morbus*.[57] Maynwaring is less concerned with antecedent causes, the Hippocratic *prophaseis*, than with the notion that disease can be traced via "series" or "trains" of causes, the next always deeper and more obscure than the last, to the vital principle. The 'grand complaint of the sick', he writes, is that physicians treat symptoms and not causes, putting patients in continual and lasting risk. Instead, he seeks the '*radix* of diseases' (34) through a method that accounts for the 'gradual progress from one disease to another, or a complication of diseases *gradatim* brought and linked together'. The 'sagacious fore-sighted Physician, seeing one disease to present it self, looks beyond that, takes a farther prospect, and discovers the train that will follow, knowing their *connexion* and *dependence* upon each other' (5).

Pain is central to his renovation of physic, since it speaks to the inadequacies of Galenic theory and practice. Pain is most commonly a 'leader; a signal...of defection or disturbance in the part where it is seated', but also a harbinger of potentially grave disorder (3). At the beginning of the work, Maynwaring offers an acute warning: if any part of the body is 'put out of its office and the rectitude of its function' by pain, all parts are 'drawn into consent' and 'by time the whole is become a sufferer' (4). He seems part of the reaction against certain aspects of Galenic medicine, a reaction which more and more frequently re-imagined the body as an ensemble of interconnected systems and parts. Maynwaring insists that the body is a series of interconnected organs that, in themselves, do not feel but are endowed with feeling by a vital force: if 'a *part* of the body decline its office and performance of duty, acts perversely or inordinately; the mischief stops not there, bother *parts* also are perverted thereby, and drawn in consent: [...] parts being thus affected and grieved, the *vital* principle residing as governor there, is hereby excited and irritated' (II, 18). This irritation (one might think of Francis Glisson here)[58] is 'the very pain and anguish that is felt in the part'. Organs are not capable of pain in themselves, he continues, 'but the *life* inhabiting and inabling the part to perform vital offices,

[57] Everard Maynwaring, *Pains Afflicting Humane Bodies. Their Various Difference, Causes, Parts Affected, Signals of Danger or Safety. Shewing the Tendency of Chronick, and Acute Diseases, for a Seasonable Prevention of Fatal Events* (London, Printed for Henry Bonwicke: 1682) 49. Further references included in parenthesis in the text.

[58] Temkin O., "The Classical Roots of Glisson's Doctrine of Irritation", in idem, *The Double Face of Janus and Other Essays in the History of Medicine* (Baltimore: 1977) 290–316.

that does *dolere* and *aestuare*' (18). Pain allows Maynwaring to imagine a notional anatomy that insists on the intimacy between affected parts, function, the sufferer's whole body, and the vital force.

The 'whole' that suffers, suffers most with pain. As he writes, of 'all *Symptoms* that attend, or are the consequents of Diseases, *Pain* is the most troublesom and irksom to bear. *Weakness* and *languishing* are tolerable evils; but *pain* is restless, tormenting and full of complaints' (36). The complaints, of course, are the patient's (and perhaps the ignorant, orthodox Galenic physician's). Pain works in mysterious ways: it is sometimes outward, on the superficies of the body, which is called 'manifest', easily discovered by the patient's directions, and sometimes inward or 'abstruse' and with 'difficulty to be certainly determined, which part is grieved' (46). In either case, congested or 'defluxed' matter accumulates in a body part (which is common medical store from Hippocrates on).[59] Pain then affects that part or parts proximate, and 'the *Spirits* resort thither, and with them the *blood* also to relieve it', which results in inflammation or tumescence (11). When one part is injured in such a way, the 'the vital principle or *Archaeus* (which hath the government and tuition) is molested and troubled therewith, and seldom lyes calm or quiet under that, that oppression, but begins to be incensed and enraged [...] and this *ira Archaei* is the *ratio formalis* of pain, the very pain it self which is felt' (12–13).

To Maynwaring, pain is several: sickness is pain, fever is pain diffused, but in the end all pains attack the vital principle or *archaeus*, a term he borrows from Van Helmont, which means the generative life force, related in some way to the potentiality and actualisation of individual parts, organs, and the body as a whole.[60] He nods to its controversial provenance – is it the *anima*, the *spiritus impetum faciens* of Hippocrates, the *archaeus* 'according to *Helmont's* doctrine'? – but demurs, suggesting the explanation would need another tract in order to distinguish it from the objections and prejudice of received doctrine (43). Clearly, though, he has Van Helmont in mind and he ventures a little farther:

> you may the better understand and have a clearer satisfaction herein (*practice* depending upon it, I mean the allay or remove of *pain*) consider

---

[59] See Bynum W.F. – Nutton V. (eds.), *Theories of Fever from Antiquity to the Enlightenment*, Medical History Supplement 1 (London: 1981).

[60] Pagel W., *Joan Baptista van Helmont* (Cambridge: 1982) 96–102. The term was Paracelsus'; see Pagel, "Van Helmont's Concept of Disease – To Be or Not To Be? The Influence of Paracelsus", *Bulletin of the History of Medicine* 46 (1972) 419–454.

> and know, that the sense of *Feeling* being spread through the whole body, is as the last or inmost covering, that does inwrap or infold the *life*; and is as it were the watch or guard upon the confines thereof. Now any thing that does stir up *Feeling*, that thus nearly and intimately approaches the *life*; if it exceed the bounds of moderation and is violent, if it be any way unnatural or injurious, it raiseth a disturbance in the *vital* principle of that part, which is pain: so that the assault first made upon the *life*, which governs and preserves unity and continuity of parts; but that *vital principle* being fretted, distracted and put by its placid, regular oeconomy and government, the *Organ* perisheth as the *life* of the part decays, or is out of course; being then unable to protect and preserve it (42).

The sense of 'feeling' is the innermost covering or wrap that encloses 'life': all pain is first and foremost an assault on the vital principle of a part, which in turn impugns the *archaeus* itself. Maywaring's primary example is the nosologically intractable fever. A fever, he writes, is pain diffused (22): this pain results from the fact that all members of the body 'consent with one another' through vessels of communication, function, or vicinity; since the *archaeus* is 'extended [...] throughout the whole fabrick of the body', we cannot suffer here or there, he argues, but the 'whole is injured, disturbed and drawn into consent, more or less, manifestly or secretly' (18). With fevers, contra the Galenists, disturbance does not arise from 'any corporal constitution or composition of the four Elements [...] but only as *effects* and *signals* discovering the *Crasis* and state of the vital principle, whether vigorous or depressed' (24). Pain, he concludes, is fever contracted.

All parts of the body wherein there is feeling are subject to pain, and pain is only proper to this sense, as seeing is to the eye, hearing to the ear, et cetera. Feeling is even 'seated' and extended through 'the Organs of all those *Senses*' (36–37), he reminds us, drawing on Aristotle's treatment of touch in *De anima*. He explains: all the symptoms of disease are objects of sense, they are discernible by some sense, usually sight, as when Donne in the *Devotions* sees maculae on his body and they indicate to him and his physicians the crisis of his disease. Pain, Maynwaring argues, 'belongs to, and is adjudged by the sense of *feeling* only; which sense has the largest capacity of all the rest; being extended throughout the body'. Seeing might discover and judge symptoms on the superficies of the body, for example, but '*feeling* takes cognisance of inside and outside, and what we cannot *see* we *feel*, and are sensible of by *pain*, even amongst the most secret and hidden parts of the body' (7–8). But only those parts endowed with feeling are capable of pain: they are invested or lined with some membrane, Maynwaring argues, 'by which the sense of feeling is communicated', making the disturbances recorded by this "*supreme*" sense grave (37). But what is the relationship between feeling and sensation? Are feelings confused thoughts, related only to touch? Drawing on a diffuse array of concepts from ancient Stoicism through to Cartesian mechanism, Maynwaring's contemporaries described sensation as a distribution of vital spirits throughout the body, which react to stimuli and which convey their reactions to the animal spirits in the brain. Serious meditation or 'recent grief', Thomas Willis avers, interrupt sensation; presumably extreme pain does as well. In fact, in Willis' Oxford lectures, we find a middle ground between mechanism and the ethico-physiology of vitalism: 'since the vital faculty supplies the material of the animal spirits and the animal faculty supplies the spirits necessary for vital motion and initiates the motion of the heart and respiration it is impossible that one of them should feel some change without the other being immediately similarly affected'.[61] Various systems of spirits are intricated, and their intimacy guarantees their vulnerability.

Maynwaring neglects to investigate sensation fully, but insists that it is seated in all parts of the body and is an 'inseparable consort with life'. It is, he concludes, a confused thought: what '*pain* is, scarce any one but can tell; and some by woful *Experience*, whereby they will consent with the definition thereof, *dolor est tristis sensatio in tactu*: pain is a trouble arising in the sense of feeling: but that which is so plainly felt, is not very easie to be understood from whence it does arise' (38). When the heart or the stomach suffers, it is feeling, 'tristis sensatio in tactu', that discovers pain (23). 'In tactu' of course suggests touch again, and Maynwaring describes violent or extreme assaults on feeling with the stock descriptors of touch: hot, cold, hard, sharp, heavy. Here is the root of sensation: it is haptic. Aristotle links touch with sleeping, aging and dying, disease and health (455a 12–b2, 435b 4–5, 648b 2–10).[62] Jean Fernel, following Galen, made pain a symptom of touch, and argued that it was not the perception of noxious qualities that constitutes pain but the affection or feeling which arose from such a situation.[63] Sensation is touch extended, diffused into the depths and recesses of the body, crucial to all its vital functions. The deepening and

[61] Dewhurst K., *Thomas Willis' Oxford Lectures* (Oxford: 1980) 68–69.

[62] See Freeland C., "Aristotle on the Sense of Touch", in Nussbaum M. – Rorty A. (eds.), *Essays on Aristotle's* De anima (Oxford: 1992) 227–248.

[63] Rey, *The History of Pain* 60–61.

extension of sensation variously appears, reconceived as irritability and "natural perception" in the work of Francis Glisson, the *archaeus* and its subsidiary *archei* in van Helomont, animism in Georg Ernst Stahl, and vitalism in the late seventeenth and early eighteenth centuries.[64] However it appears on the horizon, the extension of sensation secures the relationship between pain and imagination. As Leonard Marrande (Marandé) suggests in *The Judgment of Humane Actions* (1629), the

> number and multitude of the Senses might bee reduced to that of Feeling: for as the most delicate parts of the body feel cold or heate, good or evill, more sensibly and lively than the grosser: so Man touched with the same object, seems to be diversely touched, because his body (in her tenderest parts) receives a feeling so delicate and subtile, that it loseth the name of feeling, and then we give it another according to our fancy and opinion.[65]

Although the imagination is frequently misleading, and common opinion excreable, to 'lose the name of feeling' suggests a new language, a new set of terms for sensation: those terms emerge, it seems, in the mid- to late seventeenth century. Certainly by the 1670s and 1680s, the sensation that arises from pain, that involves the whole 'spiritual economy', was redescribed as an index of vitality, whether in terms of irritability or various conceptions of the *archaeus* or *anima*.

In its various forms, vitalism deepened the associations between the imagination and pain. While fear was crucial to early modern conceptions of illness,[66] as late as the nineteenth century vitalists thought that the mere fear of a painful operation might lead to death.[67] Writing late in the century, Théodule Ribot argues that 'pain is associated with the diminution and disorgansation of the vital functions',[68] and in the early twentieth century physicians were exploring the links between pain and

---

[64] See, for example, Haigh E.L., "The Vital Principle of Paul Joseph Barthez: the Clash between Monism and Dualism", *Medical History* 21 (1977) 1–14 and Williams E., *A Cultural History of Medical Vitalism in Enlightenment Montpellier* (Aldershot: 2003).

[65] Leonarde Marrande, *The Judgment of Humane Actions. A Most Learned & Excellent Treatise of Morrall Philosophie*, trans. John Reynolds (London: 1629) 32–33.

[66] Wear A., "Fear, Anxiety, and the Plague in Early Modern England", in *Religion, Health, and Suffering* 339–363.

[67] Travers B., *An Enquiry Concerning that Disturbed State of the Vital Functions Usually Denominated Constitutional Irritation* (London: 1826) 22, quoted in Du Moulin, "Bodily Pain in Western Man" 556, n. 54.

[68] Ribot Th., *The Psychology of the Emotions*, second edition (London: 1911) 31 ff.

imagination with vigour.[69] But in the late seventeenth century, theories of vitality were ways of treating problems of governance and function in body and soul, matter and the immaterial, that eased an increasing dependence on mechanism: one might see in Maynwaring or Willis, for example, the tendency to make all parts of the body dependent on one another, while later physicians and philosophers propose diverse means of dividing the vital principle between organs and systems, including the nerves.[70]

A social history of suffering must include, at the very least, patients, philosophers, and physicians. In my examples, the patient judges his pain via sensation; the philosopher judges sensation via pain; and the physician joins the two in order to propose new models of causation and a new affinity between parts and wholes, sensation and vitality. Much more might be written on the transition from pain as haptic to pain as a sensation moored to vitality, but at least one point is clear: Maynwaring's animadversions represent a change in the conception of pain, at least in contrast to Montaigne and Descartes. To use Montaigne's terms, physicians (or philosophers or patients) do not have a '*speculum matricis*' that would allow them to peer into the viscera. Pain must be judged by sensation: it can only be felt, described and redescribed. How should we imagine and judge pain when it is susceptible to intermittence, to remission, to its own forms of prevarication? How might diagnosis depend on imagination, on description and redescription, of something available only to feeling? The patient's experience of pain is always, in the Cartesian sense, confused; it is clear but not distinct. Thus the imagination is indispensable. As Elaine Scarry has argued, 'pain and imagining are the "framing events" within whose boundaries all other perceptual, somatic, and emotional events occur'. Between pain and imagination, then, 'the whole terrain of the human psyche' might be mapped.[71]

---

[69] See, for example, Bousfield P., *Pleasure and Pain: A Theory of the Energetic Foundation of Feeling* (London: 1926) 37–38.

[70] See Haigh, "The Vital Principle of Paul Joseph Barthez".

[71] Scarry, *The Body in Pain* 165.

Selective Bibliography

Celsus, *De medicina*, trans. W.G. Spencer, 3 vols. (Cambridge, Mass.: 1971).
Cicero M. Tullius, *Tusculan Disputations*, trl. J.E. King (London: 1966).
Cohen E., "The Animated Pain of the Body", *American Historical Review* 105,1 (2000) 36–68.
Descartes Réné, *The Passions of the Soul*, trl. S.H. Voss (Indianapolis – Cambridge: 1989).
Dewhurst K., *Thomas Willis' Oxford Lectures* (Oxford: 1980).
Donne John, *The Sermons of John Donne*, eds. E.M. Simpson and G.R. Potter, 10 vols. (Berkeley – Los Angeles: 1953–1962).
Elias N., *The Civilising Process: the History of Manners and State Formation and Civilisation* (trans. E. Jephcott) 2 vols. (Oxford: 1994).
Lössl J., "Dolor (dolere)", in Mayer C. (ed.), *Augustinus-Lexikon* 2,3 4 (Basel: 1999) 582–591.
Macdonald M., *Mystical Bedlam: Madness, Anxiety, and Healing in Seventeenth-Century England* (Cambridge: 1981).
Maynwaring Everard, *Pains Afflicting Humane Bodies. Their Various Difference, Causes, Parts Affected, Signals of Danger or Safety. Shewing the Tendency, of Chronick, and Acute Diseases, for a Seasonable Prevention of Fatal Events* (London, Henry Bonwicke: 1682).
Montaigne Michel de, *The Complete Essays of Montaigne*, trl. D.M. Frame (Stanford: 1958).
Moulin, D. Du, "A Historical-Phenomenological Study of Bodily Pain in Western Man", *Bulletin of the History of Medicine* 48 (1974) 540–570.
Pagel W., *Joan Baptista van Helmont* (Cambridge: 1982).
Porter R., "Western Medicine and Pain: Historical Perspectives", in Hinnels J.R. and Porter R. (eds.), *Religion, Health, and Suffering* (London – New York: 1999) 364–380.
Rey R., *The History of Pain*, trl. L.E. Wallace, J.A. and S.W. Cadden (Cambridge, Mass.: 1998).
Scarry E., *The Body in Pain: The Making and Unmaking of the World* (New York – Oxford: 1985).
Sepper D., *Descartes' Imagination: Proportion, Images, and the Activity of Thinking* (Berkeley – Los Angeles: 1996).
Siraisi N., *Medieval and Early Renaissance Medicine: an Introduction to Knowledge and Practice* (Chicago: 1990).
Thomas K., *Religion and the Decline of Magic* (London: 1971).
Wear A., *Knowledge and Practice in English Medicine, 1550–1680* (Cambridge: 2000).

INDEX NOMINUM

Adam 20, 206, 333, 395–396, 404
Aegidius, Petrus, *see* Gillis, Peter
Aegidius, Saint, *see* Giles
Allde, Edward 172 n. 27
Allen, William, Cardinal 75
Ambrosius, Aurelius, Saint 75 n. 51
Anisson, Jean 257 n. 7
Anthony, Saint 120, 123
Antonio Veneziano 247 n. 64
Appius Claudius (Appius Claudius Caecus, the Censor) 123
Aquinas, Thomas, *see* Thomas
Arias, Francisco 194
Ariosto, Ludovico 352
Aristotle 25–26, 35, 167–168, 171, 186, 447, 471 n. 27, 484–485, 491–492
Arnauld, Antoine 487
Ascham, Roger 39, 56, 183
Athanasius 120 n. 45
Auden, W.H. 35
Augustine, Aurelius Augustinus, Saint 278, 473–474, 485, 487
Avicenna 474
Avila, Juan of, *see* Juan
Avila, Teresa of, *see* Teresa

Bachelard, Gaston 495
Bacon, Francis 25, 178–179, 194
Bálint, Borbély 423, 435 n. 43, 436, 438 n. 47
Bálint, Orsolya 423, 427–428, 435, 438
Bankes, Lawrence 217–219
Barnaba da Modena 243
Baronio, Cesare, Cardinal 61, 63, 72, 77
Bartolomeo da Camogli 245 n. 60
Bax, Elisabeth 453
Becon, Thomas 309
Benedict XIII, Anti-Pope, *see* Luna, Peter de
Benedict, Saint 95 n. 15
Benfatti, Giacomo 227–228
Berckel, Maria van 461
Bernini, Lorenzo 11, 279–280
Beverwijck, Johan van 443, 445–448, 450–451, 453 n. 18, 454 n. 20, 463, 465
Bilney, Thomas 316–318
Bisquert, Antonio 278
Bizamano, Angelo 249 n. 67
Bodin, Jean 384
Boétie, Etienne de 259
Boileau, Jacques 257–258
Bonfadini, Bartolomeo 75 n. 53
Bor, Pieter – Christiaensz. 458 n. 24
Borcht, Pieter van der 109–110
Borlone, Giacomo 229
Borromeo, Carlo, Cardinal and Saint 258
Boyd, Zacharie 310–311
Bozio, Tommaso 66 n. 23, 78, 81, 84 n. 72, 86
Brant, Sebastian 105
Bruele, Gualterus 7–8
Brumeau, Thomas 210 n. 38
Bruni, Francesco 74
Budé, Guillaume 45
Byfield, Nicholas 300–301, 313

Calverley, Walter 330
Calvin, John 11–12, 190, 192–193, 196, 208–219, 275, 300, 303, 333–334, 351–352, 355–364
Canistris, Opicino de 223
Cano, Alonso 274
Canute (Cnut), Saint 278
Catherine of Genoa, Saint 270
Catherine of Siena, Saint 11, 268, 285 n. 47, 288 n. 50, 292, 295
Causabon, Meric 472 n. 16
Celsus, Cornelius Celsus 482
Chamberlain, John 323, 336, 344
Charles I, King of England 194, 196
Charles V, Roman Emperor 115, 117
Christ 10–13, 62, 65, 67, 72–73 n. 44, 80 n. 68, 139, 143, 146–148, 150, 152, 154, 160, 191, 197–199, 202–219, 221–223, 225–227, 228–230, 232–235, 237, 239, 242–246, 249, 250, 255, 268–272,

274–275, 276 n. 38, 281, 292–293, 295, 306, 311–312, 316, 327, 349, 351–352, 354 n. 23, 355–356, 364–365, 370–371, 373, 381, 386, 390, 405, 414
Christiaens, Jan 461
Christina of Bolsena, Saint 278
Cicero, Marcus Tullius 63, 93–94, 121, 123, 396, 473–474
Claro, Giulio 73–74
Clement VIII (Ippolito Aldobrandini), Pope 77
Clerselier, Claude 2, 464
Clitherow, Margaret 331 n. 15
Clowes, William 22, 24, 32
Collaert, Adrien 271 n. 26, 285
Comenius, Jan Amos 41
Corstyaense, Jan, *see* Christiaens, Jan
Cramoisy, Claude 81 n. 71
Crashaw, William 308–309
Crooke, Samuel 316
Cyprian, Thascius Caecilius Cyprianus 78–79, 314

Damhouder, Joos de 456
Damian, Peter (Petrus Damiani) 254
De Cheffontaines, C. 262 n. 11
De Nully, Jean 258 n. 8
Degli Antoni, Giovanni Antonio 73 n. 46
Democritus of Abdera 120, 123
Dent, Arthur 317
Descartes, René 2–4, 9, 179–180, 189–190, 219, 259, 315, 403, 406–409, 411, 416, 443, 445, 462–463, 465, 470, 473, 477, 479, 484–488, 494
Dido, Queen of Carthage 125 n. 54, 129
Didymus 120, 123
Digby, Sir Kenelm 30
Diodotus, Cicero's house philosopher 120
Donangeli, Ascanio 60 n. 4, 61 n. 11
Donangeli, Girolamo 60 n. 4, 61 n. 11
Donne, John 12, 19, 309, 323–343, 470, 476, 491
Doomer, Lambert 110
Drusus, Gaius 123
Duccio di Buoninsegna 154 n. 74
Duns Scotus 353
Dunton, John 339 n. 30
Dürer, Albrecht 105, 154, 160

Edwards, Edward 331, 336, 341
Elisabeth I, Queen of England 75
Epicurus 395–396
Erasmus, Desiderius 41–42, 45–50, 52–53, 117

Fasani, Raniero 222, 237
Featley, Daniel 314 n. 33
Fernel, Jean 336, 492
Ferrari, Gregorio de 281
Ferrer, Vincent O.P., Saint 244 n. 56, 255–256
Ficino, Marsilio 269
Floris V, Count of Holland 381, 383–385
Fowler, John 75 n. 53
Foxe, John 304–305, 317–318
Fugger, family 115

Galen 7, 9, 12, 22, 32, 34–35, 170, 326, 332, 335–338, 341–343, 445, 450–451, 465, 471 n. 27, 489–490, 492
Galle, Corneille 273 n. 26, 278 n. 43, 285
Gallonio, Antonio 14, 60–86
Gassendi, Pierre 396 n. 30
Gérard, Balthasar 76–81, 84, 86
Gerini, Niccolò di Pietro 245
Gerson, Jean 256
Giles (Aegidius), Saint 117, 278
Gillis, Peter 117
Giovanni di Corraduccio 229
Giovanni di Nicola 248 n. 65
Granada, Louis of, *see* Louis
Gregory XV, Pope 267 n. 1, 273
Gretser, James S.J. 257–258
Greville, Fulke 184
Grevius, Joannes 457 n. 24
Grey, Lady Jane 56
Grillandi, Paolo 73
Guevara, Antonio de 272
Guillemard, Jean 319
Gutschoven, Gerard van 2, 464
Gymnich, Johann 78 n. 62, 87

Hall, John 21–22, 30
Harison, Richarde 209 n. 36
Harper, Thomas 331 n. 16, 344
Harsnett, Adam 321
Haviland, John 178 n. 45
Helmont, Johannes Baptista van 488, 490

Henrietta Maria, Queen of England 194, 196, 216
Henry III, King of France 78 n. 61, 256
Henry IV of Navarre, King of France 256
Henry Jaye 194 n. 12
Heywood, Jasper 174–176
Hill, Robert 309
Hippocrates 490
Hogenberg, Frans 83
Holbein, Ambrosius 53
Holbein, Hans 53
Homer 120, 123
Honthorst, Gerard van 98
Hooft, Pieter Cornelisz. 455, 457, 460
Hopkins, Richard 193, 216–217
Huygens, Constantijn 453–454, 461–462, 465

Ignatius of Loyola S.J., Saint 190, 192, 195–196, 205, 214, 216, 218, 259, 261, 267 n. 1

James I, King of England 194, 329
John, King of Bohemia 123
Johnson, Samuel 36
Jonktys, Daniel 457, 459–460, 466
Josslin, Ralph 8 n. 13
Juan de la Miseria 285, 288
Juan of Avila, Saint 194
Judas, apostle 152
Julian, M. 262 n. 11

Kalkar, Jan Joest van 152, 154
Kalmár, Albert 423, 428
Kalmár, Margit 423, 427
Knott, Edward 196
Koning, Abraham de 454 n. 21

Laud, William, Archbishop of Canterbury 194
Le Preux, Joannes 94 n. 9
Lencsés, György 424 n. 7
Leo X, Pope 94 n. 9, 150
Lichfield, John 165 n. 2, 211 n. 39
Locke, John 51
Lodge, Thomas 168
Louis of Granada O.P. 11, 190, 192–193, 197–198, 202–204, 206, 212, 214, 216, 218–219
Loyola, *see* Ignatius
Lucan, Marcus Annaeus Lucanus 121
Lucas of Leyden 96, 98, 105, 109–110, 115
Lucretia 125 n. 54
Luke, Apostle 148, 152
Luna, Peter de, Anti-Pope Benedict XIII 256
Lupset, Thomas 307–308, 318
Luther, Martin 15, 117–118, 139, 143, 150, 160–161, 333
Luyken, Caspaares 451 n. 14
Luyken, Jan 451

Malchus 148, 152, 154, 160
Manningham, John 24
Marne, Claude 81 n. 71
Marrande, Leondard 493
Marsili, Ippolito de' 73–74
Martellini, Sebastiano 75 n. 53
Martínez, Jusepe 275
Marvell, Andrew 27–28, 33
Masolino da Panicale 244
Master of the Osservanza 139
Matthew, Toby 194, 214, 216
Maximilian I, Roman Emperor 115
Mayerne, Theodore de 329, 335
Maynwaring, Everard 9, 470, 477, 488–492, 494
Mazzaforte, Pietro di Giovanni 229
Melanchthon, Philipp 42, 484
Mersenne, Marin 180 n. 51, 462 n. 34
Meursius, Johannes 195 n. 14
Michielsz, Jacob 460
Milton, John 29–30, 35
Montaigne, Michel de 9, 26–29, 41, 67, 259, 342, 469–470, 476–484, 487–488, 494
More, Henry S.J. 195, 197
More, Thomas 45, 356 n. 27
Murillo, Geronymo 195 n. 15

Nashe, Thomas 179, 180 n. 50
Nero, Roman Emperor 110, 115, 117, 119
Newton, Thomas 172 n. 22, 176
Nicolai, Arnold 458
Nicole, Pierre 487
Noah 13, 338, 340, 379, 390–391, 393–397, 399–400
Norton, John 7 n. 11
Norton, Thomas 196, 208, 209 n. 36, 214

Oudaan, Joachim 457, 459–461, 466
Overbury, Sir Thomas 330
Ovid, Publius Ovidius Naso 70

Pacino di Buonaguida 222
Paganinus, Joannes 94 n. 9
Paleotti, Gabriele 85 n. 74, 275
Palma il Giovane 281
Paracelsus, Theophrastus Bombastus of Hohenheim 12, 333, 335
Pare, Ambroise 24
Parkhurst, Thomas 339 n. 30
Parsons, Robert 75
Paul, Apostle 212–213, 274, 285 n. 47, 294, 308, 323, 334
Pauli, Andries 115 n. 36
Pazzi, Maria Maddalena, Saint 11, 292, 294–295
Peacham, Henry 181, 183
Peña, Francisco 69 n. 32, 73–74
Perkins, William 300–301, 303, 317, 319, 321
Peter, apostle 78, 148, 150, 152, 278 n. 42
Petrarch Master 15, 91–161
Petrarch, Francis (Francesco Petrarca) 91–161
Peutinger, Conrad 115, 117
Philip II, King of Spain 76
Piero della Francesca 146
Pius V (Michele Ghislieri), Pope 69
Plaats, François vander 257 n. 7
Plato 56, 472
Plautus, Titus Maccius Plautus 63
Pliny, Gaius Plinius Secundus the Elder 63
Plutarch 46, 56
Posidonius 93–94

Quintilian, M. Fabius Quintilianus 46

Reisinger, Peter 410 n. 23
Ribera, Francisco de 272, 275
Ribot, Théodule 493
Richter, Wolfgang 73 n. 46
Robertson, Bartholomew 310
Robinson, Jonathan 339 n. 30
Rombout, Theodoor 98, 115
Roper, Margaret 45
Rubens, Peter Paul 286

Salimbeni, Jacopo 229
Salimbeni, Lorenzo 229
Samson 29–31, 454
Sanders, Nicholas 75–76
Schipper, Jan Jacobsz. 445 n. 1
Schurman, Anna Maria van 445
Schwalbe, Benedikt 154
Sebastian, Saint 278
Seneca, Lucius Annaeus Seneca 93, 95 n. 11, 144, 167–168, 170–173, 175–177, 181, 472, 488
Sennucio of Florence 144
Sercambi, Giovanni 244
Servetus, Michael (Miguel Serveto) 209
Shakespeare, William 12, 19, 21, 28, 30, 32–34, 340–341
Sidney, Philip Sir 170, 183–186
Six van Chandelier, Jan 451
Sothera, Saint 72 n. 43, 74–75
Spenser, Edmund 13
Spinello Aretino 243
Spinoza, Baruch de 403, 406, 408–412, 414–420
Stadion, Christoph von 150
Standonck, Jean 52 n. 33
Stansby, William 168 n. 12
Stijn Jansdr. 460
Studley, John 171, 173
Sturm, Johannes 42
Sydenham, Thomas 24–25

Tasso, Torquato 352
Teresa of Avila, Saint 10–11, 190, 192, 194, 196, 205, 212, 214, 219, 267
Tertullian, Quintus Septimius Florens Tertullianus 78, 379–381, 386
Theophrastus 461
Thiers, Jean-Baptiste 257
Thomas Aquinas, Saint 288 n. 50, 353, 475
Thomas of Villacastin, *see* Villacastin
Tornieri, Giacomo 78 n. 62
Tyndale, William 363–364, 367
Tyrrhenus (soldier in Lucan's epos) 121

Urban VIII, Pope 276, 293 n. 61
Ursula, Saint 278

Valdés, Fernando de, archbishop of Seville 270, 293 n. 61, 295
Valla, Lorenzo 396 n. 30
Vaughan, William 480 n. 39
Vautrollerius, Thomas 210 n. 37
Velsen, Geerardt van 381

Velsen, Machteld van 381, 383–386
Velzen, Klaeris van 384–385
Verstegan, Richard 70, 75–76
Victors, Jan 98, 109
Vieira, Antonio S.J. 292
Villacastin, Thomas of, S.J. 11, 195–198, 200, 202–203, 205–206, 211, 215, 219
Villani, Giovanni 222–223
Virgil, Publius Vergilius Maro 125 n. 54
Vitale da Bologna 229 n. 22
Vitruvius, Marcus Vitruvius Pollio 63
Vives, Juan Luis 39, 41–42, 46
Vondel, Joost van den 13, 377–400, 460 n. 28
Vosmeer, Sasbout 77

Walpole, Michael S.J. 194 n. 12
Walther, Manfred 403 n. 1
Ward, Samuel of Ipswich 299–300, 305–308, 311–312, 314–315, 320
Wear, Andrew 8, 218, 325, 332
Welser, family 115
Weston, Richard 330
White, Edward 197 n. 19
Wierix, Anton 275, 276 n. 38, 281, 288
William the Silent, Prince of Orange 76–77, 86
Willis, Thomas 492, 494
Witt, Cornelis de 459–462, 465
Witt, Johan de 459
Woerden, Herman van 381
Wolfe, Reinolde 209 n. 36
Wright, Thomas 479

Yepes, Diego de 275, 290, 293 n. 62

Zanetti, Francesco 75 n. 53

INTERSECTIONS

1. ENENKEL, K., J.L. DE JONG and J. DE LANDTSHEER (eds.). *Recreating Ancient History*. Episodes from the Greek and Roman Past in the Arts and Literature of the Early Modern Period. 2001. ISBN 90 04 12051 3
2. HOUDT, T. VAN, J.L. DE JONG, Z. KWAK, M. SPIES and M. VAN VAECK (eds.). *On the Edge of Truth and Honesty*. Principles and Strategies of Fraud and Deceit in the Early Modern Period. 2002. ISBN 90 04 12572 8
3. GELDERBLOM, A.-J., J.L. DE JONG and M. VAN VAECK (eds.). *The Low Countries as a Crossroads of Religious Beliefs*. 2004. ISBN 90 04 12288 5
4. ENENKEL, K.A.E. and W. NEUBER (eds.). *Cognition and the Book*. Typologies of Formal Organisation of Knowledge in the Printed Book of the Early Modern Period. 2005. ISBN 90 04 12450 0
5. HAMILTON, A., M.H. VAN DEN BOOGERT and B. WESTERWEEL (eds.). *The Republic of Letters and the Levant*. 2005. ISBN 90 04 14761 6
6. ENENKEL, K.A.E. and J. PAPY (eds.). *Petrarch and His Readers in the Renaissance*. 2006. ISBN 90 04 14766 7
7. ENENKEL, K.A.E. and P.J. SMITH (eds.). *Early Modern Zoology*. The Construction of Animals in Science, Literature and the Visual Arts. 2007. ISBN 978 90 04 13188 0
8. SMITH, P.J. and K.A.E. ENENKEL (eds.). *Montaigne and the Low Countries (1580-1700)*. 2007. ISBN 978 90 04 15632 6
9. GÖTTLER, C. and W. NEUBER (eds.). *Spirits Unseen*. The Representation of Subtle Bodies in Early Modern European Culture. 2008. ISBN 978 90 04 16396 6
10. MURPHY, K. and R. TODD (eds.). "*A man very well studyed*". New Contexts for Thomas Browne. 2008. ISBN 978 90 04 17173 2
11. ZITTEL, C., G. ENGEL, R. NANNI and N.C. KARAFYLLIS (eds.). *Philosophies of Technology*. Francis Bacon and his Contemporaries. 2008. ISBN 978 90 04 17050 6
12. DIJKHUIZEN, J.F VAN and K.A.E. ENENKEL (eds.). *The Sense of Suffering*. Constructions of Physical Pain in Early Modern Culture. 2009. ISBN 978 90 04 17247 0

www.brill.nl/inte

www.ingramcontent.com/pod-product-compliance
Lightning Source LLC
LaVergne TN
LVHW012050011026
849162LV00017B/33